GENE THERAPY IN LUNG DISEASE

LUNG BIOLOGY IN HEALTH AND DISEASE

Executive Editor

Claude Lenfant
Director, National Heart, Lung and Blood Institute
National Institutes of Health
Bethesda, Maryland

1. Immunologic and Infectious Reactions in the Lung, *edited by C. H. Kirkpatrick and H. Y. Reynolds*
2. The Biochemical Basis of Pulmonary Function, *edited by R. G. Crystal*
3. Bioengineering Aspects of the Lung, *edited by J. B. West*
4. Metabolic Functions of the Lung, *edited by Y. S. Bakhle and J. R. Vane*
5. Respiratory Defense Mechanisms (in two parts), *edited by J. D. Brain, D. F. Proctor, and L. M. Reid*
6. Development of the Lung, *edited by W. A. Hodson*
7. Lung Water and Solute Exchange, *edited by N. C. Staub*
8. Extrapulmonary Manifestations of Respiratory Disease, *edited by E. D. Robin*
9. Chronic Obstructive Pulmonary Disease, *edited by T. L. Petty*
10. Pathogenesis and Therapy of Lung Cancer, *edited by C. C. Harris*
11. Genetic Determinants of Pulmonary Disease, *edited by S. D. Litwin*
12. The Lung in the Transition Between Health and Disease, *edited by P. T. Macklem and S. Permutt*
13. Evolution of Respiratory Processes: A Comparative Approach, *edited by S. C. Wood and C. Lenfant*
14. Pulmonary Vascular Diseases, *edited by K. M. Moser*
15. Physiology and Pharmacology of the Airways, *edited by J. A. Nadel*
16. Diagnostic Techniques in Pulmonary Disease (in two parts), *edited by M. A. Sackner*
17. Regulation of Breathing (in two parts), *edited by T. F. Hornbein*
18. Occupational Lung Diseases: Research Approaches and Methods, *edited by H. Weill and M. Turner-Warwick*
19. Immunopharmacology of the Lung, *edited by H. H. Newball*
20. Sarcoidosis and Other Granulomatous Diseases of the Lung, *edited by B. L. Fanburg*
21. Sleep and Breathing, *edited by N. A. Saunders and C. E. Sullivan*
22. *Pneumocystis carinii* Pneumonia: Pathogenesis, Diagnosis, and Treatment, *edited by L. S. Young*
23. Pulmonary Nuclear Medicine: Techniques in Diagnosis of Lung Disease, *edited by H. L. Atkins*
24. Acute Respiratory Failure, *edited by W. M. Zapol and K. J. Falke*
25. Gas Mixing and Distribution in the Lung, *edited by L. A. Engel and M. Paiva*

26. High-Frequency Ventilation in Intensive Care and During Surgery, *edited by G. Carlon and W. S. Howland*
27. Pulmonary Development: Transition from Intrauterine to Extrauterine Life, *edited by G. H. Nelson*
28. Chronic Obstructive Pulmonary Disease: Second Edition, *edited by T. L. Petty*
29. The Thorax (in two parts), *edited by C. Roussos and P. T. Macklem*
30. The Pleura in Health and Disease, *edited by J. Chrétien, J. Bignon, and A. Hirsch*
31. Drug Therapy for Asthma: Research and Clinical Practice, *edited by J. W. Jenne and S. Murphy*
32. Pulmonary Endothelium in Health and Disease, *edited by U. S. Ryan*
33. The Airways: Neural Control in Health and Disease, *edited by M. A. Kaliner and P. J. Barnes*
34. Pathophysiology and Treatment of Inhalation Injuries, *edited by J. Loke*
35. Respiratory Function of the Upper Airway, *edited by O. P. Mathew and G. Sant'Ambrogio*
36. Chronic Obstructive Pulmonary Disease: A Behavioral Perspective, *edited by A. J. McSweeny and I. Grant*
37. Biology of Lung Cancer: Diagnosis and Treatment, *edited by S. T. Rosen, J. L. Mulshine, F. Cuttitta, and P. G. Abrams*
38. Pulmonary Vascular Physiology and Pathophysiology, *edited by E. K. Weir and J. T. Reeves*
39. Comparative Pulmonary Physiology: Current Concepts, *edited by S. C. Wood*
40. Respiratory Physiology: An Analytical Approach, *edited by H. K. Chang and M. Paiva*
41. Lung Cell Biology, *edited by D. Massaro*
42. Heart–Lung Interactions in Health and Disease, *edited by S. M. Scharf and S. S. Cassidy*
43. Clinical Epidemiology of Chronic Obstructive Pulmonary Disease, *edited by M. J. Hensley and N. A. Saunders*
44. Surgical Pathology of Lung Neoplasms, *edited by A. M. Marchevsky*
45. The Lung in Rheumatic Diseases, *edited by G. W. Cannon and G. A. Zimmerman*
46. Diagnostic Imaging of the Lung, *edited by C. E. Putman*
47. Models of Lung Disease: Microscopy and Structural Methods, *edited by J. Gil*
48. Electron Microscopy of the Lung, *edited by D. E. Schraufnagel*
49. Asthma: Its Pathology and Treatment, *edited by M. A. Kaliner, P. J. Barnes, and C. G. A. Persson*
50. Acute Respiratory Failure: Second Edition, *edited by W. M. Zapol and F. Lemaire*
51. Lung Disease in the Tropics, *edited by O. P. Sharma*
52. Exercise: Pulmonary Physiology and Pathophysiology, *edited by B. J. Whipp and K. Wasserman*
53. Developmental Neurobiology of Breathing, *edited by G. G. Haddad and J. P. Farber*
54. Mediators of Pulmonary Inflammation, *edited by M. A. Bray and W. H. Anderson*
55. The Airway Epithelium, *edited by S. G. Farmer and D. Hay*

56. Physiological Adaptations in Vertebrates: Respiration, Circulation, and Metabolism, *edited by S. C. Wood, R. E. Weber, A. R. Hargens, and R. W. Millard*
57. The Bronchial Circulation, *edited by J. Butler*
58. Lung Cancer Differentiation: Implications for Diagnosis and Treatment, *edited by S. D. Bernal and P. J. Hesketh*
59. Pulmonary Complications of Systemic Disease, *edited by J. F. Murray*
60. Lung Vascular Injury: Molecular and Cellular Response, *edited by A. Johnson and T. J. Ferro*
61. Cytokines of the Lung, *edited by J. Kelley*
62. The Mast Cell in Health and Disease, *edited by M. A. Kaliner and D. D. Metcalfe*
63. Pulmonary Disease in the Elderly Patient, *edited by D. A. Mahler*
64. Cystic Fibrosis, *edited by P. B. Davis*
65. Signal Transduction in Lung Cells, *edited by J. S. Brody, D. M. Center, and V. A. Tkachuk*
66. Tuberculosis: A Comprehensive International Approach, *edited by L. B. Reichman and E. S. Hershfield*
67. Pharmacology of the Respiratory Tract: Experimental and Clinical Research, *edited by K. F. Chung and P. J. Barnes*
68. Prevention of Respiratory Diseases, *edited by A. Hirsch, M. Goldberg, J.-P. Martin, and R. Masse*
69. *Pneumocystis carinii* Pneumonia: Second Edition, *edited by P. D. Walzer*
70. Fluid and Solute Transport in the Airspaces of the Lungs, *edited by R. M. Effros and H. K. Chang*
71. Sleep and Breathing: Second Edition, *edited by N. A. Saunders and C. E. Sullivan*
72. Airway Secretion: Physiological Bases for the Control of Mucous Hypersecretion, *edited by T. Takishima and S. Shimura*
73. Sarcoidosis and Other Granulomatous Disorders, *edited by D. G. James*
74. Epidemiology of Lung Cancer, *edited by J. M. Samet*
75. Pulmonary Embolism, *edited by M. Morpurgo*
76. Sports and Exercise Medicine, *edited by S. C. Wood and R. C. Roach*
77. Endotoxin and the Lungs, *edited by K. L. Brigham*
78. The Mesothelial Cell and Mesothelioma, *edited by M.-C. Jaurand and J. Bignon*
79. Regulation of Breathing: Second Edition, *edited by J. A. Dempsey and A. I. Pack*
80. Pulmonary Fibrosis, *edited by S. Hin. Phan and R. S. Thrall*
81. Long-Term Oxygen Therapy: Scientific Basis and Clinical Application, *edited by W. J. O'Donohue, Jr.*
82. Ventral Brainstem Mechanisms and Control of Respiration and Blood Pressure, *edited by C. O. Trouth, R. M. Millis, H. F. Kiwull-Schöne, and M. E. Schläfke*
83. A History of Breathing Physiology, *edited by D. F. Proctor*
84. Surfactant Therapy for Lung Disease, *edited by B. Robertson and H. W. Taeusch*
85. The Thorax: Second Edition, Revised and Expanded (in three parts), *edited by C. Roussos*

86. Severe Asthma: Pathogenesis and Clinical Management, *edited by S. J. Szefler and D. Y. M. Leung*
87. *Mycobacterium avium*–Complex Infection: Progress in Research and Treatment, *edited by J. A. Korvick and C. A. Benson*
88. Alpha 1–Antitrypsin Deficiency: Biology • Pathogenesis • Clinical Manifestations • Therapy, *edited by R. G. Crystal*
89. Adhesion Molecules and the Lung, *edited by P. A. Ward and J. C. Fantone*
90. Respiratory Sensation, *edited by L. Adams and A. Guz*
91. Pulmonary Rehabilitation, *edited by A. P. Fishman*
92. Acute Respiratory Failure in Chronic Obstructive Pulmonary Disease, *edited by J.-P. Derenne, W. A. Whitelaw, and T. Similowski*
93. Environmental Impact on the Airways: From Injury to Repair, *edited by J. Chrétien and D. Dusser*
94. Inhalation Aerosols: Physical and Biological Basis for Therapy, *edited by A. J. Hickey*
95. Tissue Oxygen Deprivation: From Molecular to Integrated Function, *edited by G. G. Haddad and G. Lister*
96. The Genetics of Asthma, *edited by S. B. Liggett and D. A. Meyers*
97. Inhaled Glucocorticoids in Asthma: Mechanisms and Clinical Actions, *edited by R. P. Schleimer, W. W. Busse, and P. M. O'Byrne*
98. Nitric Oxide and the Lung, *edited by W. M. Zapol and K. D. Bloch*
99. Primary Pulmonary Hypertension, *edited by L. J. Rubin and S. Rich*
100. Lung Growth and Development, *edited by J. A. McDonald*
101. Parasitic Lung Diseases, *edited by A. A. F. Mahmoud*
102. Lung Macrophages and Dendritic Cells in Health and Disease, *edited by M. F. Lipscomb and S. W. Russell*
103. Pulmonary and Cardiac Imaging, *edited by C. Chiles and C. E. Putman*
104. Gene Therapy for Diseases of the Lung, *edited by K. L. Brigham*
105. Oxygen, Gene Expression, and Cellular Function, *edited by L. Biadasz Clerch and D. J. Massaro*
106. Beta$_2$-Agonists in Asthma Treatment, *edited by R. Pauwels and P. M. O'Byrne*
107. Inhalation Delivery of Therapeutic Peptides and Proteins, *edited by A. L. Adjei and P. K. Gupta*
108. Asthma in the Elderly, *edited by R. A. Barbee and J. W. Bloom*
109. Treatment of the Hospitalized Cystic Fibrosis Patient, *edited by D. M. Orenstein and R. C. Stern*
110. Asthma and Immunological Diseases in Pregnancy and Early Infancy, *edited by M. Schatz, R. S. Zeiger, and H. N. Claman*
111. Dyspnea, *edited by D. A. Mahler*
112. Proinflammatory and Antiinflammatory Peptides, *edited by S. I. Said*
113. Self-Management of Asthma, *edited by H. Kotses and A. Harver*
114. Eicosanoids, Aspirin, and Asthma, *edited by A. Szczeklik, R. J. Gryglewski, and J. R. Vane*
115. Fatal Asthma, *edited by A. L. Sheffer*
116. Pulmonary Edema, *edited by M. A. Matthay and D. H. Ingbar*
117. Inflammatory Mechanisms in Asthma, *edited by S. T. Holgate and W. W. Busse*
118. Physiological Basis of Ventilatory Support, *edited by J. J. Marini and A. S. Slutsky*

119. Human Immunodeficiency Virus and the Lung, *edited by M. J. Rosen and J. M. Beck*

120. Five-Lipoxygenase Products in Asthma, *edited by J. M. Drazen, S.-E. Dahlén, and T. H. Lee*

121. Complexity in Structure and Function of the Lung, *edited by M. P. Hlastala and H. T. Robertson*

122. Biology of Lung Cancer, *edited by M. A. Kane and P. A. Bunn, Jr.*

123. Rhinitis: Mechanisms and Management, *edited by R. M. Naclerio, S. R. Durham, and N. Mygind*

124. Lung Tumors: Fundamental Biology and Clinical Management, *edited by C. Brambilla and E. Brambilla*

125. Interleukin-5: From Molecule to Drug Target for Asthma, *edited by C. J. Sanderson*

126. Pediatric Asthma, *edited by S. Murphy and H. W. Kelly*

127. Viral Infections of the Respiratory Tract, *edited by R. Dolin and P. F. Wright*

128. Air Pollutants and the Respiratory Tract, *edited by D. L. Swift and W. M. Foster*

129. Gastroesophageal Reflux Disease and Airway Disease, *edited by M. R. Stein*

130. Exercise-Induced Asthma, *edited by E. R. McFadden, Jr.*

131. LAM and Other Diseases Characterized by Smooth Muscle Proliferation, *edited by J. Moss*

132. The Lung at Depth, *edited by C. E. G. Lundgren and J. N. Miller*

133. Regulation of Sleep and Circadian Rhythms, *edited by F. W. Turek and P. C. Zee*

134. Anticholinergic Agents in the Upper and Lower Airways, *edited by S. L. Spector*

135. Control of Breathing in Health and Disease, *edited by M. D. Altose and Y. Kawakami*

136. Immunotherapy in Asthma, *edited by J. Bousquet and H. Yssel*

137. Chronic Lung Disease in Early Infancy, *edited by R. D. Bland and J. J. Coalson*

138. Asthma's Impact on Society: The Social and Economic Burden, *edited by K. B. Weiss, A. S. Buist, and S. D. Sullivan*

139. New and Exploratory Therapeutic Agents for Asthma, *edited by M. Yeadon and Z. Diamant*

140. Multimodality Treatment of Lung Cancer, *edited by A. T. Skarin*

141. Cytokines in Pulmonary Disease: Infection and Inflammation, *edited by S. Nelson and T. R. Martin*

142. Diagnostic Pulmonary Pathology, *edited by P. T. Cagle*

143. Particle–Lung Interactions, *edited by P. Gehr and J. Heyder*

144. Tuberculosis: A Comprehensive International Approach, Second Edition, Revised and Expanded, *edited by L. B. Reichman and E. S. Hershfield*

145. Combination Therapy for Asthma and Chronic Obstructive Pulmonary Disease, *edited by R. J. Martin and M. Kraft*

146. Sleep Apnea: Implications in Cardiovascular and Cerebrovascular Disease, *edited by T. D. Bradley and J. S. Floras*

147. Sleep and Breathing in Children: A Developmental Approach, *edited by G. M. Loughlin, J. L. Carroll, and C. L. Marcus*

148. Pulmonary and Peripheral Gas Exchange in Health and Disease, *edited by J. Roca, R. Rodriguez-Roisen, and P. D. Wagner*
149. Lung Surfactants: Basic Science and Clinical Applications, *R. H. Notter*
150. Nosocomial Pneumonia, *edited by W. R. Jarvis*
151. Fetal Origins of Cardiovascular and Lung Disease, *edited by David J. P. Barker*
152. Long-Term Mechanical Ventilation, *edited by N. S. Hill*
153. Environmental Asthma, *edited by R. K. Bush*
154. Asthma and Respiratory Infections, *edited by D. P. Skoner*
155. Airway Remodeling, *edited by P. H. Howarth, J. W. Wilson, J. Bousquet, S. Rak, and R. A. Pauwels*
156. Genetic Models in Cardiorespiratory Biology, *edited by G. G. Haddad and T. Xu*
157. Respiratory-Circulatory Interactions in Health and Disease, *edited by S. M. Scharf, M. R. Pinsky, and S. Magder*
158. Ventilator Management Strategies for Critical Care, *edited by N. S. Hill and M. M. Levy*
159. Severe Asthma: Pathogenesis and Clinical Management, Second Edition, Revised and Expanded, *edited by S. J. Szefler and D. Y. M. Leung*
160. Gravity and the Lung: Lessons from Microgravity, *edited by G. K. Prisk, M. Paiva, and J. B. West*
161. High Altitude: An Exploration of Human Adaptation, *edited by T. F. Hornbein and R. B. Schoene*
162. Drug Delivery to the Lung, *edited by H. Bisgaard, C. O'Callaghan, and G. C. Smaldone*
163. Inhaled Steroids in Asthma: Optimizing Effects in the Airways, *edited by R. P. Schleimer, P. M. O'Byrne, S. J. Szefler, and R. Brattsand*
164. IgE and Anti-IgE Therapy in Asthma and Allergic Disease, *edited by R. B. Fick, Jr., and P. M. Jardieu*
165. Clinical Management of Chronic Obstructive Pulmonary Disease, *edited by T. Similowski, W. A. Whitelaw, and J.-P. Derenne*
166. Sleep Apnea: Pathogenesis, Diagnosis, and Treatment, *edited by A. I. Pack*
167. Biotherapeutic Approaches to Asthma, *edited by J. Agosti and A. L. Sheffer*
168. Proteoglycans in Lung Disease, *edited by H. G. Garg, P. J. Roughley, and C. A. Hales*
169. Gene Therapy in Lung Disease, *edited by S. M. Albelda*
170. Disease Markers in Exhaled Breath, *edited by N. Marczin, S. A. Kharitonov, M. H. Yacoub, and P. J. Barnes*

ADDITIONAL VOLUMES IN PREPARATION

Sleep-Related Breathing Disorders: Experimental Models and Therapeutic Potential, *edited by D. W. Carley and M. Radulovacki*

Chemokines in the Lung, *edited by R. Strieter, S. L. Kunkel, and T. Standiford*

The Immunological Basis of Asthma, *edited by B. N. Lambrecht, H. C. Hoogsteden, and Z. Diamant*

Lung Volume Reduction Surgery for Emphysema, *edited by H. E. Fessler, J. J. Reilly, Jr., and D. J. Sugarbaker*

Therapeutic Targets in Airway Inflammation, *edited by N. T. Eissa and D. Huston*

Oxygen Sensing: Responses and Adaptation to Hypoxia, *edited by S. Lahiri, G. Semenza, and N. Prabhakar*

Non-Neoplastic Advanced Lung Disease, *edited by J. Maurer*

Respiratory Control and Disorders in the Newborn, *edited by O. Mathew*

Respiratory Infections in Asthma and Allergy, *edited by S. Johnston and N. Papadopoulos*

The opinions expressed in these volumes do not necessarily represent the views of the National Institutes of Health.

GENE THERAPY IN LUNG DISEASE

Edited by

Steven M. Albelda

University of Pennsylvania Medical Center
Philadelphia, Pennsylvania, U.S.A.

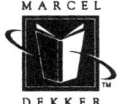

MARCEL DEKKER, INC.　　　　NEW YORK · BASEL

ISBN: 0-8247-0820-2

This book is printed on acid-free paper.

Headquarters
Marcel Dekker, Inc.
270 Madison Avenue, New York, NY 10016
tel: 212-696-9000; fax: 212-685-4540

Eastern Hemisphere Distribution
Marcel Dekker AG
Hutgasse 4, Postfach 812, CH-4001 Basel, Switzerland
tel: 41-61-260-6300; fax: 41-61-260-6333

World Wide Web
http://www.dekker.com

The publisher offers discounts on this book when ordered in bulk quantities. For more information, write to Special Sales/Professional Marketing at the headquarters address above.

Current printing (last digit):
10 9 8 7 6 5 4 3 2 1

PRINTED IN THE UNITED STATES OF AMERICA

INTRODUCTION

Gene therapy: a panacea?

In 1997, the Lung Biology in Health and Disease series introduced Volume 104, *Gene Therapy for Diseases of the Lung.* We are now presenting *Gene Therapy in Lung Disease.* Even casual observers will note that the editors and all the contributors for these two volumes are different; however, they may overlook the subtle but very significant difference in these titles. Indeed, the change in the key preposition from the inclusive "for" to the narrower "in" reflects the evolution of our understanding of, and expectations from, gene therapy.

Gene therapy as a concept, and then as a science, has been with us for a long time. The first chapter of Volume 104 retraces very well the developments of the 1960s and 1970s (1). We all remember that the first clinical applications of gene therapy were reported in the early 1990s (2,3). These first reports led to a huge research effort and, at least in some circles, optimism—and perhaps even expectation—that the cure for some conditions was in sight. We believed that gene therapy could be the hope *for* entire groups of diseases.

Since that time research has been extraordinarily productive, but each answer has led to new sets of questions. Now we have come to realize that if gene therapy ever comes to fruition, it will be applicable only *in* selected conditions, and only after much more research.

Today, at the dawn of this new decade, interest in gene therapy remains strong, as well it should, since many diseases may undoubtedly benefit from gene transfer. In some cases, pulmonary pathologies should be correctable by such an approach.

This new volume edited by Steven Albelda brings to the readership the most recent research and clinical outcomes pertaining to gene therapy in lung disease. As is quickly apparent, no definitive or even imminent cure is described, but a panoramic view of what may be expected is presented. The reader will be left with the strong feeling that we are close to something that has the potential to be very important, especially for some patients.

This volume is a valuable contribution to the Lung Biology in Health and Disease series. For this, I am very grateful to Dr. Albelda and to all the contributors.

Claude Lenfant, M.D.
Bethesda, Maryland

References

1. Anderson WF. Human gene therapy: the initial concepts. In: Brigham KL, ed. Gene Therapy for Diseases of the Lung. New York: Marcel Dekker, 1997:3–16.
2. Rosenberg SA, Aebersold P, Cornetta K, Kasid A, Morgan RA, Moen R, et al. Gene transfer into humans—immunotherapy of patients with advanced melanoma, using tumor-infiltrating lymphocytes modified by retroviral gene transduction. N Engl J Med 1990; 323:570–578.
3. Blase RM, Culver KW, Miller AD, Carter CS, Fleisher T, Cleric M, et al. T lymphocyte-directed gene therapy for ADA SCID: initial trial results after 4 years. Science 1995; 270:475–480.

PREFACE

When gene therapy became a clinical reality in the early 1990s, the possibilities seemed endless. Excitement was high and expectations were raised, leading to a generalized "suspension of disbelief." It seemed clear that the two most important pulmonary genetic diseases, cystic fibrosis and α_1-antitrypsin disease, would soon be conquered and that a cancer cure was close behind. Alas, as with the monoclonal antibody revolution of the 1970s and the molecular biology revolution of the 1980s, real and substantial translation of therapies from "bench to bedside" was a much more difficult and slow task than was originally anticipated.

Gene therapy is now in its adolescence and, like any good teenager, is suffering from the normal amount of angst and turmoil. The frenzy and hype of the early and mid-1990s were brought to a screeching halt by the general lack of successful clinical trials and by the death of a relatively normal teenager who had volunteered for a Phase I clinical trial to treat a metabolic liver disorder. Suspension of disbelief was replaced with "presumption of disbelief" and a generally negative perception.

Somewhere between these two extremes lies the truth. In actuality, gene therapy has made tremendous strides over its short 12-year lifetime. First, gene therapy techniques have been applied successfully to the study of cell biology and animal models of disease. The ability to deliver genes to animals in a controlled and specific manner has revolutionized our ability to study disease processes. Second, many clinical trials have been performed and analyzed. Although dramatic clinical efficacy has not yet been shown, almost all of the human trials conducted were dose-finding Phase I trials designed to evaluate toxicity, not responses. It is therefore not surprising that clinical success stories have been unusual to date. One major finding of the last decade is that gene therapy has proven to be a remarkably safe and nontoxic approach. Thousands of patients have undergone gene therapy with very little toxicity. Third, a great deal of research has gone into studying, characterizing, and developing new vector approaches to optimize gene transfer. These studies will define the shape of gene therapy trials in the future.

Another interesting benefit of gene therapy is that it has inspired physician-scientists, not working for pharmaceutical or drug companies, to design and conduct clinical research aimed at delivering useful treatments to patients. Many of us have dreamed of developing and testing new therapies, but for the most part, this has been within the purview of industry, not academia. Many of the early gene therapy trials were initiated and conducted by individual groups of academic investigators, with funding from the National Institutes of Health, allowing unprecedented freedom. This academic orientation has allowed researchers to define more freely the benefits and significant limitations of current technology than might be possible in a traditional pharmaceutical environment. This dissemination of knowledge about the limitations of the "first-generation" vectors has been critical in spurring the development of improved or new technologies. Thus, although the early years of gene therapy were dominated by first-generation adenoviral and retroviral vectors, more recently "gutless" third-generation adenoviruses, adeno-associated viral vectors, and lentiviral vectors have moved to center stage.

Gene therapy of lung disease has always played a central role in gene therapy and has often led the field. Although a volume of this series devoted to gene therapy for diseases of the lung was published in 1997, enough has changed since then to warrant an update. After a general historical overview, the book is divided into three parts. The first presents a detailed discussion of each of the major vector systems being used in lung gene therapy today. These include adenoviral and adeno-associated viral vectors, liposomes, and replicating vectors. Also included is an examination of advances in the targeting of gene therapy vectors. The second part focuses on the use of gene therapy to study lung disease processes (primarily in animal models) such as cytokine behavior, infection and immunity, and fibrosis. The last part describes the use of gene therapy to treat specific lung diseases such as lung cancer, mesothelioma, cystic fibrosis, pulmonary vascular diseases, α_1-antitrypsin disease, acute lung injury, and lung transplantation.

I would like to thank the chapter authors for their willingness to participate in this endeavor and for their outstanding contributions. I have been honored to work with Dr. Claude Lenfant, who asked me to edit this volume and who has been extremely supportive. I have no doubt that gene therapy will be an extremely valuable part of the therapeutic armamentarium of the 21st century. Dr. Lenfant and the authors of these chapters are the people who will ensure that this will happen.

Steven M. Albelda

CONTRIBUTORS

Eric W. F. W. Alton, M.D., F.R.C.P.　Professor, Department of Gene Therapy, Imperial College, National Heart and Lung Institute, London, England

Kunjlata M. Amin, Ph.D.　Research Assistant Professor, Department of Surgery, University of Pennsylvania School of Medicine, Philadelphia, Pennsylvania, U.S.A.

Raj K. Batra, M.D., F.C.C.P.　Assistant Professor, Division of Pulmonary and Critical Care Medicine, Department of Medicine, UCLA School of Medicine, and Veterans Administration Greater Los Angeles Healthcare System, Los Angeles, California, U.S.A.

Richard C. Boucher, M.D.　William R. Kenan Professor, Department of Medicine, and Director, Cystic Fibrosis Pulmonary Research and Treatment Center, University of North Carolina at Chapel Hill, Chapel Hill, North Carolina, U.S.A.

Mark Buchholz, M.D.　Division of Pediatric Critical Care, Department of Pediatrics, University of Colorado Health Sciences Center, and The Children's Hospital, Denver, Colorado, U.S.A.

Stephen D. Cassivi, M.D., M.Sc., F.R.C.S.C.   Assistant Professor, Division of Thoracic Surgery, Department of Surgery, Mayo Medical School, and Mayo Clinic, Rochester, Minnesota, U.S.A.

Dongsheng Duan, Ph.D.   Assistant Professor, Department of Microbiology and Immunology, University of Missouri, Columbia, Missouri, U.S.A.

Steven M. Dubinett, M.D.   Professor, Department of Medicine, and Director, UCLA Lung Cancer Research Program, UCLA School of Medicine, and Veterans Administration Greater Los Angeles Healthcare System, Los Angeles, California, U.S.A.

John F. Engelhardt, Ph.D.   Professor, Department of Anatomy and Cell Biology, and Director, Center for Gene Therapy, University of Iowa School of Medicine, Iowa City, Iowa, U.S.A.

Terence R. Flotte, M.D.   Professor, Departments of Pediatrics and Molecular Genetics and Microbiology, and Director, Powell Gene Therapy Center and University of Florida Genetics Institute, University of Florida College of Medicine, Gainesville, Florida, U.S.A.

Jack Gauldie, Ph.D.   Professor and Chair, Department of Pathology and Molecular Medicine, McMaster University, Hamilton, Ontario, Canada

Larry G. Johnson, M.D.   Associate Professor, Departments of Medicine and Pharmacology, and Cystic Fibrosis Pulmonary Research and Treatment Center, University of North Carolina at Chapel Hill, Chapel Hill, North Carolina, U.S.A.

Samer A. Kanaan, M.D.   Division of Cardiothoracic Surgery, Department of Surgery, Washington University School of Medicine, St. Louis, Missouri, U.S.A.

Martin Kolb, M.D.   Assistant Professor, Department of Medicine and Respiratory Care, Julius-Maximilian-Universität Würzburg, Würzburg, Germany

Jay K. Kolls, M.D.   Professor of Medicine and Pediatrics, Department of Medicine, and Director, Gene Therapy Program, Louisiana State University Health Sciences Center, New Orleans, Louisiana, U.S.A.

Benjamin D. Kozower, M.D.   Thoracic Surgery Research Fellow, Division of Cardiothoracic Surgery, Department of Surgery, Washington University School of Medicine, St. Louis, Missouri, U.S.A.

G. Alexander Patterson, M.D.   Joseph C. Bancroft Professor and Head, General Thoracic Surgery Section, Division of Cardiothoracic Surgery, Department of Surgery, Washington University School of Medicine, St. Louis, Missouri, U.S.A.

Perri Prellop, M.D.   Department of Medicine, Louisiana State University Health Sciences Center, New Orleans, Louisiana, U.S.A.

Paul N. Reynolds, M.B.B.S., Ph.D., F.R.A.C.P.   Senior Consultant Physician, Department of Thoracic Medicine, Royal Adelaide Hospital, Adelaide, South Australia, Australia

Thomas C. Reynolds, M.D., Ph.D.   Senior Medical Director, Zymogenetics, Seattle, Washington, U.S.A.

David M. Rodman, M.D.   Professor, Division of Pulmonary and Critical Care Medicine, Department of Medicine, University of Colorado Health Sciences Center, and The Children's Hospital, Denver, Colorado, U.S.A.

Ronald K. Scheule, Ph.D.   Scientific Director, Gene Transfer Research, Genzyme Corporation, Framingham, Massachusetts, U.S.A.

Sherven Sharma, Ph.D.   Assistant Research Professor, Division of Pulmonary and Critical Care Medicine, Department of Medicine, UCLA School of Medicine, and Veterans Administration Greater Los Angeles Healthcare System, Los Angeles, California, U.S.A.

Patricia J. Sime, M.D., F.R.C.P.(UK)   Assistant Professor, Division of Pulmonary and Critical Care Medicine, Department of Medicine, University of Rochester Medical Center, Rochester, New York, U.S.A.

Richard H. Simon, M.D.   Professor, Division of Pulmonary and Critical Care Medicine, Department of Internal Medicine, University of Michigan, Ann Arbor, Michigan, U.S.A.

Thomas H. Sisson, M.D.   Assistant Professor, Division of Pulmonary and Critical Care Medicine, Department of Internal Medicine, University of Michigan, Ann Arbor, Michigan, U.S.A.

Daniel H. Sterman, M.D.   Assistant Professor, Division of Pulmonary, Allergy, and Critical Care, Department of Medicine, University of Pennsylvania Medical Center, Philadelphia, Pennsylvania, U.S.A.

Myra Stern, Ph.D., M.B.Ch.B., M.R.C.P. Clinical Senior Lecturer, Department of Gene Therapy, Imperial College, National Heart and Lung Institute, London, England

Robert M. Strieter, M.D. Professor and Chief, Division of Pulmonary and Critical Care Medicine, and Vice Chair, Department of Medicine, UCLA School of Medicine, Los Angeles, California, U.S.A.

David Warburton, D.Sc., M.D., F.R.C.P. Professor, Developmental Biology Program, Childrens Hospital Los Angeles Research Institute, University of Southern California School of Medicine, Los Angeles, California, U.S.A.

Daniel J. Weiss, M.D., Ph.D. Division of Pulmonary and Critical Care Medicine, Department of Medicine, Vermont Lung Center, University of Vermont College of Medicine, Burlington, Vermont, U.S.A.

James West, M.D. Division of Pulmonary and Critical Care Medicine, Department of Medicine, University of Colorado Health Sciences Center, Denver, Colorado, U.S.A.

James M. Wilson, M.D., Ph.D. Director, Institute for Human Gene Therapy, University of Pennsylvania School of Medicine, Philadelphia, Pennsylvania, U.S.A.

Nelson A. Wivel, M.D. Deputy Director, Institute for Human Gene Therapy, University of Pennsylvania School of Medicine, Philadelphia, Pennsylvania, U.S.A.

Zhou Xing, M.D., Ph.D. Associate Professor, Department of Pathology and Molecular Medicine, McMaster University, Hamilton, Ontario, Canada

Yongping Yue, B.A. Research Specialist, Department of Microbiology and Immunology, University of Missouri, Columbia, Missouri, U.S.A.

CONTENTS

Introduction   Claude Lenfant   *iii*
Preface   *v*
Contributors   *ix*

1. Gene Therapy: Historical Overview and Public Oversight   1
   Nelson A. Wivel

    I.   Introduction   1
    II. Gene Delivery Systems   3
    III. Disease Targets: Clinical Trials   11
    IV. Summary of Clinical History   18
    V. Public Oversight of Human Gene Therapy   18
       References   23

Part One   VECTOROLOGY

2. **Adenoviruses as Vectors for Human Gene Therapy**   31
   James M. Wilson

   I.   Introduction   31
   II.   Biology of Adenoviruses   32
   III. Adenoviral Vectors: How Do You Make Them?   34
   IV.   Biology of E1-Deleted Adenoviruses   38
   V.   Summary   43
         References   44

3. **Adeno-Associated Virus**   51
   Dongsheng Duan, Yongping Yue, and John F. Engelhardt

   I.   Introduction   51
   II.   Basic Biology of Adeno-Associated Virus and rAAV
         Vectors   52
   III. Advances in the Use of Recombinant AAV as a Gene
         Therapy Vector   67
   IV.   Recombinant AAV–Mediated Gene Transfer to the Lung   69
   V.   Summary and Perspective   76
         References   78

4. **Cationic Lipids for Lung Gene Therapy**   93
   Ronald K. Scheule

   I.   Introduction   93
   II.   The Delivery System—Cationic Lipid:pDNA Complexes   94
   III. Cationic Lipid:pDNA Complexes and Transfection of
         the Lung   101
   IV.   Future Use of Liposomes for Lung Gene Therapy   111
         References   112

5. **Targeting Gene Delivery for Pulmonary Disease**   119
   Paul N. Reynolds

   I.   Introduction   119
   II.   Pathway of Ad Infection   120
   III. Conjugate-Based Retargeting Approaches   123
   IV.   Genetic Capsid Modifications   128
   V.   Combined Transductional and Transcriptional
         Approaches   133
   VI.   Reticuloendothelial Sequestration   135

	VII.	Targeting Approaches for Other Vectors	135
	VIII.	Conclusions	136
		References	136

6. Replicating Vectors **145**
Kunjlata M. Amin

	I.	Replicating Vectors: A Tool for Cancer Gene Therapy	145
	II.	An Ideal Targeted Replicating Vector	146
	III.	Replicating Agents	146
	IV.	Wild-Type Replicating Vectors	147
	V.	Genetically Modified Vectors	148
	VI.	Transcriptional Regulation of Early Viral Expressed Proteins	156
	VII.	Tumor Pathway Genes as Targets	159
	VIII.	Summary	160
		References	161

Part Two   USE OF GENE THERAPY TO STUDY LUNG DISEASES

7. Use of Gene Transfer to Study Lung Cytokine Biology **171**
Jack Gauldie, Martin Kolb, Patricia J. Sime, David Warburton, and Zhou Xing

	I.	Introduction	171
	II.	Gene Transfer to the Lung	172
	III.	Chemokine Function and Cell Accumulation	174
	IV.	Immune Modulation and Cytokines	175
	V.	Granulocyte-Macrophage Colony–Stimulating Factor and Lung Inflammation and Immunity	175
	VI.	Cytokines and the Allergic Airway Response	176
	VII.	Cytokines and the Pulmonary Fibrotic Response	177
	VIII.	Cytokines and Infectious Diseases	182
	IX.	Summary	184
		References	184

8. Use of Gene Therapy to Study Lung Infection and Immunity **193**
Perri Prellop and Jay K. Kolls

| | I. | Introduction | 193 |
| | II. | Candidate Genes for Immunotherapy | 194 |

	III.	DNA Vaccines	199
	IV.	Results in Disease Models	200
	V.	Summary	208
		References	208

9. Use of In Vivo Gene Transfer to Study Pulmonary Fibrosis   **219**
Thomas H. Sisson and Richard H. Simon

	I.	Introduction	219
	II.	Advantages of Using a Gene Transfer Approach to Study Lung Fibrosis	220
	III.	Elucidating the Pathogenesis of Pulmonary Fibrosis Through Gene Transfer Technology	221
	IV.	Limitations of Gene Transfer Technology in the Study of Pulmonary Fibrosis	227
	V.	Summary	228
		References	229

Part Three   **USE OF GENE THERAPY TO TREAT LUNG DISEASES**

10. Gene Therapy for Lung Cancer   **233**
Raj K. Batra, Sherven Sharma, Robert M. Strieter, and Steven M. Dubinett

	I.	Introduction	233
	II.	Human Lung Cancer	234
	III.	Preclinical Murine Models of Human Lung Cancer Utilized in Studies of Gene Therapy	236
	IV.	Gene- and Cell-Based Therapies for Lung Cancer	241
	V.	Gene Delivery for Lung Cancer Therapy	261
	VI.	Summary	265
		References	265

11. Gene Therapy for Malignant Mesothelioma   **293**
Daniel H. Sterman

	I.	Introduction	293
	II.	Suicide Gene Therapy	294
	III.	Suicide Gene Vaccines	303
	IV.	Cytokine Gene Therapy for Mesothelioma	305
	V.	Induction of Apoptosis	308
	VI.	SV40: Is There a Role in Therapy for Mesothelioma?	310
	VII.	Conclusions	311
		References	312

12. Strategies for Gene Therapy of Cystic Fibrosis   **319**
Larry G. Johnson and Richard C. Boucher

     I.   Introduction   319
   II.   Vectors for Lung Gene Transfer   320
  III.   Barriers to Airway Gene Transfer   321
  IV.   Strategies to Overcome Apical Membrane Barriers to
         Efficient Transduction   335
    V.   Conclusions   349
        References   349

**13. Use of Adeno-Associated Virus in the Treatment of
Cystic Fibrosis**   **365**
Thomas C. Reynolds

     I.   Adeno-Associated Virus for CF Gene Transfer   365
   II.   AAV-CFTR Vector Development   366
  III.   Delivery of AAV Vectors to the Lung   367
  IV.   Clinical Studies   370
    V.   Future Directions for AAV-CFTR Gene Therapy   375
        References   377

14. Use of Liposomes in the Treatment of Cystic Fibrosis   **383**
Myra Stern and Eric W. F. W. Alton

     I.   Introduction   383
   II.   Nonviral Vectors   383
  III.   Gene Therapy for Cystic Fibrosis   386
  IV.   Future Considerations   390
    V.   Conclusions   393
        References   393

15. Delivery of Genes Through the Lung Circulation   **397**
David M. Rodman, Mark Buchholz, and James West

     I.   Rationale and Therapeutic Targets   397
   II.   Cell-Based Gene Delivery   398
  III.   Nonviral Gene Delivery   399
  IV.   Viral Gene Delivery   401
    V.   Using the Airway for Gene Therapy of Pulmonary
         Hypertension   402
  VI.   Conclusions   404
        References   404

16. Gene Therapy for α₁-Antitrypsin Deficiency   407
      Terrence R. Flotte

         I. Introduction   407
        II. Retrovirus Vectors   408
       III. Recombinant Adenoviral Vectors   409
        IV. Helper-Dependent Adenoviral Vectors   410
         V. Nonviral DNA Transfer   411
        VI. Recombinant Adeno-Associated Vectors   411
       VII. Other Novel Systems   414
      VIII. Conclusions   414
             References   415

**17. Gene Therapy and Gene Transfer Approaches for Acute
      Lung Injury**   419
      Daniel J. Weiss

         I. Introduction   419
        II. Barriers to Airway Gene Delivery   420
       III. Vectors for Use in Acute Lung Injury: Airway-Based
             Delivery   422
        IV. Vectors for Use in Acute Lung Injury: Intravenous
             Delivery   428
         V. Methods of Airway Gene Delivery   429
        VI. Adjunct Methods for Airway Gene Delivery   430
       VII. Experience with Gene Transfer in Acute Lung Injury   433
      VIII. Conclusions   440
             References   440

18. Gene Therapy for Lung Transplantation   457
      Samer A. Kanaan, Benjamin D. Kozower, Stephen D. Cassivi,
      and G. Alexander Patterson

         I. Introduction   457
        II. Clinical Overview   457
       III. Therapeutic Approach Using Gene Therapy   460
        IV. Potential Human Use   466
         V. Conclusions   466
             References   467

Author Index   *475*
Subject Index   *545*

1

Gene Therapy
Historical Overview and Public Oversight

NELSON A. WIVEL

University of Pennsylvania School of Medicine
Philadelphia, Pennsylvania, U.S.A.

The goals of this chapter are to provide a historical overview of the field of gene therapy and discuss issues related to public and governmental oversight. In addition, a broad overview of the general gene delivery systems in use today and an update of gene therapy trials being conducted outside the lung will be provided. More details about each particular vector system and the use of these vectors in lung diseases will be discussed in subsequent chapters.

I. Introduction

For the past 10 years, the field of human gene therapy has received rather intense attention from the lay press because of the interest associated with clinical trials. The concept that human genetic disease can be treated at the molecular level, that is, at the level of defective genes, is of sufficient importance to attract such attention. However, as long as 40 years ago, some scientists began to postulate the ability to do gene transfer at a time when certain critical techniques in molecular genetics had not been developed (1). In 1966, Tatum hypothesized that viruses could be used as effective tools for introducing genes into cells and he outlined a set of experiments that currently would be interpreted as ex vivo transduction

(2). Lederberg predicted that it would be possible to culture germ cells in vitro, that interchange of chromosomal segments would be feasible, and that ultimately there would be the means for directly controlling nucleotide sequences (3). Shortly after Kornberg reported the in vitro synthesis of DNA, he suggested that it might be feasible to attach a gene to a harmless viral DNA and to treat monogenic deficiency diseases by putting the virus/gene complex into the patient's cells (4).

An observation in the early 1970s led to an attempt to treat arginemia. Rogers and his colleagues noted that some scientists working with the Shope papillomavirus (SPV) in the laboratory had subnormal levels of serum arginine. It was thought that SPV contained a gene encoding viral arginase and that a subclinical infection with this agent lowered the arginine levels (5). A human clinical study was initiated and wild-type SPV was administered to two young German girls who had arginase deficiency and resulting hyperargininemia. Unfortunately, no data developed to indicate that these research subjects were either improved or adversely affected as a result of this clinical experiment (6).

In 1980, the next attempt at clinical gene therapy occurred when Cline chose to treat β-thalassemia by using the calcium phosphate transfection technique to introduce the β-globin gene into bone marrow cells (7). Two patients were enrolled in this particular trial, one in Italy and one in Israel. Since this particular protocol did not receive approval from the local safety committees at the University of California at Los Angeles, the principal investigator was subjected to multiple penalties and censure. There was no report of any follow-up of these patients, and the fate of the introduced genes was unknown.

During the period of 1986–1987, there were a number of seminal discussions between French Anderson and his colleagues and members of the Human Gene Therapy Subcommittee (HGTS), a principal subcommittee of the National Institutes of Health (NIH) Recombinant DNA Advisory Committee (RAC). These discussions included the use of retroviral vectors as gene delivery agents, the use of transgenic animals in the development of preclinical data, and the proposed Food and Drug Administration (FDA) guidelines for the use of gene therapy in Phase I clinical trials. In 1987, Anderson presented a large tome to the RAC that represented an extensive collation of preclinical data. On July 29, 1988, Steven Rosenberg and French Anderson formally presented to the HGTS a request for a clinical gene transfer trial. This was not a typical gene therapy trial, but was a so-called "gene marking" trial designed to establish that retroviral vectors could be used to deliver the neomycin resistance gene to patients' cells without causing any serious adverse events. On March 30, 1990, Michael Blaese and Anderson submitted a gene therapy protocol for the study of adenosine deaminase deficiency (ADA) and by July 31, 1990, the HGTS and the RAC both approved this research proposal. On September 14, 1990, the first research subject was treated, and thus the era of clinical gene therapy was officially launched.

II. Gene Delivery Systems

A. Retroviral and Lentiviral Vectors

As early as 1981, several different research groups were successful in developing replication-defective avian and murine retroviral vectors (8–10). With the advent of such tools it was now possible to test an important proof of concept—correcting genetic defects through the transduction of normal genes into affected cells. One of the first important experiments involved the use of a retroviral vector to correct both the enzyme defect and purine metabolic abnormalities in cells taken from a patient with Lesch-Nyhan syndrome (11).

There are several characteristics of the retroviral vectors that made these entities popular as the first system for gene delivery. A key requirement in the development of a viral vector is the development of a recombinant virus that is replication defective but capable of infecting a cell. For retroviruses this has been achieved by deleting all the genes that code for viral structural proteins and then inserting either a therapeutic gene or a marker gene. The absence of approximately 80% of the viral genome reduces the likelihood that recombinational events will produce replication-competent virus as the vector is passed through a packaging cell line. Another important appeal of retroviral vectors derives from the fact that the virus integrates into the chromosomes of the host cell, thus providing the opportunity for prolonged gene expression. Two complicating characteristics of this system are the requirement for dividing cells and the fact that retroviral integration occurs randomly rather than being site specific, thus creating the potential for insertional mutagenesis. Compared to other viral systems, it is difficult to grow retroviruses to high titer, and this presents logistical problems when contemplating relatively large-scale clinical trials.

More recently, there has been an intense interest in developing vectors derived from the lentivirus subfamily Retroviridae, and the lentivirus of choice is the human immunodeficiency virus (HIV). Interest in this virus as a useful gene transfer system derives from the fact that it has the potential to integrate into nondividing cells. One vector construct using HIV is made by using a three-plasmid expression system (12). One plasmid contains a cytomegaloviral promoter, but it is defective for production of the viral envelope, and it contains substitutions that eliminate sequences essential for packaging, reverse transcription, and integration. A second plasmid encodes a heterologous envelope protein from the vesicular stomatitis virus that is used to broaden the tropism of the vector. The third plasmid contains some essential *cis*-acting sequences plus unique restriction sites for cloning of heterologous complementary DNAs. When tested in rat brains, these vectors were capable of transducing terminally differentiated neurons.

Some very recent work that has focused on developing vectors with a specificity for targeting respiratory epithelium utilizes a vector based on a Filovirus

(Ebola virus) envelope protein that is pseudotyped with an HIV vector. Pseudo-typing was chosen as a strategy since it can allow for efficient gene transfer into specific tissues via a particular cellular domain; this is based on the well-known fact that the viral envelope contributes to the tropism of the virus and determines if a virus-host cell interaction will occur. This particular vector has been shown to transduce efficiently intact airway epithelium from the apical surface in both in vitro and in vivo model systems (13).

B. Adenoviral Vectors

Much of the early work in gene therapy trials involved the ex vivo transduction of target cells and this addressed both biological and safety issues. Under ex vivo conditions, it was possible to control the target cell population by using selection methods such as introducing the neomycin resistance gene and growing the cells in G418 medium or by using fluorescence-activated cell sorting. Since it was frequently necessary to expand the cells in culture, the requisite dividing cells were provided for the retroviral vectors then in use.

In order to make the transition to in vivo gene therapy and to target termi-nally differentiated cells that divide infrequently, it was essential to develop new types of viral vectors. It was fundamentally obvious that adenoviruses had proper-ties that were relevant for in vivo gene delivery, because they could transfer transgenes into a host of different types of dividing and nondividing cells. Be-cause adenoviruses are primarily lung-trophic viruses they were first used to de-liver the cystic fibrosis transmembrane conductance regulator (CFTR) gene trans-fer in cystic fibrosis patients. As compared to retroviruses, adenoviruses can be grown to high titer (10^{12} pfu/mL); however, they are not integrating vectors and there is no potential for long-term gene expression.

One of the fundamental issues concerning adenovirus is that of the host immune response. The immune system does not distinguish between naturally occurring wild-type adenoviruses and recombinant adenoviral vectors. Similar to the parent virus, the vector is internalized by macrophages and the vector genome expresses viral proteins that are presented by major histocompatibility (MHC) class I molecules to CD8$^+$ T cells that are cytotoxic for vector-infected cells. Viral capsid proteins from the input vector are presented by MHC class II molecules to CD4$^+$ T helper cells that stimulate cytotoxic T lymphocytes that will destroy transduced target cells and provoke inflammation (14). As a part of the humoral response, B cells are activated along with certain CD4$^+$ T-cell subsets to produce neutralizing antibodies that can block adenoviral receptor sites; this immune re-sponse can effectively prevent the second administration of vector.

Two principal methodologies can be applied to address the problems asso-ciated with the immune response. One involves the development of immuno-modulatory approaches, and this work is largely confined to experimental animal models. The other requires creation of vector constructs that have additional dele-tions of structural genes. Several generations of adenoviral vectors have been produced. A first-generation recombinant had deletions of the entire E1a and part of the E1b portions of the genome (15,16). A second-generation vector was constructed by deleting the E1A and E1B genes and introducing a temperature-sensitive mutation in the E2A gene (17). One of the more useful constructs is a third-generation vector that is deleted in both E1 and E4 regions; although transgene expression is no more stable than in earlier generation vectors, the vector is more replication defective, and two recombinational events are required to produce a replication-competent virus (18). Several groups of investigators have expended considerable effort in producing adenovirus vectors that are de-leted of all viral structural genes, leaving only *cis*-acting sequences necessary for packaging and integration. Producing this type of construct requires the use of E1-deleted helper virus, but the fully deleted vector and the helper virus can be physically separated on cesium chloride density gradients. Although this class of vectors has the advantage of a large transgene capacity, and may have the advantage of prolonged expression and less toxicity than earlier generation vec-tors, the removal of helper virus is a limiting factor and results in titers that are much lower than seen in partially deleted vectors (19).

Very recent studies of innate immunity in nonhuman primates following intraportal administration of adenoviral vectors suggest some of the fundamental problems associated with the use of this particular delivery system. First-genera-tion vectors given at doses just below the level that causes severe morbidity revealed a primary distribution in macrophages and dendritic cells of the spleen and Kupffer cells of the liver. A systemic release of interleukin-6 (IL-6) occurred soon after the vector infusion. Similar findings were seen in a monkey who re-ceived an identical dose of vector in which the genes were inactivated with psor-alen and ultraviolet irradiation. Such data infer that portal infusion leads to an inadvertent targeting of antigen-presenting cells and a systemic cytokine syn-drome that could by triggered by viral capsid proteins (20). In view of these results, it is necessary to consider that use of adenoviral vectors may need to be selective; that is, their optimum advantage will occur in situations where short-term gene expression is adequate and an immune response could be useful. This strategy is typified by the adoptive immunotherapy approaches used in the study and potential treatment of various types of cancers.

C. Adeno-Associated Virus Vectors

Adeno-associated virus (AAV) has proven to be of great interest to the gene therapy community because of some of the properties of this agent. Under appro-priate experimental conditions, AAV has the capacity to efficiently transduce target cells, and there are studies documenting long-term expression of the transgene (21). Further, AAV does not appear to evoke the same type of intense immune response associated with adenoviruses, and there is an absence of toxicity with this vector, as the parent virus is not associated with any known disease in humans.

There are two very distinct components in the AAV life cycle, a latent infection that is established in cells when there is no helper virus present and a lytic infection that is initiated by adenoviral coinfection; in addition, herpesvirus can also function as a helper virus. It has been established that it is the expression of the adenoviral early region genes (E1 and E4) that is essential to triggering the lytic infection (22).

One feature of the latent infection is that AAV is integrated as a stable provirus that preferentially targets the q.13.4-ter arm of chromosome 19 (23). This property of site-specific integration is the source of considerable appeal for a vector to be used in gene therapy, as it avoids the problem of insertional mutagenesis. This stands in contrast to the retroviral vectors where insertion is a random event. However, it is not clear that the recombinant AAV vectors consistently retain the ability for site-specific integration.

There is considerable experimental data to confirm that AAV vectors can be used to transduce a wide variety of cells including both differentiated and nondifferentiated types as well as nondividing cells and hematopoietic stem cells. Much of the data were derived through the in vitro use of immortalized cell lines, and that always raises the question of relevance to in vivo conditions, a problem that applies to all vector systems.

Two characteristics of this vector system pose challenges. One involves the development of uniform standards to determine the infectious dose used in a given experiment. Different laboratories have developed sets of nomenclature to describe their results. The fact that there is a requirement for superinfection with a helper virus makes it difficult to use a simple plaque assay to measure the titer. At present, some laboratories are using a combination of techniques and compare the number of genome copies of AAV with the results of an infectious center assay. In addition to the complexities associated with assay, there are technical problems associated with the production of recombinant vectors. Although many of the current procedures have essentially removed the generation of wild-type AAV recombinants, the techniques rely on the presence of wild-type adenovirus to provide essential helper functions for recombinant AAV replication. This results in the coproduction of wild-type adenovirus along with recombinant AAV, thus creating a problem of wild-type adenovirus contamination in recombinant AAV preparations (24). In order to circumvent this problem, some investigators have replaced adenoviral helper with an adeno-helper plasmid. In effect, the method requires triple transfection but produces recombinant AAV that is free of adenoviral helper (25).

The first two clinical trials involving the application of AAV vectors were Phase I studies and enrolled cystic fibrosis patients. One trial involved the administration of an AAV-CFTR construct to the nasal and bronchial epithelium (26). In the second trial, the vector was instilled in the maxillary sinuses of patients with cystic fibrosis.

D. Herpes Simplex Viral Vectors

Because of its natural biological properties, herpes simplex virus (HSV) has generated considerable interest as a vector for gene transfer to terminally differentiated, nondividing cells of neuronal origin. Primary infection by wild-type HSV occurs by direct contact, and the virus penetrates epithelial cells of skin or mucous membrane. Replication of the virus requires expression of certain so-called immediate early (IE) genes, and late gene expression is dependent on both viral DNA synthesis and IE gene functions (27,28). During the course of lytic infection, virus comes in contact with the axon terminals of sensory neurons of the peripheral nervous system, the virus is then transported to the body of the nerve cells, and viral DNA enters the nucleus. Once in the sensory neuron, virus-induced lysis does not occur, but rather the virus enters a latent state. Expression of lytic genes is shut down and only that portion of the virus encoding latency-associated transcripts (LAT) is active (29). Several different research groups have been characterizing the promoter elements that control the expression of the LAT. The intent is to adapt these promoter sequences to drive therapeutic transgene expression during the latent state of the virus. An impressive collection of data has been developed in animal systems, and HSV will support reporter gene expression in different regions of the brain including the hippocampus, septum striatum, and the cortex. For the most part, transgene expression is limited to 1 week or less. Early vectors used in these studies were deleted in either a nonessential gene or an essential immediate early gene, but since the IE genes have been shown to be individually toxic to cells, some of the more recent constructs have been deleted for nine viral functions (30). It is thought that removal of all IE genes will eliminate HSV toxicity for cells, even at very high multiplicities of infection, since UV-irradiated particles that do not express viral functions are not cytotoxic (31).

One of the highly desirable features for all viral vector systems would be the ability to target specific cells, and this could be accomplished at the level of infection or transduction. Transductional targeting has been a popular approach and has largely involved the use of cell-specific promoters. Modulation of infection has been attempted by engineering ligands that target specific cell types by recognizing unique surface receptors. Host range of viruses has been altered by constructing pseudotype or hybrid vectors that combine elements from different virus; for example, the construction of a lentiviral vector nucleocapsid containing a vesicular stomatitis viral envelope. The engineering of hybrid HSV vectors for purposes of targeting looms as a formidable task. Even though the envelope structure and mechanisms of attachment and entry are known in some detail, the complexity of the viral envelope and the interaction of these multiple envelope glycoproteins poses some legitimate problems in deciphering structure and function.

HSV vector applications involving the nervous system have an interesting potential. For example, HSV vectors could express nerve growth factors to treat peripheral sensory neuropathies or tyrosine hydroxylase to produce L-dihydroxy-phenylalanine and dopamine in neurons of patients with Parkinson's disease. In the various other neurodegenerative diseases, the fact that the HSV latent state established in neurons is lifelong raises the possibility that a properly engineered vector could prevent the progressive loss of neurons that would otherwise occur during the course of the disease.

E. Nonviral Vectors

Direct DNA Delivery

When one considers the principal methods of nonviral mediated gene transfer, the most fundamentally obvious is the use of injected plasmid DNA or so-called "naked" DNA containing a transgene into the organ site of choice. The history of this work dates back approximately 11 years when a group of investigators systematically tested a number of organ sites using three different reporter genes: chloramphenicol acetyl transferase (CAT), beta galactosidase, and luciferase. When skeletal muscle was injected, CAT activity was detected at 48 hr after injection of the plasmid DNA, and 10–30% of the muscle cells stained positively for β-galactosidase at 7 days. A dose-response curve was established for luciferase and expression was still present at 60 days. Using a sensitivity-resistance pattern to digestion by certain restriction endonucleases, there was no evidence of integration of the DNA (32).

Unstable expression has also been observed following plasmid DNA delivery to the liver, kidney, skin, thyroid, synovium, and artery. When a reporter gene system was used to study the liver, there was a sixfold decrease in mean serum levels over a period of 2 days and a 60-fold decrease over 4 weeks (33). However, it was possible to maintain steady-state levels for 4 weeks if the animals were given both dexamethasone and cyclosporine. Although these results are likely to be due to the effects of immunosuppression, there may have been an effect on the cytomegalovirus (CMV) promoter that was a part of this plasmid construct.

One concern with naked DNA administration is the possibility of inducing anti-DNA antibodies that could lead to the development of autoimmune disorders such as systemic lupus erythematosus. One set of studies revealed that repetitive intramuscular injections of large amounts of plasmid DNA (up to 12,000 μg of pDNA) failed to elicit antinuclear antibodies (34). From other experimental work it appears that DNA needs to be denatured and complexed with a protein or an adjuvant in order to produce antinuclear antibodies.

Although there are some problems with efficiency and stability of expression, the clinical use of naked DNA is notable for its simplicity and the lack of immunogenicity; the latter issue being a recurring problem for the viral vectors. Plasmid DNA has already been used in one clinical trial in which vascular endothelial growth factor (VEGF) was delivered to skeletal muscle of the lower limbs in patients with severe occlusive vascular disease.

Liposomes

Liposomes are a heterogeneous class of compounds that can be synthesized so that they possess a wide variety of physical and chemical properties. They can consist of sheets and long cylinders of reasonably circular vesicles; such structures are the result of combining phospholipids with a fatty acid tail and hydrophilic head groups. There are two classes of these compounds that have been extensively studied as vectors for gene transfer: anionic liposomes and cationic liposomes.

In the case of anionic liposomes, the DNA must be encapsulated in the aqueous interior of the vesicle, since it cannot bind directly to the DNA. Because of this structural arrangement, there is a limitation on the packaging capacity for transgenes. Liposome vesicles have a net negative to neutral surface charge and thus they do not bind nonspecifically to the cell surface. Cellular uptake is achieved through the mechanism of receptor-mediated endocytosis. A major problem for this system resides in the fact that this lipid DNA complex is significantly shunted to endosomes containing lysosomal nucleases that degrade the plasmid-transgene DNA. There have been a number of strategies devised to achieve endosomal escape, and these include the use of a lysogenic peptide such as influenza viral hemagglutinin or a rhinoviral amphipathic capsid-n-terminal peptide. Because of endosomal shunting, DNA integration into host cell chromosomes is a rare event.

Cationic liposomes are positively charged and bind avidly with the negatively charged phosphate groups in the DNA molecule (35). Surface binding occurs as a result of nonspecific ionic interactions, and the cellular uptake mechanisms are poorly understood. Apparently they are nonreceptor mediated and may reflect a fluid endocytosis. Targeting in this system is difficult because of the nonspecific adherence to cells. Cationic liposomes may be more efficient than anionic liposomes in achieving endosomal escape, and they have a very large packaging capacity for transgene DNA (up to 50 kb).

Another challenge for this system is posed by the tendency for these lipid-DNA complexes to be ingested by reticuloendothelial cells, and this detracts from any attempts at cell targeting. In order to alleviate this problem, there have been attempts to create "stealth" liposomes by coating them with sialic acid residues so that they will not be ingested by tissue macrophages (36).

Liposomes offer the fundamental advantage of a chemical system over a biological system when one considers the necessity for large-scale preparations. In the case of the cationic liposomes, there is a much larger transgene packaging capacity when compared to any viral vector currently in use. They can be synthesized in large quantities using procedures that are uniform. Since there are no viral genes involved, the problems with acquired immune response seem to be minimal. Humoral immunity apparently does not develop and this allows for repetitive doses. However, it has recently become apparent that liposomal/DNA complexes do activate an innate immune response probably secondary to the immunogenic bacterial DNA sequences present in the plasmids. This results in cytokine release and both local and systemic inflammatory responses, an especially severe problem after intravenous administration. Although cationic liposomes are being used in a number of Phase I and II cancer trials, the fact remains that these particular nonviral vectors have a relatively low level of transduction efficiency, the gene expression is almost always very transient, and there are few mechanisms for escaping the endosomal shunt that occurs once the complex is inside the cell.

DNA-Protein Complexes

Another nonviral method of gene delivery takes advantage of the ability to combine DNA with protein complexes. Similar to the liposomes, there is the ability to administer a foreign gene on a repetitive basis in the absence of an immune response, there is a relatively large transgene capacity, and unlike the retroviruses there is no requirement for dividing cells in the target population.

Again, a principal hurdle in using this system derives from the significant degradation of the DNA that occurs when these complexes are shunted to the endosomal compartment of the cell. This problem has been attacked by conjugating polylysine to the DNA to form a binary complex, and there is suggestive evidence that polylysine can protect DNA from DNAse digestion. Agents such as chloroquine and leupeptin have been employed to disrupt endocytic trafficking, the former acting to increase endosomal stability by raising its pH (37).

It has become very clear that viruses have evolved in such a way that these agents possess the ability to circumvent the endosomal shunt. In that context, adenovirus has been complexed to polylysine-DNA to create a ternary complex that allows for more efficiency in transgene expression. It is thought that adenoviruses are able to protect their genomic DNA due to the exposure of the hydrophobic domains of the capsid proteins at a low endosomal pH. This particular reaction leads to disruption of the endosome and prevents DNA degradation by lysosomal DNAses (38). It has been demonstrated by the use of either replication-defective adenovirus or ultraviolet inactivation that virus-mediated endosomal disruption is independent of both viral replication and viral gene expression. Adenovirus can be coupled to a DNA-protein complex either by using enzymes or the biotin-avidin reaction (39).

There has been considerable experimental effort directed toward targeting specific cell populations through the use of ligands that are conjugated to poly-lysine-plasmid DNA. By using a specific ligand for the asialoglycoprotein receptor on liver cells, one could demonstrate increased targeting properties. However, if one adds adenovirus to the system to increase the efficiency of lysosomal escape, then much of the specificity is lost, as the asialoglycoprotein receptors now have to compete with the widely distributed adenovirus CAR receptors (40). This conundrum simply illustrates some of the problems associated with producing targeted vectors.

In summary, the DNA-protein complexes have several properties that are analogous to the liposomes. The transgene capacity is superior to that of viral vectors, the complex does not appear to provoke an immune response, and DNA can be successfully introduced into nondividing cells. Through the use of certain ligands it is possible to introduce cell-specific targeting characteristics. Despite all the attractive features of nonviral approaches, the fact remains that viral vector systems are much more efficient in terms of gene delivery. Viruses can infect cultured cells with nearly perfect efficiency, wherein 100 infectious viral particles containing 100 viral genomes can successfully infect almost 100 cells. To obtain similar levels of expression with nonviral vectors, it typically takes 100 million copies of plasmid DNA to transfect 100 cells (41).

III. Disease Targets: Clinical Trials

From a conceptual perspective, gene therapy stands on rather firm ground. It is ideally suited for the potential treatment of monogenic deficiency diseases in which a mutated gene is consistently associated with a defined clinical phenotype. Correction of this inborn genetic error can be potentially achieved by introducing a normal or wild-type gene that provides a normal gene product and termination of the disease pathophysiology. A review of the past 11 years of clinical experimentation reveals a pattern of disease targeting that would not have been predicted at the outset. Of the 464 protocols that have been reviewed by the NIH Recombinant DNA Advisory Committee, 290, or approximately 63%, have been devoted to the study of cancer, whereas 51, or approximately 11%, have been directed to single-gene deficiency diseases (42). Thirty-four protocols have studied AIDS, and 48 protocols have addressed a variety of diseases ranging from coronary artery disease to rheumatoid arthritis to Parkinson's disease (42). This particular pattern of research activity provides ample proof that the technology of gene transfer is an enabling technology and that it promises utility across a rather broad spectrum of diseases.

A. Monogenic Deficiency Diseases

Sixteen different diseases have been studied and essentially all of the clinical protocols have been Phase I studies. Adenosine deaminase deficiency (ADA) was the first disease to be studied, and it is noteworthy that the first two research subjects, who were treated in 1990, are doing rather well clinically. In this particular trial, both girls were subjected to leukophoresis, T lymphocytes were isolated and transduced ex vivo with the normal ADA gene, and then they were returned by intravenous catheter. Since the target cells were terminally differentiated and subject to a definitive life span, the transduction and infusion procedures had to be repeated on a periodic basis; the first research subject received 11 infusions over a 2-year period (43). Both research subjects showed multiple cellular and humoral immune responses in the normal range and both pursue a fairly normal life style. One girl contracted chickenpox in 1996 and experienced a clinical course that would be expected for a normal 10-year-old (44). Despite the desirable outcome for both these girls, the role of gene transfer remains something of an enigma. Both research subjects have received enzyme therapy with polyethylene glycol conjugated ADA (PEG-ADA) for the entire 11-year period since they were enrolled in the study. Thus, the precise role of gene transfer cannot be defined.

In addition to ADA deficiency, four other types of severe combined immune deficiency (SCID) have been under study: chronic granulomatous disease, purine nucleoside phosphorylase deficiency, X-linked SCID, and leukocyte adherence deficiency. In the 11-year history of gene therapy clinical trials there has been an absolute paucity of data suggesting efficacy, but one of the most encouraging recent results involves X-linked SCID. This particular form of SCID is characterized by an early block in T-lymphocyte and natural killer (NK) lymphocyte differentiation and is caused by mutations of the gene encoding the γc cytokine receptor subunit of IL-2, IL-4, IL-9, and IL-15 receptors. In this particular trial, ex vivo transduction of $CD34^+$ cells was done using a Moloney retroviral vector. Ten months after the experimental intervention, two research subjects showed T-, B-, and NK cell counts and function, including antigen-specific responses comparable to those of age-matched controls (45). These results document full correction of disease phenotype and a clear measure of clinical benefit.

In the relatively early phases of clinical trials, multiple groups of investigators began to study cystic fibrosis, and this is not surprising given that it is the second most common autosomal recessive disease among whites in the United States and western Europe (see Chaps. 13, 14, and 15). Three anatomical sites were targeted, the nasal mucosa, the maxillary sinus, and the lung; certainly, the lung is the site of the most serious pathology in this disease. Cystic fibrosis represents one of the first instances of in vivo gene transfer; in the United States, both adenoviral and AAV vectors were used to deliver the CFTR gene, although some of the first trials in the United Kingdom used cationic liposomes. A common challenge for gene transfer in this disease is the presence of a thick purulent mucus that fills most of the small airways of the lung and presents a formidable anatomical barrier to the pulmonary epithelial cells. Data accumulated from several studies revealed that it was possible to transduce nasal or pulmonary epithelium, but the period of CFTR gene expression was rather limited, ranging from 4 to 9 days (46,47). Given the fact that cystic fibrosis is a chronic disease, one has to postulate repeat administration of the vector in order to achieve any sort of therapeutic effect. Adenoviral vectors are not a good candidate for this approach, because of the marked immune response that occurs with the initial instillation. It remains to be determined if AAV vectors will have a significant role in the treatment of this disease.

One of the earlier studies that involved the ex vivo transduction of hepatocytes was the homozygous form of familial hypercholesterolemia. In this particular disorder, there is an absence of low-density lipoprotein (LDL) receptors in the liver parenchyma. These patients are afflicted with extremely high levels of serum LDL cholesterol and they suffer the adult consequences of severe arteriosclerosis as early as the age of 5 years. Five research subjects participated in this particular study; two of them exhibited significant reduction in LDL cholesterol levels and a third showed a measurable reduction (48). Again, the results of this study are difficult to interpret, because all the subjects were on chronic maintenance with 3-hydroxy-3-methylglutaryl-coenzyme A reductase inhibitors that are known to reduce cholesterol.

Some of the more interesting and encouraging results have been derived from the study of both hemophilia A (factor VIII deficiency) and hemophilia B (factor IX deficiency). Results from the hemophilia B study were reported first and reflect the use of an AAV vector encoding factor IX. The target site was skeletal muscle, since it was known from experimental studies in rodents and dogs that efficient transduction could occur in myocytes and that the secretory protein produced could function on release into the bloodstream. This was a dose-escalation trial, and a report was presented after a study of the first three research subjects (nine subjects were approved for the trial), since the results were sufficiently encouraging. The goal for gene therapy in hemophilia is to maintain factors greater than 1% of normal at all times; at this level many of the life-threatening bleeding complications are avoided. Although these subjects received the lowest dose of vector planned for the study, one showed a factor IX level of just above 1% and a reduction in recombinant protein usage, whereas another subject showed a reduction in hemorrhages even though the factor IX level was just below 1% (21). In the case of hemophilia A, the experimental approach was quite distinct. No viral vector was used, but instead the technique of electroporation, exposure of cells to an electrical field, was utilized to introduce the factor VIII gene into skin fibroblasts isolated from the research subject to be studied. The transduced fibroblasts were selected using G418-containing medium. Using laparoscopy, the genetically modified cells were introduced into the subject's peritoneal cavity. Of the six patients studied, four had detectable levels of factor VIII and two had levels of greater than 1% of normal, a level thought to be therapeutic (49). In the latter two patients, the use of recombinant factor decreased and the number of bleeding episodes decreased. No factor VIII inhibitors were identified in any of the subjects.

Several other trials are in progress and await completion and reporting of the data. Diseases under study include alpha$_1$-antitrypsin deficiency; Fanconi's anemia, Gaucher's disease, Hunter's syndrome, Canavan's disease, limb girdle muscular dystrophy, amyotrophic lateral sclerosis, ornithine transcarbamylase deficiency, and junctional epidermolysis bullosa.

B. Cancer

Since the majority of the clinical protocols are directed toward the study of cancer, it is instructive to analyze some of the reasons for this selected research activity. Many of the clinical trials represent a collaboration between university-based investigators and biotechnology companies, and the latter have a vested interest in patient markets that are large and broad in scope. Over the past 20–25 years, the advances in molecular biology have had a considerable influence on defining some of the mechanisms of malignant transformation, but notwithstanding this progress, the fact remains that many of the existing cancer therapies leave much to be desired. Thus, the oncology community is always on the alert to explore new approaches to cancer treatment. In view of the fact that many types of cancers are associated with an extremely poor salvage rate, it is easier to develop a defensible risk/benefit ratio when embarking on new experimental approaches that have unknown toxicities and unknown potential.

A large number of different tumor types have been targeted for study and these include acute and chronic myelogenous leukemia, breast carcinoma, hepatoma, Hodgkin's disease, non-Hodgkin's lymphoma, mesothelioma (see Chap. 12), neuroblastoma, small cell and non–small cell carcinoma of the lung (see Chap. 11), ovarian carcinoma, prostate carcinoma, and renal cell carcinoma (42). A number of diverse strategies have been designed for these various tumor types. Although there is no evidence of efficacy at this juncture, one has to accept the perspective that, for the most part, these protocols represent Phase I trials.

One of the most popular approaches encompasses the prodrug concept. This is a cytotoxic therapy and the strategy involves the introduction of a gene that is capable of inducing cell death when the appropriate drug is added to the system. In this system, normal nondividing cells are protected as long as they do not contain the gene. In the initial studies, a retroviral vector containing the herpes simplex thymidine kinase transgene (HSV*tk*) was produced in a mouse cell line and this cell line was either injected directly into the tumor mass or introduced into the tumor bed following surgical removal of the tumor. HSV*tk* can phosphorylate a nonphosphorylated nucleoside, whereas endogenous human thymidine kinase cannot. When the drug, ganciclovir, an abnormal nucleoside, is given to the patient, only HSV*tk*-containing cells will phosphorylate the drug, producing a toxic triphosphate that inhibits DNA polymerase I and kills the cell. Four mechanisms have been identified that facilitate the death of tumor cells in this setting. There is the direct effect of ganciclovir, there is a "bystander" effect in which toxic agents pass into neighboring cells through gap junctions and kill them, there is a local inflammatory response to the mouse cell line, and there is a systemic immune response (44). In more recent trials, investigators have used an adenoviral vector containing HSV*tk*, and although this virus can induce an immune response, one can avoid introducing the foreign proteins that are present in the mouse cell line. HSV*tk* vectors have been used in the study of glioblastoma multiforme, ovarian adenocarcinoma, and mesothelioma (see Chap. 12).

A recurring challenge that complicates cancer therapy is the property of malignant cells to become resistant to standard drug and radiation therapy. Alterations in the apoptotic pathway yield resistant cancer cells and restoration of apoptosis could return drug sensitivity. Several research teams are using the addition of p53 to various tumors such as non–small cell carcinoma of the lung and head and neck carcinoma in an attempt to control tumor growth (see Chap. 11). From the data available, there is no evidence of a clinical response, but there have been instances where there was evidence of local tumor regression at sites where the p53 gene was injected (50).

One of the most popular strategies for studying cancer utilizes the various techniques of adoptive immunotherapy. Many of the early protocols involved the ex vivo transduction of various cytokine genes (IL-2, IL-4, IL-7, IL-12, interferons, tumor necrosis factor [TNF], and granulocyte-macrophage colony-stimulating factor [GM-CSF]) into either autologous or allogeneic tumor cells with the aim of inducing an immune response and the production of T cells specifically targeted to the tumor. It has been suggested that this approach is analogous to creating patient-specific vaccines. Melanoma has been the most frequent tumor target and there have been studies of renal cell carcinoma. In studies with GM-CSF, some of the research subjects showed evidence of a delayed hypersensitivity reaction at the immunization site along with a suggestion of tumor regression (51,52).

Retroviral and adenoviral vectors have been used for cytokine delivery, and one group of investigators has used a plasmid containing the gene encoding the HLA-B7/β_2-microglobulin protein conjugated with a cationic liposome. The hypothesis behind this approach is that an HLA gene such as B7, which is not expressed in the tumor, will function as a foreign antigen and stimulate the immune system. Data emanating from a melanoma trial indicates that the immune system responds both to B7 antigen and other tumor cell antigens, causing immune lysis of both transduced and nontransduced tumor cells (53).

Another method of inducing antitumor immunity involves using recombinant fowlpox virus and vaccinia virus vectors that contain transgenes encoding for the melanoma defined antigens, gp 100 and MART-1. Vaccinia virus vectors have been used to deliver the CEA antigen to research subjects with metastatic adenocarcinoma of the colon and a small number of subjects did generate cytotoxic T-cell responses (54). In a related trial, research subjects with a serological recurrence of prostate cancer following radical prostatectomy are being given prostate-specific antigen (PSA) as a potential immunogen.

Although the results of the trials in gene therapy for cancer are somewhat disappointing, one has to put the results in proper perspective. It is not realistic to assume that gene transfer could be used to insert therapeutic genes into every malignant cell in a patient's body. Thus, one has to consider ways of amplifying the effects of transducing a relatively small number of cells; thus, it follows that the use of the immune system as an amplifier is a reasonable approach. Perhaps the best role for gene transfer in the treatment of cancer will come from its use as adjuvant therapy wherein the tumor burden can be reduced or held in check without the need for immunosuppression. This would allow the patient to recover from the effects of traditional chemotherapy and radiotherapy and position that individual for future interventions that are immunosuppressive.

C. Cardiovascular Disease

A recent report in the clinical literature has stimulated an intense patient interest in the use of gene transfer to treat arteriosclerosis obliterans. Nine research subjects with nonhealing ischemic ulcers due to peripheral arterial disease were enrolled in the study. They were given the gene encoding vascular endothelial growth factor (VEGF). The vector/gene construct was injected intramuscularly in the area of the lower limb where vascular occlusion had been demonstrated. Of the nine subjects who were treated, newly visible collateral blood vessels were demonstrated in seven limbs by contrast angiography, and magnetic resonance angiography revealed improved distal blood flow in eight limbs (55). The ischemic ulcer either improved or healed in four of seven limbs, and there was some temporary limb salvage in three subjects recommended for below the knee amputation. It remains to be determined how long these new networks of collateral vessels will persist, particularly since the subjects were treated only once.

Subsequent to the initial work with peripheral vascular disease there have been several studies using VEGF to stimulate angiogenesis in patients with advanced coronary arteriosclerosis. In a recent report, 13 subjects with angiographically documented heart disease were enrolled, all of whom had failed conventional therapy. Left ventricular electromechanical mapping (EMM) was used to assess the effects of gene transfer. The findings suggest improved perfusion scores calculated from single-photon emission CT-sestamibi myocardial perfusion scans (SPECT); such scans were done prospectively and 60 days after gene transfer (56). Because of the EMM results, the investigators suggested that treatment with VEGF rescued "hibernating" myocardium as a result of neovascularization. There was a significant reduction in anginal events reported by the research subjects (from 48 to 2); however, this finding must be taken with a note of caution, since this Phase I trial was not controlled and patients with cardiovascular disease are known to be predisposed to the placebo effect.

D. AIDS

There are 34 protocols designed for the study of AIDS and two principal themes have emerged. One could be called intracellular immunotherapy and the other addresses the issue of inhibition of HIV replication. In the early stages of this research, a vaccination strategy was employed. A retroviral vector containing the *env* and *rev* genes of the HIV-1 (IIIB) strain of virus was given intramuscularly with the aim of inducing cytotoxic T-lymphocyte responses and reduction in viral burden. Before this trial could be completed, protease inhibitors were introduced as key treatment agents along with reverse transcriptase inhibitors. The combination of two reverse transcriptase inhibitors and one protease inhibitor was so effective in reducing the detectable viral burden that one of the major endpoints of the vaccination study was effectively eliminated and the study was terminated.

In one of the earlier trials of immunotherapy, a very innovative approach involved the use of identical twins. CD8$^+$ T cells were removed from an uninfected identical twin, transduced with the gene encoding a universal chimeric T-cell receptor, and then infused into the HIV-infected twin. Since the twins were genetically identical, there were no problems related to histocompatibility, and one could assume that the transferred lymphocytes would survive without the danger of rejection. Preliminary data suggested evidence of a selective survival advantage for the transduced T cells that were introduced into a virus-positive environment.

One of the pathway studies of inhibition of HIV replication took advantage of the fact that the product of the *Rev* gene is essential to replication. Multiple mutations were introduced into the *Rev* gene with the result that a defective protein was produced and it functioned as a transdominant inhibitor of replication. When CD4$^+$ lymphocytes were transduced with the gene encoding the Rev M10 protein, the resulting cells developed in vitro resistance to both cloned and clinical isolates of HIV (57).

Many of the problems that confront the use of gene therapy in the study and treatment of cancer also apply to AIDS. It is not realistic to assume that all HIV-infected lymphocytes could be transduced with a therapeutic gene; the problem is further complicated by the fact that the immune system is the target of the infective agent. However, one could envision the genetic modification of a subset of early hematopoietic precursor cells (? stem cells) with the result that there would be a repopulating source of CD4$^+$ T cells resistant to HIV infection. This result in combination with drugs could serve to improve the overall treatment of these patients.

IV. Summary of Clinical History

It has been approximately 11 years since the first clinical gene therapy trial was initiated. Since then hundreds of trials have been approved and over 5000 research subjects have been enrolled. About 80% of this research activity has been conducted in the United States, but there are numerous trials in Europe and a few in Asia. Within the past 12 months there has been encouraging data suggesting some concrete evidence of efficacy in the case of hemophilia and X-linked SCID. What does the future bode? In the long-term, gene therapy will evolve into an exceedingly important element in the full mosaic of medical treatment. However, that could take 15–20 years and it would be unrealistic to suppose otherwise. One has only to look at the field of organ transplantation to find an important reference point. It is appropriate to maintain an optimistic outlook, because the field is conceptually sound; experimentation ultimately will be fruitful.

V. Public Oversight of Human Gene Therapy

A. NIH

In looking at the history of human gene therapy clinical trials, the true prologue begins with the development of recombinant DNA technology. By 1971, Paul Berg was well on the way to developing a successful recombinant viral vector, using the simian virus, SV40. His experiments had the capability of moving oncogenes or antibiotic resistance genes into bacteria that normally did not possess such foreign genes. Because of legitimate concerns in the scientific community, the first Asilomar Conference was convened in 1973. Following this conference, a voluntary moratorium was proposed and a letter was submitted to the journal *Science* with a number of active investigators in the field as cosigners (58). In February 1975, the second Asilomar Conference was held and this proved to be a signal event. Despite the natural propensity of scientists to disagree, the participants in this conference ultimately came to a consensus that there should be an organized scheme for recombinant DNA experiments that would minimize potential biohazards for the environment, the investigators, and the public. Two barriers were suggested: (1) the physical, as reflected in the design of facilities, and (2), the biological, as reflected in the engineering of microorganisms so that they would have a selective disadvantage in terms of survival outside the experimental environment.

At the conclusion of this conference, the initial meeting of the NIH Recombinant DNA Advisory Committee (RAC) was convened and its primary task was to create the "NIH Guidelines for Research Involving Recombinant DNA Molecules." This work required more than a year, and the document was published on June 23, 1976, in the *Federal Register* (59).

Over the next 4 years it became apparent that many of the postulated hazards of recombinant DNA research did not develop and the NIH Guidelines were modulated so as to be less restrictive. Human gene transfer did not really become an issue until 1980 when Martin Cline carried out his experiments on thalassemia research subjects in Italy and Israel. Because these experiments lacked the proper approval, the matter attracted the attention of both the NIH and Congress. At about the same time, a Presidential Commission was formed and it was charged with defining the major issues surrounding genetic engineering. This commission completed its work in 1982 and published a report entitled *Splicing Life* (60). One of the important conclusions contained in this document was that there were no fundamentally new social and ethical questions raised by somatic cell gene therapy. Subsequent to the commission report, congressional hearings were held and led to the precept that there was a critical need for some type of government body to oversee the development of human gene therapy research. It had been suggested by the Presidential Commission that a reconstituted RAC might be a knowledgeable oversight body for human gene therapy protocols. In 1983, the Chair of the RAC asked the members of this committee if they wished to respond to the recommendation in the *Splicing Life* report. The response was positive and a broad-based interdisciplinary working group was created for the purpose of drafting an appropriate oversight document. In 1985, a document entitled "Points to Consider in the Design of Human Gene Therapy Protocols" was published in the *Federal Register*. The full membership of the RAC accepted this document, and by February 1986 the Executive Secretary of the RAC sent a letter to all potential investigators asking for the submission of preclinical data pertaining to the development of human gene therapy protocols.

It was not until 1990 that the first human gene therapy protocol was approved, but following that signal event the number of submitted proposals increased in very rapid fashion. In this beginning period, there were two independent and parallel processes for the review of protocols, the public review process conducted by the RAC and the closed review conducted by the FDA, as mandated by their regulations. When the history of this field is written, it will probably be seen as fortuitous that the RAC accepted the responsibility for public review; in the absence of such an activity, public acceptance of this new technology could have proceeded much more slowly.

As the number of active protocols increased, there was a parallel with recombinant DNA research in its formative years; many of the fears about safety did not come to fruition. One could argue that this was due, in part, to the inefficiency in vector systems and low transduction efficiency in target cells, but the fact remains that it was 9 years before the first death attributable to gene therapy actually occurred.

By 1991, it became apparent that the two-stage national review of gene therapy was becoming redundant. Under the original format, protocols were initially reviewed by a RAC subcommittee, the Human Gene Therapy Subcommittee (HGTS), and then submitted to the full RAC. In October 1991, the RAC decided to disband the HGTS and transfer its membership to the parent body. By February 1992, the HGTS was formally disbanded, an the sole review responsibility was vested in the RAC. A further change in oversight was initiated in 1994 as a result of the formation of the National AIDS Task Force on Drug Development. Members of several AIDS activist groups were a part of this task force, and it was their contention that gene therapy had great promise as a cure for AIDS. It was their opinion that the dual agency review by the NIH and FDA imposed a serious impediment on the field. It was proposed that the RAC be abolished, but the entire membership of the task force did not accept this position. A compromise position was reached and it was predicated on the strategy of consolidated review in which both the NIH and FDA would review all new protocols simultaneously. Staff members from the two agencies would consult to determine if the new protocol represented a significant conceptual departure from previously reviewed protocols. If the protocol was absent any notable differences, it received only FDA review. This consolidated review procedure was put into place in September 1994.

In 1995, the NIH Director appointed an ad hoc review committee to evaluate the functions of the RAC and to develop recommendations about its future role in the field of human gene therapy research. This committee gave its imprimatur to the consolidated review process and it recommended that the RAC should continue to provide advice on gene therapy policy matters. In 1966, the NIH Director announced that he planned to abolish the RAC and replace it with a much smaller number of scientists and ethicists who would meet on an ad hoc basis to provide advice on public policy issues. This intent to abolish the RAC was published in the *Federal Register* and provoked a large number of negative comments. Because of this response, the NIH Director decided that the RAC would be retained, that its membership would be reduced from 25 to 15, that the approval process for gene therapy protocols would be abolished, and that the major new activity would be the organization of a series of gene therapy policy conferences to address such issues as in utero gene therapy, the use of lentiviral vectors, and use of gene transfer for enhancement.

Since 1996, the RAC has been operating under its new mandate. A number of policy conferences have been held. Selected gene therapy protocols representing new approaches or new disease targets are reviewed, but they are not approved or disapproved. Instead, the principal investigators are provided with a series of comments and suggestions; it is important to note that FDA representatives are present at these meetings and have full access to the discussions. In its current role, the RAC is functioning in a way that is complementary to the privately conducted reviews of the FDA.

B. FDA

Because of the nuances in the development of human gene therapy, the FDA found itself in a very peculiar role—that of sharing oversight of a newly emerging field of biotechnology. Since the Congress, and Representative Albert Gore in particular, had recommended that the RAC assume an oversight role in the review and approval of human gene therapy protocols, a strictly nonregulatory agency, the NIH, was thrust into the position of carrying out a quasiregulatory function. Clearly, this situation produced tensions between the two agencies. Just 3 weeks before the RAC special working group was to publish its "Points-to-Consider" document, the FDA published a statement in the *Federal Register* that defined its position in unambiguous terms. Although the FDA did acknowledge that there must be some redundancy in a dual review process, it emphasized that the existing laws and regulations were quite adequate for the oversight of human gene therapy (61).

In 1984, Frank Young was the Commissioner of the FDA, and he made a proposal that was viewed in some quarters as a method for undercutting the NIH. He proposed that a Biotechnology Science Board (BSB) be created within the office of the Assistant Secretary of Health in the Department of Health and Human Services (62). This BSB would have diminished the role of NIH. Ultimately, the proposal was referred to the White House Office of Science and Technology Policy; Bernadine Healy was the Deputy Director at that time, and since she favored a strong NIH RAC, the idea of a BSB was discarded. Subsequently, the Reagan administration established a Federal Coordinating Council for Science Engineering and Technology (FCCSET); its membership consisted of every federal government agency with a program commitment to biotechnology, but its efforts were directed at much broader issues than gene therapy and gene therapy was never an agenda item (63).

It might be overly simplistic to view the dual agency review as something of a turf battle, but the FDA made an initial effort to define its position when it issued its first draft guidance document in 1991 (64). It addressed a number of pertinent regulatory issues related to all classes of vector products for gene therapy, preclinical issues related to particular classes of vector products, preclinical issues for safety evaluation in animals of all classes of gene therapy products, and regulatory handling of modifications in vector preparations.

In January 1993, the FDA established a new Office of Therapeutics Research and Review (OTRR) and within this office a new Center for Biologicals Evaluation and Research (CBER). Within CBER was posited the Cell and Gene Therapy Branch. Shortly after it was functioning, CBER issued a second guidance document for cell and gene therapy (65). At about the same time, the Commissioner of the FDA, along with some of his staff, published a paper in the *New England Journal of Medicine* that strongly underscored the centrality of the FDA in the regulation of human gene therapy (66). However, it is interesting to note that the RAC was endorsed as having a unique role as a forum for public debate of societal and ethical issues. Thus, the FDA and the NIH were viewed as having broad complementary functions.

The evolution of the RAC has been detailed in an earlier section. Suffice it to say, the sole responsibility for approval of human gene therapy protocols now resides with the FDA, and that is entirely appropriate, since it is the only regulatory agency within the Department of Health and Human Services. Undoubtedly, the early discussions at the RAC gave the public an open window to view the field when it was in its seminal stages. However, it would be easy to overlook the fact that the FDA never changed any of its basic regulations during this 11-year period of clinical research. The Code of Federal Regulations (CFR) 21 remains unaltered. For all practical purposes, recombinant DNA has been accorded the same status as a drug. As indicated previously, numerous guidance documents have been issued, the latest addenda being published in 1996 and 1998. Even the terminology was borrowed from the RAC in that the initial issuance was entitled "Points to Consider in Human Somatic Cell Therapy and Gene Therapy." Thus, the most compelling conclusion to be drawn is that FDA oversight of gene therapy has been a process in evolution just as the RAC process was subject to frequent change. The latest chapter in this FDA evolution in oversight may have the most far-reaching and long-term effects.

With the death of a 19-year-old research subject in a clinical trial designed for the study of ornithine transcarbamylase deficiency, the field of gene therapy research entered a new era in that this was the first death attributable to gene therapy itself. Not only was there widespread publicity in the print media and on television, but a Senate hearing was conducted as well. Questions pertaining to patient safety, the informed consent process, the interpretation of preclinical data in animal model systems, and financial conflict of interest all received the utmost scrutiny.

As a result of this event, the FDA has given careful consideration to imposing very strict standards, as mandated in CFR21, on all Phase I trials in gene therapy. The reverberations from these proposed changes in policy have implications for all of clinical research. Strict adherence to standards of Good Laboratory Practices (GLP), Good Manufacturing Practices (GMP), and Good Clinical Practices (GCP) is implicit but an additional requirement will involve the monitoring of clinical trials by a Clinical Research Organization (CRO) that is independent of the Sponsor and the Principal Investigator. An obvious outgrowth of this increased regulatory stringency is an inevitable increase in costs; this is a particular problem for the academic community, because the source of such funds is not obvious. Conversely, industry can budget developmental costs, that is, regulatory costs to a given product, but the problem is not so straightforward for the academic sector where there is no primary orientation to product manufacture. The next few years will be a challenging time, particularly for gene therapy, but the ultimate driver in this scenario will be the quality of the science. As new techniques become available and more effective, this will serve as appropriate motivation to launch new clinical trials. In this setting, the issue of costs will not be a paralyzing impediment.

References

1. Wolff JA, Lederberg J. An early history of gene transfer and therapy. Gene Ther 1994; 5:469–480.
2. Tatum EL. Molecular biology, nucleic acids and the future of medicine. Perspect Biol Med 1966; 10:19–32.
3. Lederberg J. Tomorrow's Babies. Proc World Congress Fertil Steril 1968; 6:18–23.
4. Kornberg A. Remarks announcing the in vitro synthesis of DNA. In: Burnet E, ed. Genes, Dreams and Reality. New York: Basic Books, 1971:71.
5. Roger S, Lowenthal A, Terheggen HG, Columbo JP. Induction of arginase activity with the Shope papilloma virus in tissue culture cells from an argininemic patient. J Exp Med 1973; 137:1091–1096.
6. Terheggen HG, Lowenthal A, Lavinha F, Columbo JP, Rogers S. Unsuccessful trial of gene replacement in arginase deficiency. Z Kinderheilkd 1975; 119:1–3.
7. Mercola KE, Stang HD, Browne J, Salser W, Cline MJ. Insertion of a new gene of viral origin into bone marrow cells of mice. Science 1980; 208:1033–1035.
8. Shimotono K, Temin HM. Formation of infectious progeny virus after insertion of herpes simplex thymidine kinase gene into DNA of an avian retrovirus. Cell 1981; 26:67–77.
9. Wei CM, Gibson M, Spear PG, Scolnick EM. Construction and isolation of a trans-

missible retrovirus containing the src gene of Harvey murine sarcoma virus and the thymidine kinase gene of herpes simplex virus type I. J Virol 1981; 39:935–944.

10. Tabin CJ, Hoffman JW, Goff SP, Weinberg RA. Adaptation of a retrovirus as a eucaryotic vector transmitting the herpes simplex virus thymidine kinase gene. Mol Cell Biol 1982; 2:426–436.

11. Willis RC, Jolly DJ, Miller AD, Plent MM, Esty AC, Anderson PJ, Chang HC, Jones OW, Seegmiller JE, Friedmann T. Partial phenotypic correction of human Lesch-Nyhan (hypoxanthine-guanine phosphoribosyltransferase-deficient) lymphoblasts with a transmissible retroviral vector. J Biol Chem 1984; 259:7842–7849.

12. Naldini L, Blomer U, Gallay P, Ory D, Mulligan R, Gage FH, Verma IM, Trono D. In vivo gene delivery and stable transduction of nondividing cells by a lentiviral vector. Science 1996; 272:263–267.

13. Kobinger GP, Weiner DJ, Yu Q-C, Wilson JM. Filovirus-pseudotyped lentiviral vector can efficiently and stably transduce airway epithelia in vivo. Nature Biotech 2001; 19:225–230.

14. Wilson JM. Adenoviruses as gene delivery vehicles. N Engl J Med 1996; 334:1185–1187.

15. Kozarsky KF, Wilson JM. Gene therapy: adenoviral vectors. Curr Opin Genet Dev 1993; 3:499–503.

16. Krougliak V, Graham FL. Development of cell lines capable of complementing E1, E4 and protein IX defective adenovirus type 5 mutants. Hum Gene Ther 1995; 6: 1575–1586.

17. Yang Y, Nunes FA, Berencsi K, Gonczol E, Engelhardt JE, Wilson JM. Inactivation of E2a in recombinant adenoviruses improves the prospect for gene therapy in cystic fibrosis. Nat Genet 1994; 7:362–369.

18. Gao G-P, Yang Y, Wilson JM. Biology of adenovirus vectors with E1 and E4 deletions for liver-directed gene therapy. J Virol 1996; 70:8934–8943.

19. Fisher KJ, Choi H, Burda J, Chen S-J, Wilson JM. Recombinant adenovirus deleted of all viral genes for gene therapy of cystic fibrosis. J Virol 1996; 217:11–22.

20. Schnell MA, Zhang Y, Tazelaar J, Gao G-P, Yu QC, Qian R, Chen S-J, Varnavski AN, LeClair C, Raper SE, Wilson JM. Activation of innate immunity in nonhuman primates following intraportal administration of adenoviral vectors. Mol Ther 2001; 3:708–722.

21. Kay MA, Manno CS, Ragni MV, Larson PJ, Couto LB, McClelland A, Glader B, Chew AJ, Tai SJ, Heizoq RW, Arruda V, Johnson F, Scallan C, Skarsgard E, Flake AW, High KA. Evidence for gene transfer and expression of factor 1X in haemophilia B patients treated with an AAV vector. Nat Genet 2000; 24:257–261.

22. Richardson WD, Westphal H. A cascade of adenovirus early functions is required for expression of adeno-associated virus. Cell 1981; 27:133–141.

23. Kotin RM, Siniscalco R, Samulski RJ, Zhu XD, Hunter L, Laughlin CA, McLaughlin S, Muzyczka N, Rocchi M, Berns KI. Site-specific integration by adeno-associated virus. Proc Natl Acad Sci USA 1990; 87:2211–2215.

24. Samulski RJ, Sully M, Muzyczha N. Adeno-associated viral vectors. In: Friedmann T, ed. The Development of Human Gene Therapy. Cold Spring Harbor: Cold Spring Harbor Laboratory Press, 1999:131–172.

25. Gao G-P, Auricchio A, Hildinger M, Marsh J, Wang L, Wilson JM. Production and

purification of different serotypes of AAV vectors. Fourth Annual Meeting of the American Society of Gene Therapy, Seattle, WA, May 30–June 3, 2001.

26. Flotte T, Carter B, Conrad C, Guggino W, Reynolds T, Rosenstein B, Taylor G, Walden S, Wetzel R. A phase I study of an adeno-associated virus-CFTR gene vector in adult CF patients with mild lung disease. Hum Gen Ther 1996; 7:1145–1159.

27. DeLuca NA, Schaffer PA. Activation of immediate-early, early, and late promoters by temperature-sensitive and wild-type forms of herpes simplex virus type 1 protein ICP4. N Engl J Med 1985; 5:1997–2008.

28. McCarthy AM, McMahan L, Schaffer PA. Herpes simplex virus type 1 ICP27 deletion mutants exhibit altered patterns of transcription and are DNA deficient. J Virol 1989; 63:18–27.

29. Spivack JG, Fraser NW. Detection of herpes simplex virus type I transcripts during latent infection in mice. J Virol 1987; 61:3841–3847.

30. Fink DJ, Ramakrishnan R, Marconi P, Goins WF, Holland TC, Glorioso JC. Advances in the development of herpes simplex virus-based gene transfer vectors for the nervous system. Clin Neurosci 1996; 3:284–291.

31. Huard J, Akkaraju G, Watkins SC, Pike-Cavalcoli M, Glorioso JC. Lac Z gene transfer to skeletal muscle using a replication-defective herpes simplex virus type 1 mutant vector. Hum Gene Ther 1997; 8:439–452.

32. Wolff JA, Malone RW, Williams P, Chong W, Acsadi G, Jani A, Felgner PL. Direct gene transfer into mouse muscle in vivo. Science 1990; 247:1465–1468.

33. Budker V, Zhang G, Knechtle S, Wolff JA. Naked DNA delivered intraportally expresses efficiently in hepatocytes. Gene Ther 1996; 3:593–598.

34. Jiao S, Williams P, Berg RK, Hodgeman BA, Liu L, Repetto G, Wolff JA. Direct gene transfer into nonhuman primate myofibers in vivo. Hum Gene Ther 1992; 3: 21–33.

35. Felgner PL, Ringold GM. Cationic liposome-mediated transfection. Nature 1989; 337:387–388.

36. Lasic DD, Martin FJ, Gabizon A, Huang SK, Papahadjopoulos D. Sterically stabilized lyposomes: a hypothesis on the molecular origin of the extended circulation times. Biochim Biophys Acta 1991; 1070:187–192.

37. Perales JC, Ferkol T, Beegen H, Ratnoff OD, Hanson RW. Gene transfer in vivo: sustained expression and regulation of genes introduced into the liver by receptor-targeted uptake. Proc Natl Acad Sci USA 1994; 4086–4090.

38. Seth P, Fitzgerald D, Ginsberg H, Willingham M, Pastan I. Evidence that the penton base of adenovirus is involved in potentiation of toxicity of Pseudomonas exotoxin conjugated to epidermal growth factor. Mol Cell Biol 1984; 4:1528–1533.

39. Wagner E, Zatloukal K, Cotten M, Kirlappos H, Mechtler K, Curiel DT, Birnstiel ML. Coupling of adenovirus to transferrin-polylysine/DNA complexes greatly enhances receptor-mediated gene delivery and expression of transfected genes. Proc Natl Acad Sci 1992; 89:6099–6103.

40. Wu GY, Wu CH. Receptor-mediated in vitro gene transformation by a soluble DNA carrier system. J Biol Chem 1987; 262:4429–4432.

41. Felgner PL, Zelphati O, Liang X. Advances in synthetic gene-delivery system technology. In: Friedmann T, ed. The Development of Human Gene Therapy. Cold Spring Harbor: Cold Spring Harbor Laboratory Press, 1999:241–260.

42. OBA Report: Human Gene Therapy Protocols. 2001. Office of Biotechnology Activities, NIH, Bethesda, MD.
43. Blaese RM, Culver KW, Miller AD, Carter CS, Fleisher T, Clerici M, Shearer G, Chang L, Chiang Y, Tolstoshev P, Greenblatt JJ, Rosenberg SA, Klein H, Berger M, Mullen CA, Ramsey WJ, Muul L, Morgan RA, Anderson WF. T lymphocyte-directed gene therapy for ADA-SCID: initial trial results after 4 years. Science 1995; 270:475–480.
44. Anderson WF. Human gene therapy. Nature 1998; 392:25–30.
45. Cavazzana-Calvo M, Hacein-Bey S, de Saint Basile G, Gross F, Yvon E, Nusbaum P, Selz F, Hue C, Certain S, Casanova J-L, Bousso P, Le Deist FL, Fischer A. Gene therapy of human severe combined immunodeficiency (SCID)-X1 disease. Science 2000; 288:669–672.
46. Knowles MR, Hohneker KW, Zhou Z, Olsen JC, Noah TL, Hu P-C, Leigh MW, Engelhardt JF, Edwards LJ, Jones KR, Grossman M, Wilson JM, Johnson LG, Boucher RC. A controlled study of adenoviral-vector-mediated gene transfer in the nasal epithelium of patients with cystic fibrosis. N Engl J Med 1995; 333:823–831.
47. Crystal RG, McElvaney NG, Rosenfeld MA, Chu C-S, Mastrangeli A, Hay JG, Brody SL, Jaffe A, Eissa T, Danel C. Administration of an adenovirus containing the human CFTR cDNA to the respiratory tract of individuals with cystic fibrosis. Nat Genet 1994; 8:42–51.
48. Grossman M, Rader DJ, Muller DW, Kolansky DM, Kozarsky K, Clark BJ 3rd, Stein EA, Lupien PJ, Brewer HB Jr, Raper SE, Wilson JM. A pilot study of ex vivo gene therapy for homozygous familial hypercholesterolaemia. Nat Med 1995; 1: 1148–1154.
49. Roth DA, Tawa NE, O'Brien JM, Treco DA, Selden RF. Factor VIII Transkaryotic Therapy Study Group. Nonviral transfer of the gene encoding coagulation factor VIII in patients with severe hemophilia A. N Engl J Med 2001; 344:1735–1742.
50. Roth JA, Nguyen D, Lawrence DD, Kemp BL, Carrasco CH, Ferson DZ, Hong WK, Komaki R, Lee JJ, Nesbitt JC, Pisters KM, Putnam JB, Schea R, Shin DM, Walsh GL, Dolormente MM, Han CI, Martin FD, Yen N, Xu K, Stephens LC, McDonnell TJ, Mukhopadhyay T, Cai D. Retrovirus-mediated wild-type p53 gene transfer to tumors of patients with lung cancer. Nat Med 1996; 2:985–991.
51. Ellem KA, O'Rourke MG, Johnson GR, Parry G, Misko IS, Schmidt CW, Parsons PG, Burrows SR, Cross S, Fell A, Li CL, Bell JR, Dubois PJ, Moss DJ, Good MF, Kelso A, Cohen LK, Dranoff G, Mulligan RC. A case report: immune responses and clinical course of the first human use of granulocyte/macrophage-colony-stimulating-factor-transduced autologous melanoma cells for immunotherapy. Cancer Immunol Immunother 1997; 44:10–20.
52. Simons JW, Jaffee EM, Weber CE, Levitsky HI, Nelson WG, Carducci MA, Lazenby AJ, Cohen LK, Finn CC, Clift SM, Hauda KM, Beck LA, Leiferman KM, Owens AH Jr, Piantadosi S, Dranoff G, Mulligan RC, Pardoll DM, Marshall FF. Bioactivity of autologous irradiated renal cell carcinoma vaccines generated by ex vivo granulocyte-macrophage colony-stimulating factor gene transfer. Cancer Res 1997; 57:1537–1546.
53. Nabel GJ, Gordon D, Bishop DK. Immune response in human melanoma after transfer of an allogenic class I major histocompatibility complex gene with DNA-liposome complexes. Proc Natl Acad Sci USA 1996; 93:15388–15393.

54. Tsang KY, Zaremba S, Nieroda CA, Zhu MZ, Hamilton JM, Schlom J. Generation of human cytotoxic T cells specific for human carcinoembryonic antigen epitopes from patients immunized with recombinant vaccinia-CEA vaccine. J Natl Cancer Inst 1995; 87:982–990.

55. Baumgartner I, Pieczek A, Manor O, Blair R, Kearney M, Walsh K, Isner JM. Constitutive expression of phVEGF$_{165}$ after intramuscular gene transfer promotes collateral vessel development in patients with critical limb ischemia. Circulation 1998; 97:1114–1123.

56. Vale PR, Losordo DW, Milliken CE, Maysky M, Esakof DD, Symes JF, Isner JM. Left ventricular electromechanical mapping to assess efficacy of phVEGF$_{165}$ gene transfer for therapeutic angiogenesis in chronic myocardial ischemia. Circulation 2000; 102:965–974.

57. Woffendin C, Yang Z-Y, Udaykumar, Xu L, Yang N-S, Sheehy MJ, Nabel GJ. Nonviral and viral delivery of a human immunodeficiency virus protective gene into primary human T cells. Proc Natl Acad Sci USA 1994; 91:11581–11585.

58. Berg P, Baltimore D, Boyer HW, Cohen SN, Davis RW, Hogness DS, Nathans D, Robin R, Watson JD, Weissman S, Zinder ND. Potential biohazards of recombinant DNA molecules (letter). Science 1974; 185:303.

59. Guidelines for Research Involving Recombinant DNA Molecules (NIH Guidelines) Fed Reg 1976; 41:27902.

60. President's Commission for the Study of Ethical Problems in Medicine and Biomedical and Behavioral Research. Splicing Life: The Social and Ethical Issues of Genetic Engineering with Human Beings. Washington DC: U.S. Government Printing Office, 1982.

61. Food and Drug Administration. Fed Reg 1984; 49:50878.

62. Rhein R. Chem Week 10-27-1985.

63. Rhein R. Chem Eng 11-11-1985.

64. Food and Drug Administration. Fed Reg 1991; 56:61022.

65. Food and Drug Administration. Fed Reg 1993; 58:53248.

66. Kessler DA, Siegel JP, Noguchi PD, Zoon KC, Feiden KL, Woodcock J. Regulation of somatic-cell therapy and gene therapy by the food and drug administration. N Engl J Med 1993; 329:1169–1173.

Part One

VECTOROLOGY

2

Adenoviruses as Vectors for Human Gene Therapy

JAMES M. WILSON

University of Pennsylvania School of Medicine
Philadelphia, Pennsylvania, U.S.A.

I. Introduction

Human adenoviruses are well-known pathogens that cause a variety of infectious diseases. The biology of these viruses is extremely well characterized. In fact, adenoviruses have been important tools for studying the basic principles of biology including transcriptional regulation, RNA splicing, and translational control. In the early 1990s, replication-defective versions of human adenoviruses emerged as potential vectors for in vivo gene therapy. Adenoviruses have many features useful for their application as vectors including ease of production, broad tropism, and ability to transduce nondividing cells. The application of adenovirus vectors for in vivo gene therapy has taught us important paradigms, which are likely to be of broad relevance to the field.

In this review, adenoviruses will be discussed in the context of their biology and applications as vectors for human gene therapy. The goal of this chapter is to illustrate important principles, not to provide a comprehensive review of the literature.

II. Biology of Adenoviruses

Adenoviruses were first discovered in the 1950s while searching for infectious agents of respiratory diseases (1–3). These newly discovered viruses were named *adenoviruses* based on the fact that the first virus isolate was recovered from adenoid tissue (1). Infection with adenovirus occurs throughout all human populations and a number of other species. In general, diseases caused by adenoviral infections are nonlethal except in immune-suppressed hosts where disseminated and lethal infection can occur. A variety of syndromes have been described associated with adenoviral infection ranging from pharyngitis, upper respiratory tract infections, pneumonia, keratoconjunctivitis, gastroenteritis, and urinary tract infections (4).

One specific form of human adenovirus called adenovirus serotype 12 was shown to cause tumors in rodents (5). This was the first description of the formation of a tumor in animals with a human virus. However, it is important to point out that there has been no convincing association between oncogenesis in humans with human adenovirus despite intensive investigation.

One aspect of adenoviral infections that deserves further comment is acute respiratory disease of military recruits (6). This epidemic form of the virus was first described in World War II and is believed to be due to the highly infectious nature of the virus together with the close interpersonal contacts found in these congregated populations of individuals. As a result of these epidemics, the military embarked on a vaccination program using oral, enteric-coated vaccines containing infectious adenoviral serotypes 4 and 7 (7). Efficacy of the vaccine was demonstrated, although its early applications were beset by problems of manufacturing which ultimately led to discontinuation of the vaccine and the subsequent reemergence of outbreaks of acute respiratory disease in military groups (8).

The characterization of human adenoviruses is based historically on a number of serological criteria. Adenoviruses are organized into six subgroups (subgroup A–F) based on the ability of the virus to agglutinate red blood cells (9). Within each subgroup are a number of adenoviral serotypes which are defined as being distinct from one another based on the lack of neutralization with antibodies generated to other known adenoviral serotypes (10). Over 51 distinct serotypes have been identified using these criteria (11). Although this classification may have important functional implications, as discussed below, it does not discern substantial molecular heterogeneity that likely occurs within individual serotypes. The neutralizing epitopes are directed toward hexon and to a lesser extent fiber (see below) which comprises only a small fraction of the adenoviral genome (12). The advent of high-throughput DNA sequencing methods provides an opportunity to classify adenoviruses from the actual genomic structure.

Adenoviruses are icosahedral particles that measure 70–100 nm. The protein shell packages a double-stranded linear DNA genome (11). An electron mi-

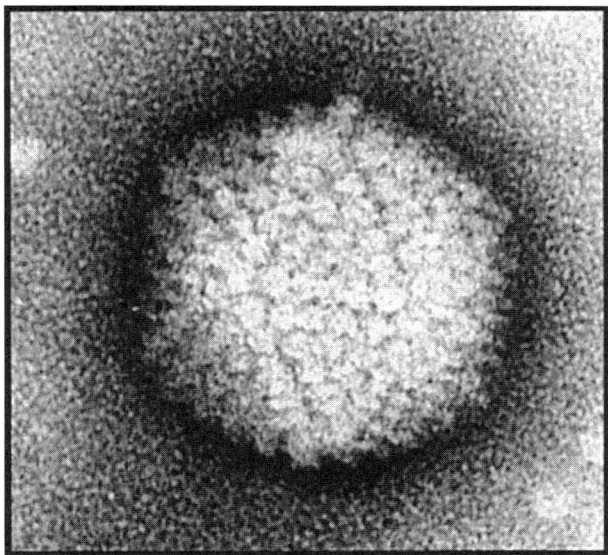

Figure 1 Electron micrograph of a human adenoviral virion. A negative stained preparation of human adenovirus was visualized under electron microscopy at 400,000 × magnification.

crographic view of a human adenovirus is presented in Figure 1. A refined structure of human adenovirus has been generated using a combination of x-ray crystallographic and electron microscopic techniques (13,14). The outer shell of the virus primarily constitutes 240 individual units comprised of hexon proteins. Incorporated into the shell are 12 penton proteins, each of which supports the fiber protein that projects out from the surface of the virus and recognizes the receptor for adenovirus called the coxsackie-adenoviral receptor (CAR) (15). Entry into the cell is a two-step process in which the fiber binds to the CAR receptor followed by interaction of the penton based with a cellular integrin that facilitates internalization (11).

The structure of the adenoviral genome and its replication has been described in detail (reviewed in Ref. 11). Figure 2 illustrates the basic transcription map of a human adenovirus. The genome for human adenoviruses spans approximately 36 kb containing a number of transcriptional units generated from both the positive and negative strands of the chromosome. Following entry of the virus into a cell and transport of the genome to the nucleus, the immediate early gene locus encoding E1A and E1B proteins is expressed. These proteins serve important functions in modulating the biology of the host as well as activating other

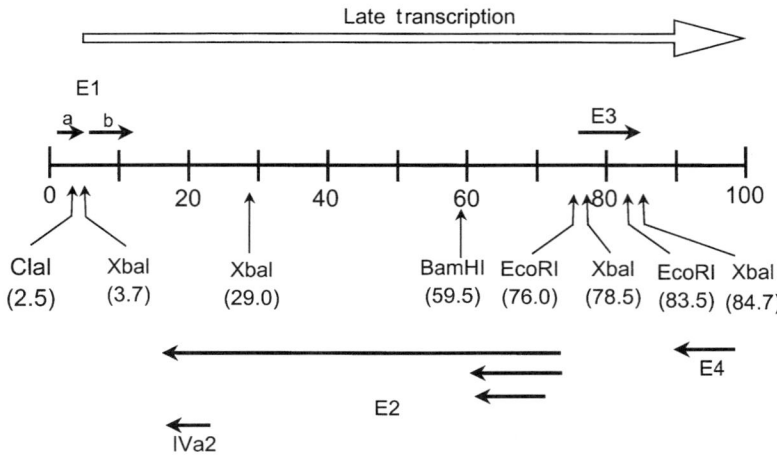

Figure 2   Transcription map of human adenovirus. (Adapted from Ref. 11.)

viral genes. The early genes, E2 and E4, play important roles in replication of the viral genome. Proteins expressed from the E3 genetic locus are not essential for propagation of the virus, although they play important roles in modulating host responses to virus-infected cells. In the first phase of the adenoviral life cycle, early genes are expressed which prepare the cell for actual replication of the viral genome and formation of progeny virus. The second phase begins with activation of the major late promoter and formation of a very long transcript encoding polypeptides involved in the formation of capsids. Coincident with the activation of transcription from the major late promoter is the onset of DNA replication. The end result of this process is the formation of a huge number of progeny virions and death of the host cell; approximately 10,000 viruses are produced from a single infected cell. Infection spreads from cell to cell forming a wave of cytopathology. The visual consequences of adenoviral infection of permissive cells in vitro is called cytopathic effect (CPE).

III.   Adenoviral Vectors: How Do You Make Them?

In creating vectors from a human adenovirus a number of issues were considered (16). The vector must be isolated as a distinct molecular entity free of contamination from adventitious agents and other undesired forms of the virus. Vector creation should be simple and scalable and yields of the resulting vector should be high. Finally, for gene replacement, it is preferable that the recombinant virus does not replicate or express viral genes.

The preferred strategy for completely disabling the adenovirus is to delete all viral open reading frames while incorporating a heterologous transcriptional unit encoding the transgene. Although this has indeed been accomplished, most applications of adenoviral vectors have focused on attenuated versions of the adenovirus made replication defective by deleting only the immediate early genes encoding E1A and E1B (16). The hypothesis is that an E1-deleted recombinant virus should be replication defective with little or no expression of the other viral genes, since their expression requires E1-encoded proteins. Critical to the rescue and propagation of an E1-deleted adenovirus is a cell line capable of *trans*-complementing the deletion of E1. Graham previously isolated a human kidney–derived cell called 293 that stably expresses E1 as a result of transfection of sheared adenoviral genomic DNA (17). This has been the "workhorse" of the early development of adenoviral vectors, although improved cell lines have now been generated.

An important concept in creating, isolating, and characterizing adenoviruses and adenoviral vectors is the isolation of distinct molecular forms of the virus. This is accomplished by infecting a monolayer of permissive cells with a low multiplicity of infection (i.e., 1–20 infectious viruses per 10^6 adherent cells). A single infectious virus will enter a cell and undergo replication yielding viral progeny that infect adjacent cells initiating the cascade of infection and a focus of cytopathology (Fig. 3). This focus is referred to as a plaque, which is usually evaluated on a monolayer of cells which have been overlaid with agarose to prevent the dissemination of virus throughout the culture. Each plaque should represent progeny from a distinct adenovirus.

Critical to the creation of engineered forms of adenoviruses is the ability to manipulate a portion of its genome within a bacterial plasmid. This was accom-

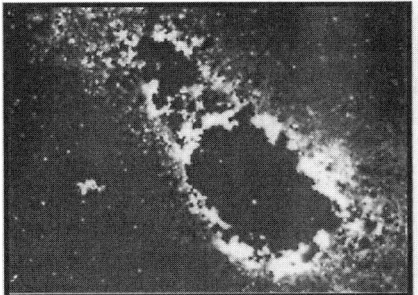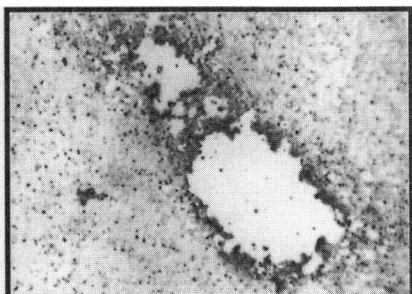

Figure 3 Plaque of human adenovirus infection. A monolayer of 293 cells was infected with a low multiplicity of infection of an E1-deleted human adenovirus vector; 10 days later the monolayer was observed by phase contrast microscopy for cytopathology.

plished for E1-deleted adenoviruses by subcloning the 5′ region of the adenoviral genome into a plasmid allowing the deletion of sequences encoding E1 and insertion of the gene of interest (18). A vector genome representing the entire chromosome of the virus except for the substituted region of E1 is generated in the following way. The subcloned and engineered plasmid containing 5′ sequence of the virus is cotransfected into 293 cells with a large fragment of the viral genome missing only a portion of 5′ sequence. If there is sufficient overlap between the 5′ viral sequence in the plasmid and the large 3′ viral chromosomal DNA, homologous recombination will occur in the cell following cotransfection leading to the generation of a vector that can replicate in E1-expressing cells.

The strategy for creating a replication-defective version of adenovirus based on homologous recombination has been used extensively, although a number of issues have emerged. The efficiency with which one can rescue the desired recombinant based on homologous recombination is low (16). Furthermore, not all of the resulting plaques represent the desired recombinant for a number of reasons including undesired rearrangements in the resulting recombinant genome and the presence of replication-competent adenovirus. Identification of the proper recombinant requires screening approximately 20 plaques.

The presence of replication-competent virus in the vector preparation is problematic, since it could be associated with increased toxicity and may facilitate the spread of the recombinant in vivo (18–20). Replication-competent adenovirus occurs by either cross contamination of the initial plaque with replication-competent virus from an adjacent plaque or reversion of the E1 deletion during the propagation of the recombinant by homologous recombination between sequences in the vector flanking the E1 deletion and the transfected E1 sequences in 293 cells.

A major advance in replication-defective adenoviruses is the development of methods for creating recombinant viruses from distinct molecular clones in which the entire genome of the vector has been subcloned into a prokaryotic or invertebrate host. This has now been accomplished in a number of systems including yeast artificial chromosomes (21), cosmids (22), and bacterial plasmids (23–25). The subsequent discussion will focus on methods in which the adenoviral genome is subcloned in its entirety into bacterial plasmids.

A number of groups have created replication-defective adenoviruses based on molecular clones of the vector in bacterial plasmids (23–25). A widely used strategy begins with a plasmid containing an E1-deleted version of the recombinant adenovirus with a multicloning site inserted in place of E1. The minigene is incorporated into this site by a two-part ligation and the desired recombinant genome is isolated following transformation of bacteria and rescue of the plasmid forming the desired recombinant genome. This plasmid is transfected into 293 cells which support the rescue of virus from the plasmid and its propagation.

Isolating recombinant adenoviruses from molecular clones has many advantages. Virus that emerges from the transfection should only represent that derived from the molecular clone, thereby eliminating the need for screening of plaques, thereby saving a substantial amount of time. We have found that rescue of virus from a clone rarely fails in contrast to the method based on homologous recombination where we are unable to isolate a recombinant approximately 20% of the time.

All strategies for creating E1-deleted adenoviruses using 293 cells are complicated by the potential emergence of replication-competent adenoviruses as a result of homologous recombination between the virus and the transfected E1 sequences as noted above (18–20). This has been circumvented by generating novel cell lines that contain stably transfected E1 gene cassettes which minimize and/or eliminate overlap sequences flanking the deletion of E1 in the vector (26,27).

Another advantage of using adenoviruses as vectors for gene therapy is the ease with which one can purify high quantities of the virus. The standard approach for isolating research-grade vector from the resulting lysate is based on sedimentation through CsCl gradients (28). The resulting preparation is highly enriched for adenovirus; analysis by SDS polyacrylamide gel electrophoresis indicates that the majority of proteins are derived from the adenoviral capsids. A number of other strategies have been developed for purifying adenovirus using liquid phase chromatography that are more practical for scale-up of clinical-grade material (29).

The recombinant virus should be subjected to a number of assays to characterize its potency and purity prior to use as a research reagent. The total number of viral particles is assessed by measurement of optical density at 260 nm which measures nucleic acid; the extinction coefficient for conversion of optical density to particles per milliliter is 1×10^{12}. The number of viruses capable of replicating in a permissive cell is determined in a plaque-forming assay. Limiting dilutions of virus are used to infect an adherent monolayer of permissive cells which are subsequently overlaid with agarose. Each single infectious virus leads to the formation of a plaque. The estimate of physical particles based on optical density exceeds that measured by functional virus in the plaque-forming assay by approximately 10- to 50-fold. This does not necessarily mean that most of the virus is nonfunctional, since the efficiency of recovery of adenovirus in a plaque-forming assay is also a function of the permissivity of the cell (30). The routine performance of the plaque-forming assay within any individual laboratory provides a common basis for assessing prep to prep variation in vector potency. Comparison of vector potency between laboratories will require a reference standard which to date does not exist. The final assay to be performed on each preparation of vector is an assessment for the presence of replication-competent adenovirus.

IV. Biology of E1-Deleted Adenoviruses

Prior to their consideration in gene therapy, replication-defective adenoviruses were used to study gene function and activity of promoters and enhancers. A seminal point in the emerging field of gene therapy was the notion of using E1-deleted adenoviruses as vectors for delivery of genes in vivo. One of the first demonstrations of in vivo gene therapy with a defective adenoviral vector was correction of the metabolic defect in mice deficient in the urea cycle gene ornithine transcarbamylase following intravenous injection of vector into newborn animals (31). The concept of in vivo gene therapy with adenoviral vectors really gained momentum for gene therapy of cystic fibrosis.

The cystic fibrosis community celebrated the isolation of the gene responsible for this disease in the fall of 1989 (32–34). Soon thereafter, Blaese and Anderson began the first human experiments in gene therapy based on ex vivo transplantation of genetically modified lymphocytes in an individual with severe combined immune deficiency (35). It was clear, however, that the ex vivo approach for gene therapy so well suited for targeting the hematopoietic system was impractical in the treatment of pulmonary disease such as that caused by cystic fibrosis. Dr. Ronald Crystal and collaborators evaluated the potential of the adenovirus as an in vivo delivery vehicle for gene therapy of cystic fibrosis. They first showed that E1-deleted versions of the adenovirus expressing the gene encoding α_1-antitrypsin did indeed target airway epithelial cells at high efficiently when vector was instilled into the airway (36). This confirmed the broad tropism of the vector and its ability to transduce nondividing cells. Subsequent studies were performed with vector expressing the normal version of the gene defective in cystic fibrosis called the cystic fibrosis transmembrane conductance regulator (CFTR) (37). These encouraging preclinical studies supported the development of a number of Phase I clinical experiments in which cystic fibrosis research subjects were administered E1-deleted vectors expressing CFTR onto the nasal mucosa or into the intrapulmonary airways (38–41).

The efficiency with which E1-deleted adenoviruses transfer genes into the airway of preclinical models was impressive relative to other vector systems available at the time. This stimulated a number of investigators to explore the use of adenoviral vectors in other applications of gene transfer. Perricaudet and colleagues showed wide dissemination of an adenoviral expressing lacZ when administered parenterally in to newborn mice (42). Crystal and colleagues showed high-level targeting of adenoviral vectors when injected into the circulation of adult rats (43). Since then, virtually every conceivable cell type amenable to in vivo and ex vivo manipulation has been targeted with adenoviral vectors.

Despite the early success of adenoviral vectors for in vivo gene therapy, a number of issues emerged. Although the efficiency of transduction in vivo is quite high, expression of the transgene eventually diminished to undetectable levels coincident with the development of inflammation at the site of gene transfer (44–50). Furthermore, most recipients became refractory to a second administration of vector; that is, the efficiency of gene transfer following an initial exposure to vector was substantially diminished (44,51–54). These problems were diminished and/or eliminated in animals deficient in T-lymphocyte functions, suggesting that antigen-specific immunity plays a critical role (47,55–59).

Through a series of experiments in a number of preclinical and clinical models, the following model has emerged for explaining the biology of adenoviral vectors delivered in vivo (Fig. 4). Loss of gene expression and the development of inflammation at the site of gene transfer is due in part to the activation of cytotoxic T lymphocytes (CTLs) directed against vector-transduced cells. The basis for recognition and destruction of the target cells is major histocompatibility (MHC) class I presentation of peptides derived from vector-encoded proteins. In the context of an E1-deleted adenoviral vector, two potential sources of antigenic epitopes exists including the transgene product as well as the products of other early and late genes that are retained in the vector. The CTL response is dependent on CD4$^+$ T helper cells that are also activated to vector-encoded antigens. MHC class II–restricted presentation of capsid-derived proteins from the input vector is an important source for CD4 T-cell activation, although one cannot rule out endogenously produced, vector-derived proteins as a source of antigen.

The second major problem is resistance of the recipient to a second engraftment of the vector-derived gene. This is caused by the activation of B cells to secreted antibodies following the initial vector administration which neutralizes any subsequent exposure to the virus. This is a CD4$^+$ T helper cell–dependent response in which B cells are activated to peptides from the capsid proteins presented in the context of MHC class II.

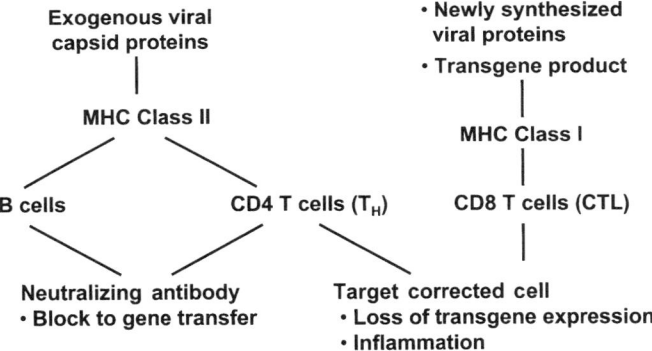

Figure 4 Antigen-specific immune responses to adenoviral vectors.

More recent studies have expanded on the model described above to explain the propensity of adenoviruses to activate T cells that is a driving step in the antigen-specific responses. The event that initiates the cascade leading to formation of CTLs and destruction of target cells is the actual recognition of the infection by the host's antigen-specific immune system which leads to the specific activation and expansion of vector-specific T cells (60). Figure 5 illustrates this process. Because of the broad tropism of adenoviruses, they infect, very efficiently, antigen-presenting cells (APCs) in addition to the desired target cells. Vector-encoded proteins expressed in the APCs are presented by MHC class I to T cells which leads to T-cell activation and amplification. This process requires a number of signaling pathways uniquely activated by molecules expressed on the surface of APCs. An obvious strategy for overcoming this problem is to engineer the virus so that it does not express proteins containing antigenic epitopes (see below).

The humoral response to vector will be more difficult to overcome, since the targets for immune activation, the capsid proteins, are critical to the formation of viable vector particles. A number of investigators have attempted to characterize the epitopes on the capsid to which the neutralizing antibodies are directed (61–63). The predominant epitopes are located in hypervariable regions of the hexon protein that are located on the surface of the capsid shell (12). Additional neutralizing epitopes may also be found on the fiber protein.

Characterization of host-vector interactions has primarily focused on activation of antigen-specific pathways. Recent studies have focused on the events that occur immediately following administration of vector. In vivo delivery of adenoviral vectors in many human trials is associated with the acute onset of fever and flu-like symptoms suggesting activation of innate immunity. Furthermore,

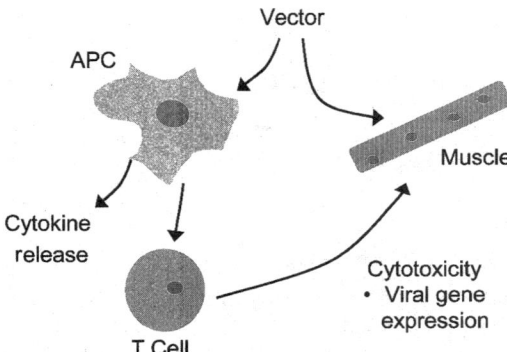

Figure 5 Interaction of adenovirus with antigen-presenting cells.

analysis of tissues in preclinical models demonstrated neutrophilic inflammatory infiltrates at the site of gene transfer that occur prior to activation of antigen-specific immunity (64). The importance of better defining the innate immune response to vector became critical during the conduct of a Phase I clinical trial of liver-directed gene transfer in patients with arnithine transcarbamylase (OTC) deficiency in which one patient developed a lethal episode of systemic inflammatory response syndrome characterized by coagulation defects and multiorgan failure (65).

In murine studies, systemic administration of adenoviral vector is associated with the production of a number of chemokines within hours of vector administration and the recruitment of neutrophils that correlates with the degree of liver injury (64). Subsequent studies suggested that the vector-induced liver damage is mediated in part through the activation of macrophages. Specifically, depletion of Kupffer's cells in mouse liver resulted in less production of tumor necrosis factor-α (TNF-α) and improved duration of transgene expression (3).

We conducted a series of experiments in mice (66) and nonhuman primates (67) to evaluate the innate immune responses to systemically administered adenovirus with the goal of understanding the systemic inflammatory response syndrome that occurred in the OTC-deficient patient (65). Our studies show that intravenous injection of adenovirus leads to targeting of macrophages and dendritic cells in liver and spleen. Activation of vector-targeted APCs results in the production of proinflammatory cytokines such as interleukin-6 (IL-6) which, in rhesus monkeys, is associated with multiorgan damage, thrombocytopenia, and coagulopathy which is reminiscent of some of the complications observed in the OTC-deficient trial.

Based on the extensive experience with adenoviral vectors in preclinical and clinical models, a number of investigators have attempted to develop modifications that improve the safety and efficacy of the system. The first approach was to minimize the activation of CTLs through the development of modified recombinant adenoviral vectors.

The premise for further modifying adenoviral vectors is that deletion of E1 is insufficient to render the remaining viral genes inactive. Endogenous transcription factors such as necrosis factor (NF) IL-6 from liver have E1-like functions that could potentially overcome the deficiency of this function in the vector. One strategy is to incorporate into the vector mutations in other essential genes that are temperature sensitive (i.e., inactive at 37°C but active at 32°C). Second-generation vectors were constructed in which the E1 locus was deleted and other essential genes such as E2A (ts125) and E2B (ts149) were rendered conditionally defective by incorporation of temperature-sensitive mutations. Analysis of these vectors in murine models demonstrated only marginal improvement in terms of safety and stability of gene expression (68,69). The next approach was to create vectors with deletions in multiple essential genes. This has now been achieved in vectors deleted of E1 in addition to E2A (70,71), E4 (72–75), and terminal protein (76). In each case, cell lines were created that stably expressed the deleted viral genes to allow isolation and propagation of the vector.

The most extensive experience has been with vectors deleted of both E1 and E4 (72–75). Four independent groups have created this type of adenoviral vector and tested its performance in murine models. In each case, toxicity related to activation of CTLs and targeting of hepatocytes (i.e., vector-induced hepatitis) was substantially diminished with these vectors as compared to E1-deleted vectors, and in most cases transgene expression was prolonged. This coincided with the desired result of significantly reduced expression of the remaining viral genes. The importance of these experiments is that it confirms the role of antigen-specific T-cell responses in the loss of transgene expression and the toxicity of systemically administered vector. These experiments, however, do not address the role of acute innate immune responses in vector performance.

An important recent advance in the field of adenoviral vectors is the development of recombinants deleted of all viral open reading frames which contain a transgene flanked by the 5' and 3' long terminal repeat sequences (77–79). The only viable strategy for isolating and propagating fully deleted vectors is to use helper viruses to rescue and expand the recombinant. The challenge with this strategy is to eliminate helper viruses in the final preparations of vectors. This is difficult, because the fully deleted vectors and the helper virus are packaged in capsids that are virtually identical. Purification is achieved by sedimentation through CsCl or by ablation of the helper virus in the production step using site-specific excision such as with cre recombinase.

Evaluation of fully deleted adenoviral vectors in preclinical models has been limited because of the difficulty in producing sufficient quantities of purified vector. The most substantial experience has been following intravenous injection for targeting liver. Beaudet and colleagues have demonstrated impressive improvements in the stability of transgene expression from fully deleted adenoviral vector in mice and baboons (77–79). The toxicity based on CTL-mediated inflammation of hepatocytes is substantially reduced. The innate immune response to fully deleted virus has not been studied. Since it appears that the innate immune response is independent of viral encoded gene expression, one would speculate that the innate immune response would proceed unabated following administration of a fully deleted adenoviral vector.

The importance of antigen-specific immune responses in the performance of adenoviral vectors suggests pharmacological strategies that modulate the activation of T and B cells may be useful. Indeed, global inhibition of T-cell activity does improve the duration of transgene expression, blunts the inflammation mediated by CTLs, and prevents the formation of neutralizing antibodies.

The CD4$^+$ T helper cell plays a critical role in both the B-cell and CTL effects. Several approaches have been developed to prevent the activation of the CD4 T cell such as blocking or depleting antibodies or reagents that interfere with necessary pathways of costimulation (47,55–59). Since MHC class II–dependent presentation of the input capsid proteins plays a dominant role in activation of the CD4 T helper cells, one could reason that interfering with its function is necessary only at the time of vector administration. In other words, chronic immune suppression may not be required. In fact, inhibition of CD4 T-cell function at the time of vector administration does extend the duration of transgene expression and prevents the development of neutralizing antibodies, although these responses become more difficult to inhibit with repeated coadministrations of vector and T-cell inhibitor.

Many applications of adenoviral vectors would benefit from more specific targeting of vector and transgene expression. Two general approaches have been pursued. A number of investigators have attempted to modify the capsid to redirect vector uptake to a specific receptor (80). Another strategy is to utilize a cell-specific promoter to drive expression of the transgene in a strategy called transcriptional targeting (81). In either case, the net effect is restriction of transgene expression to a desired cell type.

V. Summary

A number of important principles of in vivo gene transfer have emerged from preclinical and clinical studies with adenoviral vectors. Interaction of the host with the vector and vector-transduced cells dominates the biology of the vector. Antigen-specific immune responses result in destructive cellular immunity and neutralizing humoral immunity. Furthermore, high avidity of the vector for APCs not only drives the T-cell response but also activates an innate immune response that can contribute significantly to toxicity.

In light of our current knowledge of adenoviral vectors, what will be their role in clinical applications of human gene therapy? One must be very careful in any application requiring systemic delivery of the vector because of the innate immune response to the capsid proteins of the virus that can lead to lethal consequences. However, localized administration of the vector, such as intramuscular and subcutaneous delivery, should be associated with substantially less toxicity. Genetic diseases that require life-long transgene expression are not obvious candidates for adenovirus-mediated gene therapy. Despite the substantial improvement in transgene stability realized by "gutting" the adenoviral vector, the fact is that expression does diminish in a period of months to years and the recipient becomes resistant to a second administration of vector because of the formation of neutralizing antibody. Clinical applications in which transient gene expression would be therapeutic are much more attractive models. Examples include regional therapy of cancer with vectors that express antitumor cytokines and tissue remodeling such as angiogenesis, wound healing, and bone formation.

Potentially the most powerful use of adenoviral vectors is in the development of genetic vaccines. The combination of high transduction of APCs with the inherent adjuvant effect of the vector make adenoviruses ideal carriers for activating T cells to transgene products.

The one problem that remains for all in vivo applications of adenoviral vectors is that of neutralizing antibodies. A substantial portion of the human population has neutralizing antibodies as a result of naturally acquired infections that would diminish the effectiveness of vector-mediated gene transfer. Furthermore, neutralizing antibodies are generated against the vector following the first administration. The development of new and/or modified adenoviruses not recognized by humoral responses to the common existing human adenoviruses would circumvent the problem of preexisting immunity. Repeated vector administration would require the use of non–cross-reacting serotypes as well.

In conclusion, through extensive basic investigation of adenoviral vectors, important biology has been learned that will allow a more rational utilization of this technology for therapeutic applications.

Acknowledgments

This work was supported by grants from the National Institutes of Health (P01 HL59407-03 and P30 DK47757-09), Cystic Fibrosis Foundation and Juvenile Diabetes Research Foundation. The author holds equity in Targeted Genetics Corp., Seattle, Washington.

References

1. Rowe WP, Huebner RJ, Gillmore LK. Isolation of a cytopathogenic agent from human adenoids undergoing spontaneous degeneration in tissue culture. Proc Soc Exp Biol Med 1953; 84:570–573.
2. Hilleman MR, Werner JH. Recovery of new agents from patients with acute respiratory illness. Proc Soc Exp Biol Med 1954; 85:183–188.
3. Huebner RJ, Rowe WP, Ward TG. Adenoidal-pharyngoconjunctival agents. N Engl J Med 1954; 251:1077–1086.
4. Horwitz MS. Adenoviruses. In: Fields BN, Knipe DM, Howley PM, eds. Fields Virology. Vol. 2. Philadelphia: Lippincott-Raven, 1996:2149–2171.
5. Trentin JJ, Yabe Y, Taylor G. The quest for human cancer viruses. Science 1962; 137:835–849.
6. Miller LF, Rytel M, Pierce WE, Rosenbaum MJ. Epidemiology of nonbacterial pneumonia among naval recruits. JAMA 1963; 185:92–99.

7. Top FH. Control of adenovirus acute respiratory disease in U.S. army trainees. Yale J Biol Med 1975; 48:185–195.

8. Barraza EM, Ludwig SL, Gaydos JC, Brundage JF. Reemergence of adenovirus type 4 acute respiratory disease in military trainees: Report of an outbreak during a lapse in vaccination. J Infect Dis 1999; 179:1531–1533.

9. Rosen I, Hovis JF, Bell JA. Further observation of typing adenoviruses and a description of two possible additional serotypes. Proc Soc Exp Biol Med 1962; 110:710–713.

10. Norrby E. The structural and functional diversity of adenovirus capsid components. J Gen Virol 1969; 5:221–236.

11. Shenk TE. Adenoviridae: The Viruses and Their Replication. In: Fields BN, Knipe DM, Howley PM, eds. Fields Virology. Vol. 2. Philadelphia: Lippincott-Raven, 1996:2111–2148.

12. Crawford-Miksza L, Schnurr DP. Analysis of 15 adenovirus hexon proteins reveals the location and structure of seven hypervariable regions containing serotype-specific residues. J Virol 1996; 70:1836–1844.

13. Athappilly FK, Murali R, Rux JJ, Cai Z, Burnett RM. The refined crystal structure of hexon, the major coat protein of adenovirus type 2, at 209 A resolution. J Mol Biol 1994; 242:430–455.

14. Rux JJ, Burnett RM. Type-specific epitope locations revealed by X-ray crystallographic study of adenovirus type 5 hexon. Mol Ther 2000; 1:18–30.

15. Bergelson JM, Cunningham JA, Droguett G, et al. Isolation of a common receptor for coxsackie B viruses and adenoviruses 2 and 5. Science 1997; 275:1320–1323.

16. Danthinne X, Imperiale MJ. Production of first generation adenovirus vectors: a review. Gene Ther 2000; 7:1707–1714.

17. Graham FL, Smiley J, Russell WC, Nairn R. Characteristics of a human cell line transformed by DNA from human adenovirus type 5. J Gen Virol 1977; 36:59–74.

18. Schaack J, Langer S, Guo X. Efficient selection of recombinant adenoviruses by vectors that express beta-galactosidase. J Virol 1995; 69:3920–3923.

19. Munz PL, Young CS. End-joining of DNA fragments in adenovirus transfection of human cells. Virology 1991; 183:160–169.

20. Lochmuller H, Jani A, Huard J, et al. Emergence of early region 1-containing replication-competent adenovirus in stocks of replication-defective adenovirus recombinants (delta E1 + delta E3) during multiple passages in 293 cells. Hum Gene Ther 1994; 5:1485–1491.

21. Ketner G, Spencer F, Tugendreich S, Connelly C, Hieter P. Efficient manipulation of the human adenovirus genome as an infectious yeast artificial chromosome clone. Proc Natl Acad Sci USA 1994; 91:6186–6190.

22. Kojima H, Ohishi N, Yagi K. Generation of recombinant adenovirus vector with infectious adenoviral genome released from cosmid-based vector by simple procedure allowing complex manipulation. Biochem Biophys Res Commun 1998; 246:868–872.

23. Souza DW, Armentano D. Novel cloning method for recombinant adenovirus construction in Escherichia coli. Biotechniques 1999; 26:502–508.

24. Mizuguchi H, Kay MA. Efficient construction of a recombinant adenovirus vector by an improved in vitro ligation method. Hum Gene Ther 1998; 9:2577–2583.

25. Mizuguchi H, Kay MA. A simple method for constructing E1- and E1/E4-deleted recombinant adenoviral vectors. Hum Gene Ther 1999; 10:2013–2017.

26. Fallaux FJ, Bout A, van der Velde I, et al. New helper cells and matched early region 1–deleted adenovirus vectors prevent generation of replication-competent adenoviruses. Hum Gene Ther 1998; 9:1909–1917.

27. Gao GP, Engdahl RK, Wilson JM. A cell line for high-yield production of E1-deleted adenovirus vectors without the emergence of replication-competent virus. Hum Gene Ther 2000; 11:213–219.

28. Graham FL, Prevec L. Manipulation of Adenovirus Vectors. In: Murray EJ, ed. Methods in Molecular Biology: Gene Transfer and Expression Protocols. Vol. 7. Clifton, NJ: Humana Press, 1991:109–128.

29. Blanche F, Cameron B, Barbot A, et al. An improved anion-exchange HPLC method for the detection and purification of adenoviral particles. Gene Ther 2000; 7:1055–1062.

30. Hutchins B, Sajjadi N, Seaver S, et al. Working toward an adenoviral vector testing standard. Mol Ther 2000; 2:532–534.

31. Stratford-Perricaudet LD, Levrero M, Chasse JF, Perricaudet M, Briand P. Evaluation of the transfer and expression in mice of an enzyme-encoding gene using a human adenovirus vector. Hum Gene Ther 1990; 1:241–256.

32. Rommens JM, Iannuzzi MC, Kerem B, et al. Identification of the cystic fibrosis gene: chromosome walking and jumping. Science 1989; 245:1059–1065.

33. Riordan JR, Rommens JM, Kerem B, et al. Identification of the cystic fibrosis gene: cloning and characterization of complementary DNA. Science 1989; 245:1066–1073.

34. Kerem B, Rommens JM, Buchanan JA, et al. Identification of the cystic fibrosis gene: genetic analysis. Science 1989; 245:1073–1080.

35. Blaese RM, Culver KW, Miller AD, et al. T lymphocyte-directed gene therapy for ADA-SCID: initial trial results after 4 years. Science 1995; 270:475–480.

36. Rosenfeld MA, Siegfried W, Yoshimura K, et al. Adenovirus-mediated transfer of a recombinant alpha 1-antitrypsin gene to the lung epithelium in vivo. Science 1991; 252:431–434.

37. Rosenfeld MA, Yoshimura K, Trapnell BC, et al. In vivo transfer of the human cystic fibrosis transmembrane conductance regulator gene to the airway epithelium. Cell 1992; 68:143–155.

38. Zabner J, Couture LA, Gregory RJ, Graham SM, Smith AE, Welsh MJ. Adenovirus-mediated gene transfer transiently corrects the chloride transport defect in nasal epithelia of patients with cystic fibrosis. Cell 1993; 75:207–216.

39. Crystal RG, McElvaney NG, Rosenfeld MA, et al. Administration of an adenovirus containing the human CFTR cDNA to the respiratory tract of individuals with cystic fibrosis. Nat Genet 1994; 8:42–51.

40. Knowles MR, Hohneker KW, Zhou Z, et al. A controlled study of adenoviral-vector–mediated gene transfer in the nasal epithelium of patients with cystic fibrosis. N Engl J Med 1995; 333:823–831.

41. Zuckerman JB, Robinson CB, McCoy KS, et al. A phase I study of adenovirus-mediated transfer of the human cystic fibrosis transmembrane conductance regulator

gene to a lung segment of individuals with cystic fibrosis. Hum Gene Ther 1999; 10:2973–2985.

42. Stratford-Perricaudet LD, Makeh I, Perricaudet M, Briand P. Widespread long-term gene transfer to mouse skeletal muscles and heart. J Clin Invest 1992; 90:626–630.

43. Jaffe HA, Danel C, Longenecker G, et al. Adenovirus-mediated in vivo gene transfer and expression in normal rat liver. Nat Genet 1992; 1:372–378.

44. Yang Y, Li Q, Ertl HC, Wilson JM. Cellular and humoral immune responses to viral antigens create barriers to lung-directed gene therapy with recombinant adeno-viruses. J Virol 1995; 69:2004–2015.

45. Yang Y, Ertl HC, Wilson JM. MHC class I–restricted cytotoxic T lymphocytes to viral antigens destroy hepatocytes in mice infected with E1-deleted recombinant adenoviruses. Immunity 1994; 1:433–442.

46. Yang Y, Nunes FA, Berencsi K, Furth EE, Gonczol E, Wilson JM. Cellular immu-nity to viral antigens limits E1-deleted adenoviruses for gene therapy. Proc Natl Acad Sci USA 1994; 91:4407–4411.

47. Zsengeller ZK, Wert SE, Hull WM, et al. Persistence of replication-deficient adeno-virus-mediated gene transfer in lungs of immune-deficient (nu/nu) mice. Hum Gene Ther 1995; 6:457–467.

48. Tripathy SK, Black HB, Goldwasser E, Leiden JM. Immune responses to transgene-encoded proteins limit the stability of gene expression after injection of replication-defective adenovirus vectors. Nat Med 1996; 2:545–550.

49. Yao SN, Farjo A, Roessler BJ, Davidson BL, Kurachi K. Adenovirus-mediated transfer of human factor IX gene in immunodeficient and normal mice: evidence for prolonged stability and activity of the transgene in liver. Viral Immunol 1996; 9:141–153.

50. Morral N, O'Neal W, Zhou H, Langston C, Beaudet A. Immune responses to reporter proteins and high viral dose limit duration of expression with adenoviral vectors: comparison of E2a wild type and E2a deleted vectors. Hum Gene Ther 1997; 8: 1275–1286.

51. Juillard V, Villefroy P, Godfrin D, Pavirani A, Venet A, Guillet JG. Long-term humoral and cellular immunity induced by a single immunization with replication-defective adenovirus recombinant vector. Eur J Immunol 1995; 25:3467–3473.

52. Gahery-Segard H, Juillard V, Gaston J, et al. Humoral immune response to the capsid components of recombinant adenoviruses: routes of immunization modulate virus-induced Ig subclass shifts. Eur J Immunol 1997; 27:653–659.

53. Yang Y, Trinchieri G, Wilson JM. Recombinant IL-12 prevents formation of blocking IgA antibodies to recombinant adenovirus and allows repeated gene therapy to mouse lung. Nat Med 1995; 1:890–893.

54. Kozarsky KF, McKinley DR, Austin LL, Raper SE, Stratford-Perricaudet LD, Wilson JM. In vivo correction of low density lipoprotein receptor deficiency in the Watanabe heritable hyperlipidemic rabbit with recombinant adenoviruses. J Biol Chem 1994; 269:13695–13702.

55. Yang Y, Haecker SE, Su Q, Wilson JM. Immunology of gene therapy with adenovi-ral vectors in mouse skeletal muscle. Hum Mol Genet 1996; 5:1703–1712.

56. Barr D, Tubb J, Ferguson D, et al. Strain related variations in adenovirally mediated

transgene expression from mouse hepatocytes in vivo: comparisons between immunocompetent and immunodeficient inbred strains. Gene Ther 1995; 2:151–155.

57. Kass-Eisler A, Falck-Pedersen E, Elfenbein DH, Alvira M, Buttrick PM, Leinwand LA. The impact of developmental stage, route of administration and the immune system on adenovirus-mediated gene transfer. Gene Ther 1994; 1:395–402.

58. Michou AI, Santoro L, Christ M, Julliard V, Pavirani A, Mehtali M. Adenovirus-mediated gene transfer: influence of transgene, mouse strain and type of immune response on persistence of transgene expression. Gene Ther 1997; 4:473–482.

59. Yang Y, Su Q, Grewal IS, Schilz R, Flavell RA, Wilson JM. Transient subversion of CD40 ligand function diminishes immune responses to adenovirus vectors in mouse liver and lung tissues. J Virol 1996; 70:6370–6377.

60. Jooss K, Yang Y, Fisher KJ, Wilson JM. Transduction of dendritic cells by DNA viral vectors directs the immune response to transgene products in muscle fibers. J Virol 1998; 72:4212–4223.

61. Gall JGD, Crystal RG, Falck-Pederson E. Construction and characterization of hexon-chimeric adenoviruses: specification of adenovirus serotype. J Virol 1998; 72:10260–10264.

62. Ostapchuk P, Hearing P. Pseudopackaging of adenovirus type 5 genomes into capsids containing the hexon proteins of adenovirus serotypes B, D, or E. J Virol 2001; 75:45–51.

63. Roy S, Shirley PS, McClelland A, Kaleko M. Circumvention of immunity to the adenovirus major coat protein hexon. J Virol 1998; 72:6875–6879.

64. Muruve DA, Barnes MJ, Stillman IE, Libermann TA. Adenoviral gene therapy leads to rapid induction of multiple chemokines and acute neutrophil-dependent hepatic injury in vivo. Hum Gene Ther 1999; 10:965–976.

65. Raper SE, Chirmule N, Lee FS, et al. Lethal systemic inflammatory response syndrome in a patient with partial ornithine transcarbamylase deficiency following intravascular administration of recombinant adenoviral vector. Submitted.

66. Zhang Y, Chirmule N, Gao GP, et al. Acute cytokine response to systemic adenoviral vectors in mice is mediated by dendritic cells and macrophages. Mol Ther 2001; 3: 697–707.

67. Schnell MA, Zhang Y, Tazelaar J, et al. Activation of innate immunity in nonhuman primates following intraportal administration of adenoviral vectors. Mol Ther 2001; 3:708–722.

68. Engelhardt JF, Ye X, Doranz B, Wilson JM. Ablation of E2A in recombinant adenoviruses improves transgene persistence and decreases inflammatory response in mouse liver. Proc Natl Acad Sci USA 1994; 91:6196–6200.

69. Yang Y, Nunes FA, Berencsi K, Gonczol E, Engelhardt JF, Wilson JM. Inactivation of E2a in recombinant adenoviruses improves the prospect for gene therapy in cystic fibrosis. Nat Genet 1994; 7:362–369.

70. Gorziglia MI, Kadan MJ, Yei S, et al. Elimination of both E1 and E2 from adenovirus vectors further improves prospects for in vivo human gene therapy. J Virol 1996; 70:4173–4178.

71. O'Neal WK, Zhou H, Morral N, et al. Toxicological comparison of E2a-deleted and first-generation adenoviral vectors expressing alpha1-antitrypsin after systemic delivery. Hum Gene Ther 1998; 9:1587–1598.

72. Gao GP, Yang Y, Wilson JM. Biology of adenovirus vectors with E1 and E4 deletions for liver-directed gene therapy. J Virol 1996; 70:8934–8943.

73. Wang Q, Greenburg G, Bunch D, Farson D, Finer MH. Persistent transgene expression in mouse liver following in vivo gene transfer with a delta E1/delta E4 adenovirus vector. Gene Ther 1997; 4:393–400.

74. Dedieu JF, Vigne E, Torrent C, et al. Long-term gene delivery into the livers of immunocompetent mice with E1/E4-defective adenoviruses. J Virol 1997; 71:4626–4637.

75. Christ M, Louis B, Stoeckel F, et al. Modulation of the inflammatory properties and hepatotoxicity of recombinant adenovirus vectors by the viral E4 gene products. Hum Gene Ther 2000; 11:415–427.

76. Amalfitano A, Chamberlain JS. Isolation and characterization of packaging cell lines that coexpress the adenovirus E1, DNA polymerase, and preterminal proteins: implications for gene therapy. Gene Ther 1997; 4:258–263.

77. Oka K, Pastore L, Kim IH, et al. Long-term stable correction of low-density lipoprotein receptor-deficient mice with a helper-dependent adenoviral vector expressing the very low-density lipoprotein receptor. Circulation 2001; 103:1274–1281.

78. Morral N, O'Neal W, Rice K, et al. Administration of helper-dependent adenoviral vectors and sequential delivery of different vector serotype for long-term liver-directed gene transfer in baboons. Proc Natl Acad Sci USA 1999; 96:12816–12821.

79. Morral N, Parks RJ, Zhou H, et al. High doses of a helper-dependent adenoviral vector yield supraphysiological levels of alphal-antitrypsin with negligible toxicity. Hum Gene Ther 1998; 9:2709–2716.

80. Curiel DT. Strategies to adapt adenoviral vectors for targeted delivery. Ann NY Acad Sci 1999; 886:158–171.

81. Imler JL, Dupuit F, Chartier C, et al. Targeting cell-specific gene expression with an adenovirus vector containing the lacZ gene under the control of the CFTR promoter. Gene Ther 1996; 3:49–58.

3

Adeno-Associated Virus

DONGSHENG DUAN
and **YONGPING YUE**

University of Missouri
Columbia, Missouri, U.S.A.

JOHN F. ENGELHARDT

University of Iowa School of Medicine
Iowa City, Iowa, U.S.A.

I. Introduction

Over the past decade, the field of molecular medicine has witnessed a growing interest in the development of recombinant adeno-associated virus (rAAV) as a gene delivery vehicle. A large body of preclinical and clinical studies in a number of different model systems has demonstrated the promise of rAAV as a gene therapy vector for many inherited diseases (1–3). Importantly, AAV has an incredible tropism for a number of organs including the eye, brain, muscle, liver, and lung. In addition to its remarkable ability to provide long-term high-level gene expression, several outstanding features of wild-type AAV (wtAAV) have made this system even more attractive from a biosafety standpoint. First, wtAAV is not considered to be a pathogenic virus (4). Despite the fact that wtAAV has been detected in aborted fetal materials, amniotic fluid, and trophoblasts (5), there is no direct evidence that links wtAAV to any known human diseases. In fact, several studies have shown tumor-suppressive effects following wtAAV infection (6). A recent study has also suggested that wtAAV infection might prevent the development of autoimmune myositis (7). Second, all the endogenous viral genes encoding structural and replication proteins can be removed in the recombinant

51

vector. Only two terminal 145 base sequences containing inverted terminal repeats (ITRs) are required for viral replication and the generation of functional rAAV vectors. The "gutless" nature of rAAV also improves the safety of this vector system and diminishes any potential hazardous effects from viral protein expression. Third, wtAAV has evolutionarily developed a benign parasitic relationship with host cells. This cryptic life cycle (in the absence of helper virus or genotoxic stimuli) eliminates cell lytic effects seen with many other viruses such as adenovirus. Furthermore, the tendency of wtAAV to integrate in a site-specific manner also distinguishes this virus from other integrating viruses (e.g., retroviruses) which have been known to cause insertional mutagenesis.

Progress in the development of rAAV as a gene therapy vector has been made possible as a result of intensive scientific research on the basic biology of AAV. Strategies have been developed to solve several longstanding hurdles in the use of this vector system including viral production and limited packaging capacity. The identification of AAV binding receptors and coreceptors have revolutionized rAAV purification from traditional cumbersome ultracentrifugation to fast and effective methods of affinity chromatography (8). A better understanding of adenoviral helper functions has also led to the development of adenovirus-free packaging systems (9–11). Such technical achievements have been critical to the development of this vector system for large-scale clinical trials. Knowledge of the molecular mechanisms by which rAAV converts its single-stranded DNA genome into large concatamers has also led to the development of novel techniques (termed *cis*-activation and *trans*-splicing) to expand the packaging capacity of this vector system (12–15). Despite these advances, a key issue regarding the application of rAAV in the respiratory system has included a low transduction efficiency from the apical surface of the airway. Advances in this area have also begun to emerge through a systematic dissection of barriers to rAAV infection involving receptor binding, endocytic processing, nuclear trafficking, uncoating, and proviral genome conversion (16,17). In this chapter, we will review these new findings in relation to their implications for the gene therapy of lung diseases.

II. Basic Biology of Adeno-Associated Virus and rAAV Vectors

A. Physical Properties and Structure of AAV

Basic Features and Biophysical Properties

Although a recent study suggests that AAV may be categorized as an epithelial-tropic autonomous parvovirus (18), the most widely accepted classification for this single-stranded DNA virus is still the dependovirus genera of the Parvoviridae family. Phylogenetic studies indicate that AAV is a close relative to B19 and bovine parvovirus but is distantly related to rodent, canine, feline, and porcine parvoviruses (19). It has also been suggested that AAV may have evolved from a transposable element as a by-product of cellular defense mechanisms against pathogenic viruses such as adenovirus (20). In the mid 1960s, AAV was discovered as a small contaminating DNA virus in adenoviral preparations (hence the name adeno-associated virus) (21,22). Physical characterization of purified AAV particles indicates that the mature virion is an icosohedral symmetrical particle about 20–25 nm in size (Fig. 1). It has a sedimentation coefficient of 110–122S and a molecular weight of $1.5 \sim 2.2 \times 10^6$ Da. The buoyant density in CsCl gradients ranges between 1.32 and 1.45 g/mL. Viral DNA content determines the heterogeneity in density, since protein components in all AAV particles appear to be identical. Only fully packaged virions (density between $1.39 \sim 1.42$ g/mL) contain the most competent infectious viruses (normally with a physical particle to infectious particle ratio of less than 100 to 1). The lighter particles (density less than 1.39 g/mL) represent empty and/or partially packaged virions. The mo-

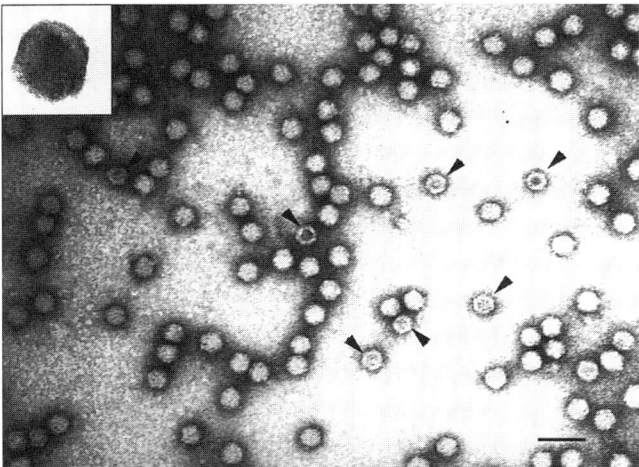

Figure 1 Transmission electron microscopy examination of purified type 2 rAAV particles. HPLC-purified type 2 rAAV particles were negatively stained with 1% aqueous uranyl acetate for 30 sec and processed for transmission electron microscopy. The image was photographed on a Hitachi H-7000 transmission electron microscope. The insert in the upper left corner is a photomicrograph of a single recombinant adenoviral particle processed under the same conditions. The arrowheads indicate the empty and/or not fully packaged rAAV particles. The 50-nm scale bar applies to both rAAV and adenovirus photomicrographs.

lecular composition of the heavy particles (1.45 g/mL) is not yet clear, but may contain an extra polypeptide (23). These high-density particles also have a much lower infectivity (24,25).

Biochemical analyses have demonstrated that the AAV virion is composed of 75–80% protein and 20–25% DNA. Either plus or minus strands of linear DNA can be encapsidated to form infectious virions (26–28). Compared to other viruses such as adenovirus, AAV is very stable and resistant to a wide range of pH (3–9) and is heat resistant (can survive 56–60°C for 1 hr). It is also moderately resistant to detergent and some proteases (29). This physical stability has aided purification strategies for separating AAV from its helper viral contaminants. However, recent studies also suggest that inappropriate storage conditions may lead to the loss of functional titer in rAAV stock. A divalent cation buffer and minimized heat exposure are recommended for long-term storage (30).

Since the discovery of the serotype-2 AAV, five additional serotypes of AAV have been isolated. Among these, AAV-6 appears to have evolved from a recombinational event between AAV-1 and AAV-2. The most common serotypes in human infection are type 2 and 3 (31–35). AAV-5 was discovered in 1984 in a penile condyloma sample and is structurally least related to all the other serotypes (36). With the exception of AAV-5, all the other AAV serotypes were discovered as adenoviral contaminants. Most of our knowledge on AAV biology is derived from studies on AAV-2. Recombinant vectors based on AAV-2 are also the most extensively tested vehicles in gene therapy experiments. Therefore, most of the data presented in this chapter refer to the AAV-2 unless otherwise specified.

A critical aspect of AAV biophysical characteristics that has been missing is the three-dimensional organization of the viral particle. Such knowledge of the AAV capsid structure will be invaluable to our understanding of AAV entry, vector-host interaction, and cellular targeting. Crystal structures for many parvoviruses (such as murine, feline and insect parvovirus) have been resolved at a very high resolution (3.5 Å). These results have provided structural insights into viral function (37). However, the ultrastructural characteristic of AAV remains unresoved. A recent 30 Å resolution cryoelectron microscopic study on AAV-5 revealed many distinctive features that are different from B19 parvovirus (38). Another study on the empty AAV-2 capsids at a 1.05 nm resolution suggests that AAV-2 may share a similar organization to the canine parvovirus in the inside of the capsids, but it has its own unique outer surface features (38a). Despite the lack of a high-resolution structure for AAV virions, studies based on antibody mapping and mutagenesis have yielded enough information to enable AAV capsid modification and retargeting (39–43). Future challenges in the biophysical characterization of AAV particles include the need for a three-dimensional structure at the high 3.5 Å resolution. Such information may lead to a better understanding of the functional requirements for infectious virions that could improve viral production and prospects for targeting rAAV vectors.

Molecular Structure

The wtAAV genome is composed of two major open reading frames (ORFs). The 5' ORF encodes Rep (replication) proteins. Four Rep proteins (Rep78, 68, 52, 48) are generated by using different promoters and alternative splicing from the same ORF. These Rep proteins have several enzymatic functions such as endonuclease and helicase activities (44,45). These proteins are responsible for viral replication and integration and may potentially be associated with mature viral particles (46,47). During latent AAV infection, low levels of Rep proteins are thought to repress transcription from both the p5 and p19 promoters in the AAV genome (48). However, under conditions permissive for viral replication, Rep proteins can also strongly activate transcription from viral promoters (49). Recent studies have suggested that Rep proteins facilitate site-specific (targeted) AAV integration at the AAVS1 locus on chromosome 19 and that the largest Rep 78 protein may also enhance the overall efficiency of integration (50,51). In contrast, the two smaller Rep proteins (52/48) appear to be critical for efficient packaging of the single-stranded viral genome (52,53).

The 3' ORF encodes three overlapping AAV capsid (Cap) proteins. The in-frame coding sequence allows for these three structural proteins to share the same C-terminal amino acids. The 68-kD VP3 (viral protein 3) is the most abundant product and accounts for 80% of protein in the mature virion capsid. It is also responsible for the attachment of the viral particle to its receptor (40,43). Each of the 72-kD VP2 and 83-kD VP1 contribute only 10% of protein in mature viral capsid. Mutagenesis studies have suggested that the N-terminal domain of the two larger capsid proteins may not be essential to viral packaging and infection. To this end, ligand insertion in this region can be used to alter the tropism of the virus (43). The 1:1:8 ratio of the three capsid proteins is essential for efficient viral packaging. This critical ratio is maintained through alternative splicing and the use of different translation starting codons for the various forms of Cap. Optimization of the Rep to Cap ratio has also been used to increase the yield of rAAV vectors (54–56).

The most essential and unique component in AAV is its inverted terminal repeats (ITRs) at both ends of the viral genome (57). In AAV-2, the ITR is composed of 145 self-complementary nucleotides (Fig. 2). This is an extremely GC (guanosine and cytosine)-rich sequence with a GC content of higher than 80% (the average GC content in human chromosomal DNA is less than 60% (58)). The overall structure of the ITR is a T-shaped hairpin with a three-way junction (Fig. 2). The A and A' fragments form a duplex stem which terminates with two small palindromes (defined as B, B' and C, C' arms). Depending on the orientation of these two small palindromes, AAV ITRs can be classified as "flip" (B arm is closer to the 3' end) or "flop" (C arm is closer to the 3' end) (29). Biophysical studies have indicated that the ITR is composed of largely

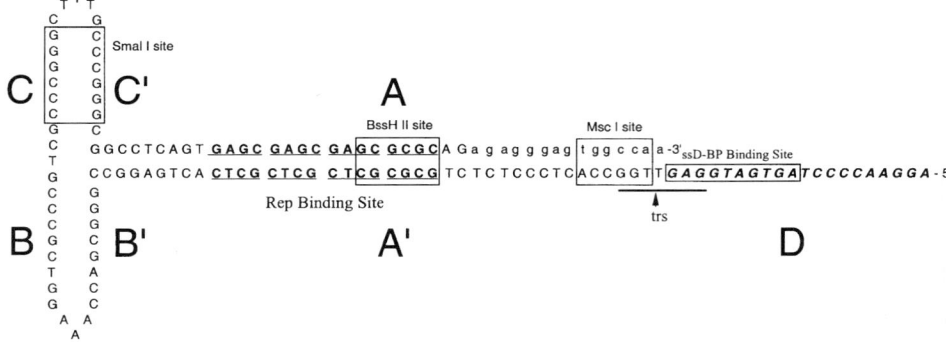

Figure 2 Structure of the flop form of type 2 AAV ITR. The 145 base AAV-2 ITR adopts a T-shaped hairpin structure due to its palindromic sequences. Only seven nucleotides at the ends of B, B′, C, and C′ sequences are not paired. The (GAGC)₃GCGC Rep binding site is underlined and in bold type. The terminal resolution site (trs) GGTTGAG is also underlined. The Rep cleavage site in the trs is indicated by an arrow. The entire D sequence is labeled in italic bold bases. The boxed nucleotides in the D sequence represent the ssD-BP binding site. The 3′ terminal 15 bases were intentionally deleted during the initial cloning of the wtAAV plasmid (28); these nucleotides are presented in small letters. Three restriction sites (boxed) including SmaI, BssHII, and MscI are commonly used to examine the intactness of the ITR sequence in proviral plasmids.

B-form DNA, and interestingly the most stable ITR structure based on biophysical assays agrees with the model predicated from primary DNA sequence (59,60).

Unique features of the ITR include a terminal resolution site (trs) and Rep binding site (RBS). The trs is the central functional component of the AAV replication origin. Under permissive conditions, nicking of this trs by endonuclease activity of Rep proteins initiates AAV DNA replication. The most amazing observations that relate to ITR structure/function comes from the analysis of the AAV integration site (AAVS1) in human chromosome 19. Detailed sequencing study of the AAVS1 locus shows a striking homology to that of the ITR. Genetic mapping of the minimal targeting site reveals a 33-nucleotide motif almost identical to that found in the A, A′ and D sequences in the ITR. In both cases, the trs is linked to the RBS by a small spacer sequence (61,62). Biochemical evidence also supports a Rep-mediated interaction between ITR and AAVS1 sequences (63).

Twenty nucleotides at the 5′ end of the ITR are defined as the D sequence. Recent studies have suggested that although this D sequence is not directly involved in the T-shaped hairpin structure of the ITR, it is crucial for efficient rescue, selective replication, and generation of single-stranded AAV genomes

(64–66). The most critical region in the D sequence lies in the 10 nucleotides proximal to the palindromic hairpin structure of the ITR. A host single-stranded D sequence binding protein (ssD-BP) has also been recently identified. Dephosphorylation of ssD-BP facilitates AAV second strand synthesis and therefore enhances rAAV transduction efficiency (67,68). Cloning of the ssD-BP has demonstrated that it is homologous to a cellular chaperone FK506 binding protein. Further elucidation of ssD-BP function in AAV transduction is being pursued by gene knockout technology.

B. Cellular and Molecular Biology of AAV

Infectious Entry Pathways for AAV

One of the most salient feature of AAV is its broad host range. This suggests that binding and entry of AAV must occur through a very common pathway. In fact, an omnipresent heparan sulfate proteoglycan (HSPG) has been identified as the primary attachment receptor for type 2 AAV (69). Cellular binding for AAV-4 and AAV-5 also involves interaction with other cell surface glycans such as N-linked and O-linked sialic acid (70). Two potential coreceptors including $\alpha V \beta 5$ integrin and human fibroblast growth factor receptor 1 (FGFR1) are thought to be critical for AAV-2 entry (71,72). Although there is dispute regarding the dependence of AAV-2 infection on these two coreceptors in certain cell types (73), it is being increasingly recognized that infectious entry pathways of AAV are considerably more complex than previously thought. For example, all known receptor and coreceptors for AAV-2 are localized in the basolateral surface in polarized airway cells, however, AAV-2 particles are still efficiently endocytosed from the apical surface (16,17). The identification and characterization of other AAV receptors and/or coreceptors will significantly influence the development of AAV-mediated gene transfer.

Following binding, the majority of AAV particles enter the cell through a dynamin-dependent process thought to involve clathrin coated pits (74,75). Molecular dissection of this process indicates that a small guanosine triphosphate (GTP) binding protein, Rac1, is also required for AAV entry (76). Subsequent activation of the phosphatidylinositol-3 (PI3) kinase pathway is also important for the movement of AAV particles to the nucleus along microtubule and/or microfilament (Fig. 3) (76). Another interesting aspect of AAV intracellular processing includes the recent finding that viral particles are ubiquitinated (17). Ubiquitination is well known as a targeting signal for endogenous or foreign protein degradation by the proteasome system. Inhibition of the ubiquitin/proteasome system with E3 ubiquitin ligase inhibitors or tripeptide proteasome inhibitors significantly enhances rAAV-mediated gene transfer. It is currently unclear exactly how ubiquitination of AAV capsid affects rAAV transduction or whether different AAV serotypes are also processed by ubiquitination.

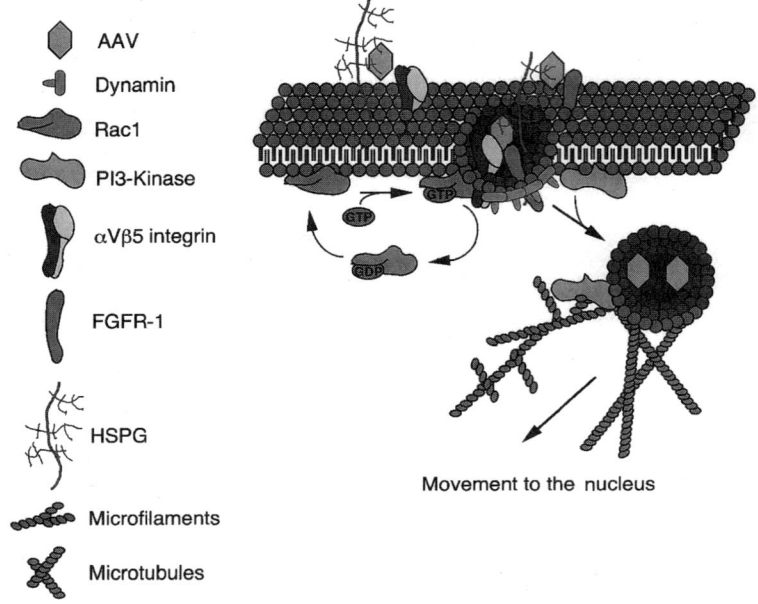

Figure 3 Mechanism of type 2 AAV endocytosis and intracellular trafficking. This schematic figure represents the major molecular mechanisms currently known to control AAV-2 infection in HeLa cells. Viral attachment is mediated through a heparan sulfate proteoglycan receptor (HSPG). Molecules involved in endocytosis of AAV-2 include αVβ5 integrin, human fibroblast growth factor receptor 1, dynamin, and a small GTP-binding protein called Rac1. In contrast, viral movement to the nucleus requires PI3-kinase activity, microtubules, and microfilaments. (Adapted from Ref. 76.)

The last stage of the AAV infectious pathway, prior to the molecular conversion of the AAV genome, involves nuclear entry and uncoating. Although the size of AAV virions might allow for free diffusion of intact viral particles through the nuclear pore complex, little is known about the molecular processes controlling AAV nuclear uptake or transport. Indirect evidence using Cy3-labeled virus suggests that AAV particles accumulate in a perinuclear region before entering into the nucleus (75,76). The importance of AAV intracellular processing and/or trafficking as a limiting barrier to efficient transduction has been increasingly appreciated. Several lines of evidence indicate that inefficient trafficking through the cytoplasm is a very significant barrier for AAV transduction (17,77,78). This barrier also appears to be uniquely regulated in airway cells by the ubiquitin/proteasome pathway (17). An increased understanding of AAV intracellular processing from the cell surface to the nucleus will undoubtedly aid in the development of strategies to overcome these endocytic barriers in AAV-mediated gene therapy.

Lytic Life Cycle

Lytic and latent life cycles are two distinctive phases of AAV replication and persistence, respectively. Productive infection occurs in the presence of helper virus (such as adenovirus, herpes virus, vaccinia virus) or genotoxic stimuli (such as ultraviolet [UV] irradiation, chemical carcinogens) (29). The propagation of both helper and AAV viruses leads to cell lysis and release of mature infectious virions. Up to 10^4 infectious AAV particles can be produced from a single cell (79).

One of the most important aspects of lytic phase growth is the production of progeny viral genomes required for virion assembly. In contrast to the well-known semiconservative mechanism involved in double-stranded DNA replication, single-stranded AAV genomes are replicated through unidirectional strand displacement. Single-strand DNA binding proteins, such Ad E2a products and HSV UL29, have been known to assist in the assembly of the replication complex on the AAV ITR (80–82). Strand elongation, leading to the formation of duplex linear molecules, begins from the 3′ end hydroxyl within the ITR. Subsequent cleavage at the trs in the parental strand creates new 3′ hydroxyl for the back replication of the ITR. The stem-loop palindromic structure of the ITR is critical for this mechanism of replication. Taken together, AAV replication is accomplished through continuous generation and resolution of head-to-head or tail-to-tail concatamers. During productive infection, up to 10^6 double-stranded viral genomes are produced per cell (25). A recent in situ localization study also suggests that AAV replication occurs in a defined subnuclear compartment called the adenoviral replication center (83). Further characterization of AAV replication loci within the nucleus may be very useful in developing more efficient AAV production systems.

The lytic AAV life cycle ends with viral particle assembly. Unlike adenoviral assembly, which is triggered by its L3 encoded cysteine protease (84), little is know about the molecular mechanisms controlling AAV assembly. In vitro expression of VP2 alone leads to virus-like particle formation. Furthermore, VP3 can be recruited into the nucleus by VP1 and VP2 (85). These data suggest that the larger capsid proteins might play a pivotal role in nuclear assembly of AAV particles. However, a recent study argues that VP1 is not essential for capsid formation and VP2 is only required for nuclear translocation of the other capsid proteins (86). Kinetic studies have suggested that building the empty capsid is not a rate-limiting step in virion assembly, but rather packaging a single-stranded genome into a preformed capsid may take several hours (85,87,88). A very intriguing finding regarding AAV capsid assembly is the involvement of nonstructural proteins. For example, Rep78 appears to be covalently linked to the mature viral particle (46). More recent studies have suggested that the interaction between Rep and structural proteins may initiate at early stages of virion assembly prior to viral genome packaging (47). A newly described "pump-in" model has also suggested the involvement of small Rep proteins (Rep52/40) in AAV genome packaging. In this model, Rep52 and Rep48 form a complex with capsid proteins in the virion. The DNA helicase activity of Rep52/48 then pumps the single-stranded AAV genome $3' \to 5'$ into the preformed empty capsid (53). Upon cell death, only a small fraction of the progeny AAV is released into culture media. The majority of the AAV particles remains as paracrystalline aggregates in the nucleus (21,89).

The latest developments in AAV assembly have arisen from studies establishing in vitro packaging systems (90,91). In these protocols, infectious AAV particles are generated in a cell-free system. Biological and physical characterizations indicate that virions produced in this manner have similar properties to those obtained from cell culture. Although, the current yield from in vitro systems is still quite low, further optimization of this system may eventually lead to industrial-scale cell-free AAV production.

Lysogenic Life Cycle

One of the unique features that distinguishes AAV from other human DNA virus is its latent integration at a site-specific locus in human chromosome 19 (19q13.3-qter) (92–96). The underlying molecular mechanisms controlling site-specific integration have yet to be fully elucidated. However, several lines of evidence suggest a deletion substitution model involving two large Rep proteins, the viral ITR, and a host AAV integration sequence (AAVS1) (95,97,98). Conclusive evidence for the involvement of AAVS1 was obtained from a series of functional assays using an Epstein-Barr virus (EBV)–based shuttle vector system (61,62,97,99–103). In this model system, the AAVS1 sequence was inserted into an EBV genome and maintained as a stable episome in 293 cells. The rescue of EBV genomes in bacteria and the analysis of clones harboring AAV sequences were used to determine the frequency of site-specific integration. Integrated AAV genomes were found only in EBV episomes carrying AAVS1 but not genomes lacking this critical sequence. These results were also confirmed by recent transgenic animal studies. In these studies, the human AAVS1 sequence was incorporated into the rat and mouse genomes that lack endogenous AAVS1 sequences. Infection with wild-type AAV or Rep-expressing vectors results in site-specific integration at the transgenic AAVS1 locus (104,105). Site-specific integration is also supported by two additional pieces of evidence. First, analysis of the human AAVS1 reveals a minisatellite sequence composed of 35-bp tandem repeats. Surprisingly, all such minisatellite sequences (about 60 total) in the human genome are clustered at chromosome 19q (101,106). Second, AAVS1 is located near a DNase I hypersensitive region. These aspects of the AAVS1 microenvironment might help to facilitate Rep-mediated integration (107).

Detailed characterization of genomic integration sites has also revealed a close linkage between AAVS1 and the muscle troponin gene (108). The significance of this relationship is not yet clear but might relate to the high efficiency of AAV transduction in muscle. A large number of AAV genomic junctional sequences have been analyzed from clonal cell lines and AAV-infected tissues (61,93,94,104,109–115). These studies suggest that most of the recombinational events occur within the ITR region. Furthermore, integration is associated with significant rearrangement of both viral and cellular sequences.

There are at least 18 sites in the human genome that share sequence homology with the Rep binding site (RBS) in AAVS1 and can mediate Rep binding using in vitro assays (105,116). Many of these contain important genes such as colony-stimulating factor-1, insulin-like growth factor binding protein-2, and perlecan (116). However, integration at these sites has yet to be reported. Interestingly, a recent in vitro experiment has demonstrated that Rep 68 is capable of cleaving trs in a supercoiled AAVS1 but not a supercoiled template from other human RBS sites (117). It is not clear whether these findings suggest the existence of additional molecular forces that drive AAV integration into chromosome 19. Furthermore, even if integration at these alternative RBS is confirmed, its biological significance still needs to be determined.

Other driving forces for AAV site-specific integration include the two large Rep proteins (Rep 78/68). This has been clearly demonstrated in numerous experiments evaluating AAV integration with Rep-deficient recombinant viruses. In these studies, integration sites of Rep-deficient rAAV were mapped either by Southern blotting, FISH (fluorescent in situ hybridization), or more accurately by recovering cellular flanking sequences (110,111,115,118–120). A common conclusion from different laboratories suggests that Rep minus AAV integrates in a random fashion. However, if Rep proteins are provided in *trans* by an expressing cDNA or as purified protein, the site specificity is restored (51,112–114,121). The direct evidence for Rep involvement comes from in vitro reconstitution experiments (103). In this study, a donor AAV molecule and an acceptor circular DNA containing the AAVS1 site were incubated together with Hela cell extract. The addition of purified Rep68 protein led to the covalent joining of donor AAV genomes with AAVS1 target in an adenosine triphosphate (ATP)–dependent manner. Consistent with previous results on AAV integration, this in vitro assay also demonstrates that recombination occurs at the RBS site within the ITR region (103).

Another yet unanswered question is the identification of cellular proteins that participate in AAV site-specific integration. According to the deletion substitution model, limited DNA replication occurs at the integration junction (103).

DNA polymerase gamma and delta (but not alpha) have been implicated in lytic phase AAV replication (122–124); however, it is not clear whether this same set of polymerases are also involved in AAV integration. At least 10 cellular proteins ranging from 24 to 180 kD have been shown to interact with Rep in different in vitro binding assays (125). Physical interaction between Rep and high-mobility group protein 1 (HMG1) has also been demonstrated to stimulate Rep activity (126). Recently, several cellular proteins that are involved in AAV DNA replication have been identified from Hela extract in the absence of adenoviral infection. These proteins include the single-stranded DNA binding protein, replication protein A (RFA), replication factor C (RFC), the 3′ primer binding complex, and proliferating cell nuclear antigen (PCNA) (124).

The recent cloning of several additional AAV serotypes has presented an additional challenge in our understanding of AAV site-specific integration. All AAV integration studies described thus far are based on type 2 AAV. Differences between AAV serotypes are not limited to viral capsids, and a significant level of dissimilarity also exists in the ITR sequence and Rep proteins, especially between AAV-5 and other serotypes. It remains to be determined whether all the AAV serotypes utilize similar mechanisms of integration or integrate into the AAVS1 locus. It is likely that at least AAV-5 has a distinct mechanism of integration given the fact that its trs is least conserved in comparison to other serotypes (127).

Mechanisms of Genome Conversion Following rAAV Vector Transduction

The molecular mechanisms underlying rAAV transduction have been a recent focus in rAAV research. The key event in rAAV-mediated transgene expression is to convert the incoming single-stranded viral DNA into a transcription-competent double-stranded molecule. The most traditional model suggests that second-strand synthesis by self-priming (similar to AAV replication during lytic phase) is the rate-limiting step for rAAV transduction (128,129). Two key pieces of evidence support this hypothesis. First, coexpression of adenoviral E1 and/or E4ORF6 products leads to several orders of magnitude enhancement in rAAV transduction. This augmentation is accompanied by increases in replication form monomer and dimer genomes as detected by Southern blot (128–130). Second, the efficiency of rAAV transduction in different cell types and tissues seems to correlate with tyrosine phosphorylation of a cellular single-strand D sequence binding protein (ssD-BP). The phosphorylation of ssD-BP by epidermal growth factor receptor protein tyrosine kinase (EGF-R PTK) promotes binding of ssD-BP to the D sequence in the ITR and blocks DNA synthesis from the 3′ hydroxyl. Dephosphorylation facilitates detachment of ssD-BP and activates second-strand synthesis by self-primering (67,68,131).

In contrast to this hypothesis, a recent study in liver suggests that, at least in hepatocytes, second-strand synthesis is not the major pathway for double-stranded DNA formation. Instead, self-annealing of the incoming plus and minus single-stranded viral genomes was suggested to be responsible for AAV transduction (132). The biological foundation for this model lies in the fact that both plus and minus single-stranded viral DNA are equally encapsidated during AAV production (26–28). This model suggests that following uncoating, complementary plus and minus viral genomes anneal to each other to form double-stranded DNA (dsDNA) in the absence of de novo DNA synthesis (132). This model is supported by the molecular analysis of AAV transduction intermediates following portal vein injection of recombinant virus. To differentiate between newly synthesized DNA and incoming viral DNA, the investigators have packaged methylated viral genomes into AAV virions. If rolling circle DNA amplification is required for double strand formation, the newly formed dsDNA will be hemi-methylated. If strand annealing were the predominant pathways for dsDNA formation, the majority of the double-stranded viral genome would be fully methylated on both DNA strands. Differential digestion with methylation-sensitive restriction enzymes DpnI, MboI, and Sau3AI confirmed that the majority of the double-stranded rAAV genomes following infection of the liver were fully methylated (132). However, additional studies are needed to solidify this hypothesis and resolve several unanswered questions. For example, this model would predict that the efficiency of transduction with rAAV is not linear with dose of input virus. Hence, at low titers of infection where each cell receives less than one virion, expression of transgenes should be absent. However, this does not appear to be the case for most model systems. Experiments evaluating transduction with physically separated plus (or minus) strand AAV particles alone or selective inhibition of DNA synthesis during the early stage of AAV infection may help to resolve mechanistic issues with this model. Furthermore, relevance of this model to tissues other than the liver remains to be determined.

A third proposed mechanism of AAV transduction suggests that formation of double-stranded circular transduction intermediates are very important for persistent transgene expression (133–135). Existence of episomal AAV genomes has been suggested for many years based on several indirect observations (136,137). However, the first conclusive evidence for the existence of circular AAV genomes was obtained using a shuttle rAAV vector containing a bacterial replication origin and an ampicillin resistance gene (133). Direct transformation of low molecular weight DNA harvested from rAAV-infected cells and tissue rescued double-stranded circular viral genomes as head-to-tail monomers and multimers. Furthermore, the formation of these circular transduction intermediates correlated with persistent transgene expression in muscle tissue in vivo and UV enhanced AAV transduction in primary cells in vitro (130,133,134). In contrast to these original reports utilizing a single shuttle viral vector, more recent studies using alternative vector design have demonstrated that circular concatamers are generated in all orientation of the viral genome (12,13,138). This alternative finding was due to a selective disadvantage for bacterial propagation of head-to-head and tail-to-tail circular concatamers with opposing origins of replication in the original reports. The formation of AAV circular intermediates has also been confirmed by independent studies from other laboratories (115,139,140). Whether circular AAV genomes represent preintegration intermediates remains to be systemically determined. However, a recent study comparing integration of circular or linear AAV-based plasmids shows that circular-form molecules integrate three times more efficiently than the linear form in the presence of Rep (141). This result lends support to circular intermediates as a precursor for integration.

Several recent studies have begun to shed light on the molecular pathway(s) controlling AAV circular intermediate formation. Structural analysis of the head-to-tail junctions in AAV circular intermediates implies the potential of joining two independent AAV molecules as the first step for concatamer formation (135). The experimental evidence for this hypothesis is provided by studies evaluating the molecular joining of two independent rAAV vectors following coinfection into murine muscle (138). Analysis of bacterially rescued circular intermediate clones demonstrated that intermolecular recombination, rather than rolling circle replication, was responsible for concatamer formation (138). A recent surprising finding was observed when proviral genomes from rAAV-infected normal BL6 and SCID mice were compared by Southern blot. Diagnostic restriction fragments for circular genomes existed only in tissues from normal BL6 mice but not from SCID mice. These data strongly suggest that DNA-dependent protein kinase (DNA-PK), which is missing in SCID mice, might catalyze circularization of the AAV genome (142). These studies also suggest that linear concatamers found in SCID mice may have a preferential capacity to integrate into the host genome of muscle as compared to circular-form genomes found in normal mice.

Latent infection can occur following infection with both wtAAV and rAAV. The lysogenic integration in chromosome 19 is responsible for wtAAV persistence. However, it is currently unclear for most tissues whether episomal or integrated forms of the rAAV genome predominate. Both episomal and integrated proviral genomes have been found in rAAV-infected tissues (133,139,142–144). Currently, both forms are thought to mediate transgene expression. The biggest difference between rAAV integration and wtAAV integration is that Rep-deficient rAAV no longer integrates site specifically at the AAVS1 locus (110,111,115,118–120,145,146). However, rAAV vectors do seem to integrate at more unstable or fragile chromosomal loci (147). Key questions include whether rAAV vectors can be adapted to restore site-specific integration at the AAVS1 loci. Such an achievement would have significant theoretical safety advantages for clinical use. The feasibility of site-specific integration of rAAV vectors has been demonstrated by codelivering Rep gene products (51,112–114,121). However, ectopic Rep expression is quite toxic and interferes with cell proliferation and leads to p53-independent caspase-activated apoptosis (148–152). Recent studies have started to define more accurately the molecular requirements for Rep-mediated AAVS1 integration. First, it has been demonstrated that transient Rep expression is sufficient to direct site-specific integration (153,154). Second, only the N-terminus of the larger Rep protein is required for this activity (155–158). It is expected that novel approaches based on these recent findings might eventually lead to AAVS1-specific integration of rAAV vectors.

C. Immunology of rAAV Vectors

Epidemiological studies have demonstrated that 70–80% of infants and 90% of adults are seropositive to AAV (31–33,96). Furthermore, the majority of seropositive subjects contain antibodies to several AAV serotypes such as AAV-1, -2, and/or -3 (31,159). However, according to a recent cohort study in normal and cystic fibrosis patients, only a third of seropositive human subjects may actually contain circulating neutralizing antibodies (34). Similar antibody profiles have also been found in mice immunized with rAAV, of which 80% developed seropositivity and 25% developed neutralizing antibodies (41). The functional significance of AAV neutralizing antibody has been disputed. Early studies in the rabbit airway have correlated the appearance of neutralizing antibody with a failure to infect following a secondary administration. The same study also concludes that the neutralizing antibodies are probably directed toward viral capsid proteins, since readministration of rAAV encoding a different reporter gene was also inhibited (160). Readministration in mouse lung is possible only if transient immunosuppression (with anti-CD40 ligand antibody or CTLA4-immunoglobulin fusion protein) is applied at the time of the initial rAAV inoculation (161). Alternatively, successful readministration can be achieved by using a different serotype AAV vector (162–164). In contrast to these results, another study in rabbit lung suggests that high levels of serum neutralizing antibody to the AAV capsid does not block repeated delivery to the lung (165). Likely explanations for this latter finding include a less traumatic viral delivery method and a lack of wtAAV contamination in recombinant viral stock. A similar study in mouse eye also suggests that a strong humoral response to viral capsid does not block transduction following repeat administration of the same rAAV vector (166). Detailed dissection of the B-cell response to AAV-2 infection in murine and nonhuman primate muscle suggests that a T-cell–dependent humoral reaction (including IgG_1 and IgG_{2a}) is responsible for neutralizing antibody production. Readministration of same type of rAAV in muscle is feasible but results in a diminished transgene expression. Transient block of the T-cell activation with anti-CD4 antibody leads to high-level gene expression following vector readministration (167). In addition to this

T-cell–dependent B-cell activation in muscle, portal vein administration of rAAV may also induce T-cell–independent responses (168). This notion is supported by the finding that transient immunosuppression with anti-CD4 or anti-CD40L at the time of vector readministration is insufficient to overcome the immune block produced by prior delivery of rAAV via the portal vein (41). Reports demonstrating a robust humoral response against transgenes following intramuscular injection, but not portal vein delivery, argues that the route of vector administration also affects the immunological consequences to the vector (169). Divergent results from different laboratories likely are also compounded by differing qualities of viral preparation and purification methods. Nevertheless, initial clinical trials should be aimed at patients lacking AAV neutralizing antibody to avoid encountering the complexities associated with preexisting immunity. Interestingly, a very recent cohort study of 85 human volunteers demonstrated that 19 and 25% of subjects had neutralizing antibodies to AAV-1 and AAV-2, respectively. Surprisingly, none of the volunteers had neutralizing antibody to the AAV-5 capsid (170). Although this finding remains to be confirmed by additional epidemiological studies, a complete appreciation of the immune reactivity to different AAV serotypes could be of clinical significance.

An often creditable feature for AAV-based vectors is its ability to evade cytotoxic T-lymphocyte (CTL) responses (1,171,172). This has been a significant obstacle for long-term transgene expression with other vectors such as adenovirus. The lack of cellular immunity to AAV vectors has been attributed to the poor infectivity of antigen-presenting cells (172) and the lack of viral genes in recombinant vectors. However, adoptive transfer of AAV-infected immature (but not mature) dendritic cells elicits a strong transgene-specific CTL response. Further analysis in CD40 ligand (CD40L)–deficient mice suggests that CD40-CD40L signaling is required for AAV-induced cellular immune response against a foreign transgene. The threshold for CTL responses might be determined by the number of AAV-infected immature dendritic cells (173). On the other hand, the type of transgenes encoded by AAV vectors likely also affects the extent to which a CTL response is mounted. For example, AAV-mediated expression of several HIV genes (including env, tat, and rev) has been shown to induce a major histocompatibility complex (MHC) class I–restricted CTL response in BALB/c mice (174). A recent study in a mouse model of gamma-sarcoglycan–deficient muscular dystrophy suggests that the employment of tissue-specific promoter could circumvent a transgene-specific CTL response and lead to persistent high-level therapeutic transgene expression (175). Since different AAV serotypes utilize distinctive cellular receptors and coreceptors for infection, immature dendritic cells might be less susceptible to infection by certain serotypes, and hence the choice of vector serotype could be used to avoid or decrease the CTL response in a given tissue (176).

III. Advances in the Use of Recombinant AAV as a Gene Therapy Vector

A. Production of rAAV

Large-scale production of highly pure rAAV stocks is a key factor that determines the ultimate clinical success of rAAV as a drug. The traditional protocol for rAAV production requires cotransfection of essential *cis* and *trans* plasmids followed by adenoviral infection (177,178). The *cis* plasmid contains the transgene expression cassette flanked by two AAV ITRs. The *trans* plasmid is a helper plasmid which provides AAV replication and viral capsid proteins. The rAAV vector is finally purified through several rounds of CsCl density gradient ultracentrifugation. This method is associated with two inherent problems. First, scale-up of viral production to meet clinical needs is not feasible. Under this vector production protocol, yields of virus on a per cell basis is approximately 10^2 viral particles. With a potential need for 10^{14} viral particles for each patient in a therapeutic application (151), the obvious inherent problems of transfecting 10^{12} cells (or 50,000 of 150-mm dishes) for each patient becomes evident. Second, viral stocks prepared by this method are often contaminated with residual adenovirus, adenoviral structure proteins, and wild-type and/or replication-competent AAV. These contaminants represent a significant biosafety concern for patients. Although an ideal clinical-grade rAAV production method remains a challenging goal, tremendous progress has been made during the last 5 years in overcoming this hurdle.

Two factors affect large-scale rAAV production: (1) the specific yield per cell from transient transfection and (2) the maximal purification capacity limits using ultracentrifugation. It has been recently demonstrated that the ratio of Rep and Cap protein expression significantly influences the efficiency of rAAV production. To achieve higher yields, numerous strategies have been explored in regulating rep and cap gene expression in the *trans* helper plasmids. These include replacing the p5 and p40 AAV promoters with heterologous promoters (including Rous sarcoma virus [RSV], cytomegalovirus [CMV], simian vacuolating virus 40 [SV40], elongation factor, parvovirus B19p6, chicken beta-actin promoter/cytomegalovirus enhancer [CAG], HIV LTR, and MMTV LTR promoters) (reviewed in Ref. 179). Additionally, insertion of an intron spacer in the AAV genome has been approached as a strategy to increase vector production (180). In summary, reduction of Rep78/68 expression and enhancement of Cap expression usually lead to higher viral yields (54,55,181). To overcome the technical limitation of the transient transfection method, several distinct AAV packaging systems have also been described. First, AAV Rep- and Cap-expressing packaging cell lines have been established (182–184). Second, hybrid adenovirus-rAAV, baculovirus-rAAV, and herpes simplex virus–AAV systems have been tested in conjunction with Rap/Cap–expressing cell lines (112,182,184–186). The beauty of these approaches is that nearly all cells in the system are making rAAV and bulk production can be easily accomplished by scaling-up cell culture.

The biggest concern for the hybrid viral systems is the helper virus contamination. Even a marginal level of adenoviral or adenoviral protein contamination could be detrimental for patients. To establish a completely virus-free system, essential adenoviral genes (including VA RNA, E2A, E4) have also been cloned into the adenoviral helper plasmids (9–11,181,187). In combination with the novel *trans* helper plasmids mentioned above, the yield of rAAV following transient transfection has increased 50~100 fold (151,179).

The development of chromatographic purification methods represents another significant stride toward clinical-scale rAAV production. Two types of chromatographic columns have been tested. The ion exchange column is based on the biophysical property, especially the surface charge, of the viral particle. Alternatively, the heparin affinity column has taken advantage of heparin sulfate proteoglycan (HSPG) as the type 2 AAV receptor (8,188–193). Both types of purification have generated biologically active rAAV stocks suitable for in vivo applications.

B. Recent Progress in the Use of rAAV Vectors in Experimental Animal Models and Human Trials

Recent preclinical trials in various animal models of disease and Phase I/II human clinical trials in patients have clearly demonstrated the increasing promise of rAAV as a therapeutic vector system. With clinical efficacy and safety as paramount considerations in the design of any gene therapy protocol, rAAV has placed itself as a leading vector of choice for molecular medicine. In neuronal systems, the most remarkable results have been achieved in Parkinson's and ocular diseases. In early studies, rAAV has been shown to mediate long-term expression of tyrosine hydroxylase and resulted in the phenotypic correction in the rat model of Parkinson's disease (194). More recently, glial cell line–derived neutrophic factor was delivered to the striatum in the rat Parkinson's disease model using rAAV, and also demonstrated persistent functional correction in the diseased nigrostriatal system (195). Clinical trials on neurodegenerative disease have also been initiated. On June 5, 2001, rAAV carrying the aspartoacylase gene was injected into a 6-year-old Canavan's disease patient. Although this 3-year, 15-patient study has just begun, it has already demonstrated some encouraging preliminary results.

From the standpoint of retinal disorders, rAAV has also demonstrated great promise in preclinical trials for Leber's congenital amaurosis (LCA). LCA is a very severe retinal degenerative disease that leads to childhood blindness. The genetic defect in LCA is the loss of a 65-kD membrane protein called RPE65.

In an effort to restore the missing protein, the Rpe65 gene was introduced into the outer retina in a canine LCA model using a rAAV vector. By 4 months postinfection, complete vision recovery was confirmed by multiple functional measurements in the diseased dog (196). This exciting result represents another landmark breakthrough in potentially treating childhood blindness with rAAV-mediated gene therapy.

Using rAAV to deliver the factor IX gene in the treatment of hemophilia B demonstrates another excellent example of the efficacy and safety of rAAV vectors. Immediately following the successful use of rAAV in murine and canine hemophilia B models, a clinical trial was initiated (197). In this dose-escalation trial, rAAV particles were injected intramuscularly to three human patients. None of the patients revealed any significant side effects to the vector. Furthermore, modest therapeutic efficacy was demonstrated in some patients. Based on these exciting findings, a second human trial with direct portal vein delivery of rAAV is currently underway.

Successful rAAV-mediated gene therapy has also proved to be efficacious in correcting pathological changes in a number of dystrophic muscular diseases. Deficiency in any components in the dystrophin-associated protein complex will result in some kind of muscular dystrophy. Limb-girdle muscular dystrophies are caused by mutations in one of the four sarcoglycan genes (alpha, beta, gamma, and delta). Direct muscular delivery of delta and gamma sarcoglycan in two different rodent models has revealed complete rescue of muscular function (198–200). Clinical trials for limb-girdle muscular dystrophy has also been proposed (201). Encouraging results have also been recently reported for rAAV-mediated gene therapy in the mouse model of Duchenne's muscular dystrophy (202,251).

Diseases that could potentially benefit from rAAV gene therapy are far greater than the limited examples mentioned above (203–205). However, when considering the utility of rAAV for gene therapy to the lung (as addressed below), this limited background provides an important reference which recognizes the broader applications of this vector system in the context of treating genetic diseases.

IV. Recombinant AAV–Mediated Gene Transfer to the Lung

A. Model Systems to Study rAAV Transduction in the Lung

Several human and nonhuman model systems have been used to study AAV-mediated gene transfer to the lung (206). A significant number of in vivo studies have been performed in rodents. In these animal models, AAV vector is delivered to the airway epithelium by nasal aspiration or intratracheal instillation (17, 207,208). One major problem associated with the use of rodent models is the divergent biology of rodent and human airways from a cellular and anatomical standpoint. For example, human airways contain goblet cells as the predominant secretory cell type, whereas mice and rats contain Clara cells and serous cells, respectively. Furthermore, the abundance and distribution of submucosal glands are also greatly different between humans and rodents (209–212). Larger animals such as rabbits, sheep, and nonhuman primates have also been used in airway gene transfer studies (160,165,167,213–215).

Although results from experimental animal models have provided extremely useful molecular insights regarding the biology and immunology of rAAV gene delivery to the airway, they lack the ability to directly predict outcomes in human patients. To this end, two extremely flexible and useful ex vivo models have been described which more closely model the human airway. One such model includes differentiated polarized human airway epithelia grown at an air-liquid interface on permeable membrane supports (206,216). Studies in this model system have demonstrated preferential infection of rAAV-2 from the basolateral surface (16,217). Ongoing studies in this model are attempting to elucidate cellular and molecular barriers to rAAV-mediated gene transfer in human airway cells (17,207,218). One drawback of the in vitro polarized airway model is that it cannot completely mirror the exact cellular compositions found in the primate airway. To overcome this problem, a human bronchial xenograft system has been developed (206,219). This model of a vascularized human airway is produced by seeding primary airway cells from human subjects onto a denuded rat trachea followed by subcutaneous grafting in athymic mice. At 4–5 weeks posttransplantation, a fully differentiated human airway epithelium has developed and bronchial xenografts are ready for gene transfer studies.

B. Overcoming Cellular Barriers to rAAV Transduction in the Lung

Unlike other organs such as liver, brain, and muscle, the mammalian conducting airway represents an ideal target for gene therapy owing to its nonintrusive accessibility for vector delivery. However, the highly polarized organization of airway epithelia and complexity of the cell surface mucous layer has created significant barriers for many gene therapy vectors such as adenovirus and retrovirus (220–225). Similar obstacles have also hindered efficient gene transfer with rAAV vectors (Fig. 4).

Excessive mucus production is a common pathological change in numerous lung diseases. Although airway surface fluid from normal humans does not appear to affect AAV transduction (16,226), thick inflammatory mucus from cystic fibrosis (CF) patients could constitute a direct barrier to block or inactivate rAAV vectors from reaching the cell membrane (226). Local application of mucolytic agents has been shown to clear this mucous barrier and increase gene transfer with adenoviral and AAV vectors (224,226). However, even if rAAV vectors make it to the airway surface, they still face a number of additional challenges before their encoded transgene can be expressed. For example, all the known

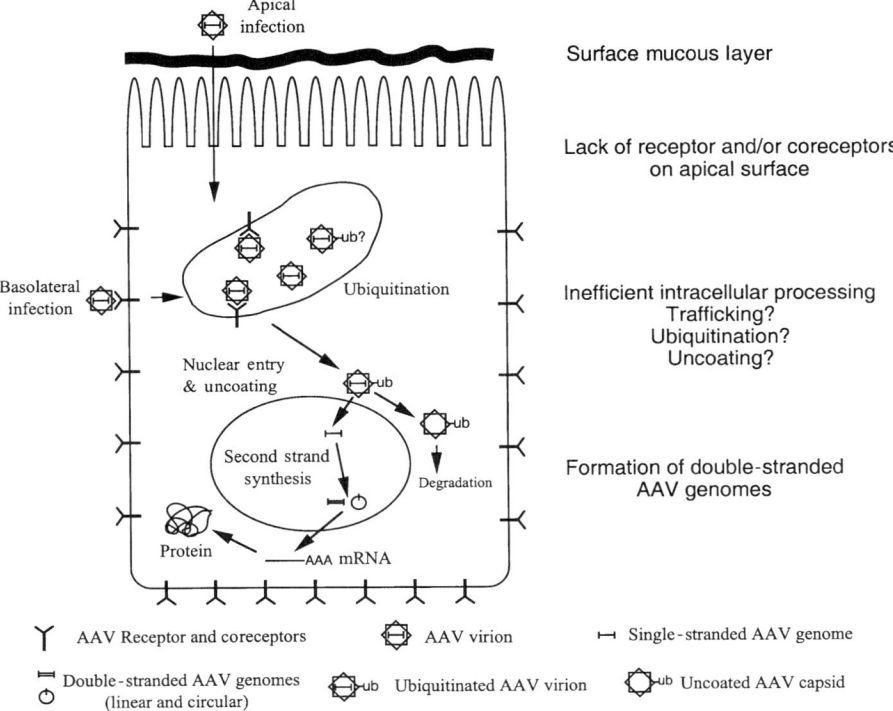

Figure 4 Barriers to rAAV-mediated gene transfer in the airway. Numerous potential barriers can hinder successful transduction from the mucosal surface of the airway. These barriers include viral binding, endocytosis, intracellular processing and trafficking, uncoating, and single-stranded viral genome conversion.

receptors and coreceptors for AAV-2 are localized to the basolateral membrane of polarized airway epithelia (217). Surprisingly, the lack of known cellular docking proteins on the apical surface does not prevent the entry of rAAV-2 from this surface. Quantitative studies with radiolabeled virus and Southern blot detection of viral DNA has indicated that rAAV-2 binding and uptake from the apical surface is only four- to fivefold less efficient than from the basolateral side (16,17). Several different strategies have been developed to enhance rAAV transduction from the apical surface of airway epithelia. First, transient disruption of tight junctions with hypotonic saline, divalent cation chelating agents (such as EGTA), or trypsin increases the accessibility of apically applied virus to basolateral receptors and leads to a 7- to 10-fold increase in transduction efficiency (16,17,227). Second, viral entry can be improved by receptor-independent pathways such as UV irradiation and calcium phosphate coprecipitation (16,207).

Using reporter gene expression as an endpoint, rAAV-2 transduction from the basolateral side is 200-fold higher than that from the mucosal surface (apical side). This 200-fold difference in expression cannot be explained by the less than fivefold difference in viral binding and uptake between these two cellular surfaces. Obviously, additional barriers to apical infection exist in polarized airway epithelia. Many chemicals that are known to augment AAV transduction at the postentry level have been evaluated. These include DNA-damaging agents, DNA synthesis and topoisomerase inhibitors, and cellular tyrosine kinase inhibitors (17,131,228–230). Limited success has been achieved in airway cells when these chemicals were added during infection. Surprisingly, however, significant levels of enhanced rAAV-2 transduction were obtained when tripeptide proteasome inhibitors (including N-Acetyl-L-Leucyl-L-Leucyl-Norleucine [LLnL] and benzyl-oxycarbonyl-Leu-Leu-l-leucinal [Z-LLL]) were administered at the time of infection (17). A greater than 200-fold enhancement in airway epithelial transduction could be achieved with these compounds following apical surface infection, an efficiency close to that from the basolateral surface. More importantly, in vivo application of proteasome inhibitors in mouse lung increases transduction with rAAV-2 from an undetectable level to an average of 10% epithelial cells in large bronchioles. Quantitative studies using a luciferase reporter gene demonstrate that this in vivo enhancement can be as high as 245-fold (Fig. 5). From a mechanistic standpoint, the first hint as to how proteasome inhibitors might augment rAAV transduction came when it was observed that AAV capsids were ubiquitinated (17). This suggested a potential link between the proteasome and rAAV transduction.

The proteasome is a major cellular clearance system for endogenous and foreign proteins (231). Proteins are targeted to the proteasome following the covalent linkage of a 76–amino acid peptide call ubiquitin. Ubiquitin can be considered to be a "zip code" which routes proteins to the proteasome for degradation. However, ubiquitination can also serve other functions in addition to signaling degradation. For example, it has been implicated in triggering endocytosis (232). It is presently unclear where and how ubiquitination alters transduction of rAAV. Mechanistic studies have suggested that proteasome inhibitors may augment rAAV transduction at several levels. First, as mentioned above, AAV capsids are ubiquitinated inside the cell. Administration of proteasome inhibitors leads to the accumulation of ubiquitinated capsid proteins, as one might expect if their degradation was blocked. Second, proteasome inhibitor treatment shifts the distribution of virus from the cytoplasm to the nucleus as demonstrated by in situ radioactive localization of AAV (17). Third, in combination with the divalent cation chelating agent EGTA, proteasome inhibitors also prevent degradation of viral particles and/or genomes (17).

The recent characterization of other AAV serotypes has led to the development of new rAAV vectors and provides additional avenues to improve rAAV

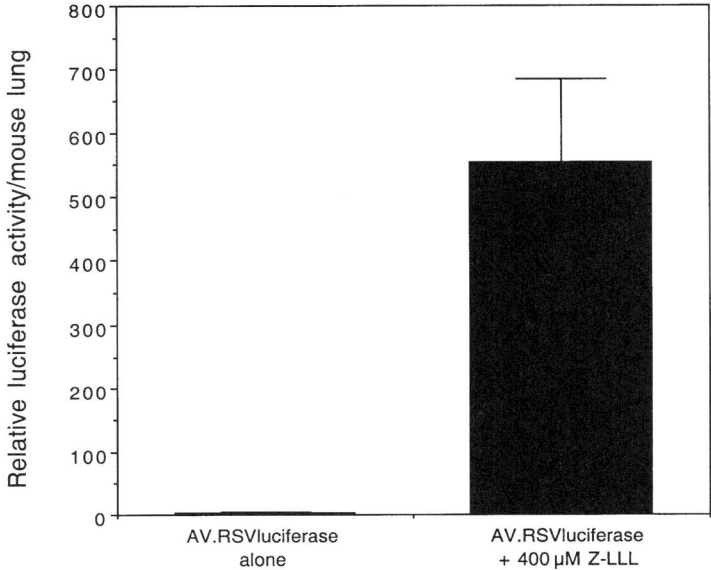

Figure 5 Quantitative analysis of tripeptide proteasome inhibitor Z-LLL on rAAV-2 transduction in mouse lung. 1×10^{11} viral particles of AV2.RSVluciferase virus was delivered into the mouse lung by nasal inhalation. To evaluate the effects of proteasome inhibitor on gene transfer, 400 μM Z-LLL (final concentration, representing 1% viral inoculation volume) was coadministrated at the time of viral infection. The entire lung was harvested at 8 months postinfection and luciferase activity was evaluated using a previously described protocol (12). The data represents the mean (±SEM) from four independent mice in each group.

transduction in airway cells. Different AAV serotypes have different capsids that may recognize different cellular receptor(s) and/or may be processed differently inside cells. Furthermore, serotype switching of rAAV vectors may be useful in circumventing neutralizing antibodies to virus following repeat administration. Most of the AAV serotypes, including AAV-2, AAV-3, AAV-4, AAV-5, and AAV-6, have been tested for lung gene transfer. Direct comparison between AAV-2, -3, and -6 shows that AAV-6 is two times better than AAV-2, whereas AAV-3 has a very low transduction efficiency in mouse lung cells (163). Furthermore, the enhancement in transduction seen with AAV-6 is primarily dependent on capsid structure, not on the ITR (164). Transduction efficiencies of AAV-2, -4, and -5 has been compared in polarized human airway epithelia cultures. Consistent with other studies, AAV-2 infection from the apical surface of airway epithelia resulted in very low transgene expression (16,17,207). AAV-4, which has greater than 90% homology to AAV-2 and -3, also demonstrates a very low transduction from the apical surface. However, AAV-5–based vectors demonstrate significantly improved transduction efficiency from the apical surface. In one study, AAV-5 was shown to transduce polarized airway cells 50 times more efficiently in vitro and 20 times more efficiently in mouse lung in vivo than that of AAV-2 (218). This enhancement correlates with a high level of AAV-5 receptor expression on the apical surface and an increased viral binding and uptake from this surface (70). At present, it is not known which serotype(s) is best suited for human lung gene transfer, and the answer to this question will likely require clinical trials directly comparing the efficacy of these serotypes.

In addition to the proteasome inhibitors, other pharmacological reagents are also being evaluated to enhance lung gene transfer (17,230). Among these chemicals, perfluorochemical (PFC) liquid, which has already been used in clinical trials for the treatment of lung diseases (233), stands out as a very promising candidate. PFC liquid is a high-density fluorinated carbon chain solution. Its low surface tension allows for the widespread distribution throughout the lung. When PFC liquid was coadministered with rAAV, a 26-fold enhancement in AAV-mediated gene transfer was achieved in rodent lungs (208). A detailed understanding of the mechanism responsible for this augmentation is lacking, but studies suggest that it may involve increased spreading and better access of rAAV to lung epithelial cells (208,234–236).

C. Overcoming Vector Limitations with rAAV

In addition to the above-mentioned cellular barriers to rAAV-mediated gene delivery in the lung, several additional aspects of this vector also limit its application for widespread clinical use. The maximal packaging capacity for rAAV is only 5 kb. This is approximately 110% of the wild-type AAV genome size (237). However, the cDNA size of many lung disease genes such as CFTR (cystic fibrosis transmembrane conductance regulator) is very close to or larger than 5 kb. If the therapeutic gene expression cassette (i.e., promoter, gene, and poly-A) is greater than 5 kb, it cannot be encapsidated into rAAV vectors. However, in certain circumstances, the ITR has been used as a weak promoter allowing for the accommodation of large genes (with a short poly-A) that just fit into the AAV vector. This strategy has been used for CFTR encoding rAAV vectors (238). Problems associated with this approach include low viral yields and poor transgene expression. Several very exciting approaches for overcoming rAAV packaging limitations have been recently reported (12–15,239). These methods were developed from the knowledge that rAAV undergoes intermolecular recombination in the formation of head-to-tail concatamers (135,138). This finding that two independent viral genomes can recombine within the cell provided the foundation for splitting large transgenes into two rAAV vectors. Assisted by engineered splicing signals, a full-length transgene can be reconstituted after coinfection with donor and acceptor rAAV vectors and subsequent "*trans*-splicing" across the intermolecular ITR junction (13–15,239). Application of this trans-splicing technology in fully differentiated human airway epithelia has demonstrated successful expression of a β-galactosidase reporter following coinfection with donor and acceptor LacZ rAAV vectors (Fig. 6). Alternatively, this same approach can be used to deliver strong tissue-specific promoters and/or enhancers that would otherwise not be able to fit into a single rAAV vector. This dual vector approach, termed *cis*-activation, allows for the covalent joining of enhancer/promoters contained within a single vector to a second transgene containing vector following coinfection and intermolecular recombination. The application of this

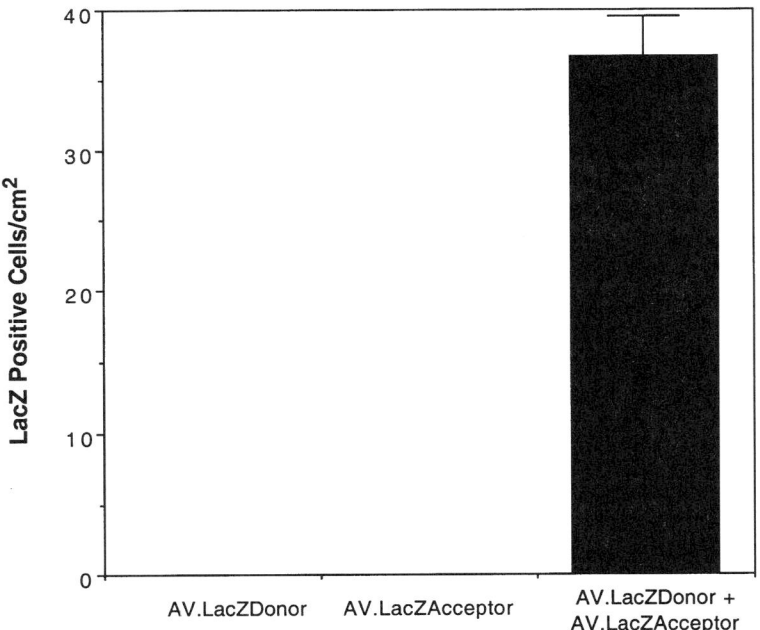

Figure 6 Reconstitution of β-galactosidase expression in polarized human airway epithelia using dual rAAV vector *trans*-splicing technology. Fully differentiated human airway epithelial cultures grown at an air-liquid interface were infected from the basolateral surface with either AV2.LacZDonor or AV2.LacZAcceptor vectors individually or together. Each of the donor and acceptor vectors contains half of the LacZ cDNA flanked by splicing sites. Cells are stained for β-galactosidase expression at 30 days postinfection. LacZ-positive cells were only detected in cultures coinfected with both donor and acceptor vectors. The data represents the mean (±SEM) from three independent experiments.

approach is ideal for genes which just fit into rAAV vectors with no space for enhancer/promoter elements (such as CFTR). This approach has been tested in muscle using a luciferase reporter gene, and it demonstrated significant enhancement of gene expression when either a minimal promoter or ITR was used to drive transgene expression (12).

An alternative method to overcome the packaging limits of rAAV vectors is to reduce the length of the transgene by deleting nonessential regions of the protein. Functional minigenes have been described for many diseases, including a 6.1-kb minidystrophin gene for the 14-kb full-length dystrophin cDNA (240). A similar approach has also been utilized to develop truncated mini-CFTR genes. A set of shortened CFTR cDNAs that are amenable to packaging in rAAV vectors with a promoter have been recently tested (241). Electrophysiological studies have demonstrated that some of these truncated mini-CFTR genes are indeed capable of correcting defective chloride channel activity following rAAV-mediated gene transfer (241,242).

D. Clinical Trials of rAAV-Mediated Gene Therapy to the Lung

Currently, cystic fibrosis is the only lung disease that has been approved for rAAV clinical trials (243–245). A Phase I study in the maxillary sinus of CF patients revealed a very promising profile with efficient and persistent gene transfer and absent or very low toxicity and immune responses (246–248) (see Chap. 14). However, initial results from lung delivery trials with CFTR rAAV have demonstrated the persistent presence of viral DNA genomes in airway epithelia but no evidence for mRNA expression. These findings are reminiscent of in vitro studies in human airway epithelium demonstrating efficient uptake of rAAV-2 and prolonged DNA persistence in the absence of gene expression (17). Whether the ubiquitin/proteasome barrier also exists in the human lung remains to be determined. Recently, AAV-based gene therapy for another lung disease, alpha$_1$-antitrypsin deficiency, has also been approved for clinical trial (see Chap. 17). It is expected that with a better understanding of AAV transduction biology and virus-host interaction, the field can anticipate a very bright future for rAAV-mediated gene therapy of lung diseases.

V. Summary and Perspective

Enthusiasm for developing rAAV vectors as therapeutic tools emerges from numerous aspects of AAV basic biology which are ideally suited for clinical application. These include high-level, long-term transduction in a broad range of cells, the potential for site-specific integration, lack of cellular immune responses to the vector, simplicity of vector design, and overall safety profile in humans. Furthermore, novel approaches based on the basic molecular biology of the AAV genome and its transduction intermediates are beginning to address some of the inherent limitation of this vector system with respect to transgene insert capacity. Several areas which require further research to improve this vector system include (1) improvement of clinical-grade rAAV production, purification, and storage protocols and establishment of viral quality control standards; (2) expanded use of alternative serotypes of AAV and a better understanding of which serotypes are best for a given disease/organ system; and (3) a better appreciation of host immune responses to rAAV.

Despite the strong interests in rAAV-mediated human gene therapy, several recent findings have suggested the need for more in-depth studies evaluating host vector interactions. The most disturbing of such issues pertain to safety. First, it was recently reported that the presence of the single-stranded AAV genome can be perceived by a host cell as a DNA-damaging signal and leads to a transient G2 phase arrest (249). It is not yet clear whether this transient cell cycling arrest may be detrimental to certain sensitive cell types. Second, although AAV has never been confirmed as being a causative agent in any human diseases, it was recently reported that in the mouse model of mucopolysaccharidosis type VII, long-term rAAV infection might be associated with hepatic cancer and angiosarcoma formation (250). When considering the safety of recombinant AAV vectors, it is important to recognize that recombinant and wild-type vector biology are not interchangeable. In the context of wild-type AAV infections, infectious titers are far lower than those used to halt genetically a disease process with the recombinant virus. Hence, some of the biological properties important for safety may be inherently different in the setting of a naturally occurring AAV infection and clinical use of rAAV vectors. As new findings emerge on vector–host interactions for rAAV, the field should take care not to become complacent in the knowledge that wild-type AAV does not produce clinical disease. Rather the field should take this opportunity to discover previously unexposed aspects of AAV biology and use this knowledge to improve the safety and efficacy of this vector system for clinical use. Despite this cautionary note, it is clear that of the recombinant viral vectors available, AAV has carved a unique niche in gene therapy and will undoubtedly prove to be an effective therapeutic vehicle for certain human diseases in the near future.

Acknowledgments

Research described in this chapter was in part supported by National Institutes of Health (NIH) grant HL58340 (J.F.E. and D.D.), the Center for Gene Therapy funded by NIH (P30 DK54759) (J.F.E.) and the Cystic Fibrosis Foundation, and a sponsored research grant from Targeted Genetics Corp., Seattle, Washington. Relevant aspects of this chapter pertaining to muscle were also supported by a research grant from the Muscular Dystrophy Association (D.D.).

References

1. Somia N, Verma IM. Gene therapy: trials and tribulations. Nat Rev Genet 2000; 1:91–99.
2. Kay MA, Glorioso JC, Naldini L. Viral vectors for gene therapy: the art of turning infectious agents into vehicles of therapeutics. Nat Med 2001; 7:33–40.
3. High KA. Gene therapy: a 2001 perspective. Haemophilia 2001; 7(Suppl) 1:23–27.
4. Berns KI, Giraud C. Adeno-associated virus (AAV) vectors in gene therapy. Current Topics in Microbiology and Immunology, 218. Berlin: Springer, 1996:vi, 173.
5. Tobiasch E, Rabreau M, Geletneky K, et al. Detection of adeno-associated virus DNA in human genital tissue and in material from spontaneous abortion. J Med Virol 1994; 44:215–222.
6. Schlehofer JR. The tumor suppressive properties of adeno-associated viruses. Mutat Res 1994; 305:303–313.
7. Tezak Z, Nagaraju K, Plotz P, Hoffman EP. Adeno-associated virus in normal and myositis human skeletal muscle. Neurology 2000; 55:1913–1917.
8. Summerford C, Samulski RJ. Viral receptors and vector purification: new approaches for generating clinical-grade reagents. Nat Med 1999; 5:587–588.
9. Xiao X, Li J, Samulski RJ. Production of high-titer recombinant adeno-associated virus vectors in the absence of helper adenovirus. J Virol 1998; 72:2224–2232.
10. Matsushita T, Elliger S, Elliger C, et al. Adeno-associated virus vectors can be efficiently produced without helper virus. Gene Ther 1998; 5:938–945.
11. Collaco RF, Cao X, Trempe JP. A helper virus-free packaging system for recombinant adeno-associated virus vectors. Gene 1999; 238:397–405.
12. Duan D, Yue Y, Yan Z, Engelhardt JF. A new dual-vector approach to enhance recombinant adeno-associated virus-mediated gene expression through intermolecular cis activation. Nat Med 2000; 6:595–598.
13. Yan Z, Zhang Y, Duan D, Engelhardt JF. From the Cover: Trans-splicing vectors expand the utility of adeno-associated virus for gene therapy. Proc Natl Acad Sci USA 2000; 97:6716–6721.
14. Sun L, Li J, Xiao X. Overcoming adeno-associated virus vector size limitation through viral DNA heterodimerization. Nat Med 2000; 6:599–602.
15. Nakai H, Storm TA, Kay MA. Increasing the size of rAAV-mediated expression cassettes in vivo by intermolecular joining of two complementary vectors (see Comments). Nat Biotechnol 2000; 18:527–532.
16. Duan D, Yue Y, Yan Z, McCray PB, Engelhardt JF. Polarity Influences the efficiency of recombinant adeno-associated virus infection in differentiated airway epithelia. Hum Gene Ther 1998; 9:2761–2776.
17. Duan D, Yue Y, Yan Z, Yang J, Engelhardt JF. Endosomal processing limits gene

transfer to polarized airway epithelia by adeno-associated virus. J Clin Invest 2000; 105:1573–1587.

18. Meyers C, Mane M, Kokorina N, Alam S, Hermonat PL. Ubiquitous human adeno-associated virus type 2 autonomously replicates in differentiating keratinocytes of a normal skin model. Virology 2000; 272:338–346.

19. Fisher RE, Mayor HD. The evolution of defective and autonomous parvoviruses. J Theor Biol 1991; 149:429–39.

20. Fisher RE, Mayor HD. Evolution of a defective virus from a cellular defense mechanism. J Theor Biol 1986; 118:395–404.

21. Atchison RW, Casto BC, Hammon WM. Electron microscopy of adenovirus-associated virus (AAV) in cell cultures. Virology 1966; 29:353–357.

22. Hoggan MD, Blacklow NR, Rowe WP. Studies of small DNA viruses found in various adenovirus preparations: physical, biological, and immunological characteristics. Proc Natl Acad Sci USA 1966; 55:1467–1474.

23. Lipps BV, Mayor HD. Characterization of heavy particles of adeno-associated virus type 1. J Gen Virol 1982; 58(Pt 1):63–72.

24. de la Maza LM, Carter BJ. Heavy and light particles of adeno-associated virus. J Virol 1980; 33:1129–1137.

25. Linden RM, Berns KI. Molecular biology of adeno-associated viruses. Contrib Microbiol 2000; 4:68–84.

26. Mayor HD, Torikai K, Melnick JL, Mandel M. Plus and minus single-stranded DNA separately encapsidated in adeno-associated satellite virions. Science 1969; 166:1280–1282.

27. Berns KI, Adler S. Separation of two types of adeno-associated virus particles containing complementary polynucleotide chains. J Virol 1972; 9:394–396.

28. Samulski RJ, Chang LS, Shenk T. A recombinant plasmid from which an infectious adeno-associated virus genome can be excised in vitro and its use to study viral replication. J Virol 1987; 61:3096–3101.

29. Muzyczka N. Use of adeno-associated virus as a general transduction vector for mammalian cells. Curr Top Microbiol Immunol 1992; 158:97–129.

30. Turnbull AE, Skulimowski A, Smythe JA, Alexander IE. Adeno-associated virus vectors show variable dependence on divalent cations for thermostability: implications for purification and handling. Hum Gene Ther 2000; 11:629–635.

31. Blacklow NR, Hoggan MD, Rowe WP. Serologic evidence for human infection with adenovirus-associated viruses. J Natl Cancer Inst 1968; 40:319–327.

32. Boucher DW, Parks WP, Melnick JL. A sensitive neutralization test for the adeno-associated satellite viruses. J Immunol 1970; 104:555–559.

33. Rosenbaum MJ, Edwards EA, Pierce WE, Peckinpaugh RO, Parks WP, Melnick JL. Serologic surveillance for adeno-associated satellite virus antibody in military recruits. J Immunol 1971; 106:711–720.

34. Chirmule N, Propert K, Magosin S, Qian Y, Qian R, Wilson J. Immune responses to adenovirus and adeno-associated virus in humans. Gene Ther 1999; 6:1574–1583.

35. Schlehofer JR, Dupressoir T. Infectiology and pathology of human adeno-associated viruses. Contrib Microbiol 2000; 4:59–67.

36. Bantel-Schaal U, zur Hausen H. Characterization of the DNA of a defective human parvovirus isolated from a genital site. Virology 1984; 134:52–63.

37. Agbandje-McKenna M, Llamas-Saiz AL, Wang F, Tattersall P, Rossmann MG. Functional implications of the structure of the murine parvovirus, minute virus of mice. Structure 1998; 6:1369–1381.

38. Walters RW, Moninger T, Olson N, et al. Structural studies of adeno-associated virus serotype 5. Mol Ther 2001; 3:S184.

38a. Kronenberg S, Kleinschmidt JA, Bottcher B. Electron cryo-microscopy and image reconstruction of adeno-associated virus type 2 empty capsids. EMBO Rep 2001; 2:997–1002.

39. Girod A, Ried M, Wobus C, et al. Genetic capsid modifications allow efficient retargeting of adeno-associated virus type 2. Nat Med 1999; 5:1052–1056.

40. Rabinowitz JE, Xiao W, Samulski RJ. Insertional mutagenesis of AAV2 capsid and the production of recombinant virus. Virology 1999; 265:274–285.

41. Moskalenko M, Chen L, van Roey M, et al. Epitope mapping of human anti–adeno-associated virus type 2 neutralizing antibodies: implications for gene therapy and virus structure. J Virol 2000; 74:1761–1766.

42. Wobus CE, Hugle-Dorr B, Girod A, Petersen G, Hallek M, Kleinschmidt JA. Monoclonal antibodies against the adeno-associated virus type 2 (AAV-2) capsid: epitope mapping and identification of capsid domains involved in AAV-2-cell interaction and neutralization of AAV-2 infection. J Virol 2000; 74:9281–9293.

43. Wu P, Xiao W, Conlon T, et al. Mutational analysis of the adeno-associated virus type 2 (AAV2) capsid gene and construction of AAV2 vectors with altered tropism. J Virol 2000; 74:8635–8647.

44. Im DS, Muzyczka N. The AAV origin binding protein Rep68 is an ATP-dependent site-specific endonuclease with DNA helicase activity. Cell 1990; 61:447–457.

45. Smith RH, Kotin RM. The Rep52 gene product of adeno-associated virus is a DNA helicase with 3′-to-5′ polarity. J Virol 1998; 72:4874–4881.

46. Prasad KM, Trempe JP. The adeno-associated virus Rep78 protein is covalently linked to viral DNA in a preformed virion. Virology 1995; 214:360–370.

47. Dubielzig R, King JA, Weger S, Kern A, Kleinschmidt JA. Adeno-associated virus type 2 protein interactions: formation of pre-encapsidation complexes. J Virol 1999; 73:8989–8998.

48. Beaton A, Palumbo P, Berns KI. Expression from the adeno-associated virus p5 and p19 promoters is negatively regulated in trans by the rep protein. J Virol 1989; 63:4450–4454.

49. Pereira DJ, McCarty DM, Muzyczka N. The adeno-associated virus (AAV) Rep protein acts as both a repressor and an activator to regulate AAV transcription during a productive infection. J Virol 1997; 71:1079–1088.

50. Balague C, Kalla M, Zhang WW. Adeno-associated virus Rep78 protein and terminal repeats enhance integration of DNA sequences into the cellular genome. J Virol 1997; 71:3299–3306.

51. Surosky RT, Urabe M, Godwin SG, et al. Adeno-associated virus Rep proteins target DNA sequences to a unique locus in the human genome. J Virol 1997; 71: 7951–9.

52. Chejanovsky N, Carter BJ. Mutagenesis of an AUG codon in the adeno-associated virus rep gene: effects on viral DNA replication. Virology 1989; 173:120–128.

53. King JA, Dubielzig R, Grimm D, Kleinschmidt JA. DNA helicase-mediated pack-

aging of adeno-associated virus type 2 genomes into preformed capsids. EMBO J 2001; 20:3282–3291.

54. Li J, Samulski RJ, Xiao X. Role for highly regulated rep gene expression in adeno-associated virus vector production. J Virol 1997; 71:5236–5243.

55. Vincent KA, Piraino ST, Wadsworth SC. Analysis of recombinant adeno-associated virus packaging and requirements for rep and cap gene products. J Virol 1997; 71: 1897–1905.

56. Salvetti A, Oreve S, Chadeuf G, et al. Factors influencing recombinant adeno-associated virus production. Hum Gene Ther 1998; 9:695–706.

57. Lusby E, Fife KH, Berns KI. Nucleotide sequence of the inverted terminal repetition in adeno-associated virus DNA. J Virol 1980; 34:402–409.

58. Zhang MQ. Statistical features of human exons and their flanking regions. Hum Mol Genet 1998; 7:919–932.

59. Ren J, Qu X, Chaires JB, Trempe JP, Dignam SS, Dignam JD. Spectral and physical characterization of the inverted terminal repeat DNA structure from adeno-associated virus 2. Nucleic Acids Res 1999; 27:1985–1990.

60. Chou SH, Tseng YY, Chu BY. Natural abundance heteronuclear NMR studies of the T3 mini-loop hairpin in the terminal repeat of the adenoassociated virus 2. J Biomol NMR 2000; 17:1–16.

61. Linden RM, Winocour E, Berns KI. The recombination signals for adeno-associated virus site-specific integration. Proc Natl Acad Sci USA 1996; 93:7966–7972.

62. Meneses P, Berns KI, Winocour E. DNA sequence motifs which direct adeno-associated virus site-specific integration in a model system. J Virol 2000; 74:6213–6216.

63. Weitzman MD, Kyostio SR, Kotin RM, Owens RA. Adeno-associated virus (AAV) Rep proteins mediate complex formation between AAV DNA and its integration site in human DNA. Proc Natl Acad Sci USA 1994; 91:5808–5812.

64. Wang XS, Ponnazhagan S, Srivastava A. Rescue and replication of adeno-associated virus type 2 as well as vector DNA sequences from recombinant plasmids containing deletions in the viral inverted terminal repeats: selective encapsidation of viral genomes in progeny virions. J Virol 1996; 70:1668–1677.

65. Wang XS, Qing K, Ponnazhagan S, Srivastava A. Adeno-associated virus type 2 DNA replication in vivo: mutation analyses of the D sequence in viral inverted terminal repeats. J Virol 1997; 71:3077–3082.

66. Xiao X, Xiao W, Li J, Samulski RJ. A novel 165–base-pair terminal repeat sequence is the sole cis requirement for the adeno-associated virus life cycle. J Virol 1997; 71:941–948.

67. Qing K, Wang XS, Kube DM, Ponnazhagan S, Bajpai A, Srivastava A. Role of tyrosine phosphorylation of a cellular protein in adeno-associated virus 2–mediated transgene expression. Proc Natl Acad Sci USA 1997; 94:10879–10884.

68. Qing K, Khuntirat B, Mah C, et al. Adeno-associated virus type 2–mediated gene transfer: correlation of tyrosine phosphorylation of the cellular single-stranded D sequence-binding protein with transgene expression in human cells in vitro and murine tissues in vivo. J Virol 1998; 72:1593–1599.

69. Summerford C, Samulski RJ. Membrane-associated heparan sulfate proteoglycan is a receptor for adeno-associated virus type 2 virions. J Virol 1998; 72:1438–1445.

70. Walters RW, Yi SM, Keshavjee S, et al. Binding of adeno-associated virus type

5 to 2,3-linked sialic acid is required for gene transfer. J Biol Chem 2001; 21:21.

71. Summerford C, Bartlett JS, Samulski RJ. AlphaVbeta5 integrin: a co-receptor for adeno-associated virus type 2 infection. Nat Med 1999; 5:78–82.

72. Qing K, Mah C, Hansen J, Zhou S, Dwarki V, Srivastava A. Human fibroblast growth factor receptor 1 is a co-receptor for infection by adeno-associated virus 2. Nat Med 1999; 5:71–77.

73. Qiu J, Mizukami H, Brown KE. Adeno-associated virus 2 co-receptors? (letter). Nat Med 1999; 5:467–468.

74. Duan D, Li Q, Kao AW, Yue Y, Pessin JE, Engelhardt JF. Dynamin is required for recombinant adeno-associated virus type 2 infection. J Virol 1999; 73:10371–10376.

75. Bartlett JS, Wilcher R, Samulski RJ. Infectious entry pathway of adeno-associated virus and adeno-associated virus vectors. J Virol 2000; 74:2777–2785.

76. Sanlioglu S, Benson PK, Yang J, Atkinson EM, Reynolds T, Engelhardt JF. Endocytosis and nuclear trafficking of adeno-associated virus type 2 are controlled by rac1 and phosphatidylinositol-3 kinase activation. J Virol 2000; 74:9184–9196.

77. Hansen J, Qing K, Kwon HJ, Mah C, Srivastava A. Impaired intracellular trafficking of adeno-associated virus type 2 vectors limits efficient transduction of murine fibroblasts. J Virol 2000; 74:992–996.

78. Hansen J, Qing K, Srivastava A. Adeno-associated virus type 2-mediated gene transfer: altered endocytic processing enhances transduction efficiency in murine fibroblasts. J Virol 2001; 75:4080–4090.

79. Carter BJ. Adeno-associated virus vectors. Curr Opin Biotechnol 1992; 3:533–539.

80. Myers MW, Laughlin CA, Jay FT, Carter BJ. Adenovirus helper function for growth of adeno-associated virus: effect of temperature-sensitive mutations in adenovirus early gene region 2. J Virol 1980; 35:65–75.

81. Mishra L, Rose JA. Adeno-associated virus DNA replication is induced by genes that are essential for HSV-1 DNA synthesis. Virology 1990; 179:632–639.

82. Weindler FW, Heilbronn R. A subset of herpes simplex virus replication genes provides helper functions for productive adeno-associated virus replication. J Virol 1991; 65:2476–2483.

83. Weitzman MD, Fisher KJ, Wilson JM. Recruitment of wild-type and recombinant adeno-associated virus into adenovirus replication centers. J Virol 1996; 70:1845–1854.

84. Greber UF. Virus assembly and disassembly: the adenovirus cysteine protease as a trigger factor. Rev Med Virol 1998; 8:213–222.

85. Ruffing M, Zentgraf H, Kleinschmidt JA. Assembly of viruslike particles by recombinant structural proteins of adeno-associated virus type 2 in insect cells. J Virol 1992; 66:6922–6930.

86. Hoque M, Ishizu K, Matsumoto A, et al. Nuclear transport of the major capsid protein is essential for adeno-associated virus capsid formation. J Virol 1999; 73: 7912–7915.

87. Myers MW, Carter BJ. Assembly of adeno-associated virus. Virology 1980; 102: 71–82.

88. Wistuba A, Weger S, Kern A, Kleinschmidt JA. Intermediates of adeno-associated virus type 2 assembly: identification of soluble complexes containing Rep and Cap proteins. J Virol 1995; 69:5311–5319.

89. Henry CJ, Merkow LP, Pardo M, McCabe C. Electron microscope study on the replication of AAV-1 in herpes-infected cells. Virology 1972; 49:618–621.
90. Ding L, Lu S, Munshi NC. In vitro packaging of an infectious recombinant adeno-associated virus 2. Gene Ther 1997; 4:1167–1172.
91. Zhou X, Muzyczka N. In vitro packaging of adeno-associated virus DNA. J Virol 1998; 72:3241–3247.
92. Kotin RM, Siniscalco M, Samulski RJ, et al. Site-specific integration by adeno-associated virus. Proc Natl Acad Sci USA 1990; 87:2211–2215.
93. Samulski RJ, Zhu X, Xiao X, et al. Targeted integration of adeno-associated virus (AAV) into human chromosome 19 (published erratum appears in EMBO J 1992; 11[3]:1228). Embo J 1991; 10:3941–3950.
94. Kotin RM, Linden RM, Berns KI. Characterization of a preferred site on human chromosome 19q for integration of adeno-associated virus DNA by non-homologous recombination. EMBO J 1992; 11:5071–5078.
95. Samulski RJ. Adeno-associated virus: integration at a specific chromosomal locus. Curr Opin Genet Dev 1993; 3:74–80.
96. Berns KI. The Gordon Wilson Lecture. From basic virology to human gene therapy. Trans Am Clin Climatol Assoc 1999; 110:75–85.
97. Dyall J, Berns KI. Site-specific integration of adeno-associated virus into an episome with the target locus via a deletion-substitution mechanism. J Virol 1998; 72:6195–6198.
98. Berns KI, Linden RM. The cryptic life style of adeno-associated virus. Bioessays 1995; 17:237–245.
99. Giraud C, Winocour E, Berns KI. Site-specific integration by adeno-associated virus is directed by a cellular DNA sequence. Proc Natl Acad Sci USA 1994; 91:10039–10043.
100. Giraud C, Winocour E, Berns KI. Recombinant junctions formed by site-specific integration of adeno-associated virus into an episome. J Virol 1995; 69:6917–6924.
101. Linden RM, Ward P, Giraud C, Winocour E, Berns KI. Site-specific integration by adeno-associated virus. Proc Natl Acad Sci USA 1996; 93:11288–11294.
102. Linden RM, Berns KI. Site-specific integration by adeno-associated virus: a basis for a potential gene therapy vector (editorial). Gene Ther 1997; 4:4–5.
103. Dyall J, Szabo P, Berns KI. Adeno-associated virus (AAV) site-specific integration: formation of AAV-AAVS1 junctions in an in vitro system. Proc Natl Acad Sci USA 1999; 96:12849–12854.
104. Rizzuto G, Gorgoni B, Cappelletti M, et al. Development of animal models for adeno-associated virus site-specific integration. J Virol 1999; 73:2517–2526.
105. Young SM, Jr., McCarty DM, Degtyareva N, Samulski RJ. Roles of adeno-associated virus Rep protein and human chromosome 19 in site-specific recombination. J Virol 2000; 74:3953–3966.
106. Das HK, Jackson CL, Miller DA, Leff T, Breslow JL. The human apolipoprotein C-II gene sequence contains a novel chromosome 19-specific minisatellite in its third intron. J Biol Chem 1987; 262:4787–4793.
107. Lamartina S, Sporeno E, Fattori E, Toniatti C. Characteristics of the adeno-associated virus preintegration site in human chromosome 19: open chromatin conformation and transcription-competent environment. J Virol 2000; 74:7671–7677.

108. Dutheil N, Shi F, Dupressoir T, Linden RM. Adeno-associated virus site-specifically integrates into a muscle-specific DNA region. Proc Natl Acad Sci USA 2000; 97:4862–4866.

109. Kotin RM, Menninger JC, Ward DC, Berns KI. Mapping and direct visualization of a region-specific viral DNA integration site on chromosome 19q13-qter. Genomics 1991; 10:831–834.

110. Rutledge EA, Russell DW. Adeno-associated virus vector integration junctions. J Virol 1997; 71:8429–8436.

111. Yang CC, Xiao X, Zhu X, et al. Cellular recombination pathways and viral terminal repeat hairpin structures are sufficient for adeno-associated virus integration in vivo and in vitro. J Virol 1997; 71:9231–9247.

112. Palombo F, Monciotti A, Recchia A, Cortese R, Ciliberto G, La Monica N, Site-specific integration in mammalian cells mediated by a new hybrid baculovirus–adeno-associated virus vector. J Virol 1998; 72:5025–5034.

113. Pieroni L, Fipaldini C, Monciotti A, et al. Targeted integration of adeno-associated virus-derived plasmids in transfected human cells. Virology 1998; 249:249–259.

114. Recchia A, Parks RJ, Lamartina S, et al. Site-specific integration mediated by a hybrid adenovirus/adeno- associated virus vector. Proc Natl Acad Sci USA 1999; 96:2615–2620.

115. Nakai H, Iwaki Y, Kay MA, Couto LB. Isolation of recombinant adeno-associated virus vector-cellular DNA junctions from mouse liver. J Virol 1999; 73:5438–5447.

116. Wonderling RS, Owens RA. Binding sites for adeno-associated virus Rep proteins within the human genome. J Virol 1997; 71:2528–2534.

117. Lamartina S, Ciliberto G, Toniatti C. Selective cleavage of AAVS1 substrates by the adeno-associated virus type 2 rep68 protein is dependent on topological and sequence constraints. J Virol 2000; 74:8831–8842.

118. Fisher-Adams G, Wong KK, Jr., Podsakoff G, Forman SJ, Chatterjee S. Integration of adeno-associated virus vectors in CD34+ human hematopoietic progenitor cells after transduction. Blood 1996; 88:492–504.

119. Kearns WG, Afione SA, Fulmer SB, et al. Recombinant adeno-associated virus (AAV-CFTR) vectors do not integrate in a site-specific fashion in an immortalized epithelial cell line. Gene Ther 1996; 3:748–755.

120. Ponnazhagan S, Erikson D, Kearns WG, et al. Lack of site-specific integration of the recombinant adeno-associated virus 2 genomes in human cells. Hum Gene Ther 1997; 8:275–284.

121. Lamartina S, Roscilli G, Rinaudo D, Delmastro P, Toniatti C. Lipofection of purified adeno-associated virus Rep68 protein: toward a chromosome-targeting nonviral particle. J Virol 1998; 72:7653–7658.

122. Handa H, Carter BJ. Adeno-associated virus DNA replication complexes in herpes simplex virus or adenovirus-infected cells. J Biol Chem 1979; 254:6603–6610.

123. Snyder RO, Im DS, Muzyczka N. Evidence for covalent attachment of the adeno-associated virus (AAV) rep protein to the ends of the AAV genome. J Virol 1990; 64:6204–6213.

124. Ni TH, McDonald WF, Zolotukhin I, et al. Cellular proteins required for adeno-associated virus DNA replication in the absence of adenovirus coinfection. J Virol 1998; 72:2777–2787.

125. Hermonat PL, Santin AD, Carter CA, Parham GP, Quirk JG. Multiple cellular proteins are recognized by the adeno-associated virus Rep78 major regulatory protein and the amino-half of Rep78 is required for many of these interactions. Biochem Mol Biol Int 1997; 43:409–420.

126. Costello E, Saudan P, Winocour E, Pizer L, Beard P. High mobility group chromosomal protein 1 binds to the adeno-associated virus replication protein (Rep) and promotes Rep-mediated site-specific cleavage of DNA, ATPase activity and transcriptional repression. EMBO J 1997; 16:5943–5954.

127. Chiorini JA, Afione S, Kotin RM. Adeno-associated virus (AAV) type 5 Rep protein cleaves a unique terminal resolution site compared with other AAV serotypes. J Virol 1999; 73:4293–4298.

128. Fisher KJ, Gao GP, Weitzman MD, DeMatteo R, Burda JF, Wilson JM. Transduction with recombinant adeno-associated virus for gene therapy is limited by leading-strand synthesis. J Virol 1996; 70:520–532.

129. Ferrari FK, Samulski T, Shenk T, Samulski RJ. Second-strand synthesis is a rate-limiting step for efficient transduction by recombinant adeno-associated virus vectors. J Virol 1996; 70:3227–3234.

130. Sanlioglu S, Duan D, Engelhardt JF. Two independent molecular pathways for recombinant Adeno-Associated virus genome conversion occur after UV-C and E4orf6 augmentation of transduction. Hum Gene Ther 1999; 10:591–602.

131. Mah C, Qing K, Khuntirat B, et al. Adeno-associated virus type 2-mediated gene transfer: role of epidermal growth factor receptor protein tyrosine kinase in transgene expression. J Virol 1998; 72:9835–9843.

132. Nakai H, Storm TA, Kay MA. Recruitment of single-stranded recombinant adeno-associated virus vector genomes and intermolecular recombination are responsible for stable transduction of liver in vivo. J Virol 2000; 74:9451–9463.

133. Duan D, Sharma P, Yang J, et al. Circular intermediates of recombinant adeno-associated virus have defined structural characteristics responsible for long term episomal persistence in muscle. J Virol 1998; 72:8568–8577.

134. Duan D, Sharma P, Dudus L, et al. Formation of adeno-associated virus circular genomes is differentially regulated by adenovirus E4 ORF6 and E2a gene expression. J Virol 1999; 73:161–169.

135. Duan D, Yan Z, Yue Y, Engelhardt JF. Structural analysis of adeno-associated virus transduction intermediates. Virology 1999; 261:8–14.

136. Flotte TR, Afione SA, Zeitlin PL. Adeno-associated virus vector gene expression occurs in nondividing cells in the absence of vector DNA integration. Am J Respir Cell Mol Biol 1994; 11:517–521.

137. Afione SA, Conrad CK, Kearns WG, et al. In vivo model of adeno-associated virus vector persistence and rescue. J Virol 1996; 70:3235–3241.

138. Yang J, Zhou W, Zhang Y, Zidon T, Ritchie T, Engelhardt JF. Concatamerization of adeno-associated viral circular genomes occurs through intermolecular recombination. J Virol 1999; 73:9468–9477.

139. Vincent-Lacaze N, Snyder RO, Gluzman R, Bohl D, Lagarde C, Danos O. Structure of adeno-associated virus vector DNA following transduction of the skeletal muscle. J Virol 1999; 73:1949–1955.

140. Musatov SA, Scully TA, Dudus L, Fisher KJ. Induction of circular episomes during

rescue and replication of adeno-associated virus in experimental models of virus latency. Virology 2000; 275:411–432.

141. Tsunoda H, Hayakawa T, Sakuragawa N, Koyama H. Site-specific integration of adeno-associated virus-based plasmid vectors in lipofected HeLa cells. Virology 2000; 268:391–401.

142. Song S, Laipis PJ, Berns KI, Flotte TR. Effect of DNA-dependent protein kinase on the molecular fate of the rAAV2 genome in skeletal muscle. Proc Natl Acad Sci USA 2001; 98:4084–4088.

143. Fisher KJ, Jooss K, Alston J, et al. Recombinant adeno-associated virus for muscle directed gene therapy. Nat Med 1997; 3:306–312.

144. Miao CH, Snyder RO, Schowalter DB, et al. The kinetics of rAAV integration in the liver (letter). Nat Genet 1998; 19:13–15.

145. Wu P, Phillips MI, Bui J, Terwilliger EF. Adeno-associated virus vector-mediated transgene integration into neurons and other nondividing cell targets. J Virol 1998; 72:5919–5926.

146. Omori F, Messner HA, Ye C, et al. Nontargeted stable integration of recombinant adeno-associated virus into human leukemia and lymphoma cell lines as evaluated by fluorescence in situ hybridization. Hum Gene Ther 1999; 10:537–543.

147. Rivadeneira ED, Popescu NC, Zimonjic DB, et al. Sites of recombinant adeno-associated virus integration. Int J Oncol 1998; 12:805–810.

148. Holscher C, Horer M, Kleinschmidt JA, Zentgraf H, Burkle A, Heilbronn R. Cell lines inducibly expressing the adeno-associated virus (AAV) rep gene: requirements for productive replication of rep-negative AAV mutants. J Virol 1994; 68: 7169–7177.

149. Clark KR, Voulgaropoulou F, Fraley DM, Johnson PR. Cell lines for the production of recombinant adeno-associated virus. Hum Gene Ther 1995; 6:1329–1341.

150. Tamayose K, Hirai Y, Shimada T. A new strategy for large-scale preparation of high-titer recombinant adeno-associated virus vectors by using packaging cell lines and sulfonated cellulose column chromatography. Hum Gene Ther 1996; 7:507–513.

151. Grimm D, Kleinschmidt JA. Progress in adeno-associated virus type 2 vector production: promises and prospects for clinical use. Hum Gene Ther 1999; 10:2445–2450.

152. Schmidt M, Afione S, Kotin RM. Adeno-associated virus type 2 Rep78 induces apoptosis through caspase activation independently of p53. J Virol 2000; 74:9441–9450.

153. Bertran J, Yang Y, Hargrove P, Vanin EF, Nienhuis AW. Targeted integration of a recombinant globin gene adeno-associated viral vector into human chromosome 19. Ann NY Acad Sci 1998; 850:163–177.

154. Satoh W, Hirai Y, Tamayose K, Shimada T. Site-specific integration of an adeno-associated virus vector plasmid mediated by regulated expression of rep based on CreloxP recombination. J Virol 2000; 74:10631–10638.

155. Davis MD, Wonderling RS, Walker SL, Owens RA. Analysis of the effects of charge cluster mutations in adeno-associated virus Rep68 protein in vitro. J Virol 1999; 73:2084–2093.

156. Rinaudo D, Lamartina S, Roscilli G, Ciliberto G, Toniatti C. Conditional site-

specific integration into human chromosome 19 by using a ligand-dependent chimeric adeno-associated virus/Rep protein. J Virol 2000; 74:281–294.

157. Cathomen T, Collete D, Weitzman MD. A chimeric protein containing the N terminus of the adeno-associated virus Rep protein recognizes its target site in an in vivo assay. J Virol 2000; 74:2372–2382.

158. Yoon M, Smith DH, Ward P, Medrano FJ, Aggarwal AK, Linden RM. Aminoterminal domain exchange redirects origin-specific interactions of adeno-associated virus rep78 in vitro. J Virol 2001; 75:3230–3239.

159. Blacklow NR, Hoggan MD, Kapikian AZ, Austin JB, Rowe WP. Epidemiology of adenovirus-associated virus infection in a nursery population. Am J Epidemiol 1968; 88:368–378.

160. Halbert CL, Standaert TA, Aitken ML, Alexander IE, Russell DW, Miller AD. Transduction by adeno-associated virus vectors in the rabbit airway: efficiency, persistence, and readministration. J Virol 1997; 71:5932–5941.

161. Halbert CL, Standaert TA, Wilson CB, Miller AD. Successful readministration of adeno-associated virus vectors to the mouse lung requires transient immunosuppression during the initial exposure. J Virol 1998; 72:9795–9805.

162. Rutledge EA, Halbert CL, Russell DW. Infectious clones and vectors derived from adeno-associated virus (AAV) serotypes other than AAV type 2. J Virol 1998; 72:309–319.

163. Halbert CL, Rutledge EA, Allen JM, Russell DW, Miller AD. Repeat transduction in the mouse lung by using adeno-associated virus vectors with different serotypes. J Virol 2000; 74:1524–1532.

164. Halbert CL, Allen JM, Miller AD. Adeno-associated virus type 6 (aav6) vectors mediate efficient transduction of airway epithelial cells in mouse lungs compared to that of aav2 vectors. J Virol 2001; 75:6615–6624.

165. Beck SE, Jones LA, Chesnut K, et al. Repeated delivery of adeno-associated virus vectors to the rabbit airway. J Virol 1999; 73:9446–9455.

166. Anand V, Chirmule N, Fersh M, Maguire AM, Bennett J. Additional transduction events after subretinal readministration of recombinant adeno-associated virus. Hum Gene Ther 2000; 11:449–457.

167. Chirmule N, Xiao W, Truneh A, et al. Humoral immunity to adeno-associated virus type 2 vectors following administration to murine and nonhuman primate muscle. J Virol 2000; 74:2420–2425.

168. Xiao W, Chirmule N, Schnell MA, Tazelaar J, Hughes JV, Wilson JM. Route of administration determines induction of T-cell–independent humoral responses to adeno-associated virus vectors. Mol Ther 2000; 1:323–329.

169. Ge Y, Powell S, Van Roey M, McArthur JG. Factors influencing the development of an anti-factor IX (FIX) immune response following administration of adeno-associated virus-FIX. Blood 2001; 97:3733–3737.

170. Hildinger M, Auricchio A, Gao G, Wang L, Chirmule N, Wilson JM. Hybrid vectors based on adeno-associated virus serotypes 2 and 5 for muscle-directed gene transfer. J Virol 2001; 75:6199–6203.

171. Hernandez YJ, Wang J, Kearns WG, Loiler S, Poirier A, Flotte TR. Latent adeno-associated virus infection elicits humoral but not cell-mediated immune responses in a nonhuman primate model. J Virol 1999; 73:8549–8558.

172. Jooss K, Yang Y, Fisher KJ, Wilson JM. Transduction of dendritic cells by DNA viral vectors directs the immune response to transgene products in muscle fibers. J Virol 1998; 72:4212–4223.

173. Zhang Y, Chirmule N, Gao G, Wilson J. CD40 ligand-dependent activation of cytotoxic T lymphocytes by adeno-associated virus vectors in vivo: role of immature dendritic cells. J Virol 2000; 74:8003–8010.

174. Xin KQ, Urabe M, Yang J, et al. A novel recombinant adeno-associated virus vaccine induces a long-term humoral immune response to human immunodeficiency virus. Hum Gene Ther 2001; 12:1047–1061.

175. Cordier L, Gao GP, Hack AA, et al. Muscle-specific promoters may be necessary for adeno-associated virus-mediated gene transfer in the treatment of muscular dystrophies. Hum Gene Ther 2001; 12:205–215.

176. Duan D, Yan Z, Yue Y, Ding W, Engelhardt JF. Enhancement of muscle gene delivery with pseudotyped AAV-5 correlates with myoblast differentiation. J Virol 2001; 75:7662–7671.

177. McLaughlin SK, Collis P, Hermonat PL, Muzyczka N. Adeno-associated virus general transduction vectors: analysis of proviral structures. J Virol 1988; 62:1963–1973.

178. Samulski RJ, Chang LS, Shenk T. Helper-free stocks of recombinant adeno-associated viruses: normal integration does not require viral gene expression. J Virol 1989; 63:3822–3828.

179. Gao GP, Wilson JM, Wivel NA. Production of recombinant adeno-associated virus. Adv Virus Res 2000; 55:529–543.

180. Cao L, Liu Y, During MJ, Xiao W. High-titer, wild-type free recombinant adeno-associated virus vector production using intron-containing helper plasmids. J Virol 2000; 74:11456–11463.

181. Grimm D, Kern A, Rittner K, Kleinschmidt JA. Novel tools for production and purification of recombinant adenoassociated virus vectors. Hum Gene Ther 1998; 9:2745–2760.

182. Gao GP, Qu G, Faust LZ, et al. High-titer adeno-associated viral vectors from a Rep/Cap cell line and hybrid shuttle virus. Hum Gene Ther 1998; 9:2353–2362.

183. Inoue N, Russell DW. Packaging cells based on inducible gene amplification for the production of adeno-associated virus vectors. J Virol 1998; 72:7024–7031.

184. Liu XL, Clark KR, Johnson PR. Production of recombinant adeno-associated virus vectors using a packaging cell line and a hybrid recombinant adenovirus. Gene Ther 1999; 6:293–299.

185. Johnston KM, Jacoby D, Pechan PA, et al. HSV/AAV hybrid amplicon vectors extend transgene expression in human glioma cells. Hum Gene Ther 1997; 8:359–370.

186. Conway JE, Zolotukhin S, Muzyczka N, Hayward GS, Byrne BJ. Recombinant adeno-associated virus type 2 replication and packaging is entirely supported by a herpes simplex virus type 1 amplicon expressing Rep and Cap. J Virol 1997; 71:8780–8789.

187. Ferrari FK, Xiao X, McCarty D, Samulski RJ. New developments in the generation of Ad-free, high-titer rAAV gene therapy vectors. Nat Med 1997; 3:1295–1297.

188. Clark KR, Liu X, McGrath JP, Johnson PR. Highly purified recombinant adeno-

associated virus vectors are biologically active and free of detectable helper and wild-type viruses. Hum Gene Ther 1999; 10:1031–1039.

189. Anderson R, Macdonald I, Corbett T, Whiteway A, Prentice HG. A method for the preparation of highly purified adeno-associated virus using affinity column chromatography, protease digestion and solvent extraction. J Virol Methods 2000; 85:23–34.

190. Debelak D, Fisher J, Iuliano S, Sesholtz D, Sloane DL, Atkinson EM. Cation-exchange high-performance liquid chromatography of recombinant adeno-associated virus type 2. J Chromatogr B Biomed Sci Appl 2000; 740:195–202.

191. O'Riordan CR, Lachapelle AL, Vincent KA, Wadsworth SC. Scaleable chromatographic purification process for recombinant adeno-associated virus (rAAV). J Gene Med 2000; 2:444–454.

192. Gao G, Qu G, Burnham MS, et al. Purification of recombinant adeno-associated virus vectors by column chromatography and its performance in vivo. Hum Gene Ther 2000; 11:2079–2091.

193. Auricchio A, Hildinger M, O'Connor E, Gao GP, Wilson JM. Isolation of highly infectious and pure adeno-associated virus type 2 vectors with a single-step gravity-flow column. Hum Gene Ther 2001; 12:71–76.

194. Kaplitt MG, Leone P, Samulski RJ, et al. Long-term gene expression and phenotypic correction using adeno-associated virus vectors in the mammalian brain. Nat Genet 1994; 8:148–154.

195. Kirik D, Rosenblad C, Bjorklund A, Mandel RJ. Long-term rAAV-mediated gene transfer of GDNF in the rat Parkinson's model: intrastriatal but not intranigral transduction promotes functional regeneration in the lesioned nigrostriatal system. J Neurosci 2000; 20:4686–4700.

196. Acland GM, Aguirre GD, Ray J, et al. Gene therapy restores vision in a canine model of childhood blindness. Nat Genet 2001; 28:92–95.

197. Kay MA, Manno CS, Ragni MV, et al. Evidence for gene transfer and expression of factor IX in haemophilia B patients treated with an AAV vector. Nat Genet 2000; 24:257–261.

198. Greelish JP, Su LT, Lankford EB, et al. Stable restoration of the sarcoglycan complex in dystrophic muscle perfused with histamine and a recombinant adeno-associated viral vector. Nat Med 1999; 5:439–443.

199. Xiao X, Li J, Tsao YP, Dressman D, Hoffman EP, Watchko JF. Full functional rescue of a complete muscle (TA) in dystrophic hamsters by adeno-associated virus vector-directed gene therapy. J Virol 2000; 74:1436–1442.

200. Cordier L, Hack AA, Scott MO, et al. Rescue of skeletal muscles of gamma-sarcoglycan-deficient mice with adeno-associated virus-mediated gene transfer. Mol Ther 2000; 1:119–129.

201. Stedman H, Wilson JM, Finke R, Kleckner AL, Mendell J. Phase I clinical trial utilizing gene therapy for limb girdle muscular dystrophy: alpha-, beta-, gamma-, or delta-sarcoglycan gene delivered with intramuscular instillations of adeno-associated vectors. Hum Gene Ther 2000; 11:777–790.

202. Wang B, Li J, Xiao X. Adeno-associated virus vector carrying human minidystrophin genes effectively ameliorates muscular dystrophy in mdx mouse model. Proc Natl Acad Sci USA 2000; 97:13714–13719.

203. During MJ, Xu R, Young D, Kaplitt MG, Sherwin RS, Leone P. Peroral gene therapy of lactose intolerance using an adeno-associated virus vector. Nat Med 1998; 4:1131–1135.

204. Lee HC, Kim SJ, Kim KS, Shin HC, Yoon JW. Remission in models of type 1 diabetes by gene therapy using a single-chain insulin analogue. Nature 2000; 408: 483–488.

205. During MJ, Symes CW, Lawlor PA, et al. An oral vaccine against NMDAR1 with efficacy in experimental stroke and epilepsy. Science 2000; 287:1453–1460.

206. Duan D, Zhang Y, Engelhardt JF. Gene delivery to the airway. In: Dracopoli NC, Haines JL, Korf BR, et al., eds. Current Protocols in Human Genetics. New York: Wiley, 1998:13.9.1–13.9.34.

207. Walters RW, Duan D, Engelhardt JF, Welsh MJ. Incorporation of adeno-associated virus in a calcium phosphate coprecipitate improves gene transfer to airway epithelia in vitro and in vivo. J Virol 2000; 74:535–540.

208. Weiss DJ, Bonneau L, Allen JM, Miller AD, Halbert CL. Perfluorochemical liquid enhances adeno-associated virus-mediated transgene expression in lungs. Mol Ther 2000; 2:624–630.

209. Engelhardt JF, Schlossberg H, Yankaskas JR, Dudus L. Progenitor cells of the adult human airway involved in submucosal gland development. Development 1995; 121:2031–2046.

210. Duan D, Sehgal A, Yao J, Engelhardt JF. Lef1 Transcription factor expression defines airway progenitor cell targets for in utero gene therapy of submucosal gland in cystic fibrosis. Am J Respir Cell Mol Biol 1998; 18:750–758.

211. Borthwick DW, West JD, Keighren MA, Flockhart JH, Innes BA, Dorin JR. Murine submucosal glands are clonally derived and show a cystic fibrosis gene-dependent distribution pattern. Am J Respir Cell Mol Biol 1999; 20:1181–1189.

212. Duan D, Yue Y, Zhou W, et al. Submucosal Gland Development in the Airway is Controlled by Lymphoid Enhancer Binding Factor-1 (Lef-1). Development 1999; 126:4441–4453.

213. Conrad CK, Allen SS, Afione SA, et al. Safety of single-dose administration of an adeno-associated virus (AAV)–CFTR vector in the primate lung. Gene Ther 1996; 3:658–668.

214. Rubenstein RC, McVeigh U, Flotte TR, Guggino WB, Zeitlin PL. CFTR gene transduction in neonatal rabbits using an adeno-associated virus (AAV) vector. Gene Ther 1997; 4:384–392.

215. Kitson C, Angel B, Judd D, et al. The extra- and intracellular barriers to lipid and adenovirus-mediated pulmonary gene transfer in native sheep airway epithelium. Gene Ther 1999; 6:534–546.

216. Zabner J, Zeiher BG, Friedman E, Welsh MJ. Adenovirus-mediated gene transfer to ciliated airway epithelia requires prolonged incubation time. J Virol 1996; 70: 6994–7003.

217. Duan D, Yue Y, Engelhardt JF. Response to "polarity influences the efficiency of recombinant adeno-associated virus infection in differentiated airway epithelia." Hum Gene Ther 1999; 10:1553–1557.

218. Zabner J, Seiler M, Walters R, et al. Adeno-associated virus type 5 (AAV5) but not AAV2 binds to the apical surfaces of airway epithelia and facilitates gene transfer. J Virol 2000; 74:3852–3858.

219. Engelhardt JF, Yang Y, Stratford-Perricaudet LD, et al. Direct gene transfer of human CFTR into human bronchial epithelia of xenografts with E1-deleted adenoviruses. Nat Genet 1993; 4:27–34.

220. Goldman MJ, Wilson JM. Expression of alpha v beta 5 integrin is necessary for efficient adenovirus-mediated gene transfer in the human airway. J Virol 1995; 69:5951–5958.

221. Zabner J, Freimuth P, Puga A, Fabrega A, Welsh MJ. Lack of high affinity fiber receptor activity explains the resistance of ciliated airway epithelia to adenovirus infection. J Clin Invest 1997; 100:1144–1149.

222. Pickles RJ, McCarty D, Matsui H, Hart PJ, Randell SH, Boucher RC. Limited entry of adenovirus vectors into well-differentiated airway epithelium is responsible for inefficient gene transfer. J Virol 1998; 72:6014–6023.

223. Walters RW, Grunst T, Bergelson JM, Finberg RW, Welsh MJ, Zabner J. Basolateral localization of fiber receptors limits adenovirus infection from the apical surface of airway epithelia. J Biol Chem 1999; 274:10219–10226.

224. Pickles RJ, Fahrner JA, Petrella JM, Boucher RC, Bergelson JM. Retargeting the coxsackievirus and adenovirus receptor to the apical surface of polarized epithelial cells reveals the glycocalyx as a barrier to adenovirus-mediated gene transfer. J Virol 2000; 74:6050–6057.

225. Wang G, Davidson BL, Melchert P, et al. Efficient gene transfer to differentiated human airway epithelia with recombinant amphotropic and xenotropic retroviruses. J Virol 1998; 72:9818–9826.

226. Virella-Lowell I, Poirier A, Chesnut KA, Brantly M, Flotte TR. Inhibition of recombinant adeno-associated virus (rAAV) transduction by bronchial secretions from cystic fibrosis patients. Gene Ther 2000; 7:1783–1789.

227. Bals R, Xiao W, Sang N, Weiner DJ, Meegalla RL, Wilson JM. Transduction of well-differentiated airway epithelium by recombinant adeno-associated virus is limited by vector entry. J Virol 1999; 73:6085–6088.

228. Alexander IE, Russell DW, Miller AD. DNA-damaging agents greatly increase the transduction of nondividing cells by adeno-associated virus vectors. J Virol 1994; 68:8282–8287.

229. Russell DW, Alexander IE, Miller AD. DNA synthesis and topoisomerase inhibitors increase transduction by adeno-associated virus vectors. Proc Natl Acad Sci USA 1995; 92:5719–5723.

230. Teramoto S, Bartlett JS, McCarty D, Xiao X, Samulski RJ, Boucher RC. Factors influencing adeno-associated virus-mediated gene transfer to human cystic fibrosis airway epithelial cells: comparison with adenovirus vectors. J Virol 1998; 72:8904–8912.

231. Baumeister W, Walz J, Zuhl F, Seemuller E. The proteasome: paradigm of a self-compartmentalizing protease. Cell 1998; 92:367–380.

232. Strous GJ, Govers R. The ubiquitin-proteasome system and endocytosis. J Cell Sci 1999; 112:1417–1423.

233. Leach CL, Greenspan JS, Rubenstein SD, et al. Partial liquid ventilation with perflubron in premature infants with severe respiratory distress syndrome. The LiquiVent Study Group. N Engl J Med 1996; 335:761–767.

234. Lisby DA, Ballard PL, Fox WW, Wolfson MR, Shaffer TH, Gonzales LW. Enhanced distribution of adenovirus-mediated gene transfer to lung parenchyma by perfluorochemical liquid. Hum Gene Ther 1997; 8:919–928.

235. Weiss DJ, Strandjord TP, Jackson JC, Clark JG, Liggitt D. Perfluorochemical liquid-enhanced adenoviral vector distribution and expression in lungs of spontaneously breathing rodents. Exp Lung Res 1999; 25:317–333.

236. Weiss DJ, Strandjord TP, Liggitt D, Clark JG. Perflubron enhances adenovirus-mediated gene expression in lungs of transgenic mice with chronic alveolar filling. Hum Gene Ther 1999; 10:2287–2293.

237. Dong JY, Fan PD, Frizzell RA. Quantitative analysis of the packaging capacity of recombinant adeno-associated virus. Hum Gene Ther 1996; 7:2101–2112.

238. Flotte TR, Afione SA, Solow R, et al. Expression of the cystic fibrosis transmembrane conductance regulator from a novel adeno-associated virus promoter. J Biol Chem 1993; 268:3781–3790.

239. Duan D, Yue Y, Yan Z, Engelhardt JF. Trans-splicing vectors expand the packaging limits of adeno-associated virus for gene therapy applications. In: Machida CA, ed. Methods in Molecular Medicine, Viral Vectors for Gene Therapy Methods and Protocols. Totowa, NJ: Humana Press, 2002. In press.

240. Phelps SF, Hauser MA, Cole NM, et al. Expression of full-length and truncated dystrophin mini-genes in transgenic mdx mice. Hum Mol Genet 1995; 4:1251–1258.

241. Zhang L, Wang D, Fischer H, et al. Efficient expression of CFTR function with adeno-associated virus vectors that carry shortened CFTR genes. Proc Natl Acad Sci USA 1998; 95:10158–10163.

242. Wang D, Fischer H, Zhang L, Fan P, Ding RX, Dong J. Efficient CFTR expression from AAV vectors packaged with promoters—the second generation. Gene Ther 1999; 6:667–675.

243. Flotte T, Carter B, Conrad C, et al. A phase I study of an adeno-associated virus-CFTR gene vector in adult CF patients with mild lung disease. Hum Gene Ther 1996; 7:1145–1159.

244. Wagner JA, Gardner P. Toward cystic fibrosis gene therapy. Annu Rev Med 1997; 48:203–216.

245. Wagner JA, Moran ML, Messner AH, et al. A phase I/II study of tgAAV-CF for the treatment of chronic sinusitis in patients with cystic fibrosis. Hum Gene Ther 1998; 9:889–909.

246. Wagner JA, Reynolds T, Moran ML, et al. Efficient and persistent gene transfer of AAV-CFTR in maxillary sinus (letter). Lancet 1998; 351:1702–1703.

247. Wagner JA, Messner AH, Moran ML, et al. Safety and biological efficacy of an adeno-associated virus vector-cystic fibrosis transmembrane regulator (AAV-CFTR) in the cystic fibrosis maxillary sinus. Laryngoscope 1999; 109:266–274.

248. Wagner JA, Nepomuceno IB, Shah N, et al. Maxillary sinusitis as a surrogate model for CF gene therapy clinical trials in patients with antrostomies. J Gene Med 1999; 1:13–21.

249. Raj K, Ogston P, Beard P. Virus-mediated killing of cells that lack p53 activity. Nature 2001; 412:914–917.

250. Donsante A, Vogler C, Muzyczka N, et al. Observed incidence of tumorigenesis in long-term rodent studies of rAAV vectors. Gene Ther 2001; 8:1343–1346.

251. Harper SQ, Hauser MA, DelloRusso C, et al. Modular flexibility of dystrophin: implications for gene therapy of Duchenne muscular dystrophy. Nat Med 2002; 8: 253–261.

4

Cationic Lipids for Lung Gene Therapy

RONALD K. SCHEULE

Genzyme Corporation
Framingham, Massachusetts, U.S.A.

I. Introduction

The lung represents an attractive target organ for gene therapy because of its relative accessibility through luminal routes and because delivery by such a route is less likely to provoke serious toxicity; that is, it is an organ that should provide a target with a reasonably high therapeutic index. Some indications that have been considered for a lung-based gene therapy approach include diseases such as cystic fibrosis (CF), asthma, cancer, pulmonary hypertension, fibrosis, and acute respiratory distress syndrome, as well as lung transplantation. Both viral and nonviral vectors are being considered for these applications; for example, both have been used in clinical trials for CF, and the advantages and disadvantages of these vectors have been well described (1–4).

Among the several types of nonviral or synthetic vectors in use, cationic lipids have perhaps been the most widely studied to date. The reader is referred to recent reviews for additional information (5,6). Other cationic systems, such as those based on cationic polymers, for example, poly-L-lysine and poly-ethyleneimine (PEI), share many of the properties of the cationic lipid systems, but they will not be described here. The reader is referred to recent reviews on these systems (7–9). Cationic lipid-based gene transfer came on the scene in the late 1980s, and since then literally hundreds of different molecular structures have been devised and evaluated (9–11).

All cationic delivery systems make use of the ionic interactions between the cationic lipid component and the negative charges of the nucleotide phosphates to help form stable complexes. This complexation also stabilizes the DNA against nuclease degradation, thereby increasing the half-life of the genetic information being delivered and increasing the potency of the cationic lipid-delivered gene relative to "naked" plasmid DNA (pDNA). The cationic lipid component no doubt serves other functions in the transit of the DNA from the delivery point to its ultimate destination in the nucleus where it can be transcribed. It should be clear, however, that the DNA compacting and stabilizing effects contributed by the cationic lipid ultimately must be balanced by the reversibility of its interactions with DNA so that transcription and gene expression can occur.

This chapter has two major goals. First, the cationic lipid vector system will be described, taking into account the properties of both the individual components and those of cationic lipid:DNA complexes. Second, the consequences of using these vector systems in the setting of the lung will be explored; that is, in vivo rather than in vitro studies will be emphasized. Systemic routes, as well as luminal routes, of delivery will be covered. Both efficacy and toxicity will be discussed, with the aim of giving the reader a grasp of the therapeutic index of these vector systems in the context of lung gene therapy. Succeeding chapters will provide more detailed examples of the uses of cationic lipids for specific clinical applications.

II. The Delivery System—Cationic Lipid:pDNA Complexes

A. Lipid Components

Cationic Lipid

The structural aspects of typical cationic lipids are depicted in Figure 1 (GL67, GL62, DOTAP, DMRIE). In general, these lipids can be thought of as being composed of three structural domains: (1) a nonpolar, lipid-like domain; (2) a polar, univalent or multivalent headgroup domain; and (3) a covalent linker domain connecting them.

The structure of the nonpolar domain mimics that of the lipids in a biological membrane, that is, it can either have a steroid-like structure, for example, a cholesterol mimetic (GL67), or it can have acyl chains (DOTAP). For acyl chain–based lipids, the two chains are generally identical, and can be either saturated or unsaturated. A commonly used unsaturated acyl chain is the dioleoyl (18:1) chain, such as that depicted in DOTAP (Fig. 1). It is important to realize that relatively small structural changes in the nonpolar domain can have significant

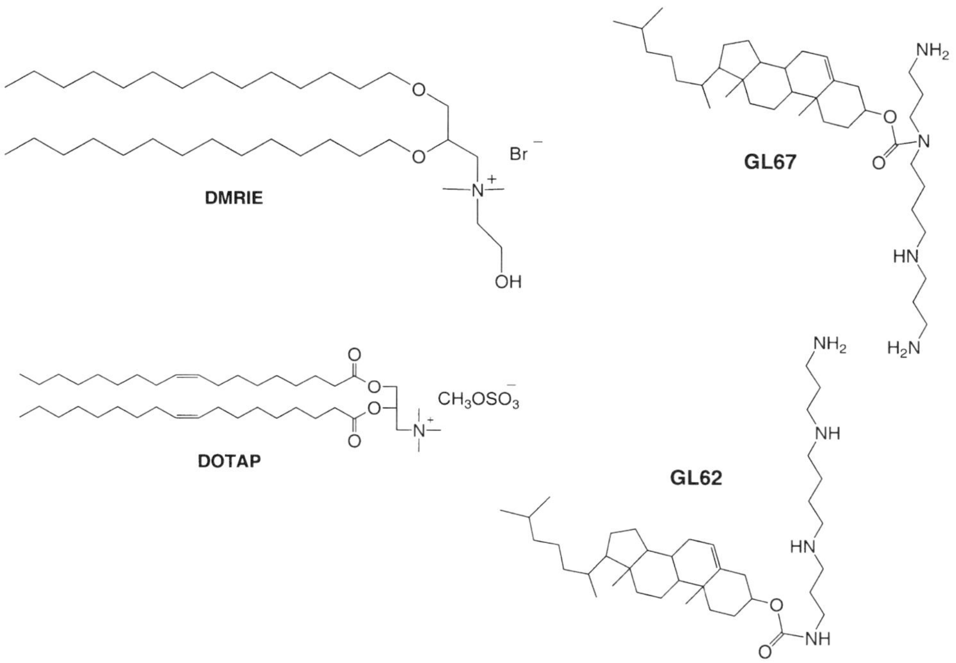

Figure 1 Structural examples of some cationic lipids.

effects on activity. For example, removing the double bond in the cholesterol moiety of GL67 entirely abrogates transfection activity in the lungs of mice (unpublished data).

The cationic headgroup domain is almost exclusively based on secondary, tertiary, or quaternary amines and can be monovalent or multivalent. For example, GL67 has what has been termed a "T-shaped" spermine headgroup; spermine is one of several naturally occurring polyamines with an affinity for DNA. The positive charge distribution and pKs of the primary and secondary amines determine the details of the headgroup-DNA interactions, and ultimately have important effects on activity. For example, cationic lipid:pDNA complexes prepared using the free base form of cationic lipids such as GL67 rather than a salt have been found to have the most in vivo activity (12). By contrast, the cationic lipid DOTAP has a quaternary amine, which is protonated independent of pH, and will therefore result in different interactions with DNA. It is also important to realize that relatively small structural changes in the headgroup can result in relatively large changes in activity. For example, attaching the spermine headgroup of GL67 through one of its primary amines (resulting in GL62) generates a cationic lipid with significantly less activity in a lung instillation model, whereas altering the methylene spacing of the amines from the natural (3,4,3) spacing also results in significant decreases in activity (12).

Joining the membrane-anchoring domain and the headgroup domain is a chemical "linker" moiety. The linker can be based on virtually any structure, but is usually restricted to functional groups, for example, esters and ethers, that are consistent with the chemical reactions necessary to couple membrane and headgroup domains. It should be emphasized that although the structure of a prototypical cationic lipid can be seen as being composed of three separate domains, it is difficult to dissociate or dissect the individual elements important for activity. Rather it is the composite cationic lipid, with all three elements, that must be optimized for activity. Thus, for example, a headgroup domain that shows good activity in the context of a sterol membrane domain may show no activity when coupled with an acyl chain–based membrane domain.

Colipids

In its simplest embodiment, a delivery system based on cationic lipids is composed solely of the cationic lipid combined with pDNA at an empirically optimized ratio. However, only a very few cationic lipids, for example, DOTAP, demonstrate significant activity when combined with DNA. For most cationic lipids it has been found necessary to include a second lipid component. This "helper" lipid is generally one that can promote nonbilayer phases due to the relatively small size and minimal hydration of its headgroup. Common examples of such lipids are dioleoylphosphatidylethanolamine (DOPE, 18:1) and cholesterol, both of which can adopt an inverted micellar, or hexagonal H_{II} lipid phase conformations. Although a mixture of a cationic lipid, which in general has a large, hydrated headgroup with a preference for bilayer phases, and a colipid such as DOPE can together form a stable bilayer, the current dogma is that the presence of DOPE in these structures leads them to become destabilized once inside the cell and facilitates escape of the DNA from membrane (bilayer)–bound compartments such as endosomes. While DOPE and cholesterol have been extensively used as colipids in cationic lipid:pDNA formulations, it is worth pointing out that significant increases in in vivo potency often can be realized by screening alternative colipids (13). In particular, diphytanoylphosphatidylethanolamine (16:0 [Me$_4$]) can be quite effective in this regard, enhancing expression 2- to 20-fold over DOPE depending on the cationic lipid (12).

Optimization

Including a second lipid component obviously introduces a new variable in the preparation of cationic lipid:DNA complexes; namely, the colipid:cationic lipid

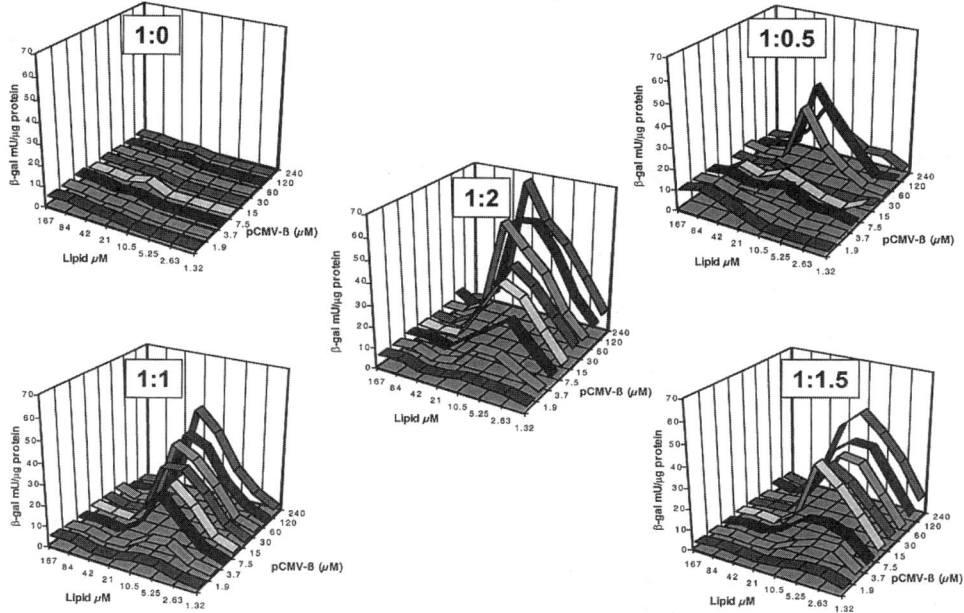

Figure 2 Optimization of the cationic lipid:colipid ratio in vitro. Variable molar (in nucleotides) amounts of plasmid DNA containing a reporter gene (β-galactosidase) were mixed with the cationic lipid GL67 formulated with different mole ratios (boxes) of the neutral lipid dioleoylphosphatidylethanolamine (DOPE) and used to transfect CFT1 epithelial cells in a 96-well plate. Expression levels were determined 2 days later, and indicate an optimal ratio of GL67:DOPE ~ 1:2 (mol:mol).

ratio. We have found that this ratio can be optimized most readily in vitro, and appears to be a function of the particular cationic lipid and neutral lipid used. Using a 96-well plate assay that varies the cationic lipid:DNA ratio, the colipid can be evaluated by using one colipid:cationic lipid ratio per plate. Figure 2 illustrates this process for GL67 and DOPE. It does not appear that this ratio has to be redetermined in vivo; in general, we have found the same optimum in vitro and in vivo (14).

B. DNA Component

Typical pDNA

The oligonucleotide component of a cationic lipid:DNA complex can consist of DNA or RNA of virtually any length. For gene transfer, however, plasmid DNA (pDNA) is generally the oligonucleotide of choice. The two-dimensional structure of a typical pDNA is illustrated in Figure 3. Of particular note are the presence of sequences necessary for growth of the plasmid in bacteria, for example, the antibiotic resistance gene (here kanamycin) and the origin for bacterial replication, as well as the presence of sequences needed for the expression of the transgene in the nucleus of the target cell, for example, the promoter (here from mammalian ubiquitin B) and the polyadenylation signal. Also included in most plasmids is an intron (here, from ubiquitin), which has been shown to enhance expression in mammalian lung (15). Many other elements, for example, multiple cloning sites, insulators, additional enhancers, such as that from cytomegalovirus (CMV in Fig. 3) can be added to this basic scheme.

Ultimately, construct choice for a given lung application will have to be decided based on the therapeutic index as well as the requirement for persistent expression. For example, a construct giving relatively low, transient expression could be adequate if the toxicity associated with delivery was low enough that multiple doses could be given to achieve the desired expression level. This con-

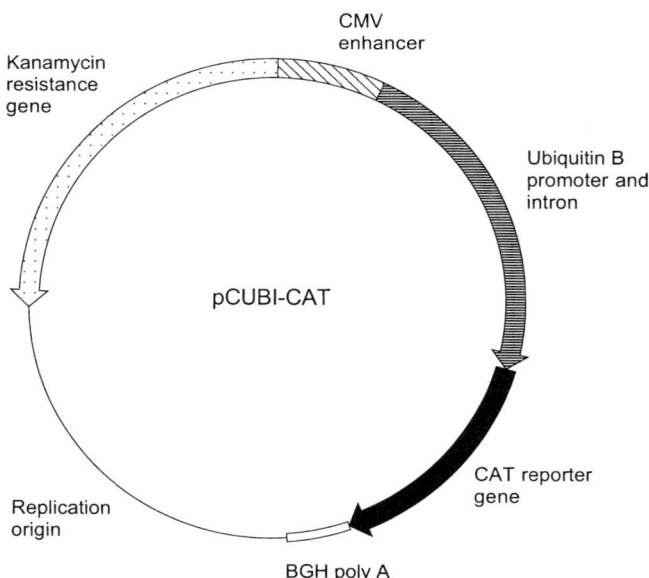

Figure 3 Schematic diagram of an expression plasmid containing the kanamycin resistance gene, origin of bacterial replication, cytomegalovirus immediate-early promoter enhancer (CMV), ubiquitin B promoter and intron, chloramphenicol acetyltransferase reporter gene (CAT), and bovine growth hormone (BGH) polyadenylation signal.

struct would have to be compared with one giving therapeutic expression levels with a single dose that might be associated with higher toxicity. For a genetic disease such as CF, a construct giving high, persistent expression (say >1 month) with minimal toxicity would be optimal. An additional criterion for a CF therapeutic agent might be the ability to transduce virtually all cell types in the small airways—a goal perhaps not readily achieved (3).

C. Cationic Lipid:pDNA Complexes

Formation

Complexation of cationic liposomes and DNA appears to be driven by the entropy gained from the loss of bound water and counterions from the lipid and DNA (16). Thus, whereas the initial association of cationic lipid and DNA results from charge-charge interactions involving cationic headgroups and DNA phosphates (17), the subsequent cooperative interaction between lipid domains is entropy driven and thermodynamically dominates the complexation reaction. Complexation appears to result in structures composed of many alternating lipid bilayers and DNA monolayers, the details of which do not appear to depend strongly on the nature of the DNA, but they do depend on variables such as the ionic strength, cationic lipid:DNA ratio, and the details of how the lipid and DNA components are mixed (16,18,19). In one model, the progressive addition of cationic liposomes to an excess of DNA leads to coating of individual liposomes by DNA followed by association of coated liposomes mediated by uncoated liposomes and an eventual rupture of the liposomes to produce the final complex consisting of alternating lipid:DNA layers (16). Conversely, the progressive addition of DNA to an excess of cationic liposomes leads to association of multiple liposomes by bridging DNA followed by liposome rupture and DNA-mediated association. Thus, the details of "mixing" of the cationic and DNA components can produce significantly different final structures.

Simple mixing of the lipid component(s) and DNA component result in what may be called first-generation cationic lipid:DNA complexes. The lipids are typically rehydrated from a dried lipid film with water or buffer to form oligolamellar or multilamellar liposomes having a relatively broad size distribution; for example, 0.1–1.0 μm; pDNA is generally in water. Complexation of lipid and DNA generally occurs over several minutes, and it results in a rather heterogenously sized population of lipid:DNA complexes (e.g., 0.1–1.0 μm). These first-generation complexes are to be compared with what may be called second-generation complexes in which the final population of complexes is significantly more homogenous in size. One example of these second-generation complexes are those prepared starting with DOTAP:cholesterol liposomes that have been extruded to generate a starting unilamellar vesicle population with a more defined size (20). When mixed with pDNA, these liposomes have been reported to encapsulate the DNA inside the liposome. A second example of these more defined, second-generation complexes are those prepared by mixing DNA with detergent-solubilized lipid components followed by dialysis to remove the detergent and induce complex formation. The resulting structures (termed stabilized plasmid-lipid particles, or SPLP) also appear to encapsulate the DNA in a bilayer lipid vesicle, and they are very homogenous in size; for example, 72 ± 5 nm in diameter (21).

Characterization

In addition to their size and size distribution, several other parameters have been used to characterize cationic lipid:pDNA complexes, such as nuclease sensitivity, dye binding (e.g., ethidium bromide binding to DNA), and zeta potentials (22). The zeta potential is a measure of the electrical field of the particle in an aqueous environment, which is determined not only by the cationic and anionic charges on the cationic lipid and pDNA but also by the counterions that are relatively tightly bound to the particle. At low molar ratios of cationic lipid to DNA (usually expressed as the molar ratio of lipid headgroup nitrogens that are positively charged around physiological pH to DNA phosphates), the zeta potential is highly negative (e.g., −40 mV). At high cationic lipid:DNA ratios, the zeta potential approaches that of cationic liposomes ∼+40 mV; at cationic lipid:DNA ratios ∼1, the particles have a zeta potential approximately zero, and tend to flocculate or precipitate. This latter phenomenon is a well-characterized, concentration-dependent property of virtually all colloids.

    The zeta potential of the lipid:DNA complex is an important determinant of its interaction with biological components such as serum proteins and cell surfaces. Since the cell membrane generally has a preponderance of negatively charged molecules on its surface (e.g., glycoproteins), it has been suggested that complexes bearing a negative zeta potential are the most effective. Although often true, this argument usually overlooks the fact that zeta potentials are most often determined in water or buffer, and may be altered significantly by the subsequent binding of extracellular proteins (e.g., serum albumin) before they reach the cell surface (23–25). Indeed, for instillation into the lung, we have found that complexes prepared with a *negative* zeta potential are the most potent (2,12).

Optimization for In Vivo Expression

Although the physical characterization of cationic lipid:DNA complexes is useful, the most important property is their transfection potency. Several groups have shown that in vivo potency is not readily predicted based on in vitro assays for activity (2,26–30) even when the in vitro assays have been carried out in a relevant cell type (e.g., alveolar epithelial cells) (2). Thus, although in vitro model systems for the lung such as primary epithelial cells grown at an air-liquid interface have yielded important activity information (31), the ultimate in vivo activity of a given formulation must be determined in the lung (32). Most investigators have found that multilamellar rather than unilamellar lipid vesicles represent the best lipid form to mix with the pDNA in terms of ultimate in vivo activity (33). Variables such as the cationic lipid:DNA ratio should be redetermined for different delivery routes (34). For example, instillation of GL67:DNA complexes into mouse lung resulted in optimal activity at a ratio of 0.6 mM GL67 to 3.6 mM DNA, whereas an optimal ratio for systemic transfection of the lung for this same lipid was determined to be 1:1 mM.

Given the polyionic nature and size of cationic lipid:pDNA complexes, it should not come as a surprise that they can bind exogenous proteins that might subsequently affect their stability and biodistribution. Indeed, several studies have pointed to the ability of complexes to bind serum proteins such as albumin (23,24,35). In addition, complexes appear to interact with cellular components in vivo such as lymphocytes (36) and red blood cells (37). Thus, although some of the effects of serum protein binding on activity might be assessed in vitro, it would be extremely difficult to mimic in vitro all the important interactions of complexes with the biological environment that would be required to predict in vivo activity.

III. Cationic Lipid:pDNA Complexes and Transfection of the Lung

A. Biodistribution and Expression

Intravenous Administration

A few minutes after an intravenous administration of cationic lipid:pDNA complexes in rodents, most of the DNA ($\sim$40% of the injected dose) is associated with the lung, with $\sim$10% being associated with the liver (38). At this same early time point, only a fraction ($\sim$10%) of the DNA can be found still circulating in the blood (38,39), and of this, most appears to be associated with blood cells. In the same time frame, platelets can be found adherent to the endothelial surface of alveolar capillaries and high endothelial venules, implying endothelial activation (36). Leukocytes as well as platelets appear to adhere to endothelium, which may be responsible for the initial apparent losses of these cells from the circulation (36). This initial biodistribution of DNA changes relatively quickly, so that by 5–10 min, the majority of the organ-associated DNA (up to 60% of the injected dose) is located in the liver; apparently largely as a result of rapid redistribution from the lung (38).

Following an intravenous administration in rodents, positively charged complexes appear to bind serum components such as albumin in a charge density–dependent manner (40), resulting in a significant and virtually immediate increase in the size of the complexes; for example, to 1–2 μm within minutes after injection (34). These aggregates appear to adhere rather more specifically to the endothelial cells of alveolar capillaries and venules rather than to those of arterioles (36). Liver, alveolar lung, and kidneys have been confirmed recently as sites of major deposition in the mouse using fluorescent DNA (41). Not surprisingly, within these organs, complexes appear to be associated with phagocytic cells of the reticular endothelial system; for example, Kupffer cells in the liver and pulmonary septal and alveolar macrophages in the lung (39). In the lung, double labeling experiments also show that DNA can be taken up by Type II cells (33).

The size of the aggregates relative to the vessel lumen is not consistent with deposition based on occlusion of the vessels. Thus, a first-pass mechanism of deposition would appear to be based on aggregation together with some element of a receptor-mediated process (36). Whether this view holds for all complexes is not clear, since at least one report detected *no* association of complexes with endothelium (39).

Following intravenous administration, gene transfer to the lung appears to be a relatively rapid process (42). Expression from cationic lipid:pDNA complexes is highest in the lung, with significantly lower levels in other organs, such as the heart and spleen (43,44). Thus, although a large proportion of the DNA subsequently localizes in the liver, most of this DNA appears to be degraded (45), and very little, if any, expression can normally be seen in the liver. In the lung, expression is seen largely in lung vascular endothelial cells of the mouse (45–47), and some expression can also be seen in intravascular monocytes and interstitial macrophages (36,45,48). Changes in formulation can lead to significant changes in the systemic expression profiles; for example, a change from DOTIM:CHOL to DOTIM:DOPE results in a shift in the bulk of expression from lung to spleen (36,45,48–51). An examination of reproductive cells in female mice following intravenous gene transfer showed no evidence of plasmid DNA or expression (28).

Luminal Administration

Instillation

When instilled into the luminal aspect of rodent lungs, cationic lipid:pDNA complexes have resulted in variable distributions of expression. This should not be too surprising, since there are multiple physical variables associated with any instillation, for examples, details of the instillation procedure (lobar, intratracheal, intranasal), volume, identity of the vehicle, rate of delivery, that are superimposed on other sources of variability, such as the identity of the cationic lipid and the lipid:pDNA ratio. Not surprisingly, intralobar instillation in rodents resulted in multifocal expression largely in the distal, alveolar aspect of the lung, presumably due to the physical pooling of the bolus instillate in this anatomical locale. Lung cells expressing the transgene under these conditions appeared to be mostly Type I alveolar epithelial cells, with some evidence of Type II cells (26). In contrast, intratracheal instillation (10 μg DNA in 30 μL) in mice resulted in expression predominantly in the trachea (52), whereas instillation of 100 μL of a DNA solution led to the majority of expression in bronchioles and terminal bronchioles, with additional amounts in the respiratory bronchioles and alveoli (33,47). Instilling 1 mL of DNA solution over 20 min in rats led to the majority of expression in bronchi and proximal bronchioles, with >70% of the epithelial cells showing expression (27). In terms of the relative level of expression that can be obtained in rodents using cationic lipid:pDNA complexes, several studies have shown that expression can be obtained that is equivalent to that seen using low multiplicities of an adenoviral vector (2,26).

Aerosol

Despite the fact that rodents are obligate nose breathers and that a large fraction of an aerosolized dose is removed before it can be deposited in the lung, several studies have demonstrated that aerosolized cationic lipid:pDNA complexes can transfect rodent lungs successfully. In addition to protecting the pDNA component from the shearing forces in a jet nebulizer by complexing it with cationic lipid, several additional important parameters are involved in aerosolizing complexes, such as the vehicle (53–55) and the nebulizer itself (55). Given estimates that less than 1% of an aerosolized dose is deposited in a rodent lung, it is important to use concentrated formulations. However, such conditions are conducive to precipitation of the complex, especially during jet nebulization. It has been found that a more concentrated dispersion of complexes can be prepared by incorporating a small percentage of a lipid containing a polyethylene glycol (PEG) headgroup (e.g., PEG coupled to phosphatidylethanolamine) (56). Using this formulation, pDNA concentrations exceeding 20 mM (measured in nucleotides) have been generated, with no loss in transfection potency. This formulation has been used successfully in clinical trials for cystic fibrosis (57,58).

In general, the kinetics of expression following an aerosol delivery of cationic lipid:pDNA complexes to rodents is similar to that seen following other delivery routes, and is likely to be most dependent on the structure of the pDNA component. In most cases, transgene expression falls rapidly to background levels over a few weeks. Because of the small amount of pDNA actually deposited, transfected cells are relatively few and difficult to visualize histologically. However, transfected cells can be seen, and are largely columnar epithelial cells of the bronchi (28).

Aerosol delivery using jet nebulizers has also demonstrated that transgene expression can be obtained in nonhuman primates (59). Thus, transgene-specific protein was found to be distributed widely throughout the airway epithelium after an aerosol delivery to rhesus monkeys (59). Importantly, aerosol clinical trials in humans have also demonstrated that vector-specific transgene expression (57), and partial correction of a genetic defect (CF), could be obtained with such an approach (58).

Targeted Complexes

For particular applications, it may be necessary to improve the therapeutic index or to alter the "tropisms" of the simple complexes. To these ends, targeting agents have been added to the simple cationic lipid: pDNA complex. For example, using a cationic lipid (DOTAP) together with a peptide consisting of a cyclic arginine-glycine-aspartic acid (RGD) domain and a DNA binding domain of 16 lysines, it has been shown possible to alter the expression pattern in rats after an intratracheal administration (60). The RGD domain was included to direct the complex to airway epithelial cells, which express the integrin target of the RGD. Compared to the untargeted complex, the RGD-targeted complex demonstrated significantly enhanced transduction of the bronchial epithelium, which is consistent with the anatomical target for CF.

The idea of targeted synthetic vectors used in an intravenous delivery mode to transduce the lung has also been evaluated by covalently attaching an antibody against platelet–endothelial cell adhesion molecule-1 (PECAM-1) to a linear polyethyleneimine (PEI) (61). The cationic PECAM-1–PEI was mixed with DNA to form a complex that when injected into the tail vein of a mouse resulted in an increase in the fraction of the injected dose localized in the lung. This increased lung delivery resulted in a significant enhancement in lung expression of the reporter gene compared to an untargeted PEI:DNA complex and also a significant decrease in the serum level of the proinflammatory cytokine tumor necrosis factor-α (TNF-α).

Tissue-Specific Expression

For some lung indications, it may be desirable to restrict transgene expression to a particular cell type. For example, CF is a disease of epithelium, not only of the lung, but of multiple organs, and it may prove to be beneficial to "target" expression by using an epithelial promoter. Using control elements, for example, promoter, polyA, from the human cytokeratin 18 (KRT18) gene to drive expression of a lacZ reporter gene, it has been shown to be possible to restrict expression to epithelial cells in which cytokeratin 18 is normally expressed, such as the lung and kidney (41). In fact "targeting" a systemically delivered cationic lipid:pDNA complex in this way led to an expression pattern consistent with that of a KRT18lacZ transgenic mouse. Thus, even though systemic delivery deposits a large amount of plasmid in the distal lung, essentially no transgene was expressed with the KRT18 construct, in contrast to the same lacZ construct driven by the more promiscuous CMV promoter, where expression in this region was apparent.

Because the operative mechanisms in a ligand-based targeting system and a tissue-specific promoter system are distinct, combining these two types of targeting into a single delivery system should lead to a synergistic effect and result in highly tissue-specific expression.

B. Toxicities Associated with Lung Gene Transfer by Cationic Lipid:pDNA Complexes

Introduction/General Comments

Historically, one of the perceived advantages of synthetic vectors in general, and cationic lipid-based systems in particular, was their lack of toxicity. Given the fact that they do not in general contain proteins, it was assumed that adaptive immune responses against the vector would not develop, as happens with virus-based gene delivery systems. This assumption has been borne out; for example, antibodies against the cationic lipid and DNA components of these vectors have not been detected (62). Predictably, however, cationic lipid:pDNA vectors are not without toxicity. Delivery of these vectors to the lung either by a luminal or systemic route has been shown to generate a characteristic spectrum of acute toxicities that sets limits on the dose of vector that can be used. In other words, like any "drug," a therapeutic index exists for cationic lipid:pDNA vectors that will inevitably determine the utility of this gene delivery system.

Toxicities Associated with Luminal Delivery to the Lung

Some early studies that delivered cationic lipid:pDNA complexes to the lungs of rodents by a luminal route reported little or no evidence of acute toxicity (27,28), perhaps because of particular aspects of dosing or administration protocols. Later work showed that instillation of complexes could cause dose-dependent acute inflammation (62,63). This inflammation was multifocal, and occurred with highest frequency at the junctions of the terminal bronchioles and alveolar ducts, locations consistent with the instillation of a fluid bolus into the distal lung. Complex instillation was also characterized by early (few hours) infiltrates of neutrophils into the luminal aspect of the lung followed by later infiltrates of macrophages and lymphocytes. Not surprisingly, these cellular infiltrates were accompanied by the acute release of proinflammatory cytokines such as interleukin-6 (IL-6), TNF-α, and interferon-γ (IFN-γ), which generally reached maximal levels in the bronchoalveolar fluid in a few days and declined to normal levels over a few weeks.

Aerosol delivery of cationic lipid:pDNA complexes to the luminal aspect of the lung would be expected to result in a more uniform deposition than instillation of a fluid bolus. In addition, since to a large degree the size of the aerosol droplet determines its site of deposition in the respiratory tract, namely, larger droplets deposit higher in the respiratory tree than smaller droplets, appropriate adjustment of the droplet size could direct deposition of complex more toward the airways and away from the alveoli. Under these conditions, aerosolizing complex to rodent lung resulted in reduced inflammation compared to instillation at equivalent levels of expression (56). Because aerosol deposition of doses equivalent to say a 100-µL instillation is experimentally difficult in a mouse, where deposited doses are more on the order of 1 µL, the possibility of aerosol toxicity at doses likely to be deposited in the human (where a much larger proportion of the inhaled dose is actually deposited), cannot be addressed adequately in rodent models.

Given that cationic lipid:pDNA complexes are composed of lipid as well as DNA, it was important to identify the source of toxicity seen following instillation in rodent models. Although the cationic lipid itself demonstrated some toxicity, the majority of the acute toxicity was found to be due to the DNA component presented to the lung in the context of a lipid complex (64). In particular, the unmethylated cytosine-guanosine deoxynucleotides (CpG) present in bacterially derived plasmid DNA were shown to be key to the observed toxicity. The frequency of unmethylated CpG motifs is roughly 20-fold higher in bacterial genomic DNA than in eukaryotic DNA, and the mammalian innate immune system has evolved an ability to recognize and respond to this structural difference (65–69). Thus, methylating the cytosines of the CpG motifs in plasmid DNA led to a significant reduction in both cellular infiltrates and inflammatory cytokines following an instillation of cationic lipid:pDNA complexes (64). Importantly, mutating 14 of the 17 consensus CpG motifs known to be most immune stimulatory in the mouse, namely, 5′-purine-purine-CG-pyrimidine-pyrimidine-3′, or 5′-RRCGYY-3′ (65), did not decrease the inflammatory cytokine response. Together with the methylation result, this result implied that additional, nonconsensus CpG motifs contributed significantly to the inflammation seen. It was subsequently shown that eliminating the majority (270/526) of the CpG motifs present in a reporter plasmid could be accomplished and did result in significantly reduced lung inflammation while preserving expression (70).

Clinical studies in CF patients demonstrated that plasmid DNA also had inflammatory consequences when aerosolized into the lung (58). Thus, aerosol delivery of cationic lipid:pDNA complexes, but not cationic liposomes, to CF subjects resulted in mild, acute flu-like symptoms in only those patients that had received the pDNA. The same clinical syndrome of fever, myalgia, and arthralgia was also seen in a second clinical trial using the same cationic lipid:pDNA complexes (57). Importantly, both of these clinical trials provided evidence of therapeutic efficacy. For example, the latter trial demonstrated the presence of wild-type cystic fibrosis transmembrane conductance regulator (CFTR) mRNA in bronchoscopic biopsies, indicating successful gene transfer and transcription.

Taken together, the clinical evidence for cationic lipid:pDNA–mediated gene transfer and the finding of pDNA-mediated toxicities in these same vectors implies that the current therapeutic index of these vectors will require significant improvement to be useful.

Toxicities Associated with Systemic Delivery to the Lung

Given the biodistribution and expression patterns of cationic lipid:pDNA complexes after systemic administration in rodents (see above), it is not surprising that significant toxicities are generated despite earlier claims to the contrary. As with luminal delivery, CpG motifs contained within the plasmid DNA were implicated in an inflammatory cytokine response—a response that could be blunted by methylation of the DNA (71). Consistent with the observations that the complexes interact with blood cells (36), the spectrum of acute toxicities seen after an intravenous administration of complex also included dose-dependent leukopenia, thrombocytopenia, and complement activation (72).

Yet another component of the toxicity was found to be the elevation of serum transaminases (e.g., aspartate aminotransferase, or AST), which is consistent with the accumulation of significant amounts of systemically administered complex in the liver (see above). These toxicities are not simply a consequence of the presence of plasmid DNA in the blood, which is rapidly degraded and much less toxic. Rather it is a consequence of the stabilization of the pDNA in the serum by cationic lipid and the subsequent interaction of this complexed DNA with host blood components and cells (72,73).

As with the pDNA-related toxicities seen after a luminal administration of complex, the systemic cytokine response can be reduced significantly while retaining lung expression by mutating and thereby eliminating vector CpG motifs (70). An alternative approach to decrease vector CpG motifs is to excise the transcriptional cassette from the bacterial plasmid. Since a large proportion of the plasmid is used only for bacterial replication (e.g., antibiotic resistance gene, bacterial origin of replication), and these sequences typically contain a large number of CpG motifs, it should be possible to decrease the number of CpG motifs per expression unit by eliminating these bacteria-specific sequences. This hypothesis was tested recently by polymerase chain reaction (PCR) amplification of the expression cassette (74), and demonstrated that significant reductions in inflammatory cytokines could be achieved without sacrificing expression.

It also has been shown that it is possible to reduce the systemic TNF-α response by sequential administration of the cationic liposome followed by naked pDNA in the mouse (75). This protocol gave an optimal increase in reporter gene expression in the lung accompanied by maximal decreases in cytokine levels when the DNA was injected a few minutes after the cationic liposomes. Indeed, most of the characteristic acute systemic toxicities noted above could be reduced by this strategy (75).

Finally, systemic administration of the anti-inflammatory steroid dexamethasone has been shown to reduce inflammatory cytokines while at the same time resulting in a significant increase in transgene expression in the lung (71). Given the similarities in the toxicity profiles following systemic and luminal delivery to the lung, it would be interesting to evaluate the effects of such anti-inflammatory agents in the context of luminal delivery models.

Overall, it is clear that the toxicities induced by cationic lipid:pDNA complexes are similar when administered by either luminal or intravenous routes. These toxicities can be traced to the recognition of bacteria-specific sequences (e.g., unmethylated CpG motifs) presented to the organism in the context of a cationic liposome. Multiple approaches, namely, elimination of CpG motifs, anti-inflammatory drugs, administration protocols, have shown promise in reducing these toxicities. It remains to be seen whether individually or together these approaches result in a vector system that possesses a therapeutic index of sufficient magnitude to be therapeutically useful.

C. General Topics/Limiting Issues

In light of the above discussion of the efficacy and toxicity attributes of cationic lipid:pDNA complexes, it is useful to ask whether there are additional characteristics of these vectors that may limit their utility for lung diseases. Two recognized limiting issues of both viral and synthetic vector systems are (1) the potential of vector administration to stimulate adaptive immune responses against the transgene product and (2) the limited persistence of transgene expression. To some extent, both of these limitations ultimately are linked to the CpG-mediated stimulation of the innate immune system, and efforts to blunt this response (see above) have borne fruit in terms of overcoming these limiting issues.

Adaptive Immune Responses Against Transgene Product

For acute lung indications where prolonged (>weeks) expression and repeat administration of the vector are not required, the stimulation of adaptive immune responses may not limit efficacy. Indeed, for diseases such as lung cancer, the generation of adaptive immune responses may even be desirable (76), and the stimulation of such responses with cationic lipid:pDNA complexes has demonstrated efficacy in several rodent tumor models (77,78). However, for genetic diseases such as cystic fibrosis, it is desirable that vector administration be as "silent" as possible to avoid the coincidence of innate immune activation and transgene expression. Especially in the case of knockouts, that is, situations in which the host immune system has not seen the transgene product, this coincidence is likely to lead to an adaptive immune response against the transgene product—clearly an undesirable outcome.

There are several potential ways to avoid or minimize the coincidence of transgene expression and immune system stimulation. First, the immune stimulatory properties of the vector can be minimized. It has been shown, for example, that by removing immune stimulatory CpG sequences from the plasmid vector the acute release of cytokines such as IFN-γ, which lead to the development of adaptive immune responses, can be significantly decreased (70). Second, immune suppression strategies (e.g., dexamethasone) also have been shown to blunt the initial immune stimulation resulting from vector administration (71). Yet another approach to decouple vector administration and expression is to target lipid:pDNA complexes *away* from antigen-presenting cells (APCs) such as macrophages (e.g., Kupffer cells) so that transgene expression does not occur in the very cells that are designed to promote adaptive immune responses. Related to this "targeting" approach is to include tissue-specific promoters (see above), so that expression in APCs can be minimized, based on the realization that even in the presence of ligand-based targeting, a significant proportion of the vector is likely to be internalized by phagocytic APCs. Obviously, by combining several of these approaches, such as immune suppression using a tissue-specific promoter as part of a CpG-reduced vector, one would hope for synergistic reductions of both acute immune stimulation and any consequent adaptive immune responses against the transgene product.

Finally, one additional approach to minimize adaptive immune responses against the transgene product is to separate in time vector administration and transgene expression. Using a small molecule as a "switch," the DNA can be engineered to include a domain responsive to the small molecule so that gene expression can be either turned on or off in response to the switch (79–81). Several examples of this strategy have been designed, and have demonstrated in principle that gene expression can be delayed until any initial, acute vector-related inflammation has subsided. Expression can then be turned on with the result that adaptive immune responses should be significantly reduced.

Persistence of Expression

A second, potentially limiting characteristic of cationic lipid:pDNA complexes for lung applications is the rapid rate at which their initial expression declines. An expression profile for a typical CMV immediate early gene promoter–driven expression cassette in mouse lung is shown in Figure 4 (82). In this example, although initial lung expression following an intranasal administration of the CMV-driven pCF1-CAT reporter gene is relatively high, it falls approximately

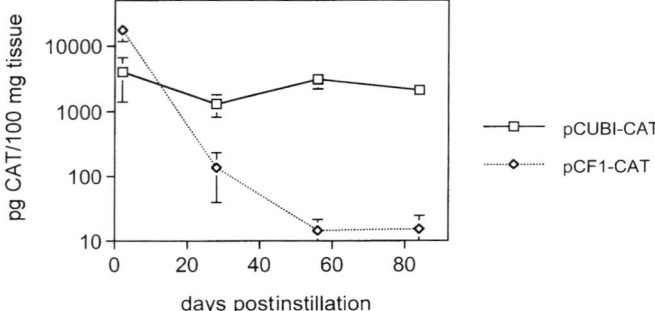

Figure 4 Comparison of lung expression profiles obtained using cytomegalovirus (pCF1; $\Diamond$) and ubiquitin B (pCUBI; $\Box$) promoters to drive CAT expression. The pCF1-CAT and pCUBI-CAT plasmids were complexed with GL67:DOPE (1:2) using a GL67:pDNA ratio of 0.6:3.6 (mol:mol) and instilled into the lungs of nude BALB/c mice. Lung expression was determined as a function of time after instillation. (From Ref. 82.)

2 logs over 3 weeks (15,45). This profile is typical of most viral expression cassettes to date, and would necessitate frequent redosing for a genetic disease such as CF. Promoter inactivation as an end result of stimulating the innate immune system appears to be a major reason for this abrupt loss of expression (82,83).

Recent efforts to improve the persistence of expression from plasmid-based vectors have included the use of (1) tissue-specific or cellular promoters (84,85), (2) linearized plasmids, which appear to form stable, nonintegrating, long-expressing concatemers (86), and (3) constructs capable of integrating into the host chromosome (e.g., "Sleeping Beauty") (87). As an indication of the improvements achievable using a mammalian promoter, Figure 4 shows a comparison of the expression profiles of a standard CMV-driven plasmid and that from a ubiquitin B–based plasmid in the lungs of mice. For mouse lung applications, coupling the human CMV immediate early gene enhancer region (−522 to −219 relative to the transcription start site) upstream of the human ubiquitin B promoter and its endogenous intron (pCUBI-CAT) led to lung expression essentially equivalent to that of the CMV-driven construct at early times (1–2 days) and persistent expression for several months at levels 2–3 logs greater than could be obtained with the parent CMV construct (82). Incorporating this construct into a CpG-depleted backbone led to not only equivalent early expression but also significantly (~1 log) *increasing* expression levels over a several month time frame (82). Clearly, the ubiquitin construct demonstrates a significant improvement in the longevity, or persistence, of expression, and represents an important advance in therapeutic utility over first-generation, virus-based promoter constructs.

IV. Future Use of Liposomes for Lung Gene Therapy

Given the limited scope of this chapter, and in light of the many related chapters designed to summarize specific disease applications for which gene therapy might be used, it is not appropriate to cover these applications here. However, it may be useful to summarize where we are presently with cationic lipid:pDNA vectors and to speculate on where they might most likely find practical use.

The past few years have seen dramatic improvements in the safety and expression profiles of these vector systems, largely due to our understanding of the biological links between the structural characteristics of the bacterially derived DNA component and the ability of the mammalian innate immune system to recognize and respond to these characteristics. As a direct consequence of this improved understanding, DNA vectors are now available with much improved persistence of expression together with reduced toxicity. Even so, use of these vectors therapeutically for lung indications still represents a challenge, especially when administered by a systemic route.

One indication that may at this time take advantage of the natural tropism of these vectors for the lung is in the systemic treatment of lung malignancies such as lung cancer. Efficacy in murine lung cancer has already been shown to respond to these vectors using a luminal delivery route (88,89). It is possible that with the judicious choice of transgene together with the immune-stimulating properties of the vector system itself, some lung cancers could be successfully treated (multiple dosing) by a systemic route. In such cases, tumor reduction might be a minimal goal, whereas stimulation of an adaptive immune response against tumor cell antigens would be the most desirable outcome (77). The systemic toxicities associated with vector delivery in this format might be acceptable and indeed even crucial to success.

Another class of indications that may deserve a renewal of effort at this juncture are those that can be approached from a luminal route. For example, additional advances have been made in our understanding of some of the factors limiting airway epithelial cell transduction and strategies for circumventing these factors (90). Thus, given the initial indications of significant efficacy following aerosol delivery of cationic lipid:pDNA complexes to CF lungs (57,58), it might prove to be illuminating to combine new "adjunct" delivery strategies (e.g., mucolytics [90]) with current vectors showing decreased toxicity and increased persistence of expression and assess the overall improvements in therapeutic index for this devastating genetic disease.

Acknowledgments

I would like to thank the Synthetic Gene Transfer Group for their unceasing efforts, and Nelson Yew and John Marshall for helping with some of the figures for this chapter.

Dedication

This chapter is dedicated respectfully to the memory of Al Fasbender, a friend and colleague who contributed much to our understanding of these vector systems, and who left us much too soon.

References

1. Zabner J, Wadsworth SC, Smith AE, Welsh MJ. Adenovirus-mediated generation of cAMP-stimulated CI transport in cystic fibrosis airway epithelium in vitro: Effects of promoter and administration method. Gene Ther 1996; 3:458–465.
2. Lee ER, Marshall J, Siegel CS, Jiang C, Yew NS, Nichols MR, Nietupski JB, Ziegler RJ, Lane MB, Wang KX, Wan NC, Scheule RK, Harris DJ, Smith AE, Cheng SH. Detailed analysis of structures and formulations of cationic lipids for efficient gene transfer to the lung. Hum Gene Ther 1996; 7(14):1701–1717.
3. Zhang Y, Jiang Q, Dudus L, Yankaskas JR, Engelhardt JF. Vector-specific complementation profiles of two independent primary defects in cystic fibrosis airways. Hum Gene Ther 1998; 9:635–648.
4. Jiang C, Finkbeiner WE, Widdicombe JH, Fang SL, Wang KX, Nietupski JB, Hehir KM, Cheng SH. Restoration of cyclic adenosine monophosphate-stimulated chloride channel activity in human cystic fibrosis tracheobronchial submucosal gland cells by adenovirus-mediated and cationic lipid-mediated gene transfer. Am J Respir Cell Mol Biol 1999; 20(6):1107–1115.
5. Scheule RK, Cheng SH. Airway delivery of cationic lipid:DNA complexes for cystic fibrosis. Adv Drug Deliv Rev 1998; 30(1–3):173–184.
6. Chesnoy S, Huang L. Structure and function of lipid-DNA complexes for gene delivery. Annu Rev Biophys Biomol Struct 2000; 29:27–47.
7. Godbey WT, Wu KK, Mikos AG. Poly(ethyleneimine) and its role in gene delivery. J Control Release 1999; 60(2–3):149–160.
8. Lemkine GF, Demeneix BA. Polyethylenemines for in vivo gene delivery. Curr Opin Mol Ther 2001; 3(2):178–182.
9. Felgner PL, Tsai YJ, Sukhu L, Wheeler CJ, Manthorpe M, Marshall J, Cheng SH. Improved cationic lipid formulations for in vivo gene therapy. Ann NY Acad Sci 1995; 772:126–139.
10. Katsel PL, Greenstein RJ. Eukaryotic gene transfer with liposomes: effect of differences in lipid structure (review). Biotechnol Annu Rev 2000; 5:197–220.
11. Lin AJ, Slack NL, Ahmad A, Koltover I, George CX, Samuel CE, Safinya CR.

Structure and structure-function studies of lipid/plasmid DNA complexes. J Drug Target 2000; 8(1):13–27.

12. Marshall J, Nietupski JB, Lee ER, Siegel CS, Rafter PW, Rudginsky SA, Chang CD, Eastman SJ, Harris DJ, Scheule RK, Cheng SH. Cationic lipid structure and formulation considerations for optimal gene transfection of the lung. J Drug Target 2000; 7(6):453–469.

13. Fasbender A, Marshall J, Moninger TO, Grunst T, Cheng S, Welsh MJ. Effect of co-lipids in enhancing cationic lipid-mediated gene transfer in vitro and in vivo. Gene Ther 1997; 4(7):716–725.

14. Cheng SH, Marshall J, Scheule RK, Smith AE. Cationic lipid formulations for intracellular gene delivery of cystic fibrosis transmembrane conductance regulator to airway epithelia. Methods Enzymol 1998; 292:697–717.

15. Yew NS, Wysokenski DM, Wang KX, Ziegler RJ, Marshall J, McNeilly D, Cherry M, Osburn W, Cheng SH. Optimization of plasmid vectors for high-level expression in lung epithelial cells. Hum Gene Ther 1997; 8:575–584.

16. Kennedy MT, Pozharshi EV, Rakhmanova VA, MacDonald RC. Factors governing the assembly of cationic phospholipid-DNA complexes. Biophys J 2000; 78:1620–1633.

17. Spink CH, Chaires JB. Thermodynamics of the binding of a cationic lipid to DNA. J Am Chem Soc 1997; 119:10920–10928.

18. Radler JO, Koltover I, Salditt T, Safinya CR. Structure of DNA-cationic liposome complexes: DNA intercalation in multilamellar membranes in distinct interhelical packing regimes. Science 1997; 275:810–814.

19. Zuidam NJ, Hirsch-Lerner D, Marguilies S, Barenholz Y. Biochim Biophys Acta 1999; 1419:207–220.

20. Templeton NS, Lasic DD, Frederik PM, Strey HH, Roberts DD, Pavlakis GN. Improved DNA: liposome complexes for increased systemic delivery and gene expression. Nat Biotechnol 1997; 15:647–652.

21. Tam P, Monck M, Lee D, Ludkovski O, Leng EC, Clow K, Stark H, Scherrer P, Graham RW, Cullis PR. Stabilized plasmid-lipid particles for systemic gene therapy. Gene Ther 2000; 7(21):1867–1874.

22. Ferrari ME, Nguyen CM, Zelphati O, Tsai Y, Felgner PL. Analytical methods for the characterization of cationic lipid-nucleic acid complexes. Hum Gene Ther 1998; 9:341–351.

23. Dash PR, Read ML, Barrett LB, Wolfert MA, Seymour LW. Factors affecting blood clearance and in vivo distribution of polyelectrolyte complexes for gene delivery. Gene Ther 1999; 6:643–650.

24. Yang J-P, Huang L. Overcoming the inhibitory effect of serum on lipofection by increasing the charge ratio of cationic liposome to DNA. Gene Ther 1997; 4:950–960.

25. Audouy S, Molema G, deLeij L, Hoekstra D. Serum as a modulator of lipoplex-mediated gene transfection: dependence of amphiphile, cell type and complex stability. J Gene Med 2000; 2:465–476.

26. Gorman CM, Aikawa M, Fox B, Fox E, Lapuz C, Michaud B, Nguyen H, Roche E, Sawa T, Wiener-Kronish JP. Efficient in vivo delivery of DNA to pulmonary cells using the novel lipid EDMPC. Gene Ther 1997; 4(9):983–992.

27. Logan JJ, Bebok Z, Walker LC, Peng S, Felgner PL, Siegal GP, Frizzell RA, Dong J, Howard M, Matalon S, et al. Cationic lipids for reporter gene and CFTR transfer to rat pulmonary epithelium. Gene Ther 1995; 2(1):38–49.
28. McLachlan G, Davidson DJ, Stevenson BJ, Dickinson P, Davidson-Smith H, Dorin JR, Porteous DJ. Evaluation in vitro and in vivo of cationic liposome-expression construct complexes for cystic fibrosis gene therapy. Gene Ther 1995; 2:614–622.
29. Fortunati E, Bout A, Zanta MA, Valerio D, Scarpa M. In vitro and in vivo gene transfer to pulmonary cells mediated by cationic liposomes. Biochim Biophys Acta 1996; 1306(1):55–62.
30. Caplen NJ, Kinrade E, Sorgi F, Gao X, Gruenert D, Gededs D, Coutelle C, Huang L, Alton EWFW, Williamson R. In vitro liposome-mediated DNA transfection of epithelial cell lines using the cationic liposome DC-Chol/DOPE. Gene Ther 1995; 2:603–613.
31. Fasbender AJ, Zabner J, Welsh MJ. Optimization of cationic lipid-mediated gene transfer to airway epithelia. Am J Physiol 1995; 269(Lung Cell Mol Physiol 13): L45–L51.
32. Wheeler CJ, Felgner PL, Tsai YJ, Marshall J, Sukhu L, Doh SG, Hartikka J, Nietupski J, Manthorpe M, Nichols M, Plewe M, Liang X, Norman J, Smith A, Cheng SH. A novel cationic lipid greatly enhances plasmid DNA delivery and expression in mouse lung. Proc Natl Acad Sci USA. 1996; 93(21):11454–11459.
33. Griesenbach U, Chonn A, Cassady R, Hannam V, Ackerley C, Post M, Tanswell AK, Olek K, O'Brodovich H, Tsui L-C. Comparison between intratracheal and intravenous administration of liposome-DNA complexes for cystic fibrosis gene therapy. Gene Ther 1998; 5:181–188.
34. Mahato RI, Anwer K, Tagliaferri F, Meaney C, Leonard P, Wadhwa MS, Logan M, French M, Rolland A. Biodistribution and gene expression of lipid/plasmid complexes after systemic administration. Hum Gene Ther 1998; 9(14):2083–2099.
35. Li S, Tseng WC, Stolz DB, Wu SP, Watkins SC, Huang L. Dynamic changes in the characteristics of cationic lipidic vectors after exposure to mouse serum: implications for intravenous lipofection. Gene Ther 1999; 6(4):585–594.
36. McLean JW, Fox EA, Baluk P, Bolton PB, Haskell A, Pearlman R, Thurston G, Umemoto EY, McDonald DM. Organ-specific endothelial cell uptake of cationic liposome-DNA complexes in mice. Am J Physiol 1997; 273(1 Pt 2):H387–H404.
37. Sakurai F, Nishioka T, Saito H, Baba T, Okuda A, Matsumoto O, Taga T, Yamashita F, Takakura Y, Hashida M. Interaction between DNA-cationic liposome complexes and erythrocytes is an important factor in systemic gene transfer via the intravenous route in mice: the role of the neutral helper lipid. Gene Ther 2001; 8(9):677–686.
38. Mahato RI, Kawabata K, Takakura Y, Hashida M. In vivo disposition characteristics of plasmid DNA complexed with cationic liposomes. J Drug Target 1995; 3:149–157.
39. Osaka G, Carey K, Cuthbertson A, Godowski P, Patapoff T, Ryan A, Gadek T, Mordenti J. Pharmacokinetics, tissue distribution, and expression efficiency of plasmid [33P]DNA following intravenous administration of DNA/cationic lipid complexes in mice: use of a novel radionuclide approach. J Pharm Sci 1996; 85(6):612–618.
40. Thierry AR, Rabinovich P, Peng B, Mahan LC, Bryant JL, Gallo RC. Characteriza-

tion of liposome-mediated gene delivery: expression, stability and pharmacokinetics of plasmid DNA. Gene Ther 1997; 4(3):226–237.

41. Koehler DR, Hannam V, Belcastro R, Steer B, Wen Y, Post M, Downey G, Transwell AK, Hu J. Targeting transgene expression for cystic fibrosis gene therapy. Mol Ther 2001; 4(1):58–65.

42. Barron LG, Gagne L, Szoka FC Jr. Lipoplex-mediated gene delivery to the lung occurs within 60 minutes of intravenous administration. Hum Gene Ther 1999; 10(10):1683–1694.

43. Song YK, Liu F, Chu S, Liu D. Characterization of cationic liposome-mediated gene transfer in vivo by intravenous administration. Hum Gene Ther 1997; 8(13):1585–1594.

44. Parker SE, Ducharme S, Norman J, Wheeler CJ. Tissue distribution of the cytofectin component of a plasmid-DNA/cationic lipid complex following intravenous administration in mice. Hum Gene Ther 1997; 8(4):393–401.

45. McClarrinon M, Gilkey L, Watral V, Fox B, Bullock C, Fradkin L, Liggitt D, Roche L, Bussey LB, Fox E, Gorman C. In vivo studies of gene expression via transient transgenesis using lipid-DNA delivery. DNA Cell Biol 1999; 18(7):533–547.

46. Hofland HE, Nagy D, Liu JJ, Spratt K, Lee YL, Danos O, Sullivan SM. In vivo gene transfer by intravenous administration of stable cationic lipid/DNA complex. Pharm Res 1997; 14(6):742–749.

47. Uyechi LS, Gagne L, Thurston G, Szoka FC Jr. Mechanism of lipoplex gene delivery in mouse lung: binding and internalization of fluorescent lipid and DNA components. Gene Ther 2001; 8(11):828–836.

48. Liu F, Qi H, Huang L, Liu D. Factors controlling the efficiency of cationic lipid-mediated transfection in vivo via intravenous administration. Gene Ther 1997; 4(6):517–523.

49. Zhu N, Liggitt D, Liu Y, Debs R. Systemic gene expression after intravenous DNA delivery into adult mice. Science 1993; 261:209–211.

50. Philip R, Liggitt D, Philip M, Dazin P, Debs R. In vivo gene delivery: Efficient transfection of T lymphocytes in adult mice. J Biol Chem 1993; 268:16087–16090.

51. Thierry AR, Lunardi-Iskandar Y, Bryant JL, Rabinovich P, Gallo RC, Mahan LC. Systemic gene therapy: biodistribution and long-term expression of a transgene in mice. Proc Natl Acad Sci USA 1995; 92:9742–9746.

52. Oudrhiri N, Vigneron JP, Peuchmaur M, Leclerc T, Lehn JM, Lehn P. Gene transfer by guanidinium-cholesterol cationic lipids into airway epithelial cells in vitro and in vivo. Proc Natl Acad Sci USA 1997; 94(5):1651–1656.

53. Guillaume C, Delepine P, Droal C, Montier T, Tymen G, Claude F. Aerosolization of cationic lipid-DNA complexes: lipoplex characterization and optimization of aerosol delivery conditions. Biochem Biophys Res Commun 2001; 286(3):464–471.

54. Pillai R, Petrak K, Blezinger P, Deshpande D, Florack V, Freimark B, Padmabandu G, Rolland A. Ultrasonic nebulization of cationic lipid-based gene delivery systems for airway administration. Pharm Res 1998; 15(11):1743–1747.

55. Eastman SJ, Tousignant JD, Lukason MJ, Murray H, Siegel CS, Constantino P, Harris DJ, Cheng SH, Scheule RK. Optimization of formulations and conditions for the aerosol delivery of functional cationic lipid:DNA complexes. Hum Gene Ther 1997; 8(3):313–322.

56. Eastman SJ, Lukason MJ, Tousignant JD, Murray H, Lane MD, St George JA, Akita GY, Cherry M, Cheng SH, Scheule RK. A concentrated and stable aerosol formulation of cationic lipid:DNA complexes giving high-level gene expression in mouse lung. Hum Gene Ther 1997; 8(6):765–773.

57. Ruiz FE, Clancy JP, Perricone MA, Bebok Z, Hong JS, Cheng SH, Meeker DP, Young KR, Schoumacher RA, Weatherly MR, Wing L, Morris JE, Sindel L, Rosenberg M, van Ginkel FW, McGhee JR, Kelly D, Lyrene RK, Sorscher EJ. A clinical inflammatory syndrome attributable to aerosolized lipid-DNA administration in cystic fibrosis. Hum Gene Ther 2001; 12(7):751–761.

58. Alton EWFW, Stern M, Farley R, Jaffe A, Chadwick SL, Phillips J, Davies J, Smith SN, Browning J, Davies MG, Hodson ME, Durham SR, Li D, Jeffery PK, Scallan M, Balfour R, Eastman SJ, Cheng SH, Smith AE, Meeker D, Geddes DM. Cationic lipid-mediated CFTR gene transfer to the lungs and nose of patients with cystic fibrosis: a double-blind placebo-controlled trial. Lancet 1999; 353:947–954.

59. McDonald RJ, Liggitt HD, Roche L, Nguyen HT, Pearlman R, Raabe OG, Bussey LB, Gorman CM. Aerosol delivery of lipid:DNA complexes to lungs of rhesus monkeys. Pharm Res 1998; 15(5):671–679.

60. Jenkins RG, Herrick SE, Meng Q-H, Kinnon C, Laurent GJ, McAnulty RJ, Hart SL. An integrin-targeted non-viral vector for pulmonary gene therapy. Gene Ther 2000; 7:393–400.

61. Li S, Tan Y, Viroonchatapan E, Pitt BR, Huang L. Targeted gene delivery to pulmonary endothelium by anti-PECAM antibody. Am J Physiol 2000; 278 (Lung Cell Mol Physiol):L504–L511.

62. Scheule RK, St George JA, Bagley RG, Marshall J, Kaplan JM, Akita GY, Wang KX, Lee ER, Harris DJ, Jiang C, Yew NS, Smith AE, Cheng SH. Basis of pulmonary toxicity associated with cationic lipid-mediated gene transfer to the mammalian lung. Hum Gene Ther 1997; 8(6):689–707.

63. Freimark BD, Blezinger HP, Florack VJ, Nordstrom JL, Long SD, Deshpande DS, Nochumson S, Petrak KL. Cationic lipids enhance cytokine and cell influx levels in the lung following administration of plasmid: cationic lipid complexes. J Immunol 1998; 160(9):4580–4586.

64. Yew NS, Wang KX, Przybylska M, Bagley RG, Stedman M, Marshall J, Scheule RK, Cheng SH. Contribution of plasmid DNA to inflammation in the lung after administration of cationic lipid:pDNA complexes. Hum Gene Ther 1999; 10(2): 223–234.

65. Krieg AM, Yi A-K, Matson S, Waldschmidt TJ, Bishop GA, Teasdale R, Koretzky G, Klinman D. CpG motifs in bacterial DNA trigger direct B-cell activation. Nature 1995; 374:546–549.

66. Krieg AM. The role of CpG motifs in innate immunity. Curr Opin Immunol 2000; 12:35–43.

67. Klinman DM, Yi AK, Beaucage SL, Conover J, Krieg AM. CpG motifs present in bacterial DNA rapidly induce lymphocytes to secrete interleukin-6, interleukin-12, and interferon-gamma. Proc Natl Acad Sci USA 1996; 93:2879–2883.

68. Janeway Jr CA. The immune system evolved to discriminate infectious nonself from noninfectious self. Immunol Today 1992; 13:11–16.

69. Matzinger P. Tolerance, danger, and the extended family. Annu Rev Immunol 1994; 12:991–1045.

70. Yew NS, Zhao H, Wu IH, Song A, Tousignant JD, Przybylska M, Cheng SH. Reduced inflammatory response to plasmid DNA vectors by elimination and inhibition of immunostimulatory CpG motifs. Mol Ther 2000; 1(3):255–262.

71. Tan Y, Li S, Pitt BR, Huang L. The inhibitory role of CpG immunostimulatory motifs in cationic lipid vector-mediated transgene expression in vivo. Hum Gene Ther 1999; 10(13):2153–2161.

72. Tousignant JD, Gates AL, Ingram LA, Johnson CL, Nietupski JB, Cheng SH, Eastman SJ, Scheule RK. Comprehensive analysis of the acute toxicities induced by systemic administration of cationic lipid:plasmid DNA complexes in mice. Hum Gene Ther 2000; 11:2493–2513.

73. Loisel S, Le Gall C, Doucet L, Ferec C, Floch V. Contribution of plasmid DNA to hepatotoxicity after systemic administration of lipoplexes. Hum Gene Ther 2001; 12(6):685–696.

74. Hofman CR, Dileo JP, Li Z, Li S, Huang L. Efficient in vivo gene transfer by PCR amplified fragment with reduced inflammatory activity. Gene Ther 2001; 8:71–74.

75. Tan Y, Liu F, Li Z, Li S, Huang L. Sequential injection of cationic liposome and plasmid DNA effectively transfects the lung with minimal inflammatory toxicity. Mol Ther 2001; 3(5):673–682.

76. Scheule RK. The role of CpG motifs in immunostimulation and gene therapy. Adv Drug Deliv Rev 2000; 44(2–3):119–134.

77. Lanuti M, Rudginsky S, Force SD, Lambright S, Siders WM, Chang MY, Amin KM, Kaiser LR, Scheule RK, Albelda SM. Cationic lipid:bacterial DNA complexes elicit adaptive cellular immunity in murine intraperitoneal tumor models. Cancer Res 2000; 60:2955–2963.

78. Dow SW, Fradkin LG, Liggitt DH, Willson AP, Heath TD, Potter TA. Lipid-DNA complexes induce potent activation of innate immune responses and antitumor activity when administered intravenously. J Immunol 1999; 163(3):1552–1561.

79. Clackson T. Controlling mammalian gene expression with small molecules. Current Opin Chem Biol 1997; 1:210–218.

80. Wang Y, DeMayo FJ, Tsai SY, O'Malley BW. Ligand-inducible and liver-specific target gene expression in transgenic mice. Nat Biotechnol 1997; 15:239–243.

81. Rivera VM, Ye X, Courage NL, Sachar J, Cerasoli Jr F, Wilson JM, Gilman M. Long-term regulated expression of growth hormone in mice after intramuscular gene transfer. Proc Natl Acad Sci USA 1999; 96:8657–8662.

82. Yew NS, Przybylska M, Ziegler RJ, Liu D, Cheng SH. High and sustained transgene expression in vivo from plasmid vectors containing a hybrid ubiquitin promoter. Mol Ther 2001; 4(1):75–82.

83. Li S, Wu SP, Whitmore M, Loeffert EJ, Wang L, Watkins SC, Pitt BR, Huang L. Effect of immune response on gene transfer to the lung via systemic administration of cationic lipidic vectors. Am J Physiol 1999; 276(5 Pt 1):L796–L804.

84. Hagstrom JN, Couto LB, Scallan C, Burton M, McCleland ML, Fields PA, Arruda VR, Herzog RW, High KA. Improved muscle-derived expression of human coagulation factor IX from a skeletal actin/CMV hybrid enhancer/promoter. Blood 2000; 95:2536–2542.

85. Koeberl DD, Bonham L, Halbert CL, Allen JM, Birkebak T, Miller AD. Persistent, therapeutically relevant levels of human granulocyte colony-stimulating factor in mice after systemic delivery of adeno-associated virus vectors. Hum Gene Ther 1999; 10(13):2133–2140.

86. Chen Z-Y, Yant SR, He C-Y, Meuse L, Shen S, Kay MA. Linear DNAs concatemerize in vivo and result in sustained transgene expression in mouse liver. Mol Ther 2001; 3(3):403–410.

87. Yant SR, Meuse L, Chiu W, Ivics Z, Izsvak Z, Kay MA. Somatic integration and long-term transgene expression in normal and haemophilic mice using a DNA transposon system. Nat Genet 2000; 25(1):35–41.

88. Zou Y, Zong G, Ling YH, Perez-Soler R. Development of cationic liposome formulations for intratracheal gene therapy of early lung cancer. Cancer Gene Ther 2000; 7(5):683–696.

89. Blezinger P, Freimark BD, Matar M, Wilson E, Singhal A, Min W, Nordstrom JL, Pericle F. Intratracheal administration of interleukin 12 plasmid-cationic lipid complexes inhibits murine lung metastases. Hum Gene Ther 1999; 10(5):723–731.

90. Ferrari S, Kitson C, Farley R, Steel R, Marriott C, Parkins DA, Scarpa M, Wainwright B, Evans MJ, Colledge WH, Geddes DM, Alton EW. Mucus altering agents as adjuncts for nonviral gene transfer to airway epithelium. Gene Ther 2001; 8(18): 1380–1386.

5

Targeting Gene Delivery for Pulmonary Disease

PAUL N. REYNOLDS

Royal Adelaide Hospital
Adelaide, South Australia, Australia

I. Introduction

There have been major advances in the understanding of the molecular pathogenesis of disease in recent years. The effective translation of this knowledge into
viable gene-based therapies is a now a major challenge. At the conceptual level,
gene therapy may be firmly established, but practical application still faces many
hurdles. Basic issues of efficiency of gene delivery, duration of gene expression,
and the toxicity of the gene delivery vectors themselves are currently areas of
intense research. An important aspect of these endeavors are strategies that seek
to incorporate specific targeting attributes into vector design, thereby optimizing
gene delivery to the appropriate target cells, avoiding gene delivery to nontarget
areas, and ideally also reducing the total dose of vector needed, thus reducing
potential vector-related toxicity. The majority of recent targeting efforts have
focused on the adenovirus (Ad, typically serotypes 2 and 5), based largely on its
relatively higher in vivo gene delivery efficiency than other agents (1,2). The
current discussion will be focused primarily on Ad; however, there has also been
some renewed interest in targeting retroviral vectors (3) as well as developments
for other viral agents (e.g., adeno-associated virus) and nonviral particles.

119

The inadequacy of gene delivery vectors for pulmonary disease became apparent in the clinical trials for cystic fibrosis (4). Despite the apparent tropism of Ad-5 for the respiratory tract (based on the spectrum of clinical disease it causes), the ability of this agent to deliver genes to respiratory epithelium was found to be inefficient. An understanding of the basic biology of Ad infection helps to explain some of the problems encountered in this and other pulmonary applications, and suggests strategies for improvement. In approaching this issue, many factors must be considered, including the natural in vivo distribution of Ad receptors, structural constraints in designing modified vectors, and the impact of nonspecific sequestration of vector by the reticuloendothelial system. The relative importance of specificity versus efficiency will be application dependent and must be factored into the overall design of the vector system.

II. Pathway of Ad Infection

The adenovirus is an unenveloped icosahedral particle with 12 fibers projecting outwardly from the vertices (5) (Fig. 1). Each fiber consists of a homotrimer of 62-kD subunits, with each subunit comprising a tail, shaft, and knob domain. During the assembly phase of viral replication, fiber monomers trimerize in the cytoplasm, and then the tail of the fiber binds to a viral penton base protein that is subsequently incorporated into the rest of the viral capsid within the cell nucleus. The knob region of the fiber is responsible for two critical functions— correct trimer formation and binding to the primary Ad cell-surface receptor (the coxsackie and adenovirus receptor, CAR (6–8)). Thus, an understanding of the biology of the knob domain and CAR is an important basis from which to consider targeting strategies.

CAR is a member of the immunoglobulin superfamily of molecules, possessing two extracellular immunoglobulin-like domains (D1 and D2) (6). The intracellular region of the molecule does not appear to be critical for Ad infection, as truncated receptors lacking this domain function as Ad receptors (9,10). Several studies of the airway epithelium have noted that CAR is located on the basolateral surface of these cells beneath the tight junctions, and is virtually absent on the accessible apical surface (11–13). This fact clearly contributes to the poor transduction efficacy noted in the cystic fibrosis trials. In addition, a relative deficiency of CAR has been noted in other Ad-resistant targets (14–18), especially tumor cells. For example, analysis of CAR levels in primary ovarian cancer cells from malignant ascites has shown that these cells are variably low in CAR expression and that this correlates to poor transducibility with Ad vectors (19). As yet, there is little direct information about CAR expression in other primary tumors, but CAR deficiency has been noted in several established and primary cell lines including melanoma, pancreas, lung, and glioma (14,20–22). In these analyses,

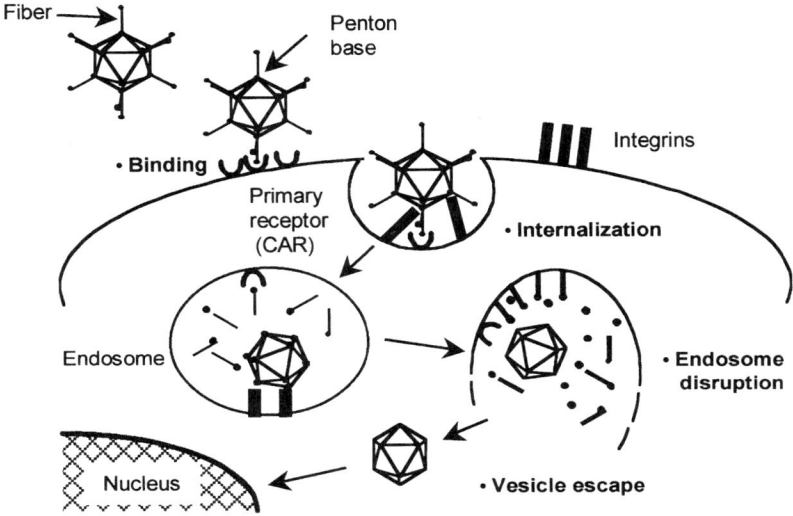

Figure 1   The pathway of adenoviral infection. Primary binding is mediated by the inter-action of the knob domain of the Ad fiber with the cellular receptor, CAR. This is followed by an interaction between RGD motifs in the penton base with cellular integrins, which mediates internalization of the virion into an endosome. Endosomal disruption occurs via mechanisms involving the penton base and the low endosomal pH. The partially disassem-bled virion particle is then transported to the nuclear membrane for release of viral DNA into the nucleus.

a direct correlation between CAR expression and transducibility with Ad vectors has been noted. In other studies using primary material, CAR deficiency has been inferred by Ad resistance to transduction, which has successfully been overcome by retargeting strategies (e.g., to head and neck tumor (16)). Recently, some evidence has been presented suggesting that the relative paucity of CAR on tu-mors may actually have functional significance, in that CAR may have some role as a tumor suppressor. Okegawa et al. (23) found a correlation between low CAR state and high rate of tumor growth. However, at this time, the normal function of CAR remains unknown and no successful generation of a CAR knockout transgenic mouse has been reported.

Although the relative lack of CAR is a problem in some tissues, high levels of CAR expression in nontarget tissues is a problem of equal importance. This is especially relevant for the liver, where high CAR levels contribute to vector sequestration in this organ after systemic administration, leading to direct vector-related toxicity as well as toxicity associated with the expression of transgenes intended for elsewhere (e.g., suicide genes intended for cancer therapy (24)).

Thus, the ability to avoid transduction of hepatocytes and other nontarget cells goes hand-in-hand with the need to achieve high-efficiency gene delivery to the target cells.

The regions of the Ad knob responsible for interacting with CAR have been determined. Roelvink et al. showed that the great majority of Ad serotypes (with the exception of those in subgroup B) had the capacity to bind to this receptor (8). Through a combination of sequence comparison and extensive mutation analysis, regions predicted to be exposed on the side of the knob domain were found to be critical for binding to CAR (25). These regions are loop structures that link together the eight B strands of the knob, which are arranged in two sheets; the V sheet faces the virion and the R sheet faces outward. The crystal structure of the complex formed between the CAR D1 domain and Ad-12 knob has also been determined (26). Furthermore, specific point mutations have been identified that enable CAR recognition to be ablated without perturbation of fiber trimerization. These mutations can be placed in loop regions, particularly the AB and DG loops. This work has since been confirmed by others (27,28) and forms an important basis for the future design of genetic tropism modification.

Following attachment, viral entry requires a second step involving an interaction between Arg-Gly-Asp (RGD) motifs in the Ad penton base and cell surface integrins (typically $\alpha_v\beta_3$ or $\alpha_v\beta_5$, but others may be used (29)), which then leads to endocytosis of the virion (30). A lack of integrins on the cell surface contributes to poor Ad transducibility for certain cells (21,31), although for cells which express high amounts of CAR, a lack of integrins is not a major impediment to transduction (32). In general, CAR deficiency seems more widespread and tends to be the dominant rate-limiting factor. In the endosome, the virus undergoes a stepwise disassembly and endosomal lysis occurs (a process mediated by the penton base and low endosomal pH), followed by transport of the viral DNA to the cell nucleus (5). This endosomolytic step is critical for efficient gene delivery, and the ability of Ad to effect endosomal escape is one of the key factors in its efficiency as a vector. In this regard, work by Curiel et al. established that the steps of cell entry and subsequent endosomal escape were functionally uncoupled, which thus allows the feasibility of achieving efficient transgene expression after Ad infection through a nonnative pathway (33). This principle was demonstrated using Ad vectors linked via a polycation (polylysine) bridge (AdpL) to plasmid DNA and to human transferrin as an alternate receptor ligand. Incorporation of Ad into the vector complex in this way achieved several orders of magnitude enhancement of transgene expression compared to plasmid-polylysine-transferrin alone, reflecting the endosomal escape properties of Ad. When a neutralizing antibody that blocked interaction of the Ad with CAR was used to ensure cell entry was restricted to the transferrin pathway, no decrement in transgene expression was seen. In contrast, efforts to target retroviral vectors through alternate cell surface receptor pathways (e.g., epidermal growth factor receptor, EGFR (34)) have been less successful, being compromised by perturbation of postbinding trafficking, leading to endosomal destruction of the vector.

From the foregoing, it can be seen that a relative deficiency or inaccessibility of either CAR or cellular integrins could potentially limit the capacity of the Ad vector to accomplish efficient gene delivery. For locoregional application of vector to the airways, nonspecific enhancement of transduction has been achieved by combining Ad with cationic liposomes (35), EGTA (36,37), calcium phosphate precipitates (38,39), and perfluorochemical liquids (40). Others have shown improvements by prior disruption of tight junctions with detergents (41). The current discussion will focus on efforts to achieve cell-specific gene delivery by tropism modification of Ad to achieve infection via specific, receptor-mediated, CAR-independent pathways.

III.   Conjugate-Based Retargeting Approaches

If one could target to receptors that are expressed on the cell surface at higher levels than CAR, improved efficiency could be achieved. Several strategies to achieve such CAR-independent gene transfer have been devised, although these can be considered in two main groups—a two-component approach in which the Ad is combined with bispecific adapter molecules and an approach involving direct genetic modification of the virion itself. In the first approach, targeting has been achieved by the development of bispecific adapters which simultaneously bind to Ad and to a cellular receptor (42) (Fig. 2). Such retargeting complexes were initially designed to achieve linkage to the Ad via an antibody, or its Fab fragment, with specific recognition for the knob domain of the Ad fiber protein. The rationality of this approach was that one could simultaneously ablate native tropism and impart new tropism, thereby potentially improving both efficiency and specificity of Ad infection. Douglas et al. (42) established this principle using an antiknob Fab linked to folate. Specific, folate-mediated binding to cells expressing the folate receptor was demonstrated. Furthermore, the magnitude of transgene expression achieved via this route was similar to that seen with native Ad infection, unlike many of the earlier efforts used to retarget retroviral vectors which had resulted in substantial losses in efficacy. These results were thus consistent with the earlier data using AdpL—that an alternate cellular entry pathway did not compromise subsequent intracellular endosomal processing.

Successful retargeting of Ad has now been achieved using a variety of chemical conjugates between an antiknob Fab and natural ligands specific for cell surface receptors (folate (42), fibroblast growth factor [FGF] (43–46), tetanus toxin fragment (47)) as well as antireceptor antibodies (including anti–epidermal growth factor receptor [EGF-R] (14),-EpCAM (48), -TAG-72 (19), and -CD40 (49)).

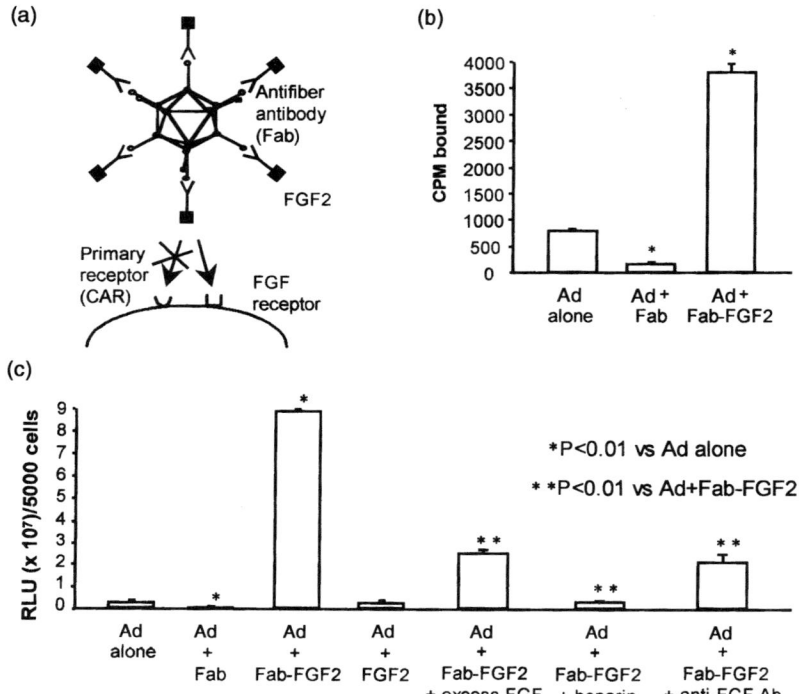

Figure 2 Conjugate-based retargeting using targeting to FGF receptors to illustrate the principle. (a) Retargeting schema. (b) [³H]-labeled Ad vector alone or after incubation with Fab or Fab-FGF2 was bound to human umbilical vein endothelial cells (HUVECs) at 4°C for 1 hr. Following washing, cell-bound radioactivity (CPM) was measured in a scintillation counter. Enhanced binding of virus to cells in the presence of conjugate is shown. (c) Anti-knob Fab alone or Fab-FGF2 was incubated with 10⁸ particles of an Ad vector carrying the luciferase reporter gene (AdCMVLuc). Thirty minutes later the complexes were added to 24-well plates containing HUVECs. After incubation for 24 hr at 37°C, cells were lysed and extracts assayed for luciferase activity. Specificity of FGF2 retargeting was confirmed by blocking with heparin, excess FGF, or anti-FGF antiserum. Free FGF2 alone had no stimulatory effect on Ad-mediated luciferase expression. (Adapted from Ref. 45.)

Employment of this retargeting approach has established several key concepts. First, it could be shown unequivocally that Ad could achieve effective gene delivery via several different CAR-independent cellular entry pathways without compromising the critical subsequent steps of endosomal escape. Second, the achievement of CAR-independent cell infection allowed augmented levels of gene transfer, sometimes by 100-fold or more, to cells naturally lacking CAR. Indeed, the concept of retargeting Ad has now been firmly established as a means generally to improve the susceptibility of target cells in vitro and, at least locoregionally, in vivo (1). Third, the new target receptor did not necessarily need intrinsic internalization capabilities, suggesting the native penton-base integrin interaction may still provide this function, thereby broadening the range of potential targets one could consider. Fourth, for those cells that lack both CAR and integrins (e.g., T lymphocytes), retargeting could achieve both of these functions (in this case, by targeting to CD3 (50) and more recently to B lymphocytes via CD70 (51)). Fifth, enhanced infectivity was shown to translate to improved therapeutic outcome (52,53). Using a locoregional murine model of ovarian carcinoma and a bispecific conjugate to target to FGF receptors, Rancourt et al. established two key principles—improved outcome at equivalent Ad dose with targeting or similar outcome at a lower dose of Ad particles when targeting was used; the latter result thus suggesting a mechanism to reduce the well-recognized dose-dependant toxicity associated with Ad vectors. Subsequent studies also indicated that retargeting could reduce ectopic hepatic transgene expression and thereby mitigate against the hepatic toxicity associated with suicide gene therapy for cancer (46). As well as demonstrating reduced toxicity, this study also showed enhanced therapeutic efficacy when the FGF retargeting approach was used to improve suicide gene delivery to a melanoma line prior to tumor implantation (although this stopped short of showing true retargeting in vivo).

In addition to benefits that directly accrue from the improvement in efficiency and/or specificity of gene delivery, the targeting moiety itself may act in a synergistic manner to improve the overall biological activity of the therapy. For example, Tillman et al. showed that use of an anti-CD40 targeting moiety to enhance gene delivery to dendritic cells not only achieved improved gene expression but also lead to maturation of the cells via CD40 cross linking, thus improving the overall efficacy of a DNA-based antitumor vaccine (53).

Despite the progress in conjugate-based approaches, this strategy has not yet demonstrated efficacy in vivo for airway epithelial gene delivery. Progress is hampered by a relative paucity of receptors suitable for targeting on the lumenal aspect of airway epithelium, and possibly by physical factors that limit Ad penetration. In this regard, Pickles et al. investigated a model system where they successfully achieved CAR expression on the apical surface of polarized epithelial cells (canine kidney cells; MDCK) in an effort to determine whether CAR accessibility was the only limiting factor (9). The cells were transduced with CAR linked to a gycosyl-phosphatidyl-inositol (GPI) anchor, which successfully directed the receptor expression to the apical membrane, as confirmed by immunohistochemistry. Subsequent infection with Ad was not enhanced until the cell surface was treated with enzymes to remove sialic acid residues in glycocalyx. The investigators hypothesized that glycocalyx may also present a barrier for airway epithelial transduction. However, in contrast, Walters et al. found that apical membrane localization of CAR in polarized human airway epithelium did allow for Ad transduction and to equivalent levels as that achieved when Ad was applied to the basal side of the cells (i.e., where native CAR is normally expressed) (10). Thus the real relevance of glycocalyx in vivo is yet to be determined. Very few specific targets have been evaluated for airway epithelial transduction. One of the few is the $P2Y_2$ receptor. In a multilayered proof-of principle approach, polarized human cells were sequentially exposed to a biotinylated $P2Y_2$ receptor ligand (UTP), then streptavidin, then biotinylated Ad (54). Enhanced transduction was reported, but data were only presented in the context of prior digestion of glycocalyx. Targeting to polarized human cells has also been achieved by the use of a novel peptide ligand identified by bacteriophage panning (55) and to the urokinase plasminogen activator (uPA) receptor using a short peptide derived from uPA (56). In both cases, the peptides were linked to Ad by the use of polyethylene glycol (PEG), and neither has been assessed in vivo. Thus, the achievement of truly specific airway epithelial transduction remains a challenge.

There has been more success in achieving targeted transduction of pulmonary endothelium than epithelium. We used a conjugate that binds to angiotensin-converting enzyme (ACE) to target Ad selectively to pulmonary vascular endothelial cells via tail vein injection in rats (57). ACE is an attractive target for several reasons, most especially its high level of expression throughout the pulmonary capillary bed (58). Although ACE is expressed on vessels elsewhere, the levels of expression are significantly lower than in the lung and, of particular relevance to Ad-targeting strategies, ACE expression is not seen on hepatic sinusoids. Furthermore, there is relevance to disease, because ACE expression is upregulated in areas of vascular remodeling associated with pulmonary hypertension, as seen in rats exposed to hypoxia, as well as in humans with primary pulmonary hypertension (PPH) (59,60). The recent discovery of the gene responsible for familial PPH, the bone morphogenetic protein receptor type 2 (BMPR2) gene (61,62), raises the possibility of a genetic therapy for this disease; thus an ACE-based targeting approach may be particularly useful in this setting. Several studies by Danilov et al. have shown the potential utility of targeting to ACE for the delivery of therapeutic agents to pulmonary endothelium. These studies are based on the use of monoclonal antibodies against ACE, especially the antibody mAb-9B9 (63). This antibody in particular has shown very good selectivity for pulmonary targeting and has been used in conjugate form to deliver agents such as superoxide dismutase and catalase to the lungs in animal models (64,65). We therefore constructed a conjugate between this antibody and the Fab fragment of the antiknob monoclonal 1D6.14. Ad infection and gene delivery via binding to ACE was confirmed in vitro using Chinese hamster ovary cells that do not express

CAR but have been stably transfected to express ACE (CHO-ACE cells) (66). Enhancement in gene delivery was specific for the ACE-expressing cells and could be blocked by an excess of free mAb-9B9. In vivo analysis was then performed. In these studies, untargeted Ad vector gave very low levels of transgene expression in the lungs, whereas the addition of the targeting conjugate improved reporter gene expression levels by over 20-fold. This effect could be substantially blocked by coinjecting an excess of free mAb-9B9, and was not seen with an irrelevant antibody conjugate or with mAb-9B9 alone. Histological analysis including immunohistochemistry, immunofluoresence, and immunoelectron microscopy confirmed that the pulmonary transgene expression was indeed in the endothelial cells. Furthermore, expression in the liver was reduced by approximately 80% compared to unconjugated virus. Thus, the twin goals of enhancement and selectivity were achieved, although in absolute terms the level of expression in the liver remained high. To determine the biodistribution of targeted Ad particles, we also assessed viral DNA distribution 90 min after injection, using quantitative real-time polymerase chain reaction (PCR). This analysis showed a 20-fold increase in Ad vector DNA localization to the lungs, which is consistent with the transgene expression results. However, no significant reduction in DNA was seen in the liver despite the reduction in hepatocyte transgene expression. We believe this discrepancy is due to the fact that a large proportion of the vector load was being taken up by Kupffer cells and degraded. Others have shown that up to 90% of an intravenously injected dose is lost in this way (67). Nevertheless, the achievement of targeted gene delivery in vivo has encouraging implications for the continued development of targeted Ad vectors, although the issue of non–receptor-mediated sequestration of vector by the reticuloendothelial system still needs to be addressed. Further, this study and those using the FGF conjugate are beginning to address one of the key concerns of the conjugate approach—whether the bond between conjugate and virus is sufficiently stable to enable systemic application. In contrast to some earlier predictions, the results so far in this regard are encouraging.

The technical development of protein complexes for Ad retargeting has progressed by a variety of methods. In addition to attachment to the Ad knob, bispecific antibodies have also been derived which bind at the penton base and reduce native tropism for CAR by steric hindrance (68,69) or attach to Ad hexon protein (70). Recombinant antibody strategies have also been used; for example, a fusion protein consisting of an antiknob single chain antibody (scFv) and EGF has been derived (71). Bi–specific single-chain antibodies have also been derived either from known monoclonal antibodies (e.g., the anti-EGFR antibody, mAb-425 (72)) or by phage panning against target cells or proteins with phage libraries displaying random scFvs. A bispecific molecule that targets to the endothelial marker endoglin has been derived in this way (73). Dmitriev et al. recently developed an alternate approach using complexes consisting of the ectodomain of CAR in fusion with retargeting ligands (74). A CAR-EGF fusion molecule achieved enhanced transduction to EGF-R-positive cells. The improved engineering involved in the development of these conjugates allows for greater control over the structure than does the cross-linking approaches used with whole antibodies. Nevertheless, production of these newer-generation agents in high quantities is not always straightforward, and as yet none has been shown to have efficacy or specificity in vivo.

Advances are also being made in the engineering of ligands per se. Phage panning approaches have been used to identify novel peptide sequences with targeting specificity (75,76). In brief, this strategy utilizes a library of bacterio-phage particles that contain random peptide sequences on their pIII coat protein. This library can be incubated with target cells or proteins, and then the nonbinding phages are washed away. Binding phage are eluted and then amplified and reapplied to the target. Several rounds of panning in this way enriches for phage-bearing peptide sequences that bind to the target. Binding clones can then be selected for DNA sequencing and determination of the peptide sequence responsible for the binding. Using this approach, one can identify ligands without prior knowledge of accessible receptors. Peptides identified in this way have been successfully incorporated into targeting conjugates and have achieved targeting fidelity in vitro (55,77,78). The libraries may be constructed to contain linear or cyclic peptide sequences and libraries also exist that express scFvs on their coat proteins. This combination of target definition with targeted delivery still further broadens the prospects for the development of improved vectors.

IV. Genetic Capsid Modifications

The use of conjugate-based targeting approaches has the advantage that a multitude of established targeting moieties can readily be incorporated into the system. Further, many Ad vectors containing different expression cassettes can quickly be combined with any targeting moiety, thereby offering a high degree of flexibility. This approach has been approved for human clinical trial involving intraperitoneal administration of the FGF targeting conjugate in patients with ovarian cancer. However, this "two-component" approach adds a degree of complexity to the system that may not be ideal for ultimate clinical application. Thus, the modification of vector tropism by genetic methods is also being pursued in an effort to produce a single targeted vector particle (2). As Ad capsid proteins are the basis of viral binding and internalization, these proteins are the focus of this approach. This work began before the means to ablate CAR-tropism genetically was discovered; thus, to date, these vectors have shown enhanced rather than specific tropism. In this regard, Wickham et al. have altered the Ad fiber gene thereby adding cell binding peptides to the carboxy-terminus of the translated protein (79). Evaluation of viruses possessing these fibers showed that enhanced infection and gene transfer could be achieved by using a limited repertoire of targeting ligands. Using a vector in which an integrin-binding RGD motif had been added to the C-terminus of the fiber, enhanced, CAR-independent, gene delivery was achieved to human vascular endothelial cells in culture and to the cortical vasculature of the rat kidney by ex vivo infusion of vector into the renal artery. In a separate study, a vector having a C-terminal poly-lysine addition to enhance binding to heparan sulfates achieved improved gene delivery to the vascular smooth muscle cells (80). Thus, these studies established the feasibility of enhanced gene delivery in vivo through genetic fiber modification.

Although carboxy-terminal modifications of fiber were able to establish an important principle, this location may be suboptimal for ligand addition. The major problem is that the upper limit of size for incorporated sequences is quite small before the structural integrity of the knob trimer is disrupted. Further, crystal structure analysis of the knob domain indicates the C-terminus is not in an ideally accessible location. Therefore, Krasnykh et al. sought to alter adenoviral tropism by exploiting an alternate locale on the fiber knob, the HI loop (Fig. 3a) (81). This choice was based upon the crystal structure of the knob domain proposed by Xia et al. (82), in which the HI loop appeared to present a locale accessible for targeting purposes. Furthermore, other aspects of the knob structure suggested its utility; specifically, the fact that the HI loop is not involved in intramolecular interactions between fiber monomers suggested that it might be altered without deleterious effects on quaternary structure. In addition, the length variability among adenoviral serotypes suggested that the HI loop did not subserve a critical function. The feasibility of using the HI loop for ligand insertion was first confirmed using a FLAG epitope as a convenient model ligand then, Dmitriev et al. inserted an integrin binding cyclic RGD sequence into this region (15). Pasqualini et al. had determined that this ligand sequence had a degree of specificity for tumor vasculature using an in vivo phage panning technique (83). Thus, this approach represented the first attempt to translate information gained by phage panning into the generation of a genetically targeted Ad. Studies of recombinant Ad fiber protein containing the ligand clearly confirmed that this motif could bind to integrins when placed at this site. The resulting Ad vector had a markedly enhanced ability to infect CAR-negative cells, as well as certain lung cancer and mesothelioma lines (Fig 3b,c). Most impressively, when this vector was evaluated using primary tumor tissue, significantly enhanced infectivity was again noted compared to the unmodified vector; in some cases, by up to three orders of magnitude (15,84). Further, the modified vector was also able to achieve gene delivery in the presence of preexisting anti-Ad antibodies in

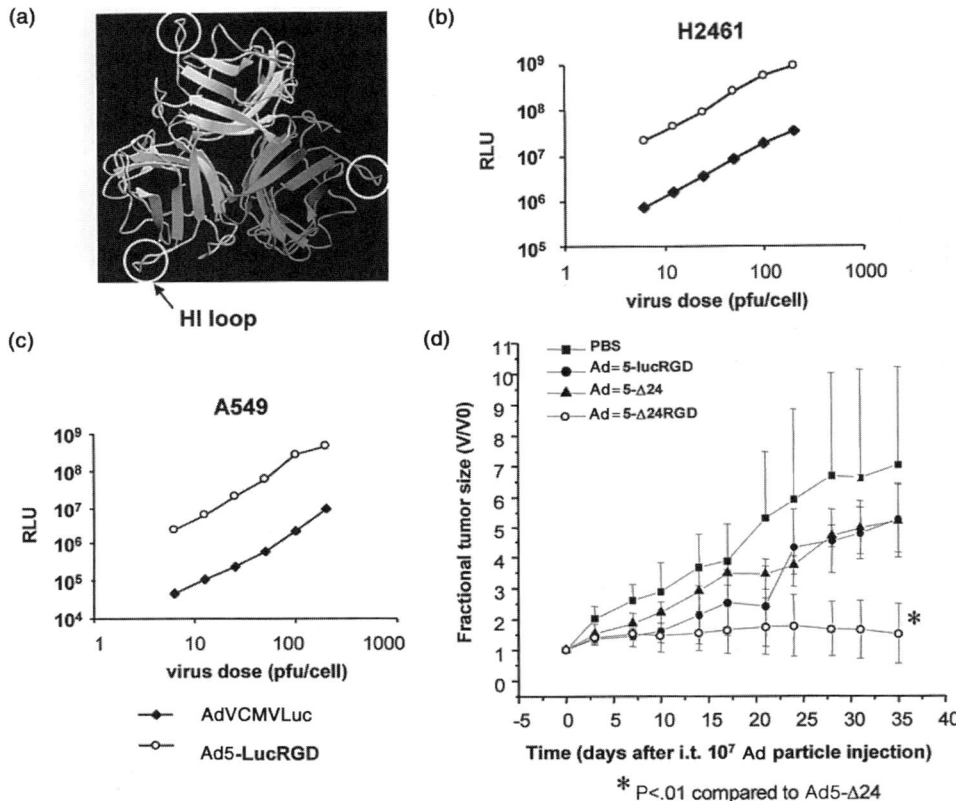

Figure 3   Enhanced infectivity by genetic modification to incorporate an integrin bind-ing RGD motif in the HI loop of knob. (a) Illustration of the knob structure according to Xia et al. (picture courtesy R. Gerard). Viewed from end-on, the propeller-like trimeric structure can be seen. HI loop is indicated. (b,c) Infection of either a mesothelioma cell line (b) or adenocarcinoma line (c) with various doses of Ad5LucRGD (containing HI loop modification) versus AdCMVLuc. Luciferase activity determined 24 hr after infection. (d) Enhanced infectivity translates to improved therapeutic outcome. A conditionally repli-cative virus (Ad-5–Δ24, which contains a deletion in the E1 Rb binding region) was com-pared to its RGD-HI–modified counterpart. A549 subcutaneous nodules were established in nude mice, which were then injected intratumorally with viruses or PBS control as indicated, and then tumor size was monitored and expressed as a percentage of size at day 1. At the low viral dose used, a substantial differential in outcome in favor of the modified vector was observed. (Adapted from Ref. 87.)

malignant ascites (85). However, although this vector had enhanced infectivity, no specificity gains with respect to tumor vasculature were seen, possibly because the vector retained the ability to bind CAR. Nevertheless, the addition of an RGD motif into the HI loop clearly altered the infection dynamics of the virus in vitro. In vivo systemic administration of vector resulted in some modification of the biodistribution of transgene expression (86). Although liver expression still predominated (consistent with the fact that this vector still recognizes CAR), relative increases in other organs, including lung, spleen, and kidney, implied that the RGD motif was available for target cell interaction in this stringent delivery context, and that the HI loop might prove to be a useful site for the introduction of more specific targeting moieties. This vector did not, however, achieve enhanced airway epithelial transduction upon intratracheal administration in mice (unpublished observations); most likely because of a lack of integrins expressed on the apical surface of these cells (11). The impact of RGD-mediated infectivity enhancement was also assessed in a conditionally replicative Ad designed to achieve tumor cell killing by viral replication and oncolysis. The enhanced vector achieved improved therapeutic outcome in subcutaneous lung tumor nodules in a murine model (Fig. 3d)(87). Subsequent studies have established that peptides of at least 63 amino acids in size can be incorporated in the HI loop without compromising the quaternary structure of the fiber or viral infection dynamics (V. Krasnykh, personal communication).

Despite the success of the RGD-HI modification, the use of other cyclic peptides defined by phage panning in tropism-modified Ad has been more difficult. The specificity of promising bicyclic ligands defined by in vivo phage panning is exquisitely dependent on correct formation of the cyclic disulfide bonds within the peptide, and whether this can be achieved in the HI loop is uncertain. In fact, to date, only three successful peptide insertions in the HI loop have been reported (15,81,88). Many peptides lose their specificity when placed in this context. To address this limitation, Pereboev et al. devised a system in which the entire knob domain of adenovirus is expressed on the pIII bacteriophage protein (89). Random peptide libraries are then inserted in the HI loop, and then panning can be performed in the knowledge that selected peptides are a priori compatible with the HI location. Furthermore, the compatibility of the insertion with knob trimerization is assessed as part of the selection process by screening clones with a monoclonal antibody that only recognizes trimeric knob.

Improving Ad infectivity via the modification of capsid proteins besides knob has also been evaluated. In this regard, Vigne et al. introduced an RGD motif into the hexon protein (90). As there are 720 hexons compared to 36 knob domains on the virus, the greater number of targeting ligands with the hexon approach might offer some advantage. However, as these moieties are located close to the virion surface, their interaction with receptors might be compromised by steric hindrance from the fibers. Nevertheless, a significant enhancement of transduction to CAR-negative cells was achieved in vitro using this approach. Shortening of fiber length to improve hexon accessibility could potentially further improve these results. A rigorous, systematic comparison of the different strategies of fiber and hexon modification with respect to the enhancements achieved has not been reported.

The foregoing genetic modification strategies have achieved enhanced infectivity, but have not improved specificity, chiefly because all of the modified vectors retained recognition for CAR. Thus, although they represent a significant advance for many disease applications where delivery can be administered locoregionally, greater specificity is required for broader application. The genetic manipulation of the Ad-5 knob to ablate its natural recognition for CAR has now been achieved (25); however, these vectors still show a high degree of tropism for the normal liver, thus indicating the need for further modifications (27,28). Mutation of the penton base to ablate the natural recognition for integrins has been achieved and combined with CAR binding ablation, but even this "doubly-ablated" construct still achieves a significant amount of transduction of hepatocytes in vivo despite the fact that transduction of primary hepatocytes in vitro is dramatically reduced (unpublished observations). The mechanism for this residual transduction is unclear, and the superimposition of a specific targeting moiety onto the background of a doubly-ablated vector is eagerly awaited. Alternate strategies to replace entirely the Ad knob domain with novel proteins that can achieve the correct trimerization of fiber as well as possess specific targeting attributes are now also being developed (91–93). These approaches are based on an extensive reengineering of the Ad fiber by totally deleting the knob domain and replacing it with an alternate trimerization motif: either the fibritin molecule from bacteriophage T4, the neck region peptide from human surfactant, or the alpha helix trimerization domain from MoMuLV envelope glycoprotein. In this way, the normal dual functions of the knob (receptor binding and fiber trimerization) are split between two new molecules—trimerization motif and ligand—thereby potentially allowing for larger, more specific ligands (such as scFvs) to be incorporated without disruption of fiber structure. These approaches hold promise, but so far only limited proof-of-principle in vitro data have been presented. Nevertheless, CAR-independent infection has been achieved using these approaches either through the use of an RGD ligand or through the use of a six-histidine (6-His) residue that targets to cell lines expressing an artificially engineered anti–6-His scFv as an artificial receptor. The 6-His/anti–6-His receptor system was designed specifically to allow the efficient propagation of Ads that lack native tropism (94). To achieve this, an E1 transcomplementing cell line (293) was stably transfected to express the anti–6-His scFv. As there is no natural receptor for 6-His, it should be possible to attach this small tag to engineered fibers without compromising the specificity of the principal targeting ligand.

V. Combined Transductional and Transcriptional Approaches

Although transductional targeting approaches are improving, the experience so far with both conjugate-based and genetic approaches in vivo with respect to residual transgene expression in nontarget sites indicates that some form of additional, complementary form of control could be advantageous. Such additional control could potentially be achieved through transcriptional regulation using cell-specific promoters. Ideally, candidate promoters would have high levels of activity in target cells but very low levels of activity in those organs in which transductional control alone is inadequate—typically the liver and spleen if vector is given systemically. Efforts to exploit cell-specific promoters have often been frustrated, because many candidate promoters lose specificity when placed

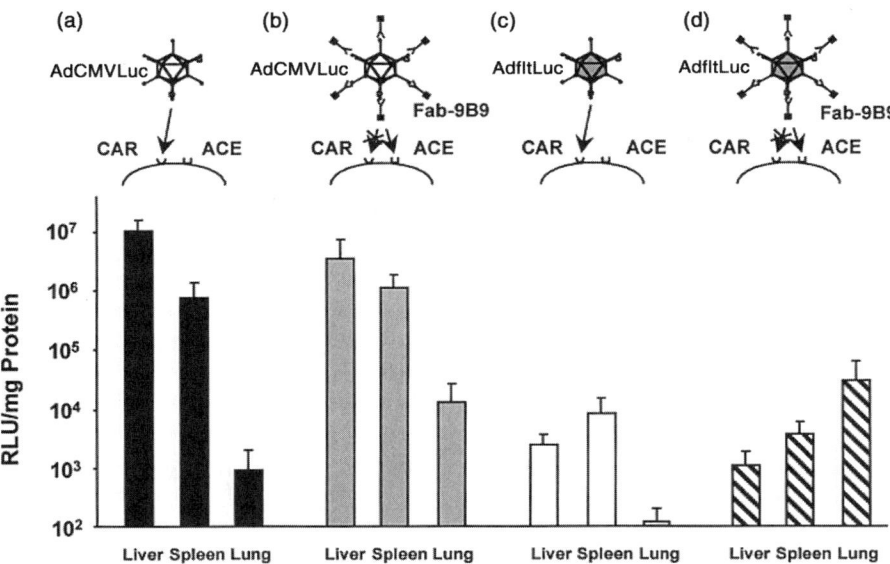

Figure 4 Combined transductional and transcriptional targeting improves the specificity of transgene expression in vivo. Stepwise improvement in transgene expression in pulmonary endothelium is shown. Rats were injected via the tail vein with vectors carrying the luciferase reporter gene and then organs were harvested and luciferase activity was determined 3 days later. (a) Untargeted vector, AdCMVLuc, showing dominant transgene expression in liver and spleen. (b) Addition of Fab-9B9 for targeting to ACE leads to enhanced pulmonary gene expression and reduction in liver expression (note log scale). (c) AdfltLuc, containing an endothelium-specific promoter results in dramatic reduction in expression in all organs. (d) AdfltLuc + Fab-9B9 restores transgene expression levels in lungs, but still further reduces expression in nontarget liver and spleen, thereby dramatically improving selectivity ratio.

in the Ad genome (95). However, promoters that do retain fidelity in this setting are emerging (96–98), and the use of insulator sequences may further expand the utility of this approach (99). We investigated a combined transductional and transcriptional targeting approach for gene delivery to the pulmonary vasculature (100). To achieve endothelium-specific transgene expression, three candidate promoters were evaluated—those for von Willebrand factor, ICAM-2, and vascular endothelial growth factor receptor 1 (flt-1) (101). The flt-1 promoter had the clear advantage in both strength and specificity when tested on a panel of cell lines in vitro, and further, had very low activity in the liver in vivo. Thus, we combined vectors containing transgenes under the control of the flt-1 promoter with the Fab-9B9 pulmonary targeting conjugate. We saw a dramatic, synergistic improvement in transgene expression ratio for the lung versus the principal non-

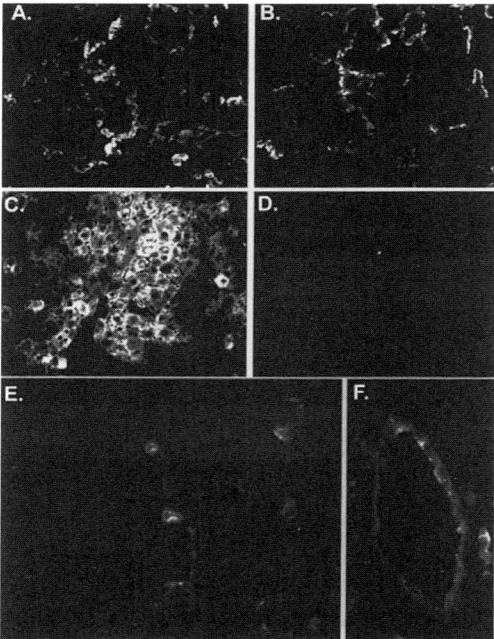

Figure 5   Immunofluorescent analysis of transgene expression with double-targeting approach. Rats were injected via the tail vein with vectors carrying the gene for carcinoembryonic antigen (CEA) as a convenient marker and then lungs were fixed in inflation four days later and paraffin sections were stained. AdCMVCEA/Fab-9B9 gave strong staining in lung (A) and liver (C). AdfltCEA/Fab-9B9 gave strong staining in lung (B), but barely detectable staining in liver (D). High-power views show staining in endothelium of alveolar capillaries (E) and a small vessel (F) with AdfltCEA/Fab-9B9.

target sites, liver and spleen (Fig. 4). At low doses of vector, luciferase reporter gene activity was 27-fold greater in the lung than in liver or spleen. At high doses, this differential improved to 200-fold; possibly as a result of the Kupffer cell saturation allowing more vector to reach the target site. Immunofluoresence confirmed that transgene expression was in endothelial cells (Fig. 5). Even at the low dose, the relative improvement in selectivity of lung versus liver compared to untargeted vector was striking: over 300,000-fold. Transgene expression in other organs, including those that express ACE in less accessible sites (e.g., testis, kidney) was at or near background levels for all vector combinations. The relatively simple concept of combined targeting had not previously been demonstrated, largely because of the lack of approaches possessing in vivo fidelity. This approach may turn out to be particularly useful for gene therapy approaches for PPH, as both flt-1 (102) and ACE (60) are increased with vascular remodeling. As technology improves for the individual transductional and transcriptional approaches, more opportunities to devise disease-relevant combinations should arise. With respect to airway epithelial expression and cystic fibrosis therapy, the cytokeratin-18 promoter shows promise (103). For lung cancer, the midkine (96) and cox-2 promoters (97) may prove to be useful.

VI. Reticuloendothelial Sequestration

In addition to issues relating to CAR and integrins, sequestration of Ad vectors by the reticuloendothelial system is a further hurdle that will need to be overcome for the optimal use of these vectors. Upon intravenous administration, the majority of vector is phagocytosed by the Kupffer cells that line the hepatic sinusoids. Up to 90% of an administered vector dose may be taken up and degraded, without leading to transgene expression (67). For airway administration a similar problem exists with alveolar macrophages (104). Recent studies have shown that uptake of Kupffer cells is a saturable phenomenon, with a threshold above which a rapid, linear increase in transgene expression can be achieved (105). Complementary approaches to block Kupffer cells (106), or the further modification of vectors into "stealth" particles, perhaps through the use of polyethylene glycol (PEG), are thus being pursued (107,108). This latter approach has shown some efficacy already in helping to reduce Ad vector inactivation by circulating antibodies.

VII. Targeting Approaches for Other Vectors

This discussion has focused primarily on Ad retargeting in view of the fact that most of the targeting efforts have concerned this vector. However, many of the basic principles can be applied more widely. The pioneering efforts to retarget retroviral vectors were compromised by changes in intracellular trafficking when the vector entered through a nonnatural pathway. However, Gordon et al. have recently developed a highly novel approach for systemic targeting with these agents. Rather than target to a cellular receptor, they have targeted to areas of exposed collagen, as is seen in vascular injury and tumor vasculature (109,110). This leads to a local accumulation of vector at the target site, but actual cellular entry is achieved via the natural retroviral entry mechanisms. In this way, transduction efficiency was preserved. Targeting efforts have also been applied to adeno-associated virus (AAV) vectors both through the use of bispecific conjugates (111) and through direct genetic modification of capsid proteins (112). In vivo efficacy has not yet been shown, however. As an evolution of the use of bacteriophage for ligand definition, there is now a growing interest in using this agent as a targeted vector per se (113). Such an approach has been compromised by complement inactivation of these particles, but recently genetically modified baculoviruses which are resistant to complement have been produced (114) and may allow for the practical development of this approach. Antibody-based targeting approaches have been used to enhance the efficacy of cationic lipid vectors by targeting to PECAM, which resulted in enhanced gene delivery to pulmonary endothelium (115).

VIII. Conclusions

Improvements in vector technology are key to the advancement of gene therapy and the development of specific targeting approaches is an important component of vector design. Significant progress has been made in recent years; however, the vast majority of this work has been limited to in vitro proof-of-principle studies. Future developments should see improvements in the basic technology of vector construction, ligand definition, and the greater use of composite approaches, which should facilitate the translation of these approaches to in vivo use. At the present time, a small repertoire of "infectivity enhanced" vectors already exists. These agents are poised to enter trials for locoregional disease in the near future.

Acknowledgments

Supported by American Heart Association, Avon Products Foundation, NIH-NIDDK P30 DK 54781.

References

1. Wickham TJ. Targeting adenovirus. Gene Ther 2000; 7:110–114.

2. Krasnykh VN, Douglas JT, van Beusechem VW. Genetic targeting of adenoviral vectors. Mol Ther 2000; 1:391–405.
3. Kasahara N, Dozy AM, Kan YW. Tissue-specific targeting of retroviral vectors through ligand-receptor interactions. Science 1994; 266:1373–1376.
4. Grubb BR, Pickles RJ, Ye H, Yankaskas JR, Vick RN, Engelhardt JF, Wilson JM, Johnson LG, Boucher RC. Inefficient gene transfer by adenovirus vector to cystic fibrosis airway epithelia of mice and humans. Nature 1994; 371:802–806.
5. Shenk T. Adenoviridae: the viruses and their replication. In: Fields BN, Knipe DM, Howley PM, eds. Fields Virology. Philadelphia: Lippincott-Raven, 1996:2111–2148.
6. Bergelson JM, Cunningham JA, Droguett G, Kurt-Jones EA, Krithivas A, Hong JS, Horwitz MS, Crowell RL, Finberg RW. Isolation of a common receptor for coxsackie B viruses and adenoviruses 2 and 5. Science 1997; 275:1320–1323.
7. Tomko RP, Xu R, Philipson L. HCAR and MCAR: the human and mouse cellular receptors for subgroup C adenoviruses and group B coxsackieviruses. Proc Natl Acad Sci USA 1997; 94:3352–3356.
8. Roelvink PW, Lizonova A, Lee JG, Li Y, Bergelson JM, Finberg RW, Brough DE, Kovesdi I, Wickham TJ. The coxsackievirus-adenovirus receptor protein can function as a cellular attachment protein for adenovirus serotypes from subgroups A, C, D, E, and F. J Virol 1998; 72:7909–7915.
9. Pickles RJ, Fahrner JA, Petrella JM, Boucher RC, Bergelson JM. Retargeting the coxsackievirus and adenovirus receptor to the apical surface of polarized epithelial cells reveals the glycocalyx as a barrier to adenovirus-mediated gene transfer. J Virol 2000; 74:6050–6057.
10. Walters RW, van't Hof W, Yi SM, Schroth MK, Zabner J, Crystal RG, Welsh MJ. Apical localization of the coxsackie-adenovirus receptor by glycosyl-phosphatidylinositol modification is sufficient for adenovirus-mediated gene transfer through the apical surface of human airway epithelia. J Virol 2001; 75:7703–7711.
11. Walters RW, Grunst T, Bergelson JM, Finberg RW, Welsh MJ, Zabner J. Basolateral localization of fiber receptors limits adenovirus infection from the apical surface of airway epithelia. J Biol Chem 1999; 274:10219–10226.
12. Pickles RJ, McCarty D, Matsui H, Hart PJ, Randell SH, Boucher RC. Limited entry of adenovirus vectors into well-differentiated airway epithelium is responsible for inefficient gene transfer. J Virol 1998; 72:6014–6023.
13. Zabner J, Freimuth P, Puga A, Fabrega A, Welsh MJ. Lack of high affinity fiber receptor activity explains the resistance of ciliated airway epithelia to adenovirus infection. J Clin Invest 1997; 100:1144–1149.
14. Miller CR, Buchsbaum DJ, Reynolds PN, Douglas JT, Gillespie GY, Mayo MS, Raben D, Curiel DT. Differential susceptibility of primary and established human glioma cells to adenovirus infection: targeting via the epidermal growth factor receptor achieves fiber receptor independent gene transfer. Cancer Res 1998; 58: 5738–5748.
15. Dmitriev I, Krasnykh K, Miller CR, Wang M, Kashentseva E, Mikheeva G, Belousova N, Curiel DT. An adenovirus vector with genetically modified fibers demonstrates expanded tropism via utilization of a coxsackievirus and adenovirus receptor–independent cell entry mechanism. J Virol 1998; 72:9706–9713.
16. Blackwell JL, Miller CR, Douglas JT, Hui L, Reynolds PN, Caroll WR, Peters

GE, Strong TV, Curiel DT. Retargeting to EGFR enhances adenovirus infection efficiency of squamous cell carcinoma. Arch Otolaryngol Head Neck Surg 1999; 125:856–863.

17. Kasono K, Blackwell JL, Douglas JT, Dmitriev I, Strong TV, Reynolds P, Kropf DA, Carroll WR, Peters GE, Bucy RP, Curiel DT, Krasnykh V. Selective gene delivery to head and neck cancer cells via an integrin targeted adenoviral vector. Clin Cancer Res 1999; 5:2571–2579.

18. Kaner RJ, Worgall S, Leopold PL, Stolze E, Milano E, Hidaka C, Ramalingam R, Hackett NR, Singh R, Bergelson J, Finberg R, Falck-Pedersen E, Crystal RG. Modification of the genetic program of human alveolar macrophages by adenovirus vectors in vitro is feasible but inefficient, limited in part by the low level of expression of the coxsackie/adenovirus receptor. Am J Resir Cell Mol Biol 1999; 20: 361–370.

19. Kelly FJ, Miller CR, Buchsbaum DJ, Gomez-Navarro J, Barnes MN, Alvarez RD, Curiel DT. Selectivity of TAG-72-targeted adenovirus gene transfer to primary ovarian carcinoma cells versus autologous mesothelial cells in vitro. Clin Cancer Res 2000; 6:4323–4333.

20. Hemmi S, Geertsen R, Mezzacasa A, Peter I, Dummer R. The presence of human coxsackievirus and adenovirus receptor is associated with efficient adenovirus-mediated transgene expression in human melanoma cell cultures. Hum Gene Ther 1998; 9:2363–2373.

21. Pearson AS, Koch PE, Atkinson N, Xiong M, Finberg RW, Roth JA, Fang B. Factors limiting adenovirus-mediated gene transfer into human lung and pancreatic cancer cell lines. Clin Cancer Res 1999; 5:4208–4213.

22. Batra RK, Olsen JC, Pickles RJ, Hoganson DK, Boucher RC. Transduction of non-small cell lung cancer cells by adenoviral and retroviral vectors. Am J Resir Cell Mol Biol 1998; 18:402–410.

23. Okegawa T, Li Y, Pong RC, Bergelson JM, Zhou J, Hsieh JT. The dual impact of coxsackie and adenovirus receptor expression on human prostate cancer gene therapy. Cancer Res 2000; 60:5031–5036.

24. Yee D, McGuire SE, Brunner N, Kozelsky TW, Allred DC, Chen SH, Woo SL. Adenovirus-mediated gene transfer of herpes simplex virus thymidine kinase in an ascites model of human breast cancer. Hum Gene Ther 1996; 7:1251–1257.

25. Roelvink PW, Mi Lee G, Einfeld DA, Kovesdi I, Wickham TJ. Identification of a conserved receptor-binding site on the fiber proteins of CAR-recognizing adenoviridae. Science 1999; 286:1568–1571.

26. Bewley MC, Springer K, Zhang YB, Freimuth P, Flanagan JM. Structural analysis of the mechanism of adenovirus binding to its human cellular receptor, CAR. Science 1999; 286:1579–1583.

27. Leissner P, Legrand V, Schlesinger Y, Hadji DA, van Raaij M, Cusack S, Pavirani A, Mehtali M. Influence of adenoviral fiber mutations on viral encapsidation, infectivity and in vivo tropism. Gene Ther 2001; 8:49–57.

28. Alemany R, Curiel DT. CAR binding ablation does not change biodistribution or toxicity of adenoviral vectors. Gene Ther 2001. In press.

29. Li E, Brown SL, Stupack DG, Puente XS, Cheresh DA, Nemerow GR. Integrin alpha(v)beta1 is an adenovirus coreceptor. J Virol 2001; 75:5405–5409.

30. Wickham TJ, Mathias P, Cheresh DA, Nemerow GR. Integrins alpha v beta 3 and alpha v beta 5 promote adenovirus internalization but not virus attachment. Cell 1993; 73:309–319.

31. Takayama K, Ueno H, Pei XH, Nakanishi Y, Yatsunami J, Hara N. The levels of integrin alpha v beta 5 may predict the susceptibility to adenovirus-mediated gene transfer in human lung cancer cells. Gene Ther 1998; 5:361–368.

32. Hautala T, Grunst T, Fabrega A, Freimuth P, Welsh MJ. An interaction between penton base and alpha v integrins plays a minimal role in adenovirus-mediated gene transfer to hepatocytes in vitro and in vivo. Gene Ther 1998; 5:1259–1264.

33. Curiel DT, Agarwal S, Wagner E, Cotten M. Adenovirus enhancement of trans-ferrin-polylysine-mediated gene delivery. Proc Natl Acad Sci USA 1991; 88:8850–8854.

34. Cosset FL, Morling FJ, Takeuchi Y, Weiss RA, Collins MK, Russell SJ. Retroviral retargeting by envelopes expressing an N-terminal binding domain. J Virol 1995; 69:6314–6322.

35. Fasbender A, Zabner J, Chillon M, Moninger TO, Puga AP, Davidson BL, Welsh MJ. Complexes of adenovirus with polycationic polymers and cationic lipids increase the efficiency of gene transfer in vitro and in vivo. J Biol Chem 1997; 272:6479–6489.

36. Wang G, Zabner J, Deering C, Launspach J, Shao J, Bodner M, Jolly DJ, Davidson BL, McCray PB, Jr. Increasing epithelial junction permeability enhances gene transfer to airway epithelia In vivo. Am J Resir Cell Mol Biol 2000; 22:129–138.

37. Chu Q, St George JA, Lukason M, Cheng SH, Scheule RK, Eastman SJ. EGTA enhancement of adenovirus-mediated gene transfer to mouse tracheal epithelium in vivo. Hum Gene Ther 2001; 12:455–467.

38. Fasbender A, Lee JH, Walters RW, Moninger TO, Zabner J, Welsh MJ. Incorporation of adenovirus in calcium phosphate precipitates enhances gene transfer to airway epithelia in vitro and in vivo. J Clin Invest 1998; 102:184–193.

39. Walters R, Welsh M. Mechanism by which calcium phosphate coprecipitation enhances adenovirus-mediated gene transfer. Gene Ther 1999; 6:1845–1850.

40. Weiss DJ, Bonneau L, Liggitt D. Use of perfluorochemical liquid allows earlier detection of gene expression and use of less vector in normal lung and enhances gene expression in acutely injured lung. Mol Ther 2001; 3:734–745.

41. Parsons DW, Grubb BR, Johnson LG, Boucher RC. Enhanced in vivo airway gene transfer via transient modification of host barrier properties with a surface-active agent. Hum Gene Ther 1998; 9:2661–2672.

42. Douglas JT, Rogers BE, Rosenfeld ME, Michael SI, Feng M, Curiel DT. Targeted gene delivery by tropism-modified adenoviral vectors. Nat Biotechnol 1996;14:1574–1578.

43. Goldman CK, Rogers BE, Douglas JT, Sosnowski BA, Ying WB, Siegal GP, Baird A, Campain JA, Curiel DT. Targeted gene delivery to Kaposi's sarcoma cells via the fibroblast growth factor receptor. Cancer Res 1997; 57:1447–1451.

44. Rogers BE, Douglas JT, Sosnowski BA, Ying W, Pierce GF, Buchsbaum DJ, Baird A, Curiel DT. Enhanced in vivo gene delivery utilizing tropism-modified adenovirus vectors. Tumor Targeting 1997; 3:25–31.

45. Reynolds PN, Miller CR, Goldman CK, Doukas J, Sosnowski BA, Rogers BE,

Gomez-Navarro J, Pierce GF, Curiel DT, Douglas JT. Targeting adenoviral infection with basic fibroblast growth factor enhances gene delivery to vascular endothelial and smooth muscle cells. Tumor Targeting 1998; 3:156–168.

46. Gu DL, Gonzalez AM, Printz MA, Doukas J, Ying W, D'Andrea M, Hoganson DK, Curiel DT, Douglas JT, Sosnowski BA, Baird A, Aukerman SL, Pierce GF. Fibroblast growth factor 2 retargeted adenovirus has redirected cellular tropism: evidence for reduced toxicity and enhanced antitumor activity in mice. Cancer Res 1999; 59:2608–2614.

47. Schneider H, Groves M, Muhle C, Reynolds PN, Knight A, Themis M, Carvajal J, Scaravilli F, Curiel DT, Fairweather NF, Coutelle C. Retargeting of adenoviral vectors to neurons using the Hc fragment of tetanus toxin. Gene Ther 2000; 7: 1584–1592.

48. Haisma HJ, Pinedo HM, Rijswijk A, der Meulen-Muileman I, Sosnowski BA, Ying W, Beusechem VW, Tillman BW, Gerritsen WR, Curiel DT. Tumor-specific gene transfer via an adenoviral vector targeted to the pan-carcinoma antigen EpCAM. Gene Ther 1999; 6:1469–1474.

49. Tillman BW, de Gruijl TD, Luykx-de Bakker SA, Scheper RJ, Pinedo HM, Curiel TJ, Gerritsen WR, Curiel DT. Maturation of dendritic cells accompanies high efficiency gene transfer by a CD40-targeted adenoviral vector. J Immunol 1999; 162: 6378–6383.

50. Wickham TJ, Lee GM, Titus JA, Sconocchia G, Bakacs T, Kovesdi I, Segal DM. Targeted adenovirus-mediated gene delivery to T cells via CD3. J Virol 1997; 71: 7663–7669.

51. Israel BF, Pickles RJ, Segal DM, Gerard RD, Kenney SC. Enhancement of adenovirus vector entry into CD70-positive B-cell lines by using a bispecific CD70-adenovirus fiber antibody. J Virol 2001; 75:5215–5221.

52. Rancourt C, Rogers BE, Sosnowski BA, Wang M, Piche A, Pierce GF, Alvarez RD, Siegel GP, Douglas JT, Curiel DT. FGF2-enhancement of adenovirus-mediated delivery of the herpes simplex virus thymidine kinase gene results in augmented therapeutic benefit in a murine model of ovarian cancer. Clin Cancer Res 1998; 4:2455–2461.

53. Tillman BW, Hayes TL, DeGruijl TD, Douglas JT, Curiel DT. Adenoviral vectors targeted to CD40 enhance the efficacy of dendritic cell-based vaccination against human papillomavirus 16-induced tumor cells in a murine model. Cancer Res 2000; 60:5456–5463.

54. Kreda SM, Pickles RJ, Lazarowski ER, Boucher RC. G-protein-coupled receptors as targets for gene transfer vectors using natural small-molecule ligands. Nat Biotechnol 2000; 18:635–640.

55. Romanczuk H, Galer CE, Zabner J, Barsomian G, Wadsworth SC, O'Riordan CR. Modification of an adenoviral vector with biologically selected peptides: a novel strategy for gene delivery to cells of choice. Hum Gene Ther 1999; 10:2615–2626.

56. Drapkin PT, O'Riordan CR, Yi SM, Chiorini JA, Cardella J, Zabner J, Welsh MJ. Targeting the urokinase plasminogen activator receptor enhances gene transfer to human airway epithelia. J Clin Invest 2000; 105:589–596.

57. Reynolds PN, Zinn KR, Gavrilyuk VD, Balyasnikova IV, Rogers BE, Buchsbaum

DJ, Wang MH, Miletich DJ, Douglas JT, Danilov SM, Curiel DT. A targetable injectable adenoviral vector for selective gene delivery to pulmonary endothelium in vivo. Mol Ther 2000; 2:562–578.

58. Danilov SM, Gavrilyuk VD, Franke FE, Pauls K, Harshaw DW, McDonald TD, Miletich DJ, Muzykantov VR. Pulmonary uptake and tissue selectivity of antibodies to surface endothelial antigens: key determinants of vascular immunotargeting. Am J Physiol (Lung Cell Mol Physiol) 2001; 280:L1335–L1347.

59. Morrell NW, Atochina EN, Morris KG, Danilov SM, Stenmark KR. Angiotensin converting enzyme expression is increased in small pulmonary arteries of rats with hypoxia-induced pulmonary hypertension (published erratum appears in J Clin Invest 1996; 97[1]:271). J Clin Invest 1995; 96:1823–1833.

60. Orte C, Polak JM, Haworth SG, Yacoub MH, Morrell NW. Expression of pulmonary vascular angiotensin-converting enzyme in primary and secondary plexiform pulmonary hypertension. J Pathol 2000; 192:379–384.

61. Lane KB, Machado RD, Pauciulo MW, Thomson JR, Phillips JA, 3rd, Loyd JE, Nichols WC, Trembath RC. Heterozygous germline mutations in BMPR2, encoding a TGF-beta receptor, cause familial primary pulmonary hypertension. The International PPH Consortium. Nat Genet 2000; 26:81–84.

62. Deng Z, Morse JH, Slager SL, Cuervo N, Moore KJ, Venetos G, Kalachikov S, Cayanis E, Fischer SG, Barst RJ, Hodge SE, Knowles JA. Familial primary pulmonary hypertension (gene PPH1) is caused by mutations in the bone morphogenetic protein receptor-II gene, Am J Hum Genet 2000; 67:737–744.

63. Danilov SM, Muzykantov VR, Martynov AV, Atochina EN, Sakharov I, Trakht IN, Smirnov VN. Lung is the target organ for a monoclonal antibody to angiotensin-converting enzyme. Lab Invest 1991; 64:118–124.

64. Muzykantov VR, Atochina EN, Ischiropoulos H, Danilov SM, Fisher AB. Immunotargeting of antioxidant enzyme to the pulmonary endothelium. Proc Natl Acad Sci USA 1996; 93:5213–5218.

65. Atochina EN, Balyasnikova IV, Danilov SM, Granger DN, Fisher AB, Muzykantov VR. Immunotargeting of catalase to ACE or ICAM-1 protects perfused rat lungs against oxidative stress. Am J Physiol 1998; 275:L806–L817.

66. Balyasnikova IV, Gavrilyuk VD, McDonald T, Berkowitz R, Miletich DJ, Danilov SM. Antibody mediated lung endothelium targeting: 1. In vitro model using a cell line expressing angiotensin converting enzyme. Tumor Targeting 1999; 4:70–83.

67. Worgall S, Wolff G, Falckpedersen E, Crystal RG. Innate immune mechanisms dominate elimination of adenoviral vectors following in vivo administration. Hum Gene Ther 1997; 8:37–44.

68. Wickham TJ, Segal DM, Roelvink PW, Carrion ME, Lizonova A, Lee GM, Kovesdi I. Targeted adenovirus gene transfer to endothelial and smooth muscle cells by using bispecific antibodies. J Virol 1996; 70:6831–6838.

69. Harari OA, Wickham TJ, Stocker CJ, Kovesdi I, Segal DM, Huehns TY, Sarraf C, Haskard DO. Targeting an adenoviral gene vector to cytokine-activated vascular endothelium via E-selection. Gene Ther 1999; 6:801–807.

70. Yoon SK, Mohr L, O'Riordan CR, Lachapelle A, Armentano D, Wands JR. Targeting a recombinant adenovirus vector to HCC cells using a bifunctional Fab-antibody conjugate. Biochem Biophys Res Commun 2000; 272:497–504.

71. Watkins SJ, Mesyanzhinov VV, Kurochkina LP, Hawkins RE. The adenobody approach to viral targeting—specific and enhanced adenoviral gene delivery. Gene Ther 1997; 4:1004–1012.
72. Haisma HJ, Grill J, Curiel DT, Hoogeland S, van Beusechem VW, Pinedo HM, Gerritsen WR. Targeting of adenoviral vectors through a bispecific single-chain antibody. Cancer Gene Ther 2000; 7:901–904.
73. Nettelbeck DM, Miller DW, Jerome V, Zuzarte M, Watkins SJ, Hawkins RE, Muller R, Kontermann RE. Targeting of adenovirus to endothelial cells by a bispecific single-chain diabody directed against the adenovirus fiber knob domain and human endoglin (CD105). Mol Ther 2001; 3:882–891.
74. Dmitriev I, Kashentseva E, Rogers BE, Krasnykh V, Curiel DT. Ectodomain of coxsackievirus and adenovirus receptor genetically fused to epidermal growth factor mediates adenovirus targeting to epidermal growth factor receptor-positive cells. J Virol 2000; 74:6875–6884.
75. Barry MA, Dower WJ, Johnston SA. Toward cell-targeting gene therapy vectors: selection of cell-binding peptides from random peptide-presenting phage libraries. Nat Med 1996; 2:299–305.
76. Pasqualini R, Ruoslahti E. Organ targeting in vivo using phage display peptide libraries. Nature 1996; 380:364–366.
77. Nicklin SA, White SJ, Watkins SJ, Hawkins RE, Baker AH. Selective targeting of gene transfer to vascular endothelial cells by use of peptides isolated by phage display. Circulation 2000; 102:231–237.
78. Trepel M, Grifman M, Weitzman MD, Pasqualini R. Molecular adaptors for vascular-targeted adenoviral gene delivery. Hum Gene Ther 2000; 11:1971–1981.
79. Wickham TJ, Tzeng E, Shears LL, Roelvink PW, Li Y, Lee GM, Brough DE, Lizonova A, Kovesdi I. Increased in vitro and in vivo gene transfer by adenovirus vectors containing chimeric fiber proteins. J Virol 1997; 71:8221–8229.
80. McDonald GA, Zhu G, Li Y, Kovesdi I, Wickham TJ, Sukhatme VP. Efficient adenoviral gene transfer to kidney cortical vasculature utilizing a fiber modified vector. J Gene Med 1999; 1:103–110.
81. Krasnykh V, Dmitriev I, Mikheeva G, Miller CR, Belousova N, Curiel DT. Characterization of an adenovirus vector containing a heterologous peptide epitope in the HI loop of the fiber knob. J Virol 1998; 72:1844–1852.
82. Xia D, Henry LJ, Gerard RD, Deisenhofer J. Crystal structure of the receptor-binding domain of adenovirus type 5 fiber protein at 1.7 A resolution. Structure 1994; 2:1259–1270.
83. Pasqualini R, Koivunen E, Ruoslahti E. Alpha v integrins as receptors for tumor targeting by circulating ligands. Nat Biotechnol 1997; 15:542–546.
84. Vanderkwaak TJ, Wang M, Gomez-Navarro J, Rancourt C, Dmitriev I, Krasnykh V, Barnes M, Siegal GP, Alvarez R, Curiel DT. An advanced generation of adenoviral vectors selectively enhances gene transfer for ovarian cancer gene therapy approaches. Gynecol Oncol 1999; 74:227–234.
85. Blackwell JL, Li H, Gomez-Navarro J, Dmitriev I, Krasnykh V, Richter CA, Shaw DR, Alvarez RD, Curiel DT, Strong TV. Using a tropism-modified adenoviral vector to circumvent inhibitory factors in ascites fluid. Hum Gene Ther 2000; 11:1657–1669.

86. Reynolds PN, Dmitriev I, Curiel DT. Insertion of an RGD motif into the HI loop of adenovirus alters the transgene expression profile of the systemically administered vector. Gene Ther 1999; 6:1336–1339.

87. Suzuki K, Fueto J, Krasnykh V, Reynolds PN, Curiel DT, Alemany R. A conditionally replicative adenovirus with enhanced infectivity shows improved oncolytic potency. Clin Cancer Res 2001; 7:120–126.

88. Xia H, Anderson B, Mao Q, Davidson BL. Recombinant human adenovirus: targeting to the human transferrin receptor improves gene transfer to brain microcapillary endothelium. J Virol 2000; 74:11359–11366.

89. Pereboev A, Pereboeva L, Curiel DT. Phage display of adenovirus type 5 fiber knob as a tool for specific ligand selection and validation. J Virol 2001; 75:7107–7113.

90. Vigne E, Mahfouz I, Dedieu JF, Brie A, Perricaudet M, Yeh P. RGD inclusion in the hexon monomer provides adenovirus type 5-based vectors with a fiber knob-independent pathway for infection. J Virol 1999; 73:5156–5161.

91. Krasnykh V, Belousova N, Korokhov N, Mikheeva G, Curiel DT. Genetic targeting of an adenovirus vector via replacement of the fiber protein with the phage T4 fibritin. J Virol 2001; 75:4176–4183.

92. van Beusechem VW, van Rijswijk AL, van Es HH, Haisma HJ, Pinedo HM, Gerritsen WR. Recombinant adenovirus vectors with knobless fibers for targeted gene transfer. Gene Ther 2000; 7:1940–1946.

93. Magnusson MK, Hong SS, Boulanger P, Lindholm L. Genetic retargeting of adenovirus: novel strategy employing "deknobbing" of the fiber. J Virol 2001; 75:7280–7289.

94. Douglas JT, Miller CR, Kim M, Dmitriev I, Mikheeva G, Krasnykh V, Curiel DT. A system for the propagation of adenoviral vectors with genetically modified receptor specificities. Nat Biotechnol 1999; 17:470–475.

95. Ring CJ, Harris JD, Hurst HC, Lemoine NR. Suicide gene expression induced in tumour cells transduced with recombinant adenoviral, retroviral and plasmid vectors containing the ERBB2 promoter. Gene Ther 1996; 3:1094–1103.

96. Adachi Y, Reynolds PN, Yamamoto M, Grizzle WE, Overturf K, Matsubara S, Muramatsu T, Curiel DT. Midkine promoter-based adenoviral vector gene delivery for pediatric solid tumors. Cancer Res 2000; 60:4305–4310.

97. Yamamoto M, Alemany R, Adachi Y, Grizzle WE, Curiel DT. Characterization of the cyclooxygenase-2 promoter in an adenoviral vector and its application for the mitigation of toxicity in suicide gene therapy of gastrointestinal cancers. Mol Ther 2001; 3:385–394.

98. Varda-Bloom N, Shaish A, Gonen A, Levanon K, Greenbereger S, Ferber S, Levkovitz H, Castel D, Goldberg I, Afek A, Kopolovitc Y, Harats D. Tissue-specific gene therapy directed to tumor angiogenesis. Gene Ther 2001; 8:819–27.

99. Vassaux G, Hurst HC, Lemoine NR. Insulation of a conditionally expressed transgene in an adenoviral vector. Gene Ther 1999; 6:1192–1197.

100. Reynolds PN, Nicklin SA, Kaliberova L, Boatman BG, Grizzle WE, Balyasnikova IV, Baker AH, Danilov SM, Curiel DT. Combined transductional and transcriptional targeting improves the specificity of transgene expression in vivo. Nat Biotechnol 2001. In press.

101. Nicklin SA, Reynolds PN, Brosnan MJ, White SJ, Curiel DT, Dominiczak AF, Baker AH. Analysis of cell-specific promoters for viral gene therapy targeted at the vascular endothelium. Hypertension 2001; 38:65–70.

102. Hirose S, Hosoda Y, Furuya S, Otsuki T, Ikeda E. Expression of vascular endothelial growth factor and its receptors correlates closely with formation of the plexiform lesion in human pulmonary hypertension. Pathol Int 2000; 50:472–479.

103. Chow YH, Plumb J, Wen Y, Steer BM, Lu Z, Buchwald M, Hu J. Targeting transgene expression to airway epithelia and submucosal glands, prominent sites of human CFTR expression. Mol Ther 2000; 2:359–367.

104. Worgall S, Leopold PL, Wolff G, Ferris B, Van Roijen N, Crystal RG. Role of alveolar macrophages in rapid elimination of adenovirus vectors administered to the epithelial surface of the respiratory tract. Hum Gene Ther 1997; 8:1675–1684.

105. Tao N, Gao GP, Parr M, Johnston J, Baradet T, Wilson JM, Barsoum J, Fawell SE. Sequestration of adenoviral vector by Kupffer cells leads to a nonlinear dose response of transduction in liver. Mol Ther 2001; 3:28–35.

106. Wolff G, Worgall S, Vanrooijen N, Song WR, Harvey BG, Crystal RG. Enhancement of in vivo adenovirus-mediated gene transfer and expression by prior depletion of tissue macrophages in the target organ. J Virol 1997; 71:624–629.

107. O'Riordan CR, Lachapelle A, Delgado C, Parkes V, Wadsworth SC, Smith AE, Francis GE. PEGylation of adenovirus with retention of infectivity and protection from neutralizing antibody in vitro and in vivo. Hum Gene Ther 1999; 10:1349–1358.

108. Croyle MA, Chirmule N, Zhang Y, Wilson JM. "Stealth" adenoviruses blunt cell-mediated and humoral immune responses against the virus and allow for significant gene expression upon readministration in the lung. J Virol 2001; 75:4792–4801.

109. Gordon EM, Zhu NL, Forney Prescott M, Chen ZH, Anderson WF, Hall FL. Lesion-targeted injectable vectors for vascular restenosis. Hum Gene Ther 2001; 12:1277–1287.

110. Gordon EM, Chen ZH, Liu L, Whitley M, Wei D, Groshen S, Hinton DR, Anderson WF, Beart RW, Jr., Hall FL. Systemic administration of a matrix-targeted retroviral vector is efficacious for cancer gene therapy in mice. Hum Gene Ther 2001; 12: 193–204.

111. Bartlett JS, Kleinschmidt J, Boucher RC, Samulski RJ. Targeted adeno-associated virus vector transduction of nonpermissive cells mediated by a bispecific F(ab'-gamma)2 antibody. Nat Biotechnol 1999; 17:181–184.

112. Girod A, Ried M, Wobus C, Lahm H, Leike K, Kleinschmidt J, Deleage G, Hallek M. Genetic capsid modifications allow efficient re-targeting of adeno-associated virus type 2. Nat Med 1999; 5:1052–1056.

113. Larocca D, Jensen-Pergakes K, Burg MA, Baird A. Receptor-targeted gene delivery using multivalent phagemid particles. Mol Ther 2001; 3:476–84.

114. Huser A, Rudolph M, Hofmann C. Incorporation of decay-accelerating factor into the baculovirus envelope generates complement-resistant gene transfer vectors. Nat Biotechnol 2001; 19:451–455.

115. Li S, Tan Y, Viroonchatapan E, Pitt BR, Huang L. Targeted gene delivery to pulmonary endothelium by anti-PECAM antibody. Am J Physiol Lung Cell Mol Physiol 2000; 278:L504–L511.

6

Replicating Vectors

KUNJLATA M. AMIN

University of Pennsylvania School of Medicine
Philadelphia, Pennsylvania, U.S.A.

I. Replicating Vectors: A Tool for Cancer Gene Therapy

Cancer gene therapy has the potential to offer selective removal of tumor cells employing a different paradigm than current surgical, chemotherapeutic, or radiotherapeutic approaches. Over the past decade, the field of cancer gene therapy has generated large amounts of information from both preclinical and clinical trials. Although there have been some successes, for the most part, progress has been modest. Evaluation of these data has revealed that the primary limitations relate more to effective delivery of vector rather than with the choice of therapeutic genes, of which there are many excellent candidates. Moreover, attempts to increase efficacy by dosage manipulation, repeat administration, or ex vivo transduction of carrier cells to enhance gene delivery have often been overshadowed by increased inflammation and immunogenic responses.

To realize the full potential of cancer gene therapy, we need an ideal targeted vector that can effectively eradicate appropriate tumor cell populations and cause minimal toxicity to the normal tissue. This goal is in keeping with the recommendations made by the landmark "Report and Recommendation of the Panel to Assess the NIH Investment in Research on Gene Therapy" (1). This report highlighted the need to design vectors that are capable of restricting cyto-pathic effects to tumors and to promote tumor destruction, especially in the clini-cal setting. To this end, the ability of a replicating vector to kill a tumor cell during the reproductive phase of its life cycle is receiving a great deal of attention: an idea that is being revisited since its first description in the middle of the last century (2,3).

II. An Ideal Targeted Replicating Vector

The first requirement for an ideal targeted replicating vector is that it replicates efficiently and selectively in tumor cells and not in normal cells, thus providing a large margin of safety. In theory, intratumoral amplification of the initial input dose makes it possible to use a less aggressive dosing regimen. The vector should be able to grow in both dividing and nondividing cancer cells, since many tumors have a high density of nondividing cells. Since tumor cell death coincides with the release of the vector, this process can be optimized for both high-potency vector production and for rapid vector uptake by surrounding cells. Such radial spread is crucial for effective tumor eradication. The vector must also be able to interact efficiently with the immune system. Ideally, it should not succumb to immune-mediated destruction, but on the other hand it should be able to help generate an antitumor immune response. From the standpoint of stability, the vector should maintain its genetic integrity both during the manufacturing process and during in vivo administration, including systemic administration. The parent (wild-type) vector should be nonpathogenic, and preferably it should not integrate into the host chromosomes. Any vector selected for cancer gene therapy must be able to be manufactured to high titers using Good Manufacturing Practice procedures. To date, such an ideal vector does not exist; however, it is useful to use this "wish list" as a way to evaluate the current vectors being developed.

III. Replicating Agents

A majority of the replicating vectors that are entering the clinic or under develop-ment in the laboratory are viruses (4). Replicating viruses that have been used in patients include Adenovirus (Ad) (5), Herpes simplex virus (HSV) (6,7), New-castle disease virus (NDV) (8), reovirus (9), vaccinia virus (10), and autonomous parvovirus (11) among others (12). All these viruses replicate selectively in tumor cells owing to an inherent tumor selectivity (i.e., NDV, reovirus, and autonomous parvovirus) or because they have been modified genetically for selective replica-tion in tumor cells (i.e., Ad, HSV). These viruses bring about cell death through many different mechanisms, the primary being cell lysis occurring at the end of their reproductive life cycle. In addition to causing direct cell lysis and apoptosis, these viruses also induce synthesis of toxic products (e.g., tumor necrosis factor-α [TNF-α]) enhance immune-mediated cell killling (T-cell–mediated and upregulation of cytokine synthesis), and sensitize tumor cells to other routinely used therapies, especially radiation and chemotherapy. For detailed descriptions of many of these viruses, the reader is directed to several excellent reviews published recently (13–23). In this chapter, the strategies adapted to targeting replicating viruses to tumor cells and their feasibility for lung cancer gene therapy will be discussed.

IV. Wild-Type Replicating Vectors

In the second half of the last century, many wild-type viruses, including adenovirus, were assessed for oncotherapy by systemically delivering virus-lysates to treat a variety of solid tumors in patients. As examples, viruses used included rabies virus for cervical carcinoma, measles virus for Burkitt's lymphoma, NDV (73-T) for melanoma, and vaccinia virus for melanoma, breast, and colon cancers (24). In general, an initial tumor response was observed; however, the response could not be sustained and regrowth of the tumors eventually led to patient demise (25). Lack of data on toxicity to normal tissues and immune reactions to the viruses has made it difficult to evaluate the effectiveness of these viruses in the clinic. In the past, versions of genetically engineered wild-type viruses (vaccinia virus and adenovirus) have also been utilized as vaccines (26,27). Thus, the properties of direct oncolysis and the ability to deliver an amplifiable transgene (as shown in vaccine technology) are currently being evaluated intensely for cancer gene therapy.

The realization that some naturally occurring viruses are better adapted to replicate in tumors because they are able to take advantage of tumor-associated defects has allowed us to widen the spectrum of approaches available for cancer virotherapy. For example, reovirus, a nonpathogenic natural human RNA virus, usurps the activated ras-signaling pathway found in many tumor cells to support its replication. In normal cells, the early transcripts of reovirus phosphorylate a double-stranded RNA-activated protein kinase (PKR), leading to inhibition of the translation initiation factor, eIF2α. This results in inhibition of viral protein translation and viral replication. In contrast, in tumor cells, activated ras inhibits PKR activation allowing viral protein synthesis and replication to proceed (28). The reovirus Dearing strain 3 has shown impressive antitumor activity in many experimental models of human tumors grown in mice after repeated local dosing and by systemic administration. However, some toxicity seen with reovirus in immunodeficient mice raises concern for its use in immunosuppressed patients (9). Currently, Reolysin (reovirus trade name) is in a Phase I clinical trial in patients with metastic disease, including head and neck cancers (4). Reolysin may prove to be effective in a subset of lung carcinomas; adenocarcinomas have a high rate of ras mutations (40–50%).

Another single-stranded RNA virus is Newcastle disease virus (NDV). Although pathogenic in chickens, NDV is harmless in humans, which has allowed its use in vaccine technology (29). It replicates in tumors that are resistant to interferon and not in normal cells (30). A Phase I clinical trial with a replication-selective NDV strain, PV701, has been conducted using patients with a variety of solid tumors, including lung, head/neck, and ovarian cancers. Using PV701 as a single agent given intravenously, some tumor responses were noted in patients with head and neck cancers, colon cancers, and mesothelioma (31). However, some side effects were noted in patients with pulmonary or liver metastatic disease.

Other vectors including polio (32), retrovirus (33), bacteria (34), and autonomous parvovirus (35) are all potential oncolytic vectors under development. Autonomous parvovirus is a nonenveloped, single-stranded DNA virus that replicates in cells in the cytoplasm of dividing and nondividing tumor cells. Its envelope can be modified, similar to retroviruses, to contain ligand moieties to target cell surface receptors. It has been used in vaccine production where it showed low toxicity in human applications (11). Currently, the H-1 strain is being evaluated in the clinic (4).

A genetically modified bacterium, *Salmonella typhimurium* (VNP20009), replicates in hypoxic solid tumor masses and not in normal cells (36). A Phase I trial of VNP20009 is now ongoing for evaluation of safety and toxicity studies in patients with advanced or metastatic disease given the bacteria systemically (34). Preclinical studies have shown that VNP20009 organisms double in quantity every 30–45 min, and they selectively accumulate (1000-fold) in solid tumors of the lung, colon, breast, prostate, liver, kidney, and in melanoma compared to normal tissues (34). However, its efficacy as a single agent is not high and it may be more effective in combination therapies or after being "armed" with additional antitumor genes.

V. Genetically Modified Vectors

Increasing understanding of the virus and cancer cell growth pathways coupled with the impressive advances made in DNA recombinant technology have given us an unprecedented opportunity to modify the wild-type virus genome for selective replication in tumor cells with minimal toxicity in normal tissue. The large number of replication-selective viruses described over the last 5 years have generally been constructed using two broad approaches. These include (1) deletion of genes required by the virus to overcome host defense systems present in normal cells (but not cancer cells) or (2) to regulate viral genes essential for replication with transcriptional elements active only in tumor.

A. Gene-Deletion Approach

To replicate effectively in a normal cell, the virus has to first subvert the host cell cycle machinery (induce S-phase) and disarm the host apoptotic defense mechanisms. The gene-deletion approach involves the removal of viral genes essential for disarming host defense systems in normal cells so that viral replication is inhibited. However, these essential viral functions are compensated in tumor cells which have a frequent cell cycle and/or apoptotic pathway defects due to a variety of biochemical and genetic abnormalities. Since genetically engineered versions of HSV-1 and Ad are in clinical trials, here I will focus on these two viruses.

B. Herpes Simplex Virus

HSV-1 is an enveloped, double-stranded DNA virus with a size of 150 kb coding over 83 genes. It has a wide host range, infects nondividing cells, can accommodate large insert sizes (30 kb), and can be generated in high titers. After HSV-1 infection, immediate early (IE, or α) genes are expressed first, which in turn induces expression of early (E, or β) genes that encode enzymes required for DNA synthesis, such as thymidine kinase (tk), and ribonucleotide reductase (RR, ICP6). The late (L, or γ) genes encode structural proteins, surface glycoproteins, and protein for virus-host interaction. The γ-34.5 gene encodes the ICP34.5 protein that promotes infection of nondividing cells, inhibits apoptosis in infected cells, and appears to be important in neurovirulence. Viruses exit the cell by exocytosis and cell lysis, often with increased cytotoxicity due to HSV proteins (37).

When the thymidine kinase, neurovirulence (γ-34.5), or ribonucleotide reductase (ICP6) genes are deleted either singly or in combinations, the replication of the HSV-1 in normal cells is markedly curtailed. However, these mutants replicate with high efficiency in many cancer cells (38). The multideleted HSV-1 virus, G207, is missing both copies of the γ-34.5 genes, and has an insertion of LacZ gene, which inactivates the ICP6 (RR) gene. A Phase I clinical trial using G207 in 21 patients with recurrent malignant glioma has been completed demonstrating direct intracranial inoculations of G207 to be safe (39). Preliminary data from another Phase I trial with nine patients administered a second HSV-1 deletion mutant, 1716 (ICP34.5 null), reveals no significant toxicity (40). Mechanisms of tumor killing are by direct oncolysis and by generation of antitumor immune responses (6,41,42). NV1020 (deleted in one copy of ICP34.5) is now in a Phase I colorectal cancer clinical trial with intrahepatic delivery (4). In preclinical studies, such HSV-1 mutants have been shown to be effective in many experimental tumor models, including lung (42) and mesothelioma cancers (43). Recently, it was demonstrated that the HSV-1 γ-34.5 deletion mutant lacking PKR activity replicates preferentially in ras-activated tumor cells—suggesting that the Ras-signaling pathway compensates for this loss (44). Thus, HSV-1 mutants could be targeted to a wide range of tumors, including the lung cancers containing ras mutations (45).

C. Adenovirus

E1A-deleted mutants: Immediately following infection by adenovirus, a key protein for viral replication, the E1A protein, is expressed. The conserved region 2 (CR2) of the E1A protein binds to the retinoblastoma (pRb) protein leading to release of E2F-1 from the pRb-E2F complexes preexisting in normal quiescent cells (46). Free E2F stimulates DNA synthesis and cell cycle progression through the S-phase, an environment suitable for viral replication. Deletion of the CR2 domain abolishes the ability of Ad to induce S-phase and viral replcation in normal cells. In contrast, the frequent mutations in the Rb gene and its upstream regulators (p16/cyclin D/cyclin) (47) in tumor cells result in high levels of free E2F, making the Rb binding function of E1A dispensable.

A "proof of concept" for an Ad-CR2 deletion mutant virus was provided by Feuyo et al., who demonstrated that the replication of the CR2-deleted virus, Ad delta24 mutant was robust in most tumor cells but was attenuated in normal fibroblasts and in tumor cells with an intact Rb gene (48). In addition, Ad delta24 exhibited a high therapeutic index in treating experimental models of glioma tumors in vivo. Although significant tumor reduction was achieved with a single low dose of virus injected into flank tumors, no comparison with wild-type virus was made. In addition, growth properties of Ad delta24 in normal cells other than fibroblasts were not reported. However, the infectivity and the tumoricidal potency was significantly increased when Arg-Gly-Asp (RGD) motif was incorporated into the fiber knob of Ad delta24, underscoring a need to have adequate adenoviral receptors (49). Heise et al. demonstrated in vivo and in vitro potency of dl922/947 (a CR2-E1A mutant Ad) to be equivalent to the wild-type virus (50). They reported effective treatment of multifocal breast metastatic disease with intravenous injection of dl922/947. Moreover, dl922/947 grew robustly in tumor cells and moderately well in proliferating normal epithelial and endothelial cells. More importantly, Ad dl922/947 did not grow or cause cytopathic effect in normal nonproliferating epithelial cells and showed a delayed and reduced induction of S-phase in these nondividing epithelial cells. The oncolytic activity of the CR2 mutants has been improved by deleting a second p300 binding site, the CR1 domain of E1A (51,52).

To circumvent the toxicity due to the low levels of E1A mutant protein expressed in normal cells, a group at ONYX Pharmaceuticals (Richmond, CA) constructed the ONYX-838 virus, in which the E2F-1 promotor controls the CR2-E1A mutant (53). Encouraging results from preclinical studies with prostate, lung, and breast tumors are currently being translated into clinical trials. Another approach with the KTB9 virus incorporates a fusion protein of pRb-E2F binding domains under the control of several copies of wild-type p53 response element. In the normal cells, wild-type p53 activates synthesis of the pRb-E2F fusion protein, which functions as a dominant negative inhibitor of E2F-responsive genes (54). Because a majority (50–60%) of the tumor cells have a defect in the p53 gene, the pRb-E2F protein is not expressed in tumors, allowing KTB9 to replicate selectively in tumors and not in normal cells.

D. E1B-Deleted Mutant

A cell responds to Ad infection by upregulating p53 to induce either G1 arrest or apoptosis. The adenoviral E1B gene, expressed early in the infection cycle, encodes two proteins, E1B 55kD and E1B 19kD. E1B 55kD binds to the p53 protein and abrogates p53-induced apoptosis and prevents early demise of the cell. Premature cell death may be detrimental for viral progeny survival, but early viral release may be beneficial for an improved lateral spread. Thus, it is hypothesized that because E1B 55kD is critical for disarming the host defense pathways; deleting it would allow the defense pathways in normal cells to remain intact and curtail any viral replication. However, tumor cells with frequent defects and mutations in the p53 pathway (often mutated in 60–70% of tumors) will be able to support viral replication.

A prime example is the E1B-deleted ONYX-015/C1-042 virus, which replicates in tumor cells with defective p53 pathways and not in normal cells, because the E1B 55 kD protein required to inactivate p53 and apoptosis is absent (55). Several studies have now outlined that this dependence on defective p53 status is not very strict, as some cells with normal p53 are able to replicate ONYX-015 (56–58). Reis et al. showed a close correlation between a defective p14[ARF] pathway, intact p53 function, and the ability of ONYX-015 to replicate (59). Such studies have highlighted the need to examine carefully all p53 functional pathways. However, ONYX-015 has been safely administered to over 240 patients enrolled in Phase I/II/III clinical trials for ovarian, lung, head and neck, pancreas, colorectal, and gastric cancers (60). Because the antitumoral efficacy has been suboptimal as a single agent, ONYX-015 is being tested in combination with chemotherapy. The potential synergy between ONYX-015 and cisplatin or 5-FU has been demonstrated in preclinical and clinical studies (61). Augmentation of ONYX-015 cytotoxicity has been achieved by inserting prodrug-

Table 1 Different Tissue- or Tumor-Specific Promoters Used to Develop Replication-Selective Adenoviral Vectors

Adenovirus	Target	Promoter–early gene	Modification	Mechanism	Reference
		Targeted Functional Pathways			
Ad E2F-1^{RC}	Overexpressed E2F-1 in lung and ovarian tumors	E2F-1-E1A	E3 deleted	E2F-1 promoter–activated in tumors	This study
ONYX-838	Deregulated pRB pathway in a panel of tumors	E2F-1-E1A-Mutant	E3 deleted	Autoregulated E2F-1 promoter and pRB binding domain deleted in E1A	53
K9TB	Deregulated p53 pathway in lung, breast, and prostate tumors	P53 response elements–E2F/pRb fusion protein	MLP-controlled E3-ADP in E3 region	Wild-type p53 activated p53 response element driven pRb-E2F fusion protein mediates inhibition of S-phase in normal cells	54
KD3-SPB–E4	Deregulated pRB pathway in lung and liver tumors	SPB-E4	MLP-controlled E3-ADP and surfactant promoter–regulated E4	pRb, p300 binding domains deleted in E1A	91

Adenovirus	Targets tumor-antigen	Promoter–early gene	Modification	Mechanism	Reference
KD3	Deregulated pRB pathway in lung and liver tumors	MLP-controlled E3/ADP	MLP-controlled Ad death protein in E3 region	pRb, p300 binding domains deleted in E1A and overexpresses E3-ADP	91
vMB27	Activated wnt pathway in colon tumors	TCF-4 controlled E1B and E2	E3 promoter–mutated	1 cf-promoter activated by transcription factor-TcF-4 and repressed by Groucho/CtBP normal cell transcription factor	89
Tumor Antigens					
AdDF3.E1	Breast/MUC-1	MUC1–E1A	Additions of GFP or TNF-α	GFP used to monitor viral spread, TNF-α to enhance apoptosis	81
Ad5ERE2	Breast/estrogen receptor	pS2 ERE–E1A	pS2-ERE regulates E4 gene also	Selective regulation of E4-ORF4 for cell lyses, pS2 induced by 17β-estradiol and inhibited by tamoxifen	70
Ad522CEA	Lung cancer/CEA	CEA–E1A	E1A promoter intact	Carcinoembryogenic antigen overexpression	90

Table 1 Continued

Adenovirus	Targets tumor-antigen	Promoter–early gene	Modification	Mechanism	Reference
		Tumor Antigens			
Ad460CEA	Lung cancer/CEA	CEA–E1A	TATA box deleted in E1A promoter	Carcinoembryogenic antigen overexpression	90
AdSLIP-1.E1A	Lung cancer/secretory leukoprotease inhibitor	SLIP1–E1A	—	SLIP1 overexpressed in non-small cell lung cancer	82
AdL-plastin–E1A	Ovarian and breast tumors/L-plastin	L-plastin–E1A	E3 deleted	L-plastin mRNA correlates with E1A activity	83
AdOC-E1A	Prostate tumors in bone/osteocalcin (OC)	OC–E1A	E3 deleted	Cotargets prostate cancer cells and supporting tissue	84
CV706	Prostate/PSA	PSE–E1A	E3 deleted	Prostate-specific antigen activates prostate-specific element	75
CV787	Metastatic prostate/PSA	Probasin–E1A	E3 intact	E3 proteins help to evade immune response and viral release	75,77
CV739	Prostate/PSA	Probasin–E1A	PSE-controlled E1B and E3 deleted	PSE regulated E1B 55 kD is not expressed in normal cells and replication is inhibited	75

CV764	Prostate/PSA	PSE–E1A	hK2-controlled E1B and E3 deleted	Basal human kallikrein 2 promoter is silent in normal cells	75
CV890	Hepatocellular carcinoma/AFP	AFP–TRE–E1A	AFP-TRE–controlled E1 and E3 intact	α-Fetoprotein–activated AFP transcriptional regulatory elements regulate biscistronic cassette of E1A and E1B linked by internal ribosomal entry site	80
AdE1A041	Hepatocellular carcinoma/AFP	AFP–E1A	AFP-controlled E4 and E3 deleted	Artificial α-Fetoprotein promoter with enhancer and silencer elements to negate expression in normal hepatocytes; E4 proteins enhance cell lyses	86
Viral Promoters					
AdRG4	Vaccine	MLP–RG	E3 deleted	Amplification of rubella glycoprotein	27
AdRG1.13	Vaccine	E3–RG	E3 deleted	Amplification of rubella glycoprotein	27
AdRG1.0	Vaccine	SV40p–RG	E3 deleted	Amplification of rubella glycoprotein	27
AdE3k	Prodrug gene delivery	E3–HSVtk	E3 deleted	Amplification of HSV tymidine kinase	65

activating transgenes such as thymidine kinase (62) or thymidine kinase–cytosine deaminase (tk-CD) fusion gene in the E1B 55kD region (63). The tk-CD virus is being used in conjunction with radiotherapy and ganciclovir and is currently being tested in a Phase I trial of reoccurring prostate cancer (64). When the pro-drug gene, tk, is inserted into the E3 region in a replication-competent virus, it appears to have no added tumoricidal benefit as demonstrated in our laboratory recently (65).

Induction of apoptosis in the late stage of viral infection can lead to an early release of the viral progeny and an improved lateral spread with increased infection of surrounding tumor cells. In this regard, deletion of the E1B 19kD gene, which has potent antiapoptotic activity generates a large-plaque phenotype, indicative of early viral release and spread (66). Moreover, this phenotype does not compromise viral yield and, in fact, tumoricidal effects are higher than wild-type virus (67). Deletion of both E1B 55kD and E1B 19kD genes results in an added selectivity without affecting potency in p53-defective cells and an increased safety in normal fibroblasts, macrophages, and lymphocytes (68). Other Ad genes that provide increased lateral spread of the virus are the E3–adenoviral death protein (ADP) and E4 proteins (69). These genes have been successfully incorporated in the KD1 (51), K9TB (54), and Ad5ERE2 (70) viruses (Table 1).

One lesson learned from these new vectors is that problems may be encountered with large deletions of essential functional genes. Many viral genes have multiple and complex functions that result in unexpected consequences when they are removed. For example, Hay and colleagues (66) found that the E1B–55 kD–deleted virus replicated poorly in p53 mutant lung cancer cells but not in p53 wild-type and normal lung fibroblasts, and they suggested that protein shutoff (mediated by 55-kD protein) may be a determinant of selectivity (66). A better approach may be to alter specific nucleotides or to delete only a specific function and leave the rest of the gene intact. However, a point mutation instead of the deletion of the whole of the E1A-CR2 domain failed to attenuate replication in normal cells (50). Whether these new E1A mutant proteins are immunogenic and still remain sensitized to radiation-induced killing remains to be determined. It is also unclear how these small mutations affect the other pleiotropic functions of the wild-type E1A protein. For true specificity with ONYX-015, consideration should be given to removal of the E4 34kD protein, which also interacts with p53 (69).

VI. Transcriptional Regulation of Early Viral Expressed Proteins

Another approach to inhibit viral replication in normal cells is to control the expression of the gene products essential for viral replication with transcriptionally controlled regions (promoters) that are active in tumor cells but not in normal cells. In theory, this strategy is very appealing, because no viral replication products are expressed in normal cells. However, in practice, promoter strength and fidelity is often a limiting factor. Transcriptionally active, *cis*-acting sequences are assembled from a combination of promoter, enhancer, and silencer elements to achieve either a constitutive, selective, or inducible transcriptionally controlled region. Identification of new tumor-specific promoters regions has been difficult in the past; however, more recently, identification has become easier with the enormous amount of data generated from functional genomics, proteomics, differential display, serial analysis of gene expression, and other comparable techniques. Selective replication of virus in tumor cells can be achieved by using (1) promoters of either aberrantly overexpressed proteins specific to tumors, including viral promoters, for temporal regulation or (2) promoters of critical genes regulating essential biochemical pathways (telomerase, metabolic pathway genes, apoptosis, Rb, or E2F-1 for cell cycle). This approach has been used most extensively for HSV-1 and Ad vectors.

A. Herpes Simplex Virus-1

To target microscopic, metastatic, and inaccessible disease, systemic modes of delivery for replicating HSV-1 need to be developed. One approach is to use transcriptional targeting to particular cancers with the use of tumor-specific promoters. For example, the HSV-1 vector, G92A, has the immediate early gene, ICP4 (which is essential for viral replication), under the control of the albumin promoter/enhancer. Since HSV-1 ICP4 null mutants cannot replicate in normal cells or tumor cells not expressing albumin, the G92A showed selective tumor growth in albumin-producing hepatoma tumors in mice but had no effect on non–albumin producing prostate tumors (71). Other, similar approaches have been described for the calponin (72) and B-myb (73) promoters for bone and brain cancers, respectively. These approaches, plus additional improvements for systemic delivery (e.g., viral formulations in dextran sulfate), that offer protection in the blood stream (74) will likely be used in clinical trials in the near future.

B. Adenovirus

Tumor-Selective Genes as Targets

As described previously, the E1A gene product is essential for viral replication. Thus, transcriptional regulation of E1A using promoters of proteins overexpressed in tumors has been an important strategy. For example, prostate cancers express the biomarker protein prostate-specific antigen (PSA) that is used widely as a diagnostic tool. The prostate specific enhancer (PSE) element of the promoter of PSA has been inserted upstream of the E1A gene by Calydon Inc. (now Cell Genesys, Foster City, CA), and has been shown preferentially to eradicate PSA-expressing cells without having significant effects on non–PSA-producing tumors (75). This selectively replicating Ad (called CN706) has been used in a Phase I clinical trial which has recently been completed (76). Results showed that CN706 administered intratumorally, as a single agent, had an acceptable safety profile. Although some histological evidence of viral replication in tumors was presented, clinical benefit was reported to be minimal.

In view of this, further modifications (see Table 1) were made to CN706. These included (1) additional regulation of E1B with PSE, (2) use of different androgen-responsive and prostate-specific promoter (probasin) regulating E1A, and (3) the inclusion of the E3 gene. Regulation of the E1B gene provides control of apoptosis in PSA-positive cells (77). This new virus, CV787, is currently being used in a Phase I/II trial for androgen refractory metastatic prostate cancer with intravenous administration. Immunoadsorption of Ad antibodies from serum of patients, prior to CV787 administration is proposed in the protocol to enhance vector stability in the blood stream. An extended persistence of CN706 has been shown in animal studies when they were depleted of Ad-neutralizing antibodies (78). In addition, CV787 exhibits antitumor synergy when combined with chemotherapeutic agents (79). In all these PSA-specific viruses, the E1A promoter was left intact. Although the genome size of the CV787 construct is 105% of the normal Ad, it had no significant effect on either the titer or cytopathic effects. Promoter size can pose a problem, particularly when used with strategies that employ insertional approaches and need to retain all viral genes including E3 gene (77). A similar α-fetoprotein–driven E1 construct (CV890) eradicated human hepatoma xenografts in mice in combination with doxorubicin without affecting normal cells (80).

In other transcriptionally regulated Ad constructs described to date, the E1A promoter has been removed and replaced with tumor or tissue-specific promoters (81–84). A list of different promoters that have been used to date is shown in Table 1. In some cases, interference from the nearby inverted terminal repeat (ITR) sequence can result in the loss of promoter strength and fidelity (85). Selectivity can be enhanced with the use of silencer (86) or insulator sequences (87). For example, the AdE1a04i virus using the artificial α-fetoprotein (AFP) promoter to express E1A needed six copies of a silencer sequence to repress the promoter activity in normal hepatocytes. This virus showed specificity and potency for hepatoma carcinoma tumors and not in non-AFP-producing cells or in normal hepatocytes (86). Interference from heterologous promoters on packaging sequences positioned close to the ITR region can lead to mispackaged progeny and a reduction in titer (88).

Transcriptional regulation of genes other than E1A can also confer tumor selectivity in certain tumors. For example, Brunori et al. constructed a replication-selective Ad, which had either the E1B or the E2 genes controlled by the Tcf4 promoter. The E2 gene product is required for viral DNA synthesis (89). In colon

tumors, the wnt (an oncogene) pathway is constitutively activated owing to mutations of the β-catenin and adenomatous polyposis coli pathway genes, with the
consequence of an upregulation of the transcription factor Tcf4. In normal cells,
Tcf4 is constitutively repressed by two factors: Groucho and CtBP. This activation and repression of the Tcf4 trascriptional element forms the basis of generating a colon cancer–specific replicating Ad. Brunori et al. demonstrated a higher
(50- to 100-fold) replication rate for the Tcf4-E2–regulated virus in colon cells
than in normal cells. Although the E1B-Tcf4 regulated virus had a reduced selectivity, it induced lower levels of inflammation in mouse lungs compared to the
wild-type virus. No in vivo tumor treatment data was presented.

Apart from *tumor*-specific promoters, often *tissue*-specific promoters,
which remain active in tumors growing in the tissue, can be utilized for a selective
replication of Ad. For example, estrogen receptors (ERs) are retained in a majority of breast tumors. Estrogen binding to the ER stimulates them to bind to estro-
gen-responsive elements (EREs) in promoters of several genes (70). Clarke's
group developed a replication-selective Ad (Ad5ERE2) by placing E1 and E4
genes under the control of a hybrid promoter consisting of a minimally active
region of the pS2 promoter (a member of the trefoil family of factors) plus two
ERE-response elements. The hybrid promoter could be activated by synthetic
estrogen (17 β-estradiol) and inhibited by the antiestrogen 4-OH–tamoxifen.
They showed that the virus in the presence of estrogen selectively replicated and
killed in ER-positive cells as well as the wild-type virus and Ad 5ERE2 was
inhibited in the presence of 4-OH–tamoxifen. This is an added safety feature to
abolish "runaway" viral replication.

VII. Tumor Pathway Genes as Targets

Using a promoter of a key gene that is a limiting step in an essential biochemical
pathway of cell growth regulation can be a powerful tool for producing a vector
with specific amplification, safety, broad applicability, and potential increased
therapeutic synergy with chemotherapy and radiotherapy. For example, the critical cell cycle regulator gene product E2F-1 plays a critical role in the transit from
G1 to S-phase and is overexpressed in tumor cells with a defective Rb pathway.
Interestingly, E2F-1 autoregulates its own transcription.

We developed Ad E2F-1^{RC}, a vector in which E1A was placed under the
control of the human E2F-1 promoter. Ad E2F-1^{RC} was as cytolytic as the wild-
type virus in a panel of tumor cells and effective in retarding tumor growth (40–
50%) of established ovarian and lung xenografts in SCID mice. Importantly,
Ad E2F-1^{RC} did not replicate in nonproliferating normal epithelial, endothelial,
or fibroblast cells. In tumor cells, the replication (titer values) of Ad E2F-1^{RC}
was comparable to wild-type virus. The E1A promoter was left intact in Ad

E2F-1^{RC} construct as described for CN706 earlier. Often with this strategy, interference from the endogenous promoter may result in loss of selectivity. In fact, we found that low levels of E1A protein were expressed in normal growth-arrested fibroblasts infected with Ad E2F-1^{RC} within 48 hr. Whether this was due to the leakiness of E2F-1 promoter or due to some residual E1A promoter activity remains to be determined.

However, in another construct, Ad CEA460, with the carcinoembryonic antigen (CEA) controlled E1A, a deletion of the E1A-TATA box resulted in an improved selectivity and a superior in vivo potency in colon and lung tumors (90). Moreover, in a preliminary study conducted in our laboratory, we demonstrated an improvement in the selectivity of Ad CEA522 virus by insulating the CEA promoter–E1 cassette with insulator sequences. To confine virus to a given population of tumor cells, multimodal approaches may prove to be effective. For example, the recent use of a partially deleted E1A mutant (unable to bind pRb and p300 cellular proteins) combined with the surfactant-B protein promoter–controlled E4 gene has demonstrated superior selectivity and potency for treating experimental models of bronchoalveolar lung cancers (91). Another approach utilizes a genetically modified adenovirus to retarget it to an abundantly expressed tumor cell surface molecule combined with transcriptional regulation of its replication with a tumor-specific promoter for targeting lung tissue (92).

VIII. Summary

Lung cancer and mesothelioma patient survival rates have not improved despite major advances in chemotherapy and radiotherapy. The new therapeutic platform of cancer gene therapy has seen rapid expansion over the last few years and offers practical promise for these tumors. Because most lung cancers are not surgically resectable at the time of diagnosis, approaches that allow either induced immune activation or systemic administration are needed. The major limiting factors for an effective oncolytic cancer therapy at present are the low gene transfer and antitumor potency. The "selective replication" platform offers an especially promising strategy. However, many obstacles still remain. Suitable animal models are not available. This is especially true with regard to replicating adenoviruses where human Ad does not replicate in mouse tissues. A recent report of a transgenic mouse model expressing CAR in all its tissues may be a start (93). Without such models, understanding the effects of the host immune system or the immune modulatory activities of the virus cannot be well studied. Even more importantly, safety studies in animals where Ad does not replicate are virtually impossible to conduct.

With respect to targeting strategies, a limiting factor that precludes the use of many promoters is the loss of promoter fidelity either due to methylation, rearrangements, deletions, interaction with viral proteins, or interference from *cis*-acting viral elements. Very little is known about the mechanisms that account for this. Additional effort needs to be invested if we are to realize the true potential of a temporally and spatially regulated, replicating virus for a targeted delivery to tumor cells.

Another problem with replicating viruses involves spread of virus within tumors. Even if a small population of tumor cells is infected, the radial spread of the virus to every tumor cell remains a rate-limiting step, in large part due to the heterogeneous microenvironment between tumor deposits and often due to a lack of appropriate receptors. The combination of replication vectors with retargeting strategies using additional cellular receptors may be a very important avenue for research.

Thus, although much has been accomplished, much remains to be done before replicating vectors can take their place in the therapeutic armamentarium for use in lung cancer and mesothelioma. Thorough preclinical studies and carefully done clinical trials are the pathways to success in this area.

Acknowledgment

I thank Dr. S. M. Albelda and all the other members of the Thoracic Oncology Research Laboratory at the University of Pennsylvania for helpful discussions.

References

1. Orkin SH, Motulsky AG. Report and recommendations of the panel to assess the NIH investment in research on gene therapy. NIH, December 1995. See *http:// nihitsii.od.nih.gov/oba/panelrep.htm*.
2. Smith R, Huebner RJ, Rowe WP, Schatten WE, Thomas LB. Studies on the use of viruses in the treatment of carcinoma of the cervix. Cancer 1956; 9:1211–1218.
3. Newman W, Southam CM. Virus treatment in advanced cancer, a pathological study of fifty-seven cases. Cancer 1954; 7:106–118.
4. Kirn D, Martuza RL, Zwiebel J. Replication-selective virotherapy for cancer: biological principles, risk management and future directions. Nat Med 2001; 7:781–787.
5. Russell WC. Update on adenovirus and its vectors. J Gen Virol 2000; 81:2573–2604.
6. Martuza RL. Conditionally replicating herpes vectors for cancer therapy. J Clin Invest 2000; 105(7):841–846.
7. Kirn DH. A tale of two trials: selectivity replicating herpesviruses for brain tumors. Gene Ther 2000; 7(10):815–816.
8. Cassel WA, Garrett RE. Newcastle virus as an antineoplastic agent. Cancer 1965; 18(52):863–869.
9. Norman KL, Lee PW. Reovirus as a novel oncolytic agent. J Clin Invest 2000; 105(8):1035–1038.

10. Mastrangelo MJ, Eisenlohr LC, Gomella L, Lattime EC. Poxvirus vectors: orphaned and under appreciated. J Clin Invest 2000; 105(8):1031–1034.

11. Palmer GA, Tattersall P. Autonomous parvoviruses as gene transfer vehicles. Contrib Microbiol 2000; 4:178–202.

12. Kirn DH. Replication-selective microbiological agents: fighting cancer with targeted germ warfare. J Clin Invest 2000; 105(7):837–839.

13. Vile RG, Russell SJ, Lemione NR. Cancer gene therapy: hard lessons and new courses. Gene Ther 2000; 7:2–8.

14. Wildner O. Oncolytic viruses as therapeutic agents. Ann Med 2001; 33:291–304.

15. Kay MA, Glorioso JC, Naldini L. Viral vectors for gene therapy: the art of turning infectious agents into vehicles of therapeutics. Nat Med 2001; 7:33–40.

16. Curiel TC. The development of conditionally explicative adenoviruses for cancer therapy. Clin Cancer Res 2000; 6:3395–3399.

17. Alemany R, Balague C, Curiel DT. Replicative adenoviruses for cancer therapy. Nat Biotechnol 2000; 18:723–727.

18. Kirn DH, McCormick F. Replicating viruses as selective cancer therapeutics. Mol Med Today 1996; 2(12):519–527.

19. Heise C, Kirn DH. Replication-selective adenoviruses as oncolytic agents. J Clin Invest 2000; 105:847–851.

20. Zweibel JA. Cancer Gene and oncolytic virus therapy. Semin Oncol 2001; 28:336–343.

21. Hermiston T. Gene delivery from replication-selective viruses: arming guided missiles in the war against cancer. J Clin Invest 2000; 105:1169–1172.

22. Wickham TJ. Targeting adenoviruses. Gene Ther 2000; 7:110–114.

23. Hallenback PL, Stevenson SC. Targetable Gene Delivery Vectors. In: Habib NA, ed. Cancer Gene Therapy: Past Achievements and Future Challenges. New York: Kluwer Academic/Plenum, 2000:37–46.

24. Southam CM. Present status of oncolytic virus studies. Ann NY Acad Sci 1960; 261:657–672.

25. Sinkovics JG, Horvath J. New developments in the virus therapy of cancer: a historical review. Intervirology 1993; 36:193–214.

26. Moss B. Genetically engineered poxviruses for recombinant gene expression, vaccination, and safety. Proc Natl Acad Sci USA 1996; 93:11341–11348.

27. Yarosh OK, Wandeler AI, Graham FL, Campbell JB, Prevec L. Human adenovirus type 5 vectors expressing rabies glycoprotein. Vaccine 1996; 4:1257–1264.

28. Coffey MC, Strong JE, Forsyth PA, Lee PW. Reovirus therapy of tumors with activated Ras pathway. Science 1998; 282(5392):1332–1334.

29. Cassel WA, Murray DR, Phillips HS. A Phase II study on the post surgical management of stage II malignant melanoma with a Newcastle disease virus oncolysate. Cancer 1983; 52(5):856–860.

30. Reichard KW, Lorence RM, Cascino CJ, Peeples ME, Walter RJ, Fernando MB, Reyes HM, Greager JA. Newcastle disease virus selectively kills human tumor cells. J Surg Res 1992; 52(5):448–453.

31. Pecora AL, Rizvi N, Cohen GI, Meropol NJ, Sterman D, Marshall J, Lorence RM. An Intravenous, Phase I Trial of a Replication-Competent Virus, PV701, in the

Treatment of Patients with Advanced Solid Cancers. Abstract No. 1009, 37th American Society of Clinical Oncologists Meeting, San Francisco, May 12–15, 2001.

32. Gromeier M, Lachmann S, Rosenfeld MR, Gutin PH, Wimmer E. Intergeneric poliovirus recombinants for the treatment of malignant glioma. Proc Natl Acad Sci USA 2000; 97(12):6803–6808.

33. Logg CR, Tai C, Logg A, Anderson FA, Kasahara N. A uniquely stable replication competent retrovirus vector achieves efficient gene delivery in vitro and in solid tumors. Hum Gene Ther 2001; 12:921–932.

34. Sznol M, Lin SL, Bermudes D, Zheng LM, King I. Use of preferentially replicating bacteria for the treatment of cancer. J Clin Invest 2000; 105(8):1027–1030.

35. Van Pachterbeke C, Tuynder M, Cosyn JP, Lespagnard L, Larsimont D, Rommelaere J. Parvovirus H-1 inhibits growth of short-term tumor-derived but not normal mammary tissue cultures. Int J Cancer 1993; 55(4):672–677.

36. Clairmont C, Lee KC, Pike J, Ittensohn M, Low KB, Pawelek J, Bermudes D, Brecher SM, Margitich D, Turnier J, Li Z, Luo X, King I, Zheng L. Biodistribution and genetic stability of the novel antitumor agent VNP20009, a genetically modified strain of *Salmonella typhimurium*. J Infect Dis 2000; 181(6):1996–2002.

37. Sears AE, Roizman B. Herpes simplex viruses and their replication. In: Fields BN, Knipe DM, eds. Virology, 2nd ed. New York: Raven Press, 1990:1795–1828.

38. Mineta T, Rabkin SD, Yazaki T, Hunter WD, Martuza RL. Attenuated multimutated herpes virus-1 for the treatment of malignant gliomas. Nat Med 1995; 1:938–943.

39. Markert JM, Medlock MD, Rabkin SD, Gillespie GY, Todo T, Hunter WD, Palmer CA, Feigenbaum F, Tornatore C, Tufaro F, Martuza RL. Conditionally replicating herpes simplex virus mutant G207 for the treatment of malignant glioma: results of a phase I trial. Gene Ther 2000; 7(10):867–874.

40. Rampling R, Cruickshank G, Papanastassiou V, Nicoll J, Hadley D, Brennan D, Petty R, MacLean A, Harland J, McKie E, Mabbs R, Brown M. Toxicity evaluation of replication-competent herpes simplex virus (ICP 34.5 null mutant 1716) in patients with recurrent malignant gliomas. Gene Ther 2000 7(10):859–866.

41. Todo T, Rabkin SD, Sundaresan P, Wu A, Meehan KR, Herscowitz HB, Martuza RL. Systemic antitumor immunity in experimental brain tumor therapy using a multimutated, replication-competent herpes simplex virus. Hum Gene Ther 1999; 10(17): 2741–2755.

42. Lambright ES, Caparrelli DJ, Abbas AE, Toyoizumi T, Coukos G, Molnar-Kimber KL, Kaiser LR. Oncolytic therapy using a mutant type-1 herpes simplex virus and the role of the immune system. Ann Thorac Surg 1999; 68(5):1756–1760; discussion 1761–1762.

43. Kucharczuk JC, Randazzo B, Chang MY, Amin KM, Elshami AA, Sterman DH, Rizk NP, Molnar-Kimber KL, Brown SM, MacLean AR, Litzky LA, Fraser NW, Albelda SM, Kaiser LR. Use of a "replication-restricted" herpes virus to treat experimental human malignant mesothelioma. Cancer Res 1997; 57(3):466–471.

44. Farassati F, Yang AD, Lee PW. Oncogenes in Ras signalling pathway dictate host-cell permissiveness to herpes simplex virus 1. Nat Cell Biol 2001; 3(8):745–750.

45. Wistuba II, Gazdar AF, Minna JD. Molecular genetics of small cell lung carcinoma. Semin Oncol 2001; 28(2 Suppl 4):3–13.

46. Nevins JR. Adenovirus E1A: transcription regulation and alteration of cell growth control. Curr Top Microbiol Immunol 1995; 199(Pt 3):25–32.

47. Rocco JW, Sidransky D. p16 (MTS-1/CDKN2/INK4a) in cancer progression. Exp Cell Res 2001; 264(1):42–55.

48. Fueyo J, Gomez-Manzano C, Alemany R, Lee PS, McDonnell TJ, Mitlianga P, Shi YX, Levin VA, Yung WK, Kyritsis AP. A mutant oncolytic adenovirus targeting the Rb pathways produces anti-glioma effect in vivo. Oncogene 2000; 19:2–12.

49. Suzuki K, Fueyo J, Krasnykh V, Reynolds PN, Curiel DT, Alemany R. A conditionally replicative adenovirus with enhanced infectivity shows improved oncolytic potency. Clin Cancer Res 2001; 7:120–126.

50. Heise C, Hermiston T, Johnson L, Brooks G, Sampson-Johannes A, Williams A, Hawkins L, Kirn D. An adenovirus E1A mutant that demonstrates potent and selective systemic anti-tumoral efficacy. Nat Med 2000; 6(10):1134–1139.

51. Doronin K, Toth K, Kuppuswamy M, Ward P, Tollefson AE, Wold WS. Tumor-specific, replication-competent adenivirus vectors overexpressing the adenovirus death protein. J Virol 2000; 74:6147–6155.

52. Howe JA, Demers GW, Johnson DE, Neugebauer SE, Perry ST, Vaillancourt MT, Faha B. Evaluation of E1-mutant adenoviruses as conditionally replicating agents for cancer therapy. Mol Ther 2000; 2:485–495.

53. Sunamura, M. Mutant adenoviruses selectively replication-competent in tumor cells. In: Habib NA, ed. Cancer Gene Therapy: Past Achievements and Further Challenges. New York: Kluwer Academic Press/Plenum, 2000:65–71.

54. Ramachandran M, Rahman A, Zou A, Vaillancourt M, Howe JA, Antelman D, Sugarman B, Demers WG, Engler H, Duane J, Shabram P. Re-engineering adenovirus regulatory pathways to enhance oncolytic specificity and efficacy. Nat Biotechnol 2001; 19:1035–1041.

55. Bischoff JR, Kern DH, Williams A, Heike C, Horn S, Mona M, Ng L, Nye JA, Sampson-Johannes A, Fattaey A, McCormick F. An adenovirus mutant that replicates selectively in p53-deficient human tumor cells. Science 1996; 274:373–376.

56. Rothmann T, Hengstermann A, Whitaker NJ, Scheffner M, zur Hausen H. Replication of ONYX-015, a potential anticancer adenovirus, is independent of p53 status in tumor cells. J Virol 1998; 72:9470–9478.

57. Hall AR, Dix BR, O'Carroll SJ, Braithwaite AW. p53-dependent cell death/apoptosis is required for a productive adenovirus infection (see comments). Nat Med 1998; 4:1068–1072.

58. Turnell AS, Grand RJ, Gallimore PH. The replicative capacities of large E1B-null group A and group C adenoviruses are independent of host cell p53 status. J Virol 1999; 73:2074–2083.

59. Ries SJ, Brandts CH, Chung AS, Biederer CH, Hann BC, Lipner EM, McCormick F, Korn WM. Loss of p14ARF in tumor cells facilitates replication of the adenovirus mutant dl1520 (ONYX-015). Nat Med 2000; 6:1128–1133.

60. Kirn D. Clinical research results with dl520 (Onyx-015), a replication-selective adenovirus for the treatment of cancer: what have we learned? Gene Ther 2001; 8:89–98.

61. Khuri FR, Nemunaitis J, Ganly I, Arseneau J, Tannock IF, Romel L, Gore M,

Ironside J, MacDougall RH, Heise C, Randlev B, Gillenwater AM, Bruso P, Kaye SB, Hong WK, Kirn DH. A controlled trial of intratumoral ONYX-015, a selectively-replicating adenovirus, in combination with cisplatin and 5-fluorouracil in patients with recurrent head and neck cancer. Nat Med 2000; 6(8):879–885.

62. Wildner O, Morris JC, Vahanian NN, Ford H Jr, Ramsey WJ, Blaese RM. Adenoviral vectors capable of replication improve the efficacy of HSVtk/GCV suicide gene therapy of cancer. Gene Ther 1999; 6:57–62.

63. Freytag SO, Rogulski KR, Paielli DL, Gilbert JD, Kim JH. A novel three-pronged approach to kill cancer cells selectively: concomitant viral, double suicide gene, and radiotherapy. Hum Gene Ther 1998; 9:1323–1333.

64. Freytag SO, Kim JH, Khil M, Menon M, Peabody J, Stricker H, Nafziger D, Pegg J, Aguilar-Cordova E. Phase I study of replication-competent adenovirus-mediated double suicide gene therapy for local recurrence of prostate cancer after definitive radiation. Abstract No. 873, 4th American Society of Gene Therapy Meeting, Seattle, May 30–June 3, 2001.

65. Lambright ES, Amin K, Wiewrodt R, Force SD, Lanuti M, Propert KJ, Kaiser LR, and Albelda SM. Inclusion of the herpes simplex thymidine kinase gene in a replicating adenovirus does not augment antitumor efficacy. Gene Ther 2001; 8:946–953.

66. Hay JG, Shapiro N, Sauthoff H, Heitner S, Phupakdi W, Rom WN. Targeting the replication of adenoviral gene therapy vectors to lung cancer cells: the importance of the adenoviral E1b-55kD gene. Hum Gene Ther 1999; 10:579–590.

67. Sauthoff H, Heitner S, Rom WN, Hay JG. Deletion of the adenoviral E1b-19kD gene enhances tumor cell killing of a replicating adenoviral vector. Hum Gene Ther 2000; 11:379–388.

68. Duque PM, Alonso C, Sanchez-Prieto R, Lleonart M, Martinez C, de Buitrago GG, Cano A, Quintanilla M, Cajal SR. Adenovirus lacking the 19-kDa and 55-kDa E1B genes exerts a marked cytotoxic effect in human malignant cells. Cancer Gene Ther 1999; 6:554–563.

69. Goodrum FD, Ornelles DA. Roles for the E4 orf6, orf3, and E1B 55-kilodalton proteins in cell cycle–independent adenovirus replication. J Virol 1999; 73(9):7474–7488.

70. Hernandez-Alcoceba R, Pihalja M, Wicha MS, Clarke MF. A novel, conditionally replicative adenovirus for the treatment of breast cancer that allows controlled replication of E1a-deleted adenoviral vectors. Hum Gene Ther 2000; 11(14):2009–2024.

71. Miyatake S, Iyer A, Martuza RL, Rabkin SD. Transcriptional targeting of herpes simplex virus for cell-specific replication. J Virol 1997; 71(7):5124–5132.

72. Yamamura H, Hashio M, Noguchi M, Sugenoya Y, Osakada M, Hirano N, Sasaki Y, Yoden T, Awata N, Araki N, Tatsuta M, Miyatake SI, Takahashi K. Identification of the transcriptional regulatory sequences of human calponin promoter and their use in targeting a conditionally replicating herpes vector to malignant human soft tissue and bone tumors. Cancer Res 2001; 61(10):3969–3977.

73. Chung RY, Saeki Y, Chiocca EA. B-myb promoter retargeting of herpes simplex virus gamma34.5 gene-mediated virulence toward tumor and cycling cells. J Virol 1999; 73(9):7556–7564.

74. Yeung S, Tufaro F, Qiang D, Zager J, Delman K, Fong Y, Horsburgh B. Dextran sulfate enhances the systemic delivery of oncolytic herpes simplex virus for treat-

ment of colorectal cancer. Abstract No. 1110, 4th American Society of Gene Therapy Meeting, Seattle, May 30–June 3, 2001.

75. Rodriguez R, Schuur ER, Lim HY, Henderson GA, Simons JW, Henderson DR. Prostate attenuated replication competent adenovirus (ARCA) CN706: a selective cytotoxic for prostate-specific antigen-positive prostate cancer cells. Cancer Res 1997; 57(13):2559–2563.

76. Simons JW, van der Poel HG, DeMarzo AM, Rodriguez R, Goemann MM, Nelson WG, Li S, Detorie N, Hamper UM, Ramakrishna N, DeWeese TL. Molecular and clinical activity of CN706, a PSA selective oncolytic Ad5 vector in a Phase I trial in locally recurrent prostate cancer following radiation therapy. Abstract No. 1804, American Society of Clinical Oncology Meeting, New Orleans, May 20–23, 2000.

77. Yu DC, Chen Y, Seng M, Dilley J, Henderson DR. The addition of adenovirus type 5 region E3 enables calydon virus 787 to eliminate distant prostate tumor xenografts. Cancer Res 1999; 59:4200–4203. (erratum in Cancer Res 2000; 60:1150.)

78. Chen Y, Yu DC, Charlton D, Henderson DR. Pre-existent adenovirus antibody inhibits systemic toxicity and antitumor activity of CN706 in the nude mouse LNCaP xenograft model: implications and proposals for human therapy. Hum Gene Ther 2000; 11:1553–1567.

79. Yu DC, Chen Y, Dilley J, Li Y, Embry M, Zhang H, Nguyen N, Amin P, Oh J, Henderson DR. Antitumor synergy of CV787, a prostate cancer-specific adenovirus, and paclitaxel and docetaxel. Cancer Res 2001; 61(2):517–525.

80. Li Y, Yu DC, Chen Y, Amin P, Zhang H, Nguyen N, Henderson DR. A hepatocellular carcinoma-specific adenovirus variant, CV890, eliminates tumor cells in combination with doxorubicin. Cancer Res 2001; 61:6428–6436.

81. Kurihara T, Brough DE, Kovesdi I, Kufe DW. Selectivity of a replication-competent adenovirus for human breast carcinoma cells expressing the MUC1 antigen. J Clin Invest 2000; 106(6):763–771.

82. Memento M, Narumi K, Saigon Y, Usual K, Kikuchi T, Tazawa R, Hagiwara K, Takahashi M, Nijitsu Y, Nukiwa T. A replication-selective adenovirus treatment for secretory leukoprotease inhibitor (SLIp1) producing lung cancer cells. Abstract No. 289, 4th American Society of Gene Therapy Meeting, Seattle, May 30–June 3, 2001.

83. Chung I, Schwartz PE, Crystal RG, Pizzorno G, Levitt HJ, Desseroth AB. Use of L-plastin promoter to develop an adenoviral system that confers transgene expression in ovarian cancer cells but not in normal mesothelial cells. Cancer Gene Ther 1999; 6:99–106.

84. Matsubara S, Wada Y, Gardner TA, Egawa M, Park MS, Hsieh CL, Zhau HE, Kao C, Kamidono S, Gillenwater JY, Chung LW. A conditional replication-competent adenoviral vector, Ad-OC-E1a, to cotarget prostate cancer and bone stroma in an experimental model of androgen-independent prostate cancer bone metastasis. Cancer Res 2001; 61(16):6012–6019.

85. Rubinchik S, Lowe S, Jia Z, Norris J, Dong J. Creation of a new transgene cloning site near the right ITR of Ad5 results in reduced enhancer interference with tissue-specific and regulatable promoters. Gene Ther 2001; 8(3):247–253.

86. Hallenbeck PL, Chang YN, Hay C, Golightly D, Stewart D, Lin J, Phipps S, Chiang YL. A novel tumor-specific replication-restricted adenoviral vector for gene therapy of hepatocellular carcinoma. Hum Gene Ther 1999; 10(10):1721–1733.

87. Vassaux G, Hurst HC, Lemoine NR. Insulation of a conditionally expressed transgene in an adenoviral vector. Gene Ther 1999; 6(6):1192–1197.

88. Shi Q, Wang Y, Worton R. Modulation of the specificity and activity of a cellular promoter in an adenoviral vector. Hum Gen Ther 1997; 8(4):403–410.

89. Brunori M, Malerba M, Kashiwazaki H, Iggo R. Replicating adenoviruses that target tumors with constitutive activation of the wnt signaling pathway. J Virol 2001; 75(6): 2857–2865.

90. Toyoizumi T, Tsukuda K, Banet G, Sandu AK, Hochberg A, Odaka M, Albelda SM, Amin K, Tykocinski MI, Kaiser LR, Molnar-Kimber KL. Deletion of E1A promoter elements enhances specificity of CEA-driven oncolytic adenoviruses. Abstract No. 986, 4th American Society of Gene Therapy Meeting, Seattle, WA, May 30–June 3, 2001.

91. Doronin K, Kuppuswamy M, Toth K, Tollefson AE, Krajcsi P, Krougliak V, Wold WS. Tissue-specific, tumor-selective, replication-competent adenovirus vector for cancer gene therapy. J Virol 2001; 75(7):3314–3324.

92. Reynolds PN, Nicklin SA, Kaliberova L, Boatman BG, Grizzle WE, Balyasnikova IV, Baker AH, Danilov SM, Curiel DT. Combined transductional and transcriptional targeting improves the specificity of transgene expression in vivo. Nat Biotechnol 2001; 19(9):838–842.

93. Tallone T, Malin S, Samuelsson A, Wilbertz J, Miyahara M, Okamoto K, Poellinger L, Philipson L, Pettersson S. A mouse model for adenovirus gene delivery. Proc Natl Acad Sci USA 2001; 98(14):7910–7915.

Part Two

USE OF GENE THERAPY TO STUDY LUNG DISEASES

7

Use of Gene Transfer to Study Lung Cytokine Biology

JACK GAULDIE and ZHOU XING

McMaster University
Hamilton, Ontario, Canada

PATRICIA J. SIME

University of Rochester Medical Center
Rochester, New York, U.S.A.

MARTIN KOLB

Julius-Maximilian-Universität Würzburg
Würzburg, Germany

DAVID WARBURTON

Childrens Hospital Los Angeles
    Research Institute
University of Southern California School of
    Medicine
Los Angeles, California, U.S.A

I. Introduction

Cytokines, chemokines, and growth factors are important mediators that allow communication between cells undergoing differentiation, response to infection, injury, and/or repair. These molecules regulate the pathobiological mechanisms involved in tissue responses to a variety of stimuli. For example, in the lung, infection with bacteria leads to release of chemotactic factors, accumulation of inflammatory cells, release of further cytokines, and stimulation of immune responses, acute phase responses, and subsequent repair responses, all involving multiple cell types, tissues, and body compartments. This cascade of events is meant to stop the injury, wall off invading organisms, initiate the immune defense system, repair and remove the damaged tissue, and return the organism to normal function. Sorting out the role for any one mediator in this complex pattern of events is very difficult, and thus the development of therapeutic interventions remains empiric at best.

This is especially so for pulmonary diseases and responses where the tissue is directly exposed to external stimuli and infectious agents, has direct and immediate contact with the circulatory system, and has a large repository of immune and inflammatory cells. This, coupled with the rapid access to the parenchyma and lumen of the lung and airway, means that determining the specific role or effect of an individual cytokine in lung pathobiology and physiology requires some unique aspects to allow reasoned and understandable interpretation. Essentially, infections, allergic reactions, or trauma/secondary injury to the lung tissue result in upregulation and release of the cytokines from multiple cell sources over a prolonged, but defined, period of time. On examination of lung tissue at any one time may reveal the presence of a cytokine, and it may even indicate that it is being released from a particular cell type(s). However, it is not possible to attribute causality to the cytokine in the ongoing process, and whether the presence of the cytokine indicates we should target this particular gene product for therapeutic intervention is a stretch.

We and others have recognized the transient and cascade-like nature of the expression of cytokines in the tissue responses. We have developed approaches to deliver genes to the lung tissue to allow expression in a tissue-restricted manner and over a suitable period of time consistent with the pathologic process (a few days or weeks). These approaches use rodent models, including the mouse, to take advantage of the unique accessibility to many immunological reagents, including gene knockout and transgenic mouse strains. Taking into account the differences in respiratory anatomy and histology of the rodent versus the human, we can interpret the data generated using these gene transfer systems to allow a better understanding of cytokine-mediated pathogenic responses and recognition of appropriate target cytokines related to specific disease processes.

II. Gene Transfer to the Lung

There has been a number of studies using transgenic mouse models of cytokine overexpression using tissue-specific promoters such as the SPC or CC10 promoter (1–3). Although such studies have provided unique and sometimes unexpected findings regarding the role of a cytokine in a disease process, without combining tissue specific promoters with conditional expression systems, such as the tetracycline transactivator (4), the transgenic approach is limited by expression during development and redundant pathways of cytokine activation being activated over a long period of time.

To overcome these limitations, we and others have developed cDNA and/ or viral vector transfection approaches, including vaccinia viral and adenoviral vectors. These approaches can limit the expression to lung tissue, can be titrated to deliver a dose response of the cytokine gene, can express over a number of days to weeks, and can be administered to animals over a wide age span and to various knockout mouse strains. In particular, the adenoviral vectors, based on recombinant, replication-deficient virus of serotype 5 and 2, have been used to transfer genes to the bronchial epithelium with high efficiency. The pulmonary epithelial cell is the natural host target for adenovirus, and many studies have shown specific infection and expression from bronchial and bronchiolar cells. Figure 1 illustrates the concept of adenoviral (Ad) vector epithelial cell infection with gene expression of cytokines, chemokines, and growth factors impacting on the lumenal contents, adjacent epithelium, interstitial cells and elements, and vascular structures in the lung. Since the gene is not integrated into the genome of the infected cell, expression remains only as long as the cell remains viable and is terminated in part by the expected immune response against the virus. Many cytokines, chemokines, growth factors, and inhibitors have been incorporated into Ad vectors and administered to the rodent lung and are detected at raised levels in BAL fluid over 7–10 days; after which the levels of cytokine gene product produced from the infection returns to normal. The construction, use, and limitations of the various gene transfer approaches have been recently reviewed elsewhere (5–10).

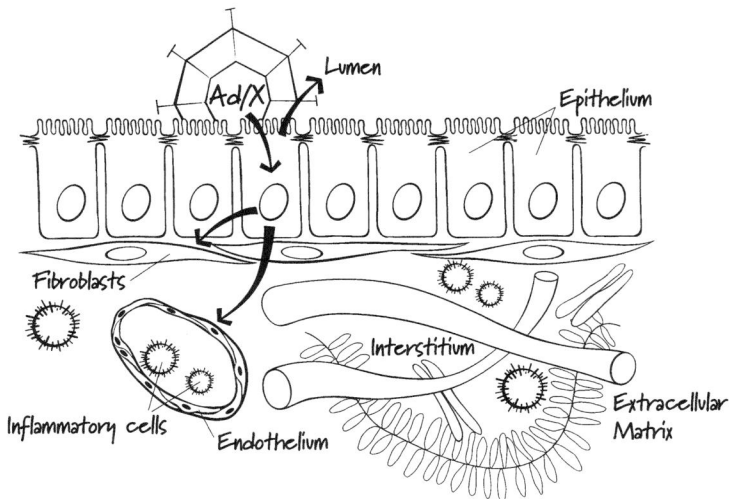

Figure 1 Ad vector cytokine gene transfer to the lung. The vector infects the epithelial cells and within 12–24 hours expresses gene product into the lumen and parenchyma of the lung. The expressed cytokines have effects on the interstitium and vasculature as well as influencing the microenvironment of luminal cells. The direct effect of expressed cytokine genes can be augmented by paracrine stimulation of other lung cells in a cascade of events.

III. Chemokine Function and Cell Accumulation

One of the early events in the acute respiratory distress syndrome (ARDS) is the marked accumulation of neutrophils to the lung in response to infection or other traumatic injury. A useful model for study of this disease has been the instillation of gram-negative bacterium-derived lipopolysaccharide (LPS) resulting in transient accumulation of polymorphonuclear cells, presumably through the release of chemokines, such as the C-X-C factors macrophage inflammatory protein-2 (MIP-2) and cytokine-induced neutrophil chemoattractant (KCs) in the rodent (11) and other cytokines in the inflammatory cascade (12), including tumor necrosis factor-α (TNF-α), interleukin-1β (IL-1β), and IL-6 (13). However, there is little evidence of severe alveolar damage or progression to fibrosis in the LPS model, making it distinct from the normal sequelae of ARDS (14). When we expressed several C-X-C and C-C cytokines in the lung by Ad vector, there was a general response common to all chemokines: As long as gene was being expressed (7–10 days), there was dramatic evidence of specific cell accumulation, but after the gene was switched off, there was no permanent change to the tissue and no evidence of progressive fibrosis. Overexpression of RANTES (regulated on activation, normal T cell expressed and secreted) leads primarily to mononuclear cell accumulation (15), whereas Ad vector expression of the non-ELR chemokines IP-10 and MIG induces mononuclear cell accumulation with attendant presence of neutrophils. In this case, the accumulation of neutrophils was dependent on the release of chemokines from the accumulated lymphocytes as the presence of neutrophils was absent in nude mice treated with the Ad vectors (16). In neither case was subsequent chronic tissue changes seen. The most dramatic changes in accumulation of neutrophils come with the Ad vector expression of MIP-2 in the rodent. Marked tissue and bronchoalveolar lavage (BAL) neutrophilia is evident, which is reminiscent of acute bacterial pneumonia (17). Remarkably, as the gene expression lessens and is subsequently turned off, the neutrophils disappear and the lung returns to normal with no evidence of residual tissue changes. In each case, reduction of inflammatory cells is likely to proceed through apoptosis (therefore, no general inflammatory response is generated) as seen in reduction of lung neutrophilia after LPS treatment (18) and as suggested from the earlier work on macrophage engulfment of apoptotic neutrophils (19).

It appears from these studies that chemokines by themselves serve to bring the specific cell to the tissue. Although some activation of the accumulated cell can be seen, likely as a result of transition from circulation into the parenchyma, there is no obvious cell degranulation and no evidence of extensive tissue destruction. It seems likely that a "second hit" is needed to cause the accumulated cells to become fully activated and cause tissue destruction resulting in fibrotic sequelae. In the absence of this second hit, the cells undergo apoptosis and are removed from the tissue by noninflammatory macrophage-dependent mechanisms.

IV. Immune Modulation and Cytokines

One of the most prominent cytokines involved in both acute inflammation and immune regulation is IL-6 (20). Others, such as IL-5 and IL-4 are able to modulate immune responses, particularly in T helper cell type 2 (TH2)–related pathways. Overexpression of IL-6 by Ad vector results in accumulation of lymphocytes, probably through local proliferation, and induction of altered immune responses, such as those in the lung against the Ad vector itself (21). There is an enhanced IgA response to the vector (22,23), and pulmonary transfer to IL-6–deficient animals can restore immune function and control inflammation in the lung (13). These changes were similar to those seen with pulmonary transfer of IL-6 using vaccinia viral vectors (24).

In a second approach to modulation of immunity, transfer of the gene for IL-4 to the lung by Ad vector in a mouse sensitized to purified protein derivative (PPD) and reactive through the TH1 pathway causes the lung environment to resemble a TH2 condition and changes the outcome of antigen challenge to a more TH2-like response (25). However, there was no change in this model in the primary pathway of memory immunity, remaining as a TH1-sensitized animal.

There have been several studies using gene transfer to the lung to modulate an immune response or to inhibit an inflammatory response. Delivery of the gene for viral IL-10 or transforming growth factor-$\beta 1$ (TGF-$\beta 1$) by liposome plasmid transfection of the isolated lung prior to transplantation can result in an attenuated host immune response to allograft (26,27). Plasmid gene transfer of IL-10 also reduces inflammatory responses to challenge in the lung (28). These latter data complement others showing systemic levels of IL-10 can suppress the lung reactivity to LPS challenge (29) and indicate that local expression of inhibitory factors such as IL-10 or IL-1 receptor antagonist (IL-1RA) by gene transfer to the lung can modulate inflammation and/or regulate immunity (30). Such modulation can represent stimulation when gene transfer is used to express immune stimulatory cytokines, such as IL-12, where enhanced immune responses are required in protective action against tumor metastases (31). Expression of other factors, such as those involved in angiogenesis or angiostasis, elicit effects consistent with the known action of these cytokines. Thus, Ad vector expression of vascular endothelial growth factor (VEGF) in the lung protects against hyperoxic pulmonary hypertension in rats (32), whereas local transfer of angiostatin interferes with new vessel growth and protects from lung metastatic growth of tumor (33).

V. Granulocyte-Macrophage Colony–Stimulating Factor and Lung Inflammation and Immunity

In the case of the lung, granulocyte-macrophage colony-stimulating factor (GM-CSF), initially thought to be a primary hemopoietic cytokine, can influence a number of pathogenic and physiological responses dependent on the duration and extent of expression after vector transfection. In the case of limited but prolonged overexpression through transgenic lung-specific manipulation, GM-CSF can correct the alveolar proteinosis seen in GM-CSF–deficient mice, possibly related to the alveolar type II epithelial cell hyperplasia seen in these lung-specific transgenic animals (34,35). Moreover, lung transfer by Ad vector of low levels of GM-CSF to granulocytopenic mice with low proliferative alveolar macrophage was able to expand macrophage numbers and function, thus restoring innate immunity in an otherwise immune-compromised individual (36).

On the other hand, when GM-CSF is overexpressed through an Ad vector to the lung, remarkably different sequelae appear. The levels of GM-CSF expressed under these conditions are logarithmically greater than those described above. Under these heightened conditions, the lung undergoes accumulation of monocytes, alveolar macrophage expansion, granuloma formation, and accumulation of myofibroblasts (37,38). Subsequent development of fibrosis is seen along with generation of TGF-β as described below. Thus overexpression of a potent hemopoietic cytokine will lead to dramatically different outcomes in the lung dependent on the extent and duration of the expression. This is not true for all cytokines we have examined.

VI. Cytokines and the Allergic Airway Response

Over the past few years, considerable progress has been made in understanding the role of cytokines in the pathogenesis of asthma and other airway allergic diseases. This has been achieved through the use of mouse models and airway allergen challenges, which, although not equating exactly to the human condition, allows detailed temporal and environmental examination of the sensitization and challenge pathways giving rise to the eosinophilic inflammation and hyperresponsive state of the airway. A number of transgenic lung tissue–specific models of cytokine overexpression have indicated that factors expected to be involved in the pathogenesis of asthma, such as IL-4 and IL-5, clearly influence the microenvironment and physiology of the lung, including mucin hypersecretion and goblet cell hyperplasia along with heightened airway responsiveness (1,39,40). Other studies indicate that cytokines not previously considered to be part of the pathogenic cascade of sensitization or activation of the asthmatic response may play a role in airway physiology. These include IL-11 and IL-6, thought to play roles primarily in the acute phase and immune response (3,4,41), but whether these studies reflect the natural development of the disease or represent changes seen on long-term and/or in utero expression of the gene is not clear.

More realistic are the studies involving gene transfer of cytokines to the adult normal airway/lung and development of models of allergic airway disease.

Allergic sensitization of mice can be achieved by intraperitoneal (IP) presentation of antigen in association with alum adjuvant followed by aerosolized challenge with allergen (42,43) and can lead to appropriate airway inflammation, including accumulation of eosinophils, and to hyperresponsiveness. This model can be further manipulated to demonstrate the impact of local (lung) expression of cytokines through gene transfer by Ad vectors of cytokines with inhibitory (IL-10) or stimulatory (IL-18) properties (44–46). This model has also been used to show the necessity of local, but not systemic, IL-5, achieved by administration of IL-5 gene to the lung of IL-5-/-mice, in the development of the eosinophilic response upon antigen challenge (42,47).

However, presentation of antigen through the IP route is not expected to reflect the normal route of sensitization. The use of Ad vectors to transfer GM-CSF to the lung during airway exposure of allergen (ovalbumin [OVA] as a model allergen) have more direct implication for the role of cytokines in the induction of allergic airway disease (48). The model in which GM-CSF is overexpressed in the lung at the time of airway inhalation of allergen (OVA) seems to be more physiological in development and is more amenable to experimental manipulation. Such conditioning of the lung microenvironment by GM-CSF has an effect on the development of antigen-presenting cells, dendritic cells, in the lung (49) and modifies the immune response from one of no reaction to one of a TH2 pathway of sensitization (50). This appears to reflect the conditions present during allergen exposure and may be more typical of human sensitization. Indeed, by modifying the lung microenvironment through delivery and transfer of additional cytokines by Ad vector gene transfer, it can be shown that altering the lung microenvironment during the sensitization stage of the model leads to either an inhibition of the allergic reactivity by IL-10 (51) or directs the reaction toward a TH1 pathway in the presence of IL-12 (52). The local expression of GM-CSF was shown to impact on airway eosinophilia, but only if there were adequate levels of systemic GM-CSF or IL-5 to mobilize the progenitor cells from the bone marrow (37,42). Similar approaches have shown that local expression of IL-4 and TNF are needed to upregulate vascular cell adhesion molecule-1 (VCAM-1) expression by pulmonary endothelium, a requirement for lung accumulation of eosinophils after allergen challenge (53).

VII. Cytokines and the Pulmonary Fibrotic Response

After lung injury, acute inflammation and tissue repair mechanisms are engaged to halt the injurious stimulus, remove infectious organisms, and initiate immediate repair to crucial membranes that function to provide gas exchange for survival. Usually, this results in return of the organ to normal function. However, in chronic tissue injury, with repeat episodes of inflammation, many of the control mehanisms involved in this otherwise well-orchestrated process are bypassed. Continued repair results in remodeling of the tissue-distorted matrix deposition, mesenchymal cell proliferation, and alteration of normal lung structure with compromised gas exchange. This overall process is known as fibrosis, and in cases where the initiating event is known, such as with postradiation fibrosis or with asbestos- or silica-induced injury, the pathogenesis seems to follow the inflammatory response. In the majority of cases of pulmonary fibrosis, however, an unknown initiating event is recognized and idiopathic pulmonary fibrosis (IPF) is diagnosed (54). It has long been thought that IPF is a process of chronic repair resulting from persistent inflammation with attendant activation of inflammatory cells and the local presence of cytokines and growth factors capable of activating mesenchymal cells with enhanced matrix production and deposition.

A number of experimental models of pulmonary fibrosis have been used to determine the presence of multiple inflammatory cytokines and growth factors during the initiation and propagation of chronic tissue remodeling associated with progressive and irreversible fibrosis, particularly those associated with IPF. Intratracheal administration of bleomycin, silica, or asbestos particles elicits many aspects of response seen in human IPF (55–57). All models suffer from the underlying issue of our profound lack of knowledge about the natural history of IPF. Nonetheless, we are now aware that some cytokines are more involved than others in this process. Through examination of these models, cytokines such as TNF and IL-1 are involved in the early phase of inflammatory response and others such as GM-CSF and TGF-β are involved in the repair and fibrogenic phase of the disease (58–62). The demonstration of cytokines present in the lung in these models coincides with findings in human tissue (63–65) and further supports the preposition that these factors are involved in the pathogenesis of the fibrotic response. Inflammation is usually defined through the use of morphology and the demonstration of accumulation of inflammatory cells, including neutrophils and/or eosinophils and mast cells in biopsy material. All of these criteria need to be satisfied in the models if relevance to the human condition is to be applied.

Direct implication of a functional role for cytokines in the fibrogenic process has come from studies involving gene transfer to the lung of suspect cytokines. Transgenic lung-specific studies have indicated that overexpression of TGF-α or TNF-α can induce the presence of chronic inflammation (although not typical of that occurring in human disease) and accumulation of myofibroblasts and matrix deposition (2,66). Other cytokines cannot be tested in this way, as transgenic overexpression is embryonic lethal, such as for TGF-β1. These limitations can be overcome through the use of Ad vector cytokine gene transfer to the lung of adult rodents.

Crucial to the suggested interaction of epithelium and mesenchyme in fibrosis is the growth factor TGF-β. This factor is involved in normal alveolar development and regulation of repair processes in addition to its broad activities in regulating the immune response (67,68). Most important is the demonstration that it is an integral component of fibrotic tissue in IPF (62,63), with a known role in causing the differentiation of myofibroblasts, a critical element in tissue repair and fibrosis (69).

There have been a number of studies in which specific cytokine transgenes have been transferred to rodent lungs to determine the effects on the induction of fibrosis. Examination immediately and over several months after transfer has included morphology to detect inflammation and extent of fibrosis and matrix deposition, immunohistochemistry for α smooth muscle actin (αSMA) to detect the accumulation of myofibroblasts, and hydroxyproline content to measure increased matrix production. Gene transfer of chemokines such as MIP-2, the IL-8 bioequivalent in the rodent, results in dramatic and prolonged accumulation of the targeted inflammatory cells to the lung; in this case neutrophils. However, there is little evidence of tissue destruction and no evidence of a progression to fibrosis. The inflammatory response resembles acute bacterial pneumonia, but there is no progression to fibrotic sequelae, with the lung returning to normal structure and function after the gene is switched off (17). Gene transfer of TNF-α results in marked accumulation of inflammatory cells, neutrophils, and mononuclear cells over 4–6 days. There are increased levels of other cytokines in BAL fluid, with remarkably little evidence of tissue damage or apoptosis despite very high levels of TNF-α in the tissue (70). TGF-β levels were raised and some αSMA-positive myofibroblasts were present. However, there was only slight residual fibrosis after 10–14 days and only patchy evidence of fibrosis persisted for several months. When GM-CSF was expressed at high levels in the lung (in contrast to the low levels of expression used in the allergic airway sensitization approach (48), there was evidence of alveolar macrophage activation and mononuclear cell accumulation (37–38). Levels of TGF-β in BAL were higher than those seen with TNF-α transfer, and there was the presence of multinucleate giant cells, presumably derived from alveolar macrophages under the influence of GM-CSF. Granuloma formation was evident over 14–21 days, and significant accumulations of myofibroblasts were seen. These findings were consistent with the fact that fibrosis was seen throughout the experiment (65 days) and was distributed in a patchy fashion throughout the lung. Gene transfer of IL-1β results in profound inflammation and tissue destruction in the lung at early times (2–6 days after administration) (71). This is followed by increased levels of TGF-β in the BAL fluid and concomitant accumulation of myofibroblasts with extensive fibrosis and matrix production and deposition. This process continues well past the time when inflammation has subsided and it progresses independent of IL-1β gene expression. Finally, gene transfer of active TGF-β1, and not the full-length latent form, resulted in very early (within 2 days) evidence of expansion of parenchymal cells, induction of myofibroblasts throughout the lung, and induction of very high endogenous levels of TGF-β1. This is not accompanied by any real evidence of tissue destruction, and rather there is an appearance of tissue remodeling in the absence of inflammation. Marked matrix production accompanies the expanded and altered phenotype of the parenchyma, and the process of fibrosis is both progressive and aggressive in this rodent model (72). Of approximately 25 different cytokines that have been examined by this gene transfer approach, only these 4 appear to have effects on the fibrogenic process in vivo.

Thus, it can be seen that remodeling can occur subsequent to acute tissue destruction and inflammation, as seen with gene transfer of IL-1β (71), or independent of inflammation, as seen with gene transfer of active TGF-β1 (72). Overexpression of other factors identified as being profibrogenic exhibit acute inflammation with minimal remodeling, as with TNF-α (70), or both acute and chronic inflammation with moderate remodeling, as with GM-CSF (37). The common theme is the generation of active TGF-β and the extent of fibrosis and myofibroblast induction appears related to the level of TGFβ present (Table 1).

Consistent with the role of TGF-β in fibrogenesis, as seen in both experimental fibrotic and gene transfer models, transfer of an inhibitor of TGF-β signaling, Smad 7, by Ad vector, prevents bleomycin-induced fibrosis in the mouse (73). Confirmation that TGF-β is critical in the induction of fibrosis comes from recent data from our laboratory showing that Smad 3 -/- knockout mice do not demonstrate a fibrogenic response when TGF-β gene is transferred to the lung by Ad vector administration (Gauldie et al., unpublished). Moreover, when the gene for decorin, a proteoglycan with known inhibitory activity for TGF-β (74), was transferred by Ad vector in a bleomycin model, there was inhibition of the fibrotic sequelae. This inhibition was not seen when the gene for biglycan, a second proteoglycan that binds, but does not inhibit TGF-β, was transferred (75,76).

An interesting twist to the investigation of cytokine roles in IPF makes use of Ad vector gene transfer to lung tissue ex vivo in embryonic lung culture to determine cytokine roles in development of the lung. These studies showed

Table 1 Transfer of Cytokine Transgene by Adenovirus Vector to the Lung of Rodent Lung in the Investigation of Fibrosis

Cytokine	Level of inflammation	TGF β in BAL fluid	αSMA myofibroblasts	Extent of fibrosis
MIP-2/IL-8	Acute ++++	None detected	None	None
TNFα	Acute +++	150 pg/μL	+	+
GM-CSF	Acute ++	600 pg/μL	++	++
IL-1β	Acute +++ alveolar destruction	400 pg/μL	+++	++++
TGFβ1	−	>50 ng/μL	++++	++++

that transfer of active TGF-β1 to the embryonic epithelium causes inhibition of branching morphogenesis, similar to effects seen in the embryonic lethal transgenic studies (77). However, there was no evidence that fibrosis was initiated, as expected from similar gene transfer of active TGF-β1 to the adult lung (72). Moreover, Ad vector–mediated transfer to embryonic epithelial cells of a gene coding for a dominant negative form of the TGF-β receptor showed that the epithelial cell is the target for TGF-β signaling for alveolar branching during development (78). These conclusions were drawn from the known inhibitory activity of the decoy receptor and from the fact that Ad vectors administered in this way (intratracheal microinfusion) will only infect epithelial cells and not parenchyma. This communication by cytokines between the epithelium and parenchyma, the formation of an epithelial-mesenchymal trophic unit, is crucial in development and appears to be equally important in tissue remodeling and fibrosis (79,80). In addition to demonstration of cytokine function specific to age of development of the lung tissue, the same system of gene transfer to the embryonic lung ex vivo has been used to demonstrate inhibition of TGF-β function through

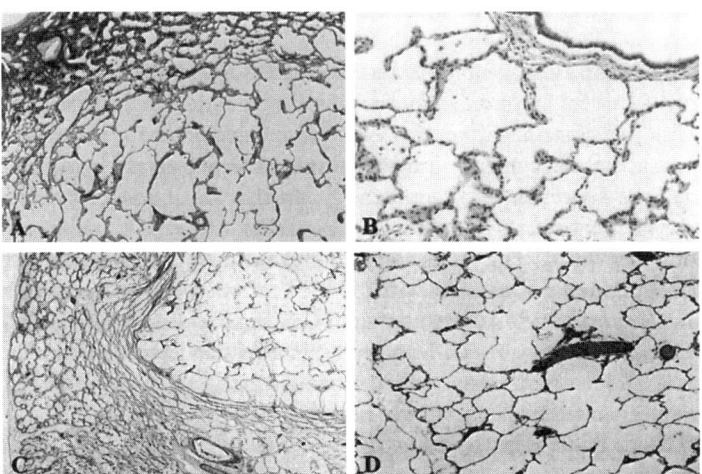

Figure 2 Neonatal rat model of bronchopulmonary dysplasia reproduces the human disease. (A) EvG stain for matrix deposition and (B) H&E stain in rat lung 28 days after treatment with Ad vector expressing active TGF-β1 (29 days old). (A) demonstrates a combination of fibrosis (dark stain) and large alveoli and (B) demonstrates inhibition of alveolarization with large alveoli and a lack of any interstitial infiltrate. (C) and (D) H&E stain of human infant, (C) 120 days old and (D) 790 days old, showing midstage (C) and late-stage (D) BPD with combination of fibrosis and enlarged alveoli. A,B, 100× magnification; C, 20×; D50× (C and D from Ref. 96.)

gene transfer of decorin (81), resulting in enhanced alveolar branching as the lung develops ex vivo.

Consistent with the findings of altered/blocked alveolar development in the embryo and induction of fibrosis in the adult, transfer of Ad vector TGF-β1 to rat neonatal lung tissue induces an interesting combination of pathologies. Newborn rat lung is still under development and does not reach full alveolar maturity for several weeks. Transfer and overexpression of TGF-β1 to the lung by Ad vector from day 1 of birth causes areas of the lung to demonstrate blunted alveolar development with excessive large alveolar spaces adjacent to areas that exhibit distinct fibrotic changes. Thus, the development of pathologies in a tissue depends on the age and maturity of the organ at the time of gene transfer and expression. This combination of changes in the newborn mimics very well the changes seen in human bronchopulmonary dysplasia (BPD) and suggests that the human disorder is caused by expression of TGF-β due to hyperoxic challenge or some other insult during the postnatal development period in the neonate. These morphological similarities are shown in Figure 2.

VIII.   Cytokines and Infectious Diseases

There is an increasing morbidity and mortality of acute bacterial pneumonia throughout the world. Among the most frequent organisms found as agents of this process are gram-negative *Escherichia coli* and *Pseudomonas aeruginosa*. In addition, acute and chronic viral infections cause pulmonary damage and may elicit airway and parenchymal remodeling, and chronic pulmonary infection with mycobacteria, particularly *Mycobacterium tuberculosis*, is a growing concern throughout the world. This is because there are now drug-resistant strains of *M. tuberculosis* and coinfection with HIV is common in those from the lower socioeconomic areas of the world (82,83). A number of experimental models of infection and endotoxin challenge have shown that cytokines are prominent participants in host responses to infection and may be targets for therapeutic intervention in addition to antimicrobial administration (83–85). Understanding the cellular and molecular events and the nature of the key cytokines involved in the host response to infection should help design appropriate prophylactic and/or therapeutic vaccines. This would include recombinant viral or cDNA vaccines, especially for drug-resistant or latent infections. Such vaccines are notorious in the difficulty of inducing potent, long-lasting, and locally acting defences. Knowledge of the cytokine involvement can identify cytokines suited for gene transfer to the lung as vaccine adjuvants for the induction of mucosal immunity. In this regard, administration of recombinant interferon-γ (IFN-γ) as an aerosol in patients infected with *M. tuberculosis* has shown some efficacy (86), and may indicate a role for cytokine gene therapy as an economical and efficient way to boost immune responses.

Several recent studies have transferred the IFN-γ gene to the lung by Ad vector and shown an impact on clearance of *P. aeruginosa* in mice (87,88). These investigators also showed that IFN-γ gene transfer could enhance the clearance of *Pneumocystis carinii* from immune compromised (CD4-/- depleted) mice; data that could have a direct impact on therapeutic intervention in human HIV patients (89). This also suggests an impact on innate as well as adaptive immunity through this administration. This was shown through effects on the alveolar macrophage with upregulation of major histocompatibility complex class (MHC) II expression and activation to subsequent challenge with LPS (88). That IFN-γ gene transfer could also enhance lung host response to viral infection was shown by plasmid intranasal administration. When challenged with respiratory syncytial virus (RSV), there was decreased epithelial cell damage, lower infiltration of inflammatory cells, and decreased RSV replication (90). Equally important are the data from a study showing enhanced protection against fatal mycobacterial infection in SCID beige mice by gene transfer of IFN-γ; again by Ad vector administration (91). In this immune-compromised strain, IFN-γ gene expression directly affected the lung macrophage, causing MHC-enhanced expression, release of type I cytokines (IFN-γ and IL-12), and nitric oxide release. All of these changes suggest that cytokine gene transfer to the lung of IFN-γ has a profound impact on the innate immune response and can enhance protection from bacterial, viral, and mycobacterial infection. Although these effects all appear to be beneficial, one must have caution, as a separate study using conditional expression of IFN-γ in a transgenic animal, with inducible promoters being used to protect the embryo and developing lung, showed the development of emphysema with alveolar enlargement and an imbalance in pulmonary protease/antiprotease levels (92). These differences indicate the complexity of altering the normal genome expression and possible different pathways of activation being engaged.

A second cytokine pathway involved in the host response is TNF-α, a pleotropic cytokine that has been implicated in the pathogenesis of endotoxic shock, but known also to be crucial in host defense against intracellular pathogens. In a model of gram-negative bacterial pneumonia caused by infection with *Klebsiella pneumoniae*, transfer of the gene for murine TNF-α to the lung caused enhanced clearance of the organism from the lung and resulted in significantly increased survival (93). The beneficial role of TNF-α was also shown in a mouse model of *P. aeruginosa* by gene transfer of a potent inhibitor of TNF-α, a chimeric protein made up of the mouse IgG heavy-chain linked to the 55-kD TNF receptor extracellular domain. This soluble inhibitor impaired bacterial killing, although it also served to decrease the acute inflammatory response associated with release of TNF-α (94). The role of innate immunity and the induction of a protective immune response depends on suitable antigen recognition and processing with subsequent presentation through antigen-presenting cells, such as the dendritic cell, to the lymphocyte population. Crucial in this set of reactions is the cytokine IL-12. Although this cytokine is thought to be a type I or TH1 cytokine, and important in host response to viral infection and other intracellular pathogens, studies in bacterial pneumonia have shown its importance in resistance to extra-cellular bacterial diseases as well. In the *Klebsiella pneumoniae* mouse model of infection, gene transfer of IL-12 through Ad vector administration resulted in significant survival from a lethal challenge (95), presumably through activation of the innate immune response, as this is required for clearance of gram-negative and gram-positive bacterial organisms.

IX. Summary

During normal development or as a result of infection or trauma to the lung, cytokines are often expressed in a transient but prolonged period and participate in a cascade of events involved in inflammation and immunity. These changes most often occur on a normal host background, and for most chronic disorders, the changes occur in the normal adult. Although stable transgenic expression can be tissue directed and the use of complicated regulatory promoters can achieve some degree of local control of expression, the use of transient transgene approaches for the overexpression of cytokines and their modifiers would seem more desirable for studies of cytokine function in vivo. The use of liposome and viral vectors to transfer the genes for cytokines has been quite successful in defining the role of some cytokines in host protection and chronic inflammation. In particular, the use of Ad vectors, which have a natural affinity for bronchial epithelium, have been proven to be most informative. These model systems can help define those cytokines involved in initiation of inflammation and immunity, as well as those involved in the chronicity of inflammation. Such studies will provide model systems in which therapeutic targets can be identified and drug regimens tested in the development of further therapies for pulmonary diseases.

References

1. Rankin JA, Picarella DE, Geba GP, Temann U-A, Prasad B, DiCosmo B, Tarallo A, Stripp B, Whitsett J, Flavell RA. Phenotypic and physiologic characterization of transgenic mice expressing interleukin 4 in the lung: lymphocytic and eosinophilic inflammation without airway hyperreactivity. Proc Natl Acad Sci USA 1996; 93: 7821–7825.
2. Korfhagen TR, Swantz RJ, Wert SE, McCarty JM, Keriakian CB, Glasser SW, Whitsett JA. Respiratory epithelial cell expression of human transforming growth factor-α induces lung fibrosis in transgenic mice. J Clin Invest 1994; 93:1691–1699.

3. Tang W, Geba GP, Zheng T, Ray P, Homer RJ, Kuhn III C, Flavell RA, Elias JA. Targeted expression of IL-11 in the murine airway causes lymphocytic inflammation, bronchial remodeling, and airways obstruction. J Clin Invest 1996; 98:2845–2853.

4. Ray P, Tang W, Wang P, Homer R, Kuhn III C, Flavell RA, Elias JA. Regulated overexpression of interleukin 11 in the lung. Use to dissociate development-dependent and -independent phenotypes. J Clin Invest 1997; 100:2501–2511.

5. Bramson JL, Graham FL, Gauldie J. The use of adenoviral vectors for gene therapy and gene transfer in vivo. Curr Opin Biotechnol 1995; 6:590–595.

6. Gauldie J, Graham F, Xing Z, Braciak T, Foley R, Sime PJ. Adenovirus vector mediated cytokine gene transfer to lung tissue. Ann NY Acad Sci 1996; 796:235–244.

7. Hitt MM, Gauldie J. Gene vectors for cytokine expression in vivo. Curr Pharm Des 2000; 6:613–632.

8. Sime PJ, Xing Z, Foley R, Graham FL, Gauldie J. Transient gene transfer and expression in the lung. Chest 1997; 111:89S–94S.

9. Xing Z, Braciak T, Ohkawara Y, Sallenave JM, Foley R, Sime PJ, Jordana M, Graham FL, Gauldie J. Gene transfer for cytokine functional studies in the lung: the multifunctional role of GM-CSF in pulmonary inflammation. J Leukoc Biol 1996; 59:481–488.

10. Xing Z, Stämpfli MR, Gauldie J. Transient transgenic approaches for investigating the role of GM-CSF in pulmonary inflammatory and immune diseases. In: Chung KF, Adcock I, eds. Methods in Molecular Medicine. Totowa, NJ: Humana Press, 2000:161–178.

11. Huang S, Paulauskis JD, Goodleski JJ, Kobzik L. Expression of MIP-2 and KC mRNA in pulmonary inflammation. Am J Pathol 1992; 141:981–988.

12. Friedland JS, Griffin GE. Cytokines and bacterial infection. In: Kunkel SL, Remick DG, eds. Cytokines in Health and Disease, New York: Marcel Dekker, 1992:165–180.

13. Xing Z, Gauldie, J, Cox G, Baumann H, Jordana M, Lei XF, Achong MK. IL-6 is an anti-inflammatory cytokine required for controlling local or systemic acute inflammatory responses. J Clin Invest 1998; 101:311–320.

14. Bachofen M, Weibel ER. Alterations of the gas exchange apparatus in adult respiratory insufficiency associated with septicemia. Am Rev Respir Dis 1977; 116:589–615.

15. Braciak TA, Bacon K, Xing Z, Torry DJ, Graham FL, Schall TJ, Richards CD, Croitoru K, Gauldie J. Overexpression of RANTES using a recombinant adenovirus vector induces the tissue-directed recruitment of monocytes to the lung. J Immunol 1996; 157:5076–5084.

16. Palmer K, Emtage PCR, Strieter RM, Gauldie J. Transient gene transfer of non-ELR chemokines to rodent lung induces mononuclear cell accumulation and activation. J Interferon Cytokine Res 1999; 19:1381–1390.

17. Foley R, Driscoll K, Wan Y, Braciak T, Howard B, Xing Z, Graham F, Gauldie J. Adenoviral gene transfer of macrophage inflammatory protein-2 in rat lung. Am J Pathol 1996; 149:1395–1403.

18. Cox G, Crossley J, Xing Z. Macrophage engulfment of apoptotic neutrophils contrib-

utes to the resolution of acute pulmonary inflammation in vivo. Am J Respir Cell Mol Biol 1995; 12:232–237.

19. Savill J, Fadok V, Henson PM, Haslett C. Phagocyte recognition of cells undergoing apoptosis. Immunol Today 1993; 14:131–136.

20. Baumann H, Gauldie J. The acute phase response. Immunol Today 1994; 15:74–80.

21. Xing Z, Braciak T, Jordana M, Croitoru K, Graham FL, Gauldie J. Adenovirus-mediated cytokine gene transfer at tissue sites: overexpression of IL-6 induces lymphocytic hyperplasia in the lung. J Immunol 1994; 153:4059–4069.

22. Braciak TA, Gallichan WS, Graham FL, Richards CD, Ramsay AJ, Rosenthal KL, Gauldie J. Recombinant adenovirus vectors expressing interleukin-5 and -6 specifically enhance mucosal immunoglobulin A responses in the lung. Immunology 2000; 101:388–396.

23. Xing Z, Braciak T, Chong D, Feng X, Schroeder JA, Gauldie J. Adenoviral-mediated gene transfer of interleukin-6 in rat lung enhances antiviral immunoglobulin A and G responses in distinct tissue compartments. Biochem Biophys Res Commun 1999; 258:332–335.

24. Ramsay AJ, Husband AJ, Ranshaw IA, Bao S, Matthaei KI, Koehler G, Kopf M. The role of interleukin-6 in mucosal IgA antibody responses in vivo. Science 1994; 264:561–563.

25. Lukacs NW, Addison CL, Gauldie J, Graham F, Simpson K, Strieter RM, Warmington K, Chensue SW, Kunkel SL. Transgene-induced production of IL-4 alters the development and collagen expression of T helper cell 1-type pulmonary granulomas. J Immunol 1997; 158:4478–4484.

26. Itano H, Mora BN, Zhang W, Ritter JH, McCarthy TJ, Yew NS, Mohanakumar T, Patterson GA. Lipid-mediated ex vivo gene transfer of viral interleukin 10 in rat lung allotransplantation. J Thorac Cardiovasc Surg 2001; 122:29–38.

27. Mora BN, Boasquevisque CH, Boglione M, Ritter JM, Scheule RK, Yew NS, Debruyne L, Qin L, Bromberg JS, Patterson GA. Transforming growth factor-β1 gene transfer ameliorates acute lung allograft rejection. J Thorac Cardiovasc Surg 2000; 119:913–920.

28. Dokka S, Malanga CJ, Shi X, Chen F, Castranova V, Rojanasakul Y. Inhibition of endotoxin-induced lung inflammation by interleukin-10 gene transfer in mice. Am J Physiol Lung Cell Mol Physiol 2000; 279:L872–877.

29. Xing Z, Ohkawara Y, Jordana M, Graham FL, Gauldie J. Adenoviral vector–mediated IL-10 expression in vivo: intramuscular gene transfer inhibits cytokine responses in endotoxemia. Gene Ther 1997; 4:140–149.

30. McCoy RD, Davidson BL, Roessler BJ, Huffnagle GB, Simon RH. Expression of human interleukin-1 receptor antagonist in mouse lungs using a recombinant adenovirus: effects on vector-induced inflammation. Gene Ther 1995; 2:437–442.

31. Worth LL, Jia SF, Zhou Z, Chen L, Kleinerman ES. Intranasal therapy with an adenoviral vector containing the murine interleukin-12 gene eradicates osteosarcoma lung metastases. Clin Cancer Res 2000; 6:3713–3718.

32. Partovian C, Adnot S, Raffestin B, Louzier V, Levame M, Mavier IM, Lemarchand P, Eddahibi S. Adenovirus-mediated lung vascular endothelial growth factor overex-

pression protects against hypoxic pulmonary hypertension in rats. Am J Respir Cell Mol Biol 2000; 23:762–771.

33. Gyorffy S, Palmer K, Gauldie J. Adenoviral vector expressing murine angiostatin inhibits a model of breast cancer metastatic growth in the lungs of mice. Am J Pathol 2001; 159:1137–1147.

34. Huffman JA, Hull WM, Dranoff G, Mulligan RC, Whitsett JA. Pulmonary epithelial cell expression of GM-CSF corrects the alveolar proteinosis in GM-CSF-deficient mice. J Clin Invest 1996; 97:649–655.

35. Huffman Reed JA, Rice WR, Zsengeller ZK, Wert SE, Dranoff G, Whitsett JA. GM-CSF enhances lung growth and causes alveolar type II epithelial cell hyperplasia in transgenic mice. Am J Physiol 1997; 273:L715–L725.

36. Santosuosso M, Divangahi M, Zganiacz A, Xing Z. Reduced tissue macrophage population in the lung by anti-cancer agent cyclophosphamide: restoration by local GM-CSF gene transfer. Blood 2002; 99:1246–1252.

37. Xing Z, Ohkawara Y, Jordana M, Graham FL, Gauldie J. Transfer of granulocyte-macrophage colony-stimulating factor gene to rat lung induces eosinophilia, mono-cytosis and fibrotic reactions. J Clin Invest 1996; 97:1102–1110.

38. Xing Z, Tremblay GM, Sime PJ, Gauldie J. Overexpression of granulocyte-macro-phage colony-stimulating factor induces pulmonary granulation tissue formation and fibrosis by induction of transforming growth factor-$\beta 1$ and myofibroblast accumula-tion. Am J Pathol 1997; 150:59–66.

39. Temann U-A, Prasad G, Gallup MW, Basbaum C, Ho SB, Flavell RA, Rankin JA. A novel role for murine IL-4 in vivo: induction of MUC5AC gene expression and mucin hypersecretion. Am J Respir Cell Mol Biol 1997; 16:471–478.

40. Lee JJ, McGarry MP, Farmer SC, Denzler KL, Larson KA, Carrigan PE, Brenneise IE, Horton MA, Haczku A, Gelfand EW, Leikauf GD, Lee NA. Interleukin-5 expres-sion in the lung epithelium of transgenic mice leads to pulmonary changes pathogno-monic of asthma. J Exp Med 1997; 185:2143–2156.

41. DiCosmo BF, Geba GP, Picarella D, Elias JA, Rankin JA, Stripp BR, Whitsett JA, Flavell RA. Airway epithelial cell expression of interleukin-6 in transgenic mice. Uncoupling of airway inflammation and bronchial hyperreactivity. J Clin Invest 1994; 94:2028–2035.

42. Wang J, Palmer K, Lotvall J, Milan S, Lei XF, Matthaei KI, Gauldie J, Inman MD, Jordana M, Xing Z. Circulating, but not local lung, IL-5 is required for the develop-ment of antigen-induced airways eosinophilia. J Clin Invest 1998; 102:1132–1141.

43. Hamelmann E, Takeda K, Haczku A, Cieslewicz G, Shultz L, Hamid Q, Xing Z, Gauldie J, Gelfand EW. Interleukin (IL)-5 but not immunoglobulin E reconstitutes airway inflammation and airway hyperresponsiveness in IL-4–deficient mice. Am J Respir Cell Mol Biol 2000; 23:327–334.

44. Ohkawara Y, Xing Z, Gauldie J, Jordana M. Adenovirus vector–mediated gene transfer of murine IL-10 inhibits antigen-induced airways inflammation in sensitized mice. Am J Respir Crit Care Med 1996; 153:A143.

45. Wiley R, Palmer K, Gajewska B, Stämpfli M, Alvarez D, Coyle A, Gutierrez-Ramos J, Jordana M. Expression of the Th1 chemokine IFN-gamma–inducible protein 10 in the airway alters mucosal allergic sensitization in mice. J Immunol 2001; 166: 2750–2759.

46. Walter DM, Wong CP, DeKruyff RH, Berry GJ, Levy S, Umetsu DT. IL-18 gene transfer by adenovirus prevents the development of and reverses established allergen-induced airway hyperreactivity. J Immunol 2001; 166:6392–6398.

47. Foster PS, Hogan SP, Ramsay AJ, Matthaei KI, Young IG. IL-5 deficiency abolishes eosinophilia, airways hyperreactivity and lung damage in a mouse asthma model. J Exp Med 1996; 183:195–201.

48. Lei XF, Ohkawara Y, Stämpfli MR, Gauldie J, Croitoru K, Jordana M, Xing Z. Compartmentalized transgene expression of granulocyte-macrophage colony-stimulating factor (GM-CSF) in mouse lung enhances allergic airways inflammation. Clin Exp Immunol 1998; 113:157–165.

49. Wang J, Snider D, Hewlett B, Lukacs N, Gauldie J, Liang H, Xing Z. Transgenic expression of GM-CSF induces the differentiation and activation of a novel dendritic cell population in the lung. Blood 2000; 95:2337–2345.

50. Stämpfli MR, Wiley RE, Neigh GS, Gajewska BU, Lei X-F, Snider DP, Xing Z, Jordana M. GM-CSF transgene expression in the airway allows aerosolized ovalbumin to induce allergic sensitization in mice. J Clin Invest 1998; 102:1704–1714.

51. Stämpfli MR, Cwiartka M, Gajewska BU, Alvarez D, Ritz SA, Inman MD, Xing Z, Jordana M. Interleukin-10 gene transfer to the airway regulates allergic mucosal sensitization in mice. Am J Respir Cell Mol Biol 1999; 21:586–596.

52. Stämpfli MR, Neigh SG, Wiley RE, Cwiartka M, Ritz SA, Hitt MM, Xing Z, Jordana M. Regulation of allergic mucosal sensitization by interleukin-12 gene transfer to the airway. Am J Respir Cell Mol Biol 1999; 21:317–326.

53. Lei XF, Ohkawara Y, Stämpfli MR, Mastruzzo C, Marr RA, Snider D, Xing Z, Jordana M. Disruption of antigen-induced inflammatory responses in CD40 ligand knock-out mice. J Clin Invest 1998; 101:1342–1353.

54. Ward PA, Hunninghake GW. Lung inflammation and fibrosis. Am J Respir Crit Care Med 1998; 157:S123–S129.

55. Piguet PF, Collart MA, Grau GE, Sappino A-P, Vassalli P. Requirements of TNF for development of silica-induced pulmonary fibrosis. Nature 1990; 344:245–247.

56. Selman M, King TE, Pardo A. Idiopathic pulmonary fibrosis: prevailing and evolving hypothesis about its pathogenesis and implications for therapy. Ann Intern Med 2001; 134:136–151.

57. Idiopathic pulmonary fibrosis: diagnosis and treatment. International consensus statement. Am J Respir Crit Care Med 2000; 161:646–664.

58. Piguet PF, Collart MA, Grau GE, Kapanci Y, Vassalli P. TNF/cachectin plays a key role in bleomycin-induced pneumopathy and fibrosis. J Exp Med 1989; 170: 655–663.

59. Piguet PF. Pulmonary fibrosis induced by silica, asbestos and bleomycin. In: Schook LB, Laskin DL, eds. Xenobiotics and Inflammation. New York: Academic Press, 1994:283–300.

60. Phan SH, Kunkel SL. Lung cytokine production in bleomycin-induced pulmonary fibrosis. Exp Lung Res 1992, 18:29–43.

61. Raghow R, Irish P, Kang AH. Coordinate regulation of TGF beta gene expression and cell proliferation in hamster lungs undergoing bleomycin-induced pulmonary fibrosis. J Clin Invest 1989; 84:1836–1842.

62. Santana A, Saxena B, Noble NA, Gold LI, Marshall BC. Increased expression of

TGF beta isoforms (beta1, beta2, beta3) in bleomycin-induced pulmonary fibrosis. Am J Respir Cell Mol Biol 1995; 13:34–44.

63. Broekelmann TJ, Limper AH, Colby TV, McDonald JA. Transforming growth factor β1 is present at sites of extracellular matrix gene expression in human pulmonary fibrosis. Proc Natl Acad Sci USA 1991; 88:6642–6646.

64. Coker RK, Laurent GJ, Shahzeidi S, Lympany PA, du Bois RM, Jeffery PK, McAnulty RJ. TGFβ1, β2, β3 stimulate fibroblast procollagen production in vitro but are differentially expressed during bleomycin-induced lung fibrosis. Am J Pathol 1997; 150:981–991.

65. Khalil N, O'Connor RN, Flanders KC, Unruh H. TGF-β1, but not TGF-β2 or TGF-β3, is differentially present in epithelial cells of advanced pulmonary fibrosis: an immunohistochemical study. Am J Respir Cell Mol Biol 1996; 14:131–138.

66. Miyazaki Y, Araki K, Vesin C, Garcia I, Kapanci Y, Whitsett JA, Piguet P-F, Vassalli P. Expression of a tumor necrosis factor-α transgene in murine lung causes lymphocytic and fibrosing alveolitis. A mouse model of progressive pulmonary fibrosis. J Clin Invest 1995; 96:250–259.

67. Kelly J. TGFβ. In: Kelly, J, ed. Cytokines of the Lung. New York: Marcel Dekker, 1993:101–137.

68. Letterio JJ, Roberts AB. Molecule of the month. TGFβ: A key modulator of immune cell function. Clin Immunol Immunopathol 1997; 84:244–250.

69. Desmouliere A, Geinoz A, Gabbiani F, Gabbiani G. Transforming growth factor-β1 induces α-smooth actin expression in granulation tissue myofibroblasts and in quiescent and growing cultured fibroblasts. J Cell Biol 1993; 122:103–111.

70. Sime PJ, Marr RA, Gauldie D, Xing Z, Hewlett BR, Graham FL, Gauldie J. Transfer of TNFα to rat lung induces severe pulmonary inflammation and patchy interstitial fibrogenesis with induction of TGF-β1 and myofibroblasts. Am J Pathol 1998; 153:825–832.

71. Kolb M, Margetts PJ, Anthony DC, Pitossi F, Gauldie J. Transient expression of IL-1β induces acute lung injury and chronic repair leading to pulmonary fibrosis. J Clin Invest 2001; 107:1529–1536.

72. Sime PJ, Xing Z, Graham FL, Csaky KG, Gauldie J. Adenovector-mediated gene transfer of active TGF-β1 induces prolonged severe fibrosis in rat lung. J Clin Invest 1997; 100:768–776.

73. Nakao A, Fujii M, Matsumura R, Kumano K, Saito Y, Miyazono K. Iwamoto I. Transient gene transfer and expression of Smad7 prevents bleomycin-induced lung fibrosis in mice. J Clin Invest 1999; 104:5–11.

74. Isaka Y, Brees DK, Ikegaya K, Kaneda Y, Imai E, Noble NA, Border WA. Gene therapy by skeletal muscle expression of decorin prevents fibrotic disease in rat kidney. Nat Med 1996; 2:418–423.

75. Kolb M, Margetts PJ, Galt T, Sime PJ, Xing Z, Schmidt M, Gauldie J. Transient transgene expression of decorin in the lung reduces the fibrotic response to bleomycin. Am J Respir Crit Care Med 2001; 163:770–777.

76. Kolb M, Margetts PJ, Sime PJ, Gauldie J. Proteoglycans decorin and biglycan differentially modulate TGFβ-mediated fibrotic responses in the lung. Am J Physiol Lung Cell Mol Physiol 2001; 280:L1327–L1334.

77. Zhao J, Sime PJ, Bringas P, Tefft JD, Buckley S, Bu D, Gauldie J, Warburton D.

Spatial-specific TGF-β1 adenoviral expression determines morphogenetic phenotypes in embryonic mouse lung. Eur J Cell Biol 1999: 78:715–725.

78. Zhao J, Sime PJ, Bringas P, Gauldie J, Warburton D. Epithelium-specific adenoviral
transfer of a dominant-negative mutant TGF-β type II receptor stimulates embryonic
lung branching morphogenesis in culture and potentiates EGF and PDGF-AA. Mech
Dev 1998; 72:89–100.

79. Warburton D, Schwartz M, Tefft D. Flores-Delgado G, Anderson KD, Cardoso WV.
The molecular basis of lung morphogenesis. Mech Dev 2000; 92:55–81.

80. Holgate ST, Davies DE, Lackie PM, Wilson SJ, Puddicombe SM, Jordan JL. The
epithelial-mesenchymal trophic unit. J Allergy Clin Immunol 2000; 105:193–204.

81. Zhao J, Sime PJ, Bringas P, Gauldie J, Warburton D. Adenovirus-mediated decorin
gene transfer prevents TGF-β–induced inhibition of lung morphogenesis. Am J
Physiol 1999; 277:L412–L422.

82. Cooper AM, Flynn JL. The protective immune response to Mycobacterium tuberculosis. Curr Opin Immunol 1995; 7:512–516.

83. Standiford TJ, Huffnagle GB. Cytokines in host defense against pneumonia. J Invest
Med 1997; 45:335–345.

84. Xing Z, Wang J. Consideration of cytokines as therapeutic agents or targets. Curr
Pharm Des 2000; 6:599–611.

85. Munk ME, Emoto M. Functions of T-cell subsets and cytokines in mycobacterial
infections. Eur Respir J 1995; 8:668s–675s.

86. Condos R, Rom WN, Schluger NW. Treatment of multidrug-resistant pulmonary
tuberculosis with IFN gamma via aerosol. Lancet 1997; 349:1513–1515.

87. Kolls JK, Lei D, Nelson S, Summer WR, Shellito JE. Adenoviral-mediated murine
IFN gene transfer compartmentally activates alveolar macrophages and enhances
bacterial clearance. Chest 1997; 111:104S.

88. Lei D, Lancaster JR Jr, Joshi MS, Nelson S, Stolz D, Bagby GJ, Odom G, Shellito
JE, Kolls JK. Activation of alveolar macrophages and lung host defenses using transfer of the interferon-γ gene. Am J Physiol 1997; 272:L852–L859.

89. Kolls JK, Habetz S, Shean MK, Vazquez C, Brown JA, Lei D, Schwarzenberger P,
Ye P, Nelson S, Summer WR, Shellito JE. IFN-γ and CD8+ T cells restore host
defenses against pneumocystis carinii in mice depleted of CD4+ T cells. J Immunol
1999; 162:2890–2894.

90. Kumar M, Behera AK, Matsuse H, Lockey RF, Mohapatra SS. Intranasal IFN-
gamma gene transfer protects BALB/c mice against respiratory syncytial virus infection. Vaccine 1999; 18:558–567.

91. Xing Z, Zganiacz A, Wang J, Sharma SK. Enhanced protection against fatal mycobacterial infection in SCID beige mice by reshaping innate immunity with IFN-γ
transgene. J Immunol 2001; 167:375–383.

92. Wang Z, Zheng T, Zhu Z, Homer RJ, Riese RJ, Chapman HA Jr, Shapiro SD, Elias
JA. Interferon γ induction of pulmonary emphysema in the adult murine lung. J Exp
Med 2000; 192:1587–1599.

93. Standiford TJ, Wilkowski JM, Sisson TH, Hattori N, Mehrad B, Bucknell KA,
Moore TA. Intrapulmonary tumor necrosis factor gene therapy increases bacterial
clearance and survival in murine gram-negative pneumonia. Hum Gene Ther 1999;
10:899–909.

94. Kolls JK, Lei D, Nelson S, Summer WR, Greenberg S, Beutler B. Adenovirus-mediated blockade of tumor necrosis factor in mice protects against endotoxic shock yet impairs pulmoary host defense. J Infect Dis 1995; 171:570–575.

95. Greenberger MJ, Kunkel SL, Strieter RM, Lukacs NW, Bramson J, Gauldie J, Graham FL, Hitt M, Danforth JM, Standiford TJ. IL-12 gene therapy protects mice in lethal Klebsiella pneumonia. J Immunol 1996; 157:3006–3012.

96. Erickson AM, de la Monte SM, Moore GW, Hutchins GM. The progression of morphological changes in bronchopulmonary dysplasia. Am J Pathol 1987; 127:474–484.

8

Use of Gene Therapy to Study Lung Infection and Immunity

PERRI PRELLOP and JAY K. KOLLS

Louisiana State University Health Sciences Center
New Orleans, Louisiana, U.S.A.

I. Introduction

The lung has a vast array of host defense mechanisms to cope with inhaled or aspirated pathogens (1). The alveolar macrophage is the predominant cell occupying the alveolar space in healthy individuals, and it therefore plays a critical role on the front line of host defense against invading organisms. Alveolar macrophages phagocytize bacteria, process antigen, and secrete several cytokines that recruit inflammatory cells into the lung and serve as amplifiers of the host defense response (2–4). Using monoclonal antibodies or knockout mice to abrogate specific cytokines, it has become clear that these secretory products are essential for normal host defense against a variety of pathogens (5–11). However, what may be more clinically applicable is the role of recombinant cytokines in upregulating in vivo host defenses in normal or immunocompromised hosts.

The administration of recombinant cytokines or cytokine receptors in experimental animal models of infection has proven to be a powerful tool to study the biological effects of specific cytokine mediators. However, cytokine-based immunotherapy is often complicated by significant toxicity, especially when cytokines or cytokine antagonists are given systemically. This is particularly true

193

for cytokines such as tumor necrosis factor (TNF), interleukin-2 (IL-2), and IL-12, which are often associated with substantial hemodynamic instability and end organ injury when administered intravenously (12–14). Therefore, in instances where the disease process is localized, as in most lung infections, it seems reasonable that delivery of specific immunotherapy may have a higher therapeutic index than systemic treatment. Gene therapy, which can be delivered in a local and compartmentalized manner, has provided a robust instrument effectively to study cytokine biology. Moreover, gene therapy offers a means for constitutive or regulated production of a cytokine and thus may optimize the ability to observe an effect of the cytokine gene product.

Although much of the work in the area of gene delivery to pulmonary infectious disease has focused specifically on cytokine or chemokine delivery, some noncytokine gene targets have also been examined. Novel immunomodulators in the form of converting enzymes, receptor ligands, and viral proteins are being exploited for potential therapies in the lung. Moreover, DNA vaccines for several pulmonary infections are being investigated. In this chapter, we will review the current candidate cytokine and noncytokine genes that have been delivered to the lungs of experimental animal models of infection, and the candidate diseases, such as bacterial pneumonia and tuberculosis, which represent potential therapeutic targets.

II. Candidate Genes for Immunotherapy

A. Cytokines

Although numerous cytokines/chemokines are involved in host defense against both intracellular and extracellular pathogens, this chapter will focus on those that have been delivered as genes to the lung. There are, namely, interferon-γ (IFN-γ), IL-12, macrophage inflammatory protein-2 (MIP-2), TNF, IL-17, and IL-10 (Table 1). We will give an overview of their biology and then their use in the context of gene delivery for pulmonary infections.

1. Interferon-γ

Interferon-γ, a cytokine that is produced by T cells and natural killer (NK) cells, has a broad range of biological effects. IFN-γ activates the alveolar macrophage in vitro and in vivo and increases the surface expression of IgG Fc receptors and class II histocompatibility antigens (15,16). Furthermore, IFN-γ primes the macrophage for increased release of oxygen radicals (17) and TNF in response to lipopolysaccharide (18) and overcomes the suppressive effects of dexamethasone (19) and ethanol (20) on TNF production. IFN-γ also has intrinsic antiviral activity and enhances antimicrobial activity against intracellular parasites, bacteria, fungi, and mycobacteria (21–24). Studies using recombinant IFN-γ (rIFN-γ)

Table 1 Candidate Genes

Gene	Biological Function in the Lung
IFN-γ	Macrophage activation
	Increased neutrophil recruitment
IL-12	T-cell development
	Stimulation of IFN-γ secretion from T and NK cells
MIP-2	Neutrophil recruitment and activation
TNF	Stimulation of neutrophils and macrophages
IL-17	Macrophage stimulation
	Neutrophil recruitment and activation
	Granulopoiesis
IL-10	Inhibition of TH1 cytokine secretion
TACE	Release of mature TNF-α from membrane-bound TNF-α
	p55 and p75 TNF receptor shedding
	L-selectin shedding
CD40L	Development of humoral responses to T-cell–dependent antigens
M3	Chemokine binding and subsequent blocking from cellular receptors

or anti-IFN in vivo demonstrate that IFN-γ is a pivotal factor for normal host defense against a variety of pulmonary pathogens including *Pseudomonas, Histoplasma, Candida, Mycoplasma, Toxoplasma, Haemophilus, Legionella, Chlamydia, Listeria,* and *Pneumocystis carinii* infections (6,21,25–30).

2. Interleukin-12

Interleukin-12 is a heterodimeric protein consisting of two subunits (p35 and p40) that promotes TH1 phenotype immune responses (31). Specifically, IL-12 promotes the development of TH1 T cells, increases the cytolytic activity of CD8$^+$ cells and NK cells, and, importantly, serves as the major inducer of IFN-γ production from T cells and NK cells (32). The administration of IL-12 systemically to mice has been shown to increase host resistance to a number of intracellular pathogens, including *Leishmania major, Toxoplasma gondii, Listeria monocytogenes, Mycobacterium tuberculosis, Cryptococcus neoformans,* and *Plasmodium chabaudi* (33–38). More recently, IL-12 has been identified as being an integral component of lung antibacterial host defenses. In CBA/J mice challenged with *Klebsiella pneumoniae*, administration of an anti–IL-12 antibody resulted in an increased lung bacterial burden and decreased overall survival (39). Similarly, BALB/c mice given an anti–IL-12 antibody during the course of *Chla-*

mydia pneumoniae infection showed higher bacterial load and longer recovery times as compared to controls (40).

3. Macrophage Inflammatory Protein-2

Macrophage inflammatory protein-2 (MIP-2) is a C-X-C chemokine that possesses potent neutrophilic chemotactic and activating properties (41). Recently, it has been shown that MIP-2 is an important component of the immune response to certain pulmonary infections. In murine *Klebsiella* pneumonia, the neutralization of MIP-2 in vivo results in impaired lung neutrophilic recruitment, bacterial clearance, and decreases in early but not long-term survival (42). In a murine model of *Legionella* pneumonia, the blockade of the CXC chemokine receptor-2 (CXCR-2), a common receptor for CXC chemokines, resulted in a 67% decrease in neutrophilic recruitment and markedly enhanced mortality (43). Further investigations of the role of MIP-2 and other chemokines in pulmonary infections are warranted.

4. Tumor Necrosis Factor

Tumor necrosis factor is a proinflammatory cytokine secreted principally by macrophages. TNF stimulates both neutrophils and macrophages, which leads to increased protease release, stimulation of the respiratory burst, and enhanced leukocyte phagocytic and microbicidal activity (44,45). Early studies revealed that TNF is a critical mediator of septic shock (46,47), autoimmune disorders (48,49), and graft-versus-host disease (50), but there is now clear evidence that TNF is also necessary for pulmonary and systemic host defenses (46,51,52). After an intratracheal challenge with gram-negative or gram-positive bacteria, there is an abrupt rise in TNF in the bronchoalveolar lavage fluid (BALF) (53,54). If this TNF release is blocked by prechallenge administration of an anti-TNF antibody, polymorphonuclear (PMN) recruitment and pulmonary bactericidal activity are significantly suppressed (53). Other studies using anti-TNF antibodies have also confirmed the importance of TNF in pulmonary host defense against infections caused by *Legionella pneumophilia* (55), *Pneumocystis carinii* (56), and pulmonary granuloma formation in *M. bovis* (BCG strain) infection (5) and *M. tuberculosis* infection (57).

5. Interleukin-10

Interleukin-10 is a cytokine produced by T cells, B cells, monocytes, and macrophages that possesses both proinflammatory and anti-inflammatory activities (58). IL-10's anti-inflammatory activities include the inhibition of the production of several cytokines; namely, IFN-γ and TNF-α (59–61). In contrast, IL-10 functions as a proinflammatory agent by stimulating B-cell proliferation and Ig secretion (62). Overexpression of IL-10 to exploit its anti-inflammatory properties has been investigated as a therapy for many disease processes including cardiac and hepatic transplantation (63,64), rheumatoid arthritis (65), bronchiolititis obliterans (66), and endotoxemia (67). Recently, the anti-inflammatory properties of IL-10 were also studied in a *Pseudomonas aeruginosa* pneumonia model. Systematically administered IL-10 to mice with a cytotoxic strain of *Pseudomonas* pneumonia significantly decreased lung injury and mortality (68). Conversely, in both *Klebsiella* and *Streptococcus pneumoniae* models, neutralization of IL-10 by a blocking antibody led to enhanced pulmonary production of proinflammatory cytokines, reduced bacterial growth, and improved survival in mice (69,70). These results imply that the specific approach used for IL-10 treatment of pulmonary infections, whether agonistic or antagonistic, may be dependent on the characteristics of the particular pathogen. More investigations are needed to define better these relationships.

6. Interleukin-17

Interleukin-17 is predominantly secreted by activated CD4$^+$ lymphocytes. IL-17 can elicit granulopoiesis in vitro (71) and in vivo (72) and can induce an array of proinflammatory cytokines in human macrophages, including TNF, IL-1β, IL-6, and IL-12 (73). Moreover, two reports show that IL-17 can result in neutrophilic recruitment in the lung by augmenting chemokine expression (74) and by the release of tachykinins (75). It has also been observed that IL-17 can also activate neutrophils in association with their recruitment into the airway in vivo (76). Recently, we have shown IL-17 receptor signaling is required for normal chemokine secretion in the lung in response to *K. pneumoniae* infection (77). As IL-17 is principally elaborated by CD4$^+$ T cells, this may represent one mechanism by which HIV-infected individuals with diminished CD4$^+$ T cells are predisposed to bacterial pneumonia.

B. Other Genes

1. TNF-α Converting Enzyme

TNF-α converting enzyme (TACE) is a newly discovered enzyme in the disintegrin and metalloproteinase (ADAM) family (78). This enzyme releases the 17-kD mature TNF-α from membrane-bound TNF-α by cleaving Ala 76 and Val 77 linkage. TACE has also been shown to be involved with other cell surface protein shedding events such as the p55 and p75 TNF-α receptors (79). Our laboratory has previously shown that acute administration of alcohol (EtOH) to rats suppresses TNF-α production posttranscriptionally in the lung and blood (20,80). Recently, we have further defined the mechanism of TNF-α inhibition by EtOH, which revealed that suppression of TACE enzymatic activity might play a role in this process. Using Mono Mac 6 cells exposed to EtOH, we have observed an accumulation of cell-associated TNF-α compared to secreted TNF-α as well as suppression of TNF p75 receptor shedding, a process mediated by TACE (81). We therefore postulated that EtOH possibly interferes with TACE/substrate interactions in the cell membrane, which then results in suppression of TNF-α secretion and ectodomain shedding (81). Since alcohol has long been recognized as an immunosuppressive drug and a risk factor for bacterial pneumonias, perhaps through its effect on TNF, restitution of TACE activity through gene therapy may be an alternative approach for treating bacterial pneumonias in alcoholics.

2. CD40 Ligand

CD40 is a 50-kD surface glycoprotein expressed on B lymphocytes (82), cytokine-activated monocytes (82), and follicular dendritic cells (83) and plays a key role in the survival, growth, and differentiation of B cells. CD40 ligand (CD40L) is expressed on activated CD4$^+$ T cells and interaction between T and B cells (Fig. 1) through the linkage of CD40L with CD40 is crucial for the development of humoral responses to T-cell–dependent antigens (84,85). Studies using recombinant CD40L, agonistic anti-CD40 antibodies, or anti-CD40L antibodies have shown that CD40L is critical in the host defense against an array of pathogens including *Toxoplasma*, *Mycobacterium*, *Trypanosoma*, and *Leishmania* (86–89).

Hyper-IgM syndrome is an X-linked immunodeficiency that is caused by mutations in the gene coding for the CD40L (90). This disease is characterized by a lack of germinal centers, immunoglobulin isotype switching, and affinity maturation of B cells, as well as defects in T-cell activation, making these individuals highly susceptible to pulmonary infections including *Pn. carinii*. The administration of recombinant CD40L to rats at the onset of dexamethasone immunosuppression was protective against *Pn. carinii* pneumonia (PCP) (91). Moreover, the administration of anti-CD40L antibody to SCID mice reconstituted with immunocompetent spleen cells resulted in unresolved PCP (92). In a *Streptococcus pneumoniae* model, treatment of mice with an anti-CD40L antibody resulted in markedly reduced antibody responses upon immunization with the whole bacteria (93). Thus, CD40L appears to be an attractive molecule for lung-directed gene therapy to augment host defense.

3. M3 Protein

It has been established that several DNA viruses secrete proteins that are able to intercept cytokines as a means to modulate the host immune response (94–96). Recently, it has been discovered that the murine gammaherpesvirus 68 M3 gene encodes a secreted 44-kD protein that binds a wide range of chemokines (97,98). The M3 protein binds chemokines from all four subfamilies of chemokines including murine macrophage inflammatory protein-1α (MIP-1α), IL-8, murine monocyte chemoattractant protein-1 (MCP-1), and human regulated

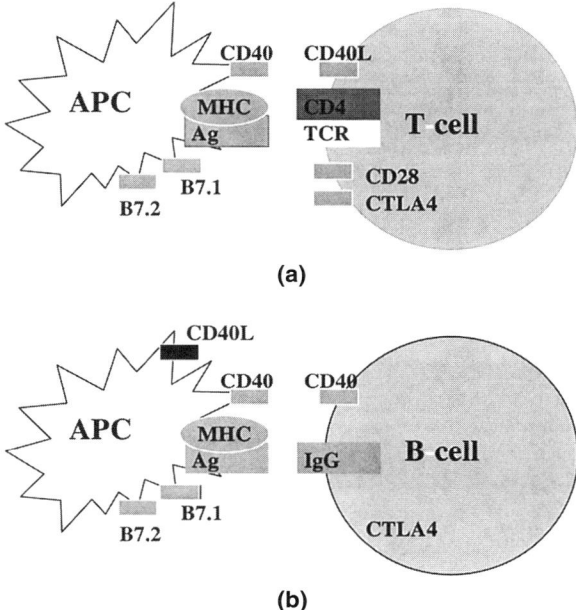

Figure 1 CD40-CD40L interactions. (a) An antigen-presenting cell (APC), such as a dendritic cell, captures antigens and presents the processed antigens in association with class II major histocompatibility complex (MHC) molecules. After interaction of the MHC-antigen complex with the T-cell receptor (TCR) on resting T cells, the T cell becomes activated and expresses CD40L. CD40L-CD40 interaction between T cells and APCs further activates the APC and results in upregulation of the expression of costimlatory molecules on the APC such as B7.1 and B7.2. The ligation of CD40L on T cells with CD40 on B cells results in B-cell proliferation, differentiation, and lg production. (b) Modifying APCs to express CD40L enables the APC to interact with specific antigens and directly activate B cells to produce specific antibodies without CD4$^+$ T-cell help.

upon activation of normal T-cell expressed and secreted (RANTES) (98). The M3 protein blocks the binding of chemokines with cellular receptors and abolishes chemokine-induced calcium signaling within the cell. These anti–anti-inflammatory functions of the M3 protein may be beneficial to downregulate overexuberant inflammatory response in the context of lung injury or lung infection.

III. DNA Vaccines

DNA vaccines are typically plasmids carrying the gene of a pathogen under the control of an active promoter such as the CMV promoter. Upon injection into

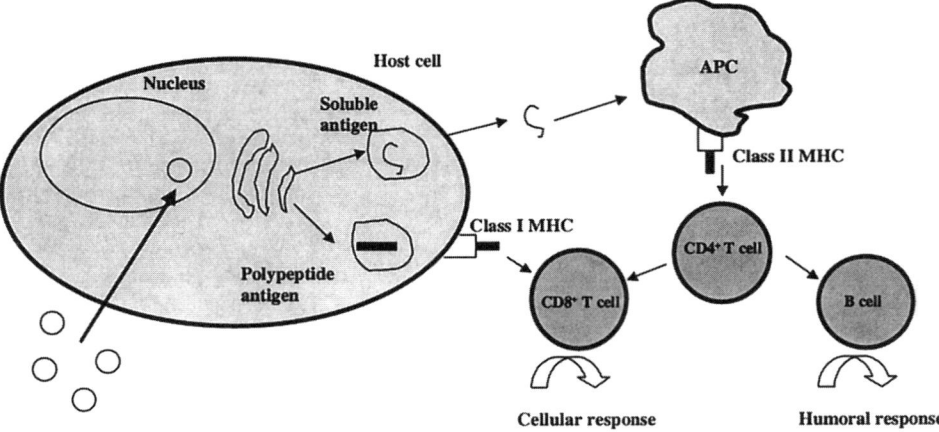

Figure 2   DNA vaccines. The DNA vaccine traverses the plasma membrane and uses the cellular machinery to translate the encoded proteins. The plasmid-encoded proteins are processed intracellularly and are presented in association with MHC class I molecules. The antigen can then activate the cellular immune response by interaction with CD8$^+$ T cells. In addition, soluble or secreted vaccine antigen can be phagocytosed by an antigen-presenting cell (APC) and presented by MHC class II molecules. Through the exogenous pathway, CD4$^+$ T cells can further activate the cellular immune response through CD8$^+$ T cells and also activate the humoral response through the B-cell pathway.

the muscle or skin, the DNA vaccine enters host cells and directs synthesis of its polypeptide antigen. The antigen is processed and presented by transfected cells, which results in the activation of cellular and humoral immune responses (Fig. 2). Low dosage requirements, inability to revert into virulence, easy manipulation of plasmid vectors, and longer shelf life are a few of the many advantages of genetic immunization over traditional vaccines (99). In this chapter, we will discuss the use of DNA vaccines for the prevention of *M. tuberculosis* and *Chlamydia pneumoniae* infections.

IV.   Results in Disease Models

A.   *Klebsiella pneumoniae*

K. pneumoniae is a gram-negative pathogen that causes both community acquired and nosocomial pneumonia. Mice pretreated with a recombinant adenovirus encoding either IL-12 (100) or TNF (101) showed improved survival that was associated with enhanced clearance of bacteria. Despite the beneficial effects observed with these genes, upregulation of MIP-2 utilizing adenovirus-mediated gene

transfer (AdMIP-2) of the rat MIP-2 gene which results in augmented PMN recruitment to the lung resulted in decreased survival in the *K. pneumoniae* model
(102). A likely explanation of these unpredicted results is that MIP-2 overexpression results in exuberant PMN influx and/or activation culminating in excessive
lung injury. Alternatively, the expression of a rat cytokine in the mouse may
have contributed to immune-mediated lung injury and increased mortality.

K. *pneumoniae* has a particularly strong association with alcohol consumption, and it is likely that the predisposition of alcoholics to infection is related
in part to cytokine suppression (20,80). An earlier study done by our laboratory
showed that in a model of acute ethanol intoxication, adenovirus-mediated gene
transfer of the IFN-γ gene resulted in significantly augmented host defenses
against *K. pneumoniae* (103). Recently, a related study utilized IL-17 to again
investigate the effect of vector-mediated cytokine release in mice on an alcohol-
containing diet. Mice were maintained on 20% ethanol in the drinking water for
2 weeks and then subsequently challenged with *K. pneumoniae*. Ethanol consumption resulted in suppressed release of IL-17 into lung tissue, decreased neutrophilic
recruitment, and increased mortality whereas in vivo administration of a recombinant adenovirus encoding murine IL-17 (AdmIL-17) to the lung resulted in a
normalization of neutrophil recruitment and mortality (Fig. 3) (104). These results
demonstrate that IL-17 is suppressed by chronic EtOH and its restoration could
represent a useful adjunct to treat lung infections in patients with EtOH abuse.

B. *Pseudomonas aeruginosa*

Ps. aeruginosa is a frequent cause of nosocomial pneumonia as well as a frequent
pathogen isolated from sputa in patients with bronchiectasis or cystic fibrosis
(105). Moreover, gram-negative nosocomial pneumonia has a 30–50% mortality

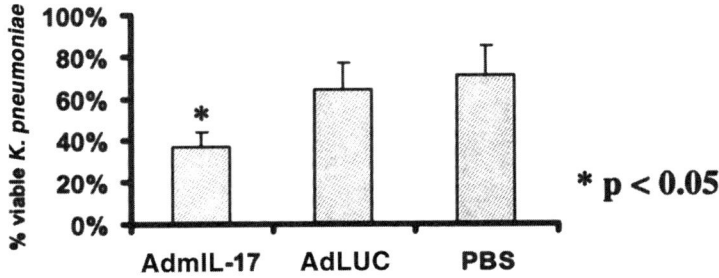

Figure 3 Reduced *K. pneumoniae* burden in ethanol-treated mice receiving AdmIL-17.
BALB/c mice were maintained on alcohol in drinking water or control mice were inoculated intratracheally with AdIL-17 or AdLuc and inoculated with *K. pneumoniae*. Mice
were sacrificed at 0 or 4 h to determine bacterial clearance. Mice receiving AdIL-17 had
a significant decrease in viable *K. pneumoniae* as compared to controls (p <.05).

in most series (106). Macrophage activation and neutrophils are required for eradication in the normal lung, and cytokine gene therapy in an experimental animal
model of *Pseudomonas* pneumonia has been shown to be beneficial in augmenting lung host defense against this pathogen. AdIFN administration intratracheally to rats results in activation of the alveolar macrophage and upregulation
of the pulmonary response upon stimulation with endotoxin and an enhanced
clearance of *Ps. aeruginosa* (107). In a murine sepsis model, adenovirus-mediated
expression of TNF improved survival from *Ps. aeruginosa* pneumonia from 25%
in controls to 91% in the vector-treated animals. This improved survival was
accompanied by enhanced cytokine expression and alveolar macrophage phagocytic activity (108).

Dendritic cells (DCs) are antigen-presenting cells (APCs) that capture antigens in the periphery and travel to the lymphoid organs to present the antigens
to CD4$^+$ T lymphocytes. Interaction with the DCs stimulates the CD4$^+$ T cells
to express CD40L among other surface activation proteins. The interaction of
CD40L on T cells with CD40 on B cells is essential in enabling B cells to generate
antigen-specific antibodies. A recent study has investigated the possibility of circumventing CD4$^+$ T cells in the pathway to specific antibody production. In this
study, DCs were transduced with an adenoviral vector that encodes the murine
CD40L (AdmCD40L) and subsequently pulsed with heat-killed *Ps. aeruginosa*.
In vitro, coculture of AdmCD40L-modified DCs with B cells resulted in B-cell
proliferation (Fig. 4). CD4$^{-/-}$ mice were then administered the modified DCs and
challenged with a lethal dose of *Ps. aeruginosa*. The CD4$^{-/-}$-immunized mice
were capable of developing anti-*Ps. aeruginosa* antibodies and were completely
protected from *Ps. aeruginosa*, as were wild-type immunized mice (109). The

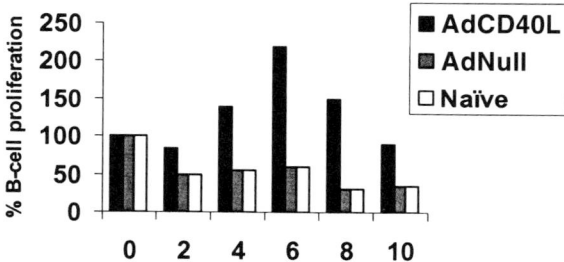

Figure 4   Enhanced B-cell proliferation by coculture of AdCD40L-modified DCs and
syngeneic B cells. DCs purified from bone marrow were transduced with AdCD40L or
AdNull and then cocultured with nonspecific B cells. Coculture of irradiated AdCD40L
transduced DCs (AdCD40L) with B cells resulted in the proliferation of the B cells,
whereas AdNull-modified DCs (AdNull) or naïve DCs (Naïve) induced no B-cell proliferation.

results show that in a situation of CD4$^+$ T-cell deficiency, such as HIV infection, DCs can be stimulated to serve as an alternate route in the pathway to pathogen-specific humoral immunity.

C. *Pneumocystis carinii*

Pn. carinii is a ubiquitous organism that causes no disease in immunocompetent individuals but is the cause of a severe pneumonia in many HIV-infected individuals. Despite current strategies to treat HIV infection and its complications, *Pn. carinii* pneumonia remains a common clinical problem. Though the relationship between CD4$^+$ cells and the risk of *Pn. carinii* infection is well established (110,111), the role of mononuclear phagocytes, CD8$^+$ cells, NK cells, and their secreted cytokines in host defense against this infection has not been well defined. Previous studies from our laboratory have demonstrated that aerosolized, rIFN-γ can ameliorate *Pn. carinii* infection in mice depleted of CD4$^+$ T cells (21). Based on these data, we hypothesized that in mice depleted of CD4$^+$ T cells, overexpression of IFN-γ in the lung would substitute for CD4$^+$ T lymphocytes and mediate clearance of *Pn. carinii* pneumonia. Intratracheally administered AdIFN to CD4$^+$ and CD4-depleted mice resulted in prolonged levels of IFN in CD4-depleted mice as compared with AdLuc-transduced controls (Fig. 5). The administration

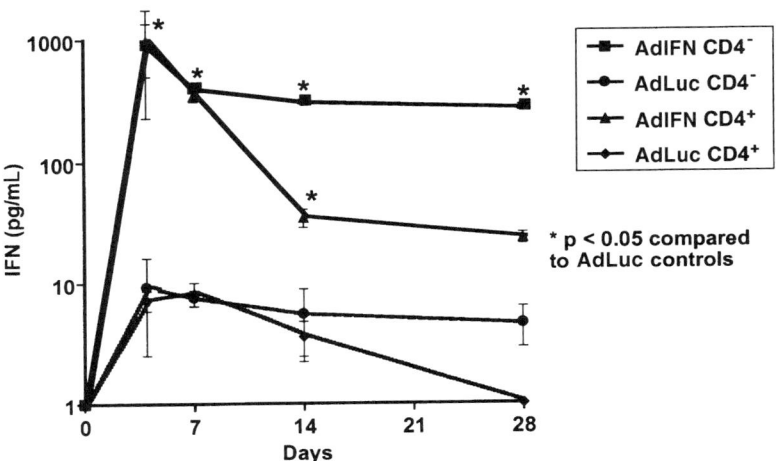

Figure 5 IFN-γ pharmacokinetics after adenovirus-mediated lung gene transfer with AdIFN in both CD4$^+$ and CD4$^-$ mice. BALB/c mice were transduced with either 10^9 plaque-forming units of AdIFN or AdLuc. AdIFN resulted in significantly higher IFN-γ levels in CD4$^+$ and CD4-depleted mice and prolonged levels of CD4-depleted mice as compared with controls (n = 4–6).

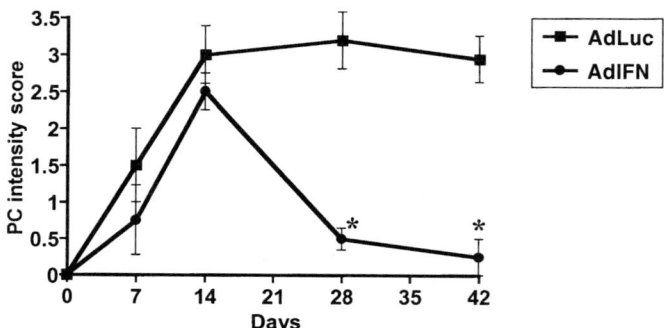

Figure 6 AdIFN-mediated clearance of *Pn. carinii* in CD4 mice. CD4-depleted BALB/c mice were pretreated with AdIFN or AdLuc intratracheally and subsequently challenged with 2×10^5 *Pn. carinii* cysts. Control CD4-depleted mice developed a progressive, severe infection, whereas CD4-depleted mice that received AdIFN developed a moderate *Pn. carinii* infection over the first 2 weeks that was cleared within 4–6 weeks (n = 6–8/time point). * p < 0.01 compared to AdLuc.

of AdIFN to CD4-depleted mice subsequently challenged with *Pn. carinii* resulted in a moderate *Pn. carinii* infection at 2 weeks but the infection was cleared by 4–6 weeks, whereas control mice developed a severe, progressive infection that was not cleared at 6 weeks (Fig. 6). Clearance of infection observed in CD4-depleted mice treated with AdIFN was associated with significant recruitment of CD8$^+$ T cells and NK cells into the lung (112). To determine whether recruited CD8$^+$ T cells associated with AdIFN were effector cells in AdIFN-induced clearance of *Pn. carinii*, we administered AdIFN to mice depleted of both CD4$^+$ and CD8$^+$ T cells. CD8 T-cell depletion completely abrogated the effect of AdIFN in CD4-depleted mice, demonstrating that CD8 cells are critical to the beneficial effect of AdIFN immunotherapy in *Pn. carinii*. Moreover, lung CD8$^+$ T cells from CD4-depleted mice treated with AdIFN have a significant increased precursor frequency of IFN clones, suggesting that cytokine gene transfer can polarize the T-cell response based on the class of cytokine delivered (112).

D. *Coccidioides immitis*

Co. immitis is a dimorphic fungus that causes the disease coccidioidomycosis, which ranges from a benign, self-limited pulmonary infection to a severe progressive extrapulmonary disease (113). Recovery from primary infection with *Co. immitis* affords lifelong immunity that is associated with the acquisition of a delayed-type hypersensitivity response and the production of certain cytokines such as IFN-γ and IL-2 (114–118). The cytokine IL-12 is a potent inducer of TH1-associated cytokines, notably IFN-γ, and has been shown to play a critical role in host defense against *Co. immitis* (119). Based on these data, it was postulated that vector-delivered IL-12 would prove to be protective against lethal pulmonary challenge with *Co. immitis*. J774 macrophages were transduced with a retroviral construct encoding the p40 and p35 subunits of IL-12. The transduced macrophages were then administered intraperitoneally to BALB/c mice that had been infected with 60 arthroconidia via a pulmonary route. Mice treated with the J774 macrophages showed a significant decrease in the number of pathogens in the lungs accompanied by an increase in IFN-γ in both the serum and the lung (120).

E. *Chlamydia pneumoniae*

Ch. pneumoniae, a gram-negative intracellular pathogen, is a common cause of pneumonia, sinusitis, and bronchitis. *Ch. pneumoniae* infection has also been linked to asthma, atherosclerosis, and acute myocardial infarction (121,122). Thus, there is an interest in developing a protective vaccine against *Ch. pneumoniae* and recent studies have focused on DNA immunization. Studies of experimental animal models of *Ch. pneumoniae* have shown that protection from this bacterium is largely dependent on the CD8$^+$ cytotoxic T lymphocyte (CTL) response (123,124). Identification of antigens able to elicit this CD8$^+$ response is crucial to the development of effective DNA vaccines.

Nasal administration of a plasmid encoding the heat shock protein 60 (pHSP-60) gene of *Ch. pneumoniae* to C56BI/6 mice resulted in 5- to 20-fold reduction of bacteria in lungs and a decreased severity of disease but did not lead to the production of specific antibodies. Administration of pHSP-60 to genetically deficient mice (major histocompatibility complex [MHC] class II$^{-/-}$, CD4$^{-/-}$, CD8$^{-/-}$, and CD4$^{-/-}$CD8$^{-/-}$) showed that induced protection was dependent on CD4$^+$ and CD8$^+$ T cells and IFN-γ secretion. However, immune CD4$^+$ T cells in the absence of CD8$^+$ T cells led to a worsening of infection. It was postulated that CD8$^+$ T cells might protect against infection while also hampering a deleterious CD4$^+$ T-cell–mediated response (125).

Another study investigated plasmids encoding three different *Ch. pneumoniae* genes: major outer membrane protein (MOMP), cysteine-rich outer membrane protein-2 (Omp-2), or heat shock protein-60 (HSp-60) (126). Intramuscular DNA immunization with pmomp or PHSp-60 showed 1.2–1.5 log reduction in the mean lung bacterial counts after challenge, but immunization with any of the three vaccines did not reduce the severity of histologically assessed pneumonia. However, the lymphoid reaction score was higher in the DNA-vaccinated mice, suggesting that the DNA vaccination was able to induce immunological memory resembling that seen after repeated infection.

Finally, a study testing eight DNA immunization constructs showed that those encoding MOMP or ADP/ATP translocase (Npt1$_{CP}$) can elicit protective immune responses as indicated by a reduced lung burden of *Ch. pneumoniae* after challenge (127). Collectively, these data provide important information by defining protective antigens and their role in the immune response to *Ch. pneumoniae*. Although not yet clinically applicable, DNA vaccination is a promising possibility for protection against *Ch. pneumoniae* infection.

F. *Mycobacterium tuberculosis*

It has been estimated that approximately one-third of the world's population in 1990 (1.7 billion individuals) were infected with *M. tuberculosis* affecting mostly people living in developing countries, and that with the global control measures in place at that time, 30 million people were expected to die due to tuberculosis by the year 2000 (128). The most effective vaccine against tuberculosis in humans is the BCG (Bacillus Calmette-Guérin) vaccine, an attenuated substrain of *M. bovis* that has been used for more than 50 years worldwide. However, this vaccine is very erratic in conferring protection, varying as much as 0–80% in separate clinical trials (129). In countries with a lower incidence of tuberculosis, such as the United States, the emergence of multidrug-resistant strains threatens control measures with antimycobacterial drugs. It is apparent that current immunotherapeutic and chemotherapeutic approaches for the control of tuberculosis need to be improved.

Through studying IFN-γ knockout mice, it has been determined that this cytokine plays a pivotal role in protective immunity to *M. tuberculosis* (130–132). To further define this relationship, a replication-deficient adenoviral vector designed to deliver IFN-γ (AdIFN) was delivered intratracheally into the lungs of BALB/c mice, which were subsequently challenged with a sublethal aerosol of *M. tuberculosis* (133). AdIFN-γ–treated mice showed improved containment of infection as compared to control, but this protective effect was short-lived such that the load of viable bacilli in AdIFN-γ–treated lungs reached levels similar to the controls by 30 days of infection. Enhanced expression of genes encoding interferon regulatory factor-1 (IRF-1), IRF-2, IFN-γ, and the chemokine macrophage inflammatory protein-1β (MIP-1β) was also observed. However, other cytokines, which were functionally linked to an IFN-γ response in the host response, were not affected, including IL-12, IP-10, IL-2, and inducible nitric oxide synthase (iNOS). Preliminary analysis of such data would suggest that AdIFN treatment enhanced the early control of *M. tuberculosis*–infected mice through virus-mediated expression of IFN-γ in the lung. Such control was accompanied by increased expression of the interferon-responsive factors, IRF-1 and IRF-2. However, the expression of all macrophage-activation genes, which are responsible to these factors, were not enhanced by such treatment.

Being that *M. tuberculosis* is an intracellular pathogen, cell-mediated immunity is vital in the control of the bacterial replication and subsequent protection against tuberculosis. DNA vaccines are powerful inducers of cellular immune responses (99), making them an attractive approach to the prevention of tuberculosis. Proteins produced and secreted by *M. tuberculosis* bacilli, referred to as culture filtrate (CF) proteins, have been recognized as the key antigens in the protective immune response (134–137), and an array of DNA vaccines have been constructed using genes encoding various CF proteins. Testing of these DNA vaccines in animal models has shown partial protection against challenge that is equivalent but not consistently superior to the protection conferred by BCG (138–141). However, studies are ongoing further to define protective antigens and to develop mechanisms to enhance the immunogenicity of DNA vaccines for tuberculosis (142–144).

In addition to their protective effect, DNA vaccines have also been shown to have an impressive therapeutic effect on *M. tuberculosis* infections. Recently, investigators hypothesized that the cellular immune responses induced by DNA vaccines would augment the innate immune response to *M. tuberculosis*. When BALB/c mice infected with *M. tuberculosis* were administered a plasmid expressing the HSp-65, the numbers of live bacteria in the spleen and lungs declined rapidly. This therapeutic effect of DNA vaccination was associated with a switch from a predominantly TH2 to a predominantly TH1 response (145). Administration of DNA vaccines in conjunction with conventional chemotherapeutic antibacterial drugs might result in more efficient treatment of *M. tuberculosis* in humans.

G. Respiratory Syncytial Virus

Respiratory syncytial virus (RSV), a negative-stranded RNA virus, is the most important viral agent of serious respiratory disease in the pediatric population worldwide. Ongoing efforts to develop an effective vaccine to RSV have been unsuccessful. In the 1960s, a formalin-inactivated RSV vaccine (FI-RSV) given to infants resulted in enhanced disease upon subsequent natural infection (146,147). Ensuing investigations have identified differences in the T-cell response to FI-RSV immunization versus live RSV infection. FI-RSV immunization induces a TH2-biased response that causes enhanced lung pathology upon challenge (148,149) (150), whereas live RSV infection results in predominant secretion of TH1 cytokines and confers protective immunity (151,152). Thus, a vaccine that discriminates toward a TH1 response would seem to be favorable.

Recently, several live attenuated and subunit vaccine candidates have been constructed using an RSV infectious clone. However, striking a balance between immunogenicity and attenuation has proved to be difficult, since any augmentation of attenuation usually results in decreased immunogenicity. Two separate studies have investigated the effects of coexpressing immunomodulator genes with viral vaccine candidates. The immunomodulators CD40L and IFN-γ were not only chosen for their immune-enhancing capabilities but also for their predisposition to induce the TH1 subset of cytokines. Nasal administration of an infectious recombinant human RSV that encodes murine IFN-γ (rRSV/mIFN-γ) to BALB/c mice induced titers of total IgG against RSV F protein and RSV-neutralizing serum antibodies that were higher than that induced by wild-type RSV. In addition, mice immunized with rRSV/mIFN-γ were highly resistant to RSV challenge (153). A related study investigated the effect of CD40L on RSV immunity by infecting mice simultaneously with RSV and an adenoviral vector expressing CD40L or coimmunizing mice with plasmid DNA vectors expressing CD40L and RSV F and/or G proteins and subsequently challenging the mice with RSV. In mice infected with RSV and AVCD40L, an augmented production of IFN-γ, enhanced virus clearance, and a higher frequency of RSV-specific CTLs in the lung, was observed. In the mice coimmunized with plasmid DNA vectors expressing CD40L and RSV glycoproteins, the addition of CD40L resulted in moderate enhancement of anti-RSV antibody responses when coexpressed with the F subunit and combined F/G subunit and a striking seven-fold increase in response to the G subunit vector (154).

V. Summary

Our increasing knowledge of DNA has given us powerful tools to study the role of various genes in infectious pulmonary diseases. In the past several years, immunomodulation in the lung has expanded from cytokine gene therapy to noncytokine gene targets and DNA vaccination. As we continue to piece together the picture of infection and immunity in the lung, we will hopefully come closer to developing immunotherapy that can be used in the clinical setting and advance DNA vaccines further into clinical trials.

References

1. Reynolds HY. Host defense impairments that may lead to respiratory infections. Clin Chest Med 1987; 8(3):339–358.
2. Fels AOS, Cohn ZA. The alveolar macrophage. J Appl Physiol 1986; 60:353–369.
3. Sibille Y, Reynolds HY. Macrophages and polymorphonuclear neutrophils in lung defense and injury. Am Rev Respir Dis 1990; 141:471–501.
4. Nathan CF. Secretory products of macrophages. J Clin Invest 1987; 79:319–326.
5. Kindler V, Sappino A-P, Grau GE, Piguet P-F, Vassalli P. The inducing role of

tumor necrosis factor in the development of bactericidal granulomas during BCG infection. Cell 1989; 56:731–740.

6. Lai WC, Bennett M, Pakes SP, Kumar V, Steutermann D, Owusu I, et al. Resistance to *Mycoplasma pulmonis* mediated by activated natural killer cells. J Infect Dis 1990; 161:1269–1275.

7. Nikaido Y, Yoshida S, Goto Y, Mizuguchi Y, Kuroiwa A. Macrophage-activating T-cell factor(s) produced in an early phase of *Legionella pneumophila* infection in guinea pigs. Infect Immun 1989; 57(11):3458–3465.

8. Ebrahimi B, Dutia BM, Brownstein DG, Nash AA. Murine gammaherpesvirus-68 infection causes multi-organ fibrosis and alters leukocyte trafficking in interferon-gamma receptor knockout mice. Am J Pathol 2001; 158(6):2117–2125.

9. Li C, Corraliza I, Langhorne J. A defect in interleukin-10 leads to enhanced malarial disease in *Plasmodium chabaudi* infection in mice. Infect Immun 1999; 67(9): 4435–4442.

10. Zhang Y, Denkers EY. Protective role for interleukin-5 during chronic *Toxoplasma gondii* infection. Infect Immun 1999; 67(9):4383–4392.

11. Wei XQ, Leung BP, Niedbala W, Piedrafita D, Feng GJ, Sweet M, et al. Altered immune responses and susceptibility to *Leishmania major* and *Staphylococcus aureus* infection in IL-18–deficient mice. J Immunol 1999; 163(5):2821–2828.

12. Tracey KJ, Beutler B, Lowry SF, Merryweather J, Wolpe S, Milsark IW, et al. Shock and tissue injury induced by recombinant human cachectin. Science 1986; 234:470–474.

13. Rosenberg SA, Lotze MT, Muul LM, Chang AE, Avis FP, Leitman S, et al. A progress report on the treatment of 157 patients with advanced cancer using lymphokine-activated killer cells and interleukin-2 or high-dose interleukin-2 alone. N Engl J Med 1987; 316(15):889–897.

14. Cohen J. IL-12 deaths: explanation and a puzzle (news). Science 1995; 270(5238): 908.

15. Nathan CF, Prendergast TJ, Wiebe ME, Stanley ER, Platzer E, Remold HG, et al. Activation of human macrophages. Comparison of other cytokines with interferon-gamma. J Exp Med 1984; 160:600–605.

16. Black CM, Catterall JR, Remington JS. In vivo and in vitro activation of alveolar macrophages by recombinant interferon-gamma. J Immunol 1987; 138:491–495.

17. Nathan CF, Murray HW, Wiebe ME, Rubin BY. Identification of interferon-gamma as the lymphokine that activates human macrophage oxidative metabolism and antimicrobial activity. J Exp Med 1983; 158:670–689.

18. Collart MA, Belin D, Vassalli JD, de Kossodo S, Vassalli P. Gamma interferon enhances macrophage transcription of the tumor necrosis factor/cachectin, interleukin 1, and urokinase genes, which are controlled by short-lived repressors. J Exp Med 1986; 164:2113–2118.

19. Luedke C, Cerami A. Interferon-gamma overcomes glucocorticoid suppression of cachectin/tumor necrosis factor biosynthesis by murine macrophages. J Clin Invest 1990; 86:1234–1240.

20. Kolls JK, Xie J, Lei D, Greenberg S, Summer WR, Nelson S. Differential effects of in vivo ethanol on LPS-induced TNF and nitric oxide production in the lung. Am J Physiol Lung Cell Mol Physiol 1995; 268:L991–L998.

21. Beck JM, Liggit HD, Brunette EN, Fuchs HJ, Shellito JE, Debs RJ. Reduction in intensity of *Pneumocystis carinii* pneumonia in mice by aerosol administration of interferon-gamma. Infect Immun 1991; 59:3859–3862.

22. Murray HW. Interferon-gamma, the activated macrophage, and host defense against antimicrobial challenge. Ann Intern Med 1988; 108:595–608.

23. Murray HW, Gellene RA, Libby DM, Rothermel CD, Rubin BY. Activation of tissue macrophages from AIDS patients: in vitro response of AIDS alveolar macrophages to lymphokines and interferon-gamma. J Immunol 1985; 135:2374–2377.

24. Vecchiarelli A, Todisco T, Puliti M, Dottorini M, Bistoni F. Modulation of anti-candida activity of human alveolar macrophages by interferon-gamma or interleu-kin-1-alpha. Am J Respir Cell Mol Biol 1989; 1:49–55.

25. Wu-Hsieh B. Relative susceptibilities of inbred mouse strains C57BL/6 and A/J to infection with *Histoplasma capsulatum.* Infect Immun 1989; 57:3788–3792.

26. Zhong G, Peterson EM, Czarniecki CW, Schrieber RD, De La Maza LM. Role of endogenous gamma interferon in host defense against *Chlamydia trachomatis* infections. Infect Immun 1989; 57:152–157.

27. Chiang Y-W, Roth JA, Andrews JJ. Influence of recombinant interferon gamma and dexamethasone on pneumonia attributable to *Heamophilus somnus* in calves. Am J Vet Res 1990; 51:759–762.

28. Suzuki Y, Joh K, Kobayashi A. Tumor necrosis factor-independent protective effect of recombinant IFN-gamma against acute toxoplasmosis in T-cell deficient mice. J Immunol 1991; 147:2728–2733.

29. Skerrett SJ, Martin TR. Intratracheal interferon-gamma augments pulmonary de-fenses in experimental legionellosis. Am J Respir Crit Care Med 1994; 149:50–58.

30. Steinmuller C, Franke-Ullmann G, Lohmann-Matthes ML, Emmendorffer A. Local activation of nonspecific defense against a respiratory model infection by applica-tion of interferon-gamma: comparison between rat alveolar and interstitial lung macrophages. Am J Respir Cell Mol Biol 2000; 22(4):481–490.

31. Brunda MJ. Interleukin-12 (Review). J Leukoc Biol 1994; 55(2):280–288.

32. Kobayashi M, Fitz L, Ryan M, Hewick RM, Clark SC, Chan et al. Identification and purification of natural killer cell stimulatory factor (NKSF), a cytokine with multiple biologic effects on human lymphocytes. J Exp Med 1989; 170(3):827–845.

33. Heinzel FP, Schoenhaut DS, Rerko RM, Rosser LE, Gately MK. Recombinant in-terleukin 12 cures mice infected with Leishmania major. J Exp Med 1993; 177(5):1505–1509.

34. Flynn JL, Goldstein MM, Triebold KJ, Sypek J, Wolf S, Bloom BR. IL-12 increases resistance of BALB/c mice to *Mycobacterium tuberculosis* infection. J Immunol 1995; 155(5):2515–2524.

35. Stevenson MM, Tam MF, Wolf SF, Sher A. IL-12-induced protection against blood-stage *Plasmodium chabaudi* AS requires IFN-gamma and TNF-alpha and occurs via a nitric oxide–dependent mechanism. J Immunol 1995; 155(5):2545–2556.

36. Wagner RD, Steinberg H, Brown JF, Czuprynski CJ. Recombinant interleukin-12

enhances resistance of mice to *Listeria monocytogenes* infection. Microb Pathogen 1994; 17(3):175–186.

37. Cooper AM, Roberts AD, Rhoades ER, Callahan JE, Getzy DM, et al. The role of interleukin-12 in acquired immunity to *Mycobacterium tuberculosis* infection. Immunology 1995; 84(3):423–432.

38. Zhou P, Sieve MC, Bennett J, Kwon-Chung KJ, Tewari RP, Gazzinelli RT, et al. IL-12 prevents mortality in mice infected with Histoplasma capsulatum through induction of IFN-gamma. J Immunol 1995; 155(2):785–795.

39. Greenberger MJ, Kunkel SL, Strieter RM, Lukacs NW, Bramson J, Gauldie J, et al. IL-12 gene therapy protects mice in lethal *Klebsiella pneumonia* J Immunol 1996; 157(7):3006–3012.

40. Geng Y, Berencsi K, Gyulai Z, Valyi-Nagy T, Gonczol E, Trinchieri G. Roles of interleukin-12 and gamma interferon in murine *Chlamydia pneumoniae* infection. Infect Immun 2000; 68(4):2245–2253.

41. Wolpe SD, Sherry B, Juers D, Davatelis G, Yurt RW, Cerami A. Identification and characterization of macrophage inflammatory protein 2. Proc Natl Acad Sci USA 1989; 89(2):612–616.

42. Greenberger MJ, Strieter RM, Kunkel SL, Danforth JM, Laichalk LL, McGillicuddy DC, et al. Neutralization of macrophage inflammatory protein-2 attenuates neutrophil recruitment and bacterial clearance in murine *Klebsiella* pneumonia. J Infect Dis 1996; 173:159–165.

43. Tateda K, Moore TA, Newstead MW, Tsai WC, Zeng X, Deng JC, et al. Chemokine-dependent neutrophil recruitment in a murine model of Legionella pneumonia: potential role of neutrophils as immunoregulatory cells. Infect Immun 2001; 69(4): 2017–2024.

44. Gamble JR, Harlan JM, Klebanoff SJ, Vadas MA. Stimulation of the adherence of neutrophils to umbilical vein endothelium by human recombinant tumor necrosis factor. Proc Natl Acad Sci USA 1985; 82(24):8667–8671.

45. Beutler B, Cerami A. Cachectin: more than a tumor necrosis factor. N Engl J Med 1987; 316:379–385.

46. Beutler B, Milsark I, Cerami A. Passive immunization against cachectin/tumor necrosis factor (TNF) protects mice from the lethal effect of endotoxin. Science 1985; 229:869–871.

47. Bonavida B, Paubert-Braquet M, Hosford D, Braquet P. The involvement of platlet-actiating factor (PAF)–induced monocyte activation and tumor necrosis factor production in shock. Prog Clin Biol Res 1989; 308:485–489.

48. Jacob CO. Tumor necrosis factor alpha in autoimmunity: pretty girl or old witch. Immunol Today 1992; 13:122–125.

49. Jacob CO, McDevitt HO. Tumor necrosis factor-alpha in autoimmune 'lupus' nephritis. Nature 1988; 331:356–358.

50. Piquet P-F, Grau GE, Allet B, Vassalli P. Tumor necrosis factor/cachectin is an effector of skin and gut lesions of the acute graft-versus-host disease. J Exp Med 1987; 166:1280–1289.

51. Bonavida B. Immunomodulatory effect of tumor necrosis factor. Biotherapy 1991; 3:127–133.

52. Cerami A, Beutler B. The role of cachectin/TNF in endotoxin shock and cachexia. Immunol Today 1988; 9:28–31.

53. Kolls JK, Nelson S, Summer WR. Recombinant cytokines and pulmonary host defense. Am J Med Sci 1993; 306(5):330–335.

54. Nelson S, Bagby GJ, Bainton B, Wilson LA, Thompson JJ, Summer WR. Compartmentalization of intraalveolar and systemic lipopolysaccharide-induced tumor necrosis factor and the pulmonary inflammatory response. J Infect Dis 1989; 159: 189–194.

55. Blanchard DK, Djeu JY, Klein TW, Friedman M, Stewart WE. Protective effects of tumor necrosis factor in experimental *Legionella pneumophila* infections of mice via activation of PMN function. J Leukoc Biol 1988; 4342:429–435.

56. Chen W, Havell EA, Harmsen A. Importance of endogenous tumor necrosis factor-alpha and gamma interferon in host resistance against *Pneumocystis carinii* infection. Infect Immun 1992; 60:1279–1284.

57. Adams LB, Mason CM, Kolls JK, Scollard D, Krahenbuhl JL, Nelson S. Exacerbation of acute and chronic murine tuberculosis by administration of a TNF receptor expressing adenovirus. J Infect Dis 1995; 171:400–405.

58. Moore KW, O'Garra A, de Waal MR, Vieira P, Mosmann TR. Interleukin-10. Annu Rev Immunol 1993; 11:165–190.

59. de Waal Malefyt R, Abrams J, Bennett B, Figdor CG, de Vries JE. Interleukin 10 (IL-10) inhibits cytokine synthesis by human monocytes: an autoregulatory role of IL-10 produced by monocytes. J Exp Med 1991; 174:1209–1220.

60. Fiorentino DF, Zlotnik A, Mosmann TR, Howard M, O'Garra A. IL-10 inhibits cytokine production by activated macrophages. J Immunol 1991; 147(11):3815–3822.

61. Gerard C, Bruyns C, Marchant A, Abramowicz D, Vandenabeele P, Delvaux A, et al. Interleukin 10 reduces the release of tumor necrosis factor and prevents lethality in experimental endotoxemia. J Exp Med 1993; 177(2):547–550.

62. Rousset F, Garcia E, Defrance T, Peronne C, Vezzio N, Hsu DH, et al. Interleukin 10 is a potent growth and differentiation factor for activated human B lymphocytes. Proc Natl Acad Sci USA 1992; 89(5):1890–1893.

63. Qin L, Ding Y, Pahud DR, Robson ND, Shaked A, Bromberg JS. Adenovirus-mediated gene transfer of viral interleukin-10 inhibits the immune response to both alloantigen and adenoviral antigen. Hum Gene Ther 1997; 8(11):1365–1374.

64. Drazan KE, Wu L, Olthoff KM, Jurim O, Busuttil RW, Shaked A. Transduction of hepatic allografts achieves local levels of viral IL-10 which suppress alloreactivity in vitro. J Surg Res 1995; 59(1):219–223.

65. Apparailly F, Verwaerde C, Jacquet C, Auriault C, Sany J, Jorgensen C. Adenovirus-mediated transfer of viral IL-10 gene inhibits murine collagen-induced arthritis. J Immunol 1998; 160(11):5213–5220.

66. Boehler A, Chamberlain D, Xing Z, Slutsky AS, Jordana M, Gauldie J, et al. Adenovirus-mediated interleukin-10 gene transfer inhibits post-transplant fibrous airway obliteration in an animal model of *Bronchiolitis obliterans*. Hum Gene Ther 1998; 9(4):541–551.

67. Xing Z, Ohkawara Y, Jordana M, Graham FL, Gauldie J. Adenoviral vector–medi-

ated interleukin-10 expression in vivo: intramuscular gene transfer inhibits cytokine responses in endotoxemia. Gene Ther 1997; 4(2):140–149.

68. Sawa T, Corry DB, Gropper MA, Ohara M, Kurahashi K, Wiener-Kronish JP. IL-10 improves lung injury and survival in *Pseudomonas aeruginosa* pneumonia. J Immunol 1997; 159(6):2858–2866.

69. Greenberger MJ, Strieter RM, Kunkel SL, Danforth JM, Goodman RE, Standiford TJ. Neutralization of IL-10 increases survival in a murine model of *Klebsiella pneumonia*. J Immunol 1995; 155(2):722–729.

70. van der Poll T, Marchant A, Keogh CV, Goldman M, Lowry SF. Interleukin-10 impairs host defense in murine pneumococcal pneumonia. J Infect Dis 1996; 174(5):994–1000.

71. Fossiez F, Djossou O, Chomarat P, Flores-Romo L, Ait-Yahia S, Maat C, et al. T cell interleukin-17 induces stromal cells to produce proinflammatory and hematopoietic cytokines (see comments). J Exp Med 1996; 183(6):2593–2603.

72. Schwarzenberger P, La R, V, Miller A, Ye P, Huang W, Zieske A, et al. IL-17 stimulates granulopoiesis in mice: use of an alternate, novel gene therapy-derived method for in vivo evaluation of cytokines. J Immunol 1998; 161(11):6383–6389.

73. Jovanovic DV, Di Battista JA, Martel-Pelletier J, Jolicoeur FC, He Y, Zhang M, et al. IL-17 stimulates the production and expression of proinflammatory cytokines, IL-beta and TNF-alpha, by human macrophages. J Immunol 1998; 160(7):3513–3521.

74. Laan M, Cui ZH, Hoshino H, Lotvall J, Sjostrand M, Gruenert DC, et al. Neutrophil recruitment by human IL-17 via C-X-C chemokine release in the airways. J Immunol 1999; 162(4):2347–2352.

75. Hoshino H, Lotvall J, Skoogh BE, Linden A. Neutrophil recruitment by interleukin-17 into rat airways in vivo. Role of tachykinins. Am J Respir Crit Care Med 1999; 159(5 Pt 1):1423–1428.

76. Hoshino H, Laan M, Sjostrand M, Lotvall J, Skoogh BE, Linden A. Increased elastase and myeloperoxidase activity associated with neutrophil recruitment by IL-17 in airways in vivo. J Allergy Clin Immunol 2000; 105(1 Pt 1):143–149.

77. Ye P, Rodriguez FH, Kanaly S, Stocking KL, Schurr J, Schwarzenberger P, et al. Requirement of interleukin 17 receptor signaling for lung CXC chemokine and granulocyte colony-stimulating factor expression, neutrophil recruitment, and host defense. J Exp Med. In press.

78. Black RA, Rauch CT, Kozlosky CJ, Peschon JJ, Slack JL, Wolfson MF, et al. A metalloproteinase disintegrin that releases tumour-necrosis factor-alpha from cells. Nature 1997; 385:729–733.

79. Peschon JJ, Slack JL, Reddy P, Stocking KL, Sunnarborg SW, Lee DC, et al. An essential role for ectodomain shedding in mammalian development (see comments). Sci 1998; 282(5392):1281–1284.

80. Nelson S, Bagby G, Summer WR. Alcohol suppresses lipopolysaccharide-induced tumor necrosis factor activity in serum and lung. Life Sci 1989; 44:673–676.

81. Zhang Z, Cork J, Ye P, Lei D, Schwarzenberger PO, Summer WR, et al. Inhibition of TNF-alpha processing and TACE-mediated ectodomain shedding by ethanol. J Leukoc Biol 2000; 67(6):856–862.

82. Wang CY, Fu SM, Kunkel HG. Isolation and immunological characterization of a major surface glycoprotein (gp54) preferentially expressed on certain human B cells. J Exp Med 1979; 149(6):1424–1437.

83. Caux C, Massacrier C, Vanbervliet B, Dubois B, Van Kooten C, Durand I, et al. Activation of human dendritic cells through CD40 cross-linking. J Exp Med 1994; 180(4):1263–1272.

84. Armitage RJ, Fanslow WC, Strockbine L, Sato TA, Clifford KN, Macduff BM, et al. Molecular and biological characterization of a murine ligand for CD40. Nature 1992; 357(6373):80–82.

85. Spriggs MK, Armitage RJ, Strockbine L, Clifford KN, Macduff BM, Sato TA, et al. Recombinant human CD40 ligand stimulates B cell proliferation and immunoglobulin E secretion. J Exp Med 1992; 176(6):1543–1550.

86. Subauste CS, Wessendarp M, Sorensen RU, Leiva LE. CD40-CD40 ligand interaction is central to cell-mediated immunity against *Toxoplasma gondii*: patients with hyper IgM syndrome have a defective type 1 immune response that can be restored by soluble CD40 ligand trimer. J Immunol 1999; 162(11):6690–6700.

87. Hayashi T, Rao SP, Meylan PR, Kornbluth RS, Catanzaro A. Role of CD40 ligand in *Mycobacterium avium* infection. Infect Immun 1999; 67(7):3558–3565.

88. Chaussabel D, Jacobs F, de Jonge J, de Veerman M, Carlier Y, Thielemans K, et al. CD40 ligation prevents *Trypanosoma cruzi* infection through interleukin-12 upregulation. Infect Immun 1999; 67(4):1929–1934.

89. Gurunathan S, Irvine KR, Wu CY, Cohen JI, Thomas E, Prussin C, et al. CD40 ligand/trimer DNA enhances both humoral and cellular immune responses and induces protective immunity to infectious and tumor challenge. J Immunol 1998; 161(9):4563–4571.

90. Grewal IS, Flavell RA. CD40 and CD154 in cell-mediated immunity. Annu Rev Immunol 1998; 16:111–135.

91. Oz HS, Hughes WT, Rehg JE, Thomas EK. Effect of CD40 ligand and other immunomodulators on *Pneumocystis carinii* infection in rat model. Microb Pathogen 2000; 29(3):187–190.

92. Wiley JA, Harmsen AG. CD40 ligand is required for resolution of *Pneumocystis carinii* pneumonia in mice. J Immunol 1995; 155(7):3525–3529.

93. Hwang Y, Nahm MH, Briles DE, Thomas D, Purkerson JM. Acquired, but not innate, immune responses to *Streptococcus pneumoniae* are compromised by neutralization of CD40L. Infect Immun 2000; 68(2):511–517.

94. Spriggs MK. One step ahead of the game: viral immunomodulatory molecules. Annu Rev Immunol 1996; 14:101–130.

95. Smith GL, Symons JA, Khanna A, Vanderplasschen A, Alcami A. Vaccinia virus immune evasion. Immunol Rev 1997; 159:137–154.

96. Alcami A, Smith GL. Cytokine receptors encoded by poxviruses: a lesson in cytokine biology. Immunol Today 1995; 16(10):474–478.

97. Parry CM, Simas JP, Smith VP, Stewart CA, Minson AC, Efstathiou S, et al. A broad spectrum secreted chemokine binding protein encoded by a herpes virus. J Exp Med 2000; 191(3):573–578.

98. van B, V, Barrett J, Tiffany HL, Fremont DH, Murphy PM, McFadden G, et al.

Identification of a gammaherpesvirus selective chemokine binding protein that inhibits chemokine action. J Virol 2000; 74(15):6741–6747.

99. Shedlock DJ, Weiner DB. DNA vaccination: antigen presentation and the induction of immunity. J Leukoc Biol 2000; 68(6):793–806.

100. Gilliand G, Perrin S, Blanchard K, Bunn HF. Analysis of cytokine mRNA and DNA: detection and quantition by competitive polymerase chain reaction. Proc Natl Acad Sci USA 1992; 87:2725–2729.

101. Standiford TJ, Wilkowski JM, Sisson TH, Hattori N, Mehrad B, Bucknell KA, et al. Intrapulmonary tumor necrosis factor gene therapy increases bacterial clearance and survival in murine gram-negative pneumonia. Hum Gene Ther 1999; 10(6): 899–909.

102. Foley R, Driscoll K, Wan Y, Braciak T, Howard B, Xing, et al. Adenoviral gene transfer of macrophage inflammatory protein-2 in rat lung. Am J Pathol 1996; 149(4):1395–1403.

103. Kolls JK, Lei D, Stoltz D, Zhang P, Schwarzenberger PO, Ye P, et al. Adenoviral-mediated interferon-gamma gene therapy augments pulmonary host defense of ethanol-treated rats. Alcohol Clin Exp Res 1998; 22(1):157–162.

104. Shellito JE, Zheng M, Ye P, Ruan S, Shean MK, Kolls J. Effect of alcohol consumption on host release interleukin-17 during pulmonary infection with Klebsiella pneumoniae. Alcohol Clin Exp Res 2001; 25(6):872–881.

105. Bodey GP, Bolivar R, Fainstein V, Jadeja L. Infections caused by *Pseudomonas aeruginosa*. Rev Infect Dis 1983; 5(2):279–313.

106. Bowton DL. Nosocomial pneumonia in the ICU—year 2000 and beyond. Chest 1999; 115(3 Suppl):28S–33S.

107. Lei D, Lancaster JR, Jr, Joshi MS, Nelson S, Stoltz D, Bagby GJ, et al. Activation of alveolar macrophages and lung host defenses using transfer of the interferon-gamma gene. Am J Physiol Lung Cell Mol Physiol 1997; 272(5):L852–L859.

108. Chen GH, Reddy RC, Newstead MW, Tateda K, Kyasapura BL, Standiford TJ. Intrapulmonary TNF gene therapy reverses sepsis-induced suppression of lung antibacterial host defense. J Immunol 2000; 165(11):6496–6503.

109. Kikuchi T, Worgall S, Singh R, Moore MA, Crystal RG. Dendritic cells genetically modified to express CD40 ligand and pulsed with antigen can initiate antigen-specific humoral immunity independent of CD4+ T cells. Nat Med 2000; 6(10): 1154–1159.

110. Fauci AS, Macher AM, Longo DL, Lane HC, Rook AH, Masur H, et al. NIH Conference. Acquired immunodeficiency syndrome: epidemiologic, clinical, immunologic, and therapeutic considerations. Ann Intern Med 1984; 100:92–106.

111. Phair J, Munoz A, Detels R, Kaslow R, Rinaldo C, Saahet A. The risk of *Pneumocystis carinii* pneumonia among men infected with human immunodeficiency virus type I. N Engl J Med 1990; 322:155–161.

112. Kolls JK, Habetz S, Shean MK, Vazquez C, Brown JA, Lei D, et al. IFN-gamma and CD8+ T cells restore host defenses against Pneumocystis carinii in mice depleted of CD4+ T cells. J Immunol 1999; 162(5):2890–2894.

113. Stevens DA. Coccidioidomycosis. N Engl J Med 1995; 332(16):1077–1082.

114. Ampel NM, Bejarano GC, Salas SD, Galgiani JN. In vitro assessment of cellular

immunity in human coccidioidomycosis: relationship between dermal hypersensitivity, lymphocyte transformation, and lymphokine production by peripheral blood mononuclear cells from healthy adults. J Infect Dis 1992; 165(4):710–715.

115. Beaman L, Pappagianis D, Benjamini E. Significance of T cells in resistance to experimental murine coccidioidomycosis. Infect Immun 1977; 17(3):580–585.

116. Corry DB, Ampel NM, Christian L, Locksley RM, Galgiani JN. Cytokine production by peripheral blood mononuclear cells in human coccidiodomycosis. J Infect Dis 1996; 174(2):440–443.

117. Cox RA, Kennell W, Boncyk L, Murphy JW. Induction and expression of cell-mediated immune responses in inbred mice infected with *Coccidioides immitis*. Infect Immun 1988; 56(1):13–17.

118. Cox RA, Magee DM. Protective immunity in coccidioidomycosis. Res Immunol 1998; 149(4–5):417–428.

119. Magee DM, Cox RA. Interleukin-12 regulation of host defenses against *Coccidioides immitis*. Infect Immun 1996; 64(9):3609–3613.

120. Jiang C, Magee DM, Cox RA. Construction of a single-chain interleukin-12–expressing retroviral vector and its application in cytokine gene therapy against experimental coccidioidomycosis. Infect Immun 1999; 67(6):2996–3001.

121. Hahn DL, Dodge RW, Golubjatnikov R. Association of *Chlamydia pneumoniae* (strain TWAR) infection with wheezing, asthmatic bronchitis, and adult-onset asthma. JAMA 1991; 266(2):225–230.

122. Saikku P, Leinonen M, Mattila K, Ekman MR, Nieminen MS, Makela PH, et al. Serological evidence of an association of a novel Chlamydia, TWAR, with chronic coronary heart disease and acute myocardial infarction. Lancet 1988; 2(8618):983–986.

123. Starnbach MN, Beven MJ, Lampe MF. Protective cytotoxic T lymphocytes are induced during murine infection with *Chlamydia trachomatis*. J Immunol 1994; 153(11):5183–5189.

124. Lampe MF, Wilson CB, Bevan MJ, Starnbach MN. Gamma interferon production by cytotoxic T lymphocytes is required for resolution of *Chlamydia trachomatis* infection. Infect Immun 1998; 66(11):5457–5461.

125. Svanholm C, Bandholtz L, Castanos-Velez E, Wigzell H, Rottenberg ME. Protective DNA immunization against *Chlamydia pneumoniae*. Scand J Immunol 2000; 51(4):345–353.

126. Penttila T, Vuola JM, Puurula V, Anttila M, Sarvas M, Rautonen N, et al. Immunity to *Chlamydia pneumoniae* induced by vaccination with DNA vectors expressing a cytoplasmic protein (Hsp60) or outer membrane proteins (MOMP and Omp2). Vaccine 2000; 19(9–10):1256–1265.

127. Murdin AD, Dunn P, Sodoyer R, Wang J, Caterini J, Brunham RC, et al. Use of a mouse lung challenge model to identify antigens protective against *Chlamydia pneumoniae* lung infection. J Infect Dis 2000; 181(Suppl 3):S544–S551.

128. Dolin PJ, Raviglione MC, Kochi A. Global tuberculosis incidence and mortality during 1990–2000. Bull WHO 1994; 72(2):213–220.

129. Sudre P, ten DG, Kochi A. Tuberculosis: a global overview of the situation today. Bull WHO 1992; 70(2):149–159.

130. Cooper AM, Dalton DK, Stewart TA, Griffin JP, Russell DG, et al. Disseminated

tuberculosis in interferon gamma gene–disrupted mice. J Exp Med 1993; 178(6): 2243–2247.

131. Flynn JL, Chan J, Triebold KJ, Dalton DK, Stewart TA, Bloom BR. An essential role for interferon gamma in resistance to *Mycobacterium tuberculosis* infection. J Exp Med 1993; 178(6):2249–2254.

132. Tascon RE, Stavropoulos E, Lukacs KV, Colston MJ. Protection against *Mycobacterium tuberculosis* infection by CD8+ T cells requires the production of gamma interferon. Infect Immun 1998; 66(2):830–834.

133. Rodriguez FH, Nelson S, Kolls JK. Cytokine therapeutics for infectious diseases. Curr Pharm Des 2000; 6(6):665–680.

134. Andersen P. Effective vaccination of mice against *Mycobacterium tuberculosis* infection with a soluble mixture of secreted mycobacterial proteins. Infect Immun 1994; 62(6):2536–2544.

135. Hubbard RD, Flory CM, Collins FM. Immunization of mice with mycobacterial culture filtrate proteins. Clin Exp Immunol 1992; 87(1):94–98.

136. Pal PG, Horwitz MA. Immunization with extracellular proteins of *Mycobacterium tuberculosis* induces cell-mediated immune responses and substantial protective immunity in a guinea pig model of pulmonary tuberculosis. Infect Immun 1992; 60(11):4781–4792.

137. Roberts AD, Sonnenberg MG, Ordway DJ, Furney SK, Brennan PJ, Belisle JT, et al. Characteristics of protective immunity engendered by vaccination of mice with purified culture filtrate protein antigens of *Mycobacterium tuberculosis*. Immunology 1995; 85(3):502–508.

138. Morris S, Kelley C, Howard A, Li Z, Collins F. The immunogenicity of single and combination DNA vaccines against tuberculosis. Vaccine 2000; 18(20):2155–2163.

139. Kamath AT, Feng CG, Macdonald M, Briscoe H, Britton WJ. Differential protective efficacy of DNA vaccines expressing secreted proteins of *Mycobacterium tuberculosis*. Infect Immun 1999; 67(4):1702–1707.

140. Baldwin SL, D'Souza C, Roberts AD, Kelly BP, Frank AA, Lui MA, et al. Evaluation of new vaccines in the mouse and guinea pig model of tuberculosis. Infect Immun 1998; 66(6):2951–2959.

141. Huygen K, Content J, Denis O, Montgomery DL, Yawman AM, Deck RR, et al. Immunogenicity and protective efficacy of a tuberculosis DNA vaccine. Nat Med 1996; 2(8):893–898.

142. McShane H, Brookes R, Gilbert SC, Hill AV. Enhanced immunogenicity of CD4(+) t-cell responses and protective efficacy of a DNA-modified vaccinia virus Ankara prime-boost vaccination regimen for murine tuberculosis. Infect Immun 2001; 69(2):681–686.

143. Tanghe A, D'Souza S, Rosseels V, Denis O, Ottenhoff TH, Dalemans W, et al. Improved immunogenicity and protective efficacy of a tuberculosis DNA vaccine encoding Ag85 by protein boosting. Infect Immun 2001; 69(5):3041–3047.

144. Delogu G, Howard A, Collins FM, Morris SL. DNA vaccination against tuberculosis: expression of a ubiquitin-conjugated tuberculosis protein enhances antimycobacterial immunity. Infect Immun 2000; 68(6):3097–3102.

145. Lowrie DB, Tascon RE, Bonato VL, Lima VM, Faccioli LH, Stavropoulos E, et

al. Therapy of tuberculosis in mice by DNA vaccination. Nature 1999; 400(6741): 269–271.

146. Kim HW, Canchola JG, Brandt CD, Pyles G, Chanock RM, Jensen K et al. Respiratory syncytial virus disease in infants despite prior administration of antigenic inactivated vaccine. Am J Epidemiol 1969; 89(4):422–434.

147. Kapikian AZ, Mitchell RH, Chanock RM, Shvedoff RA, Stewart CE. An epidemiologic study of altered clinical reactivity to respiratory syncytial (RS) virus infection in children previously vaccinated with an inactivated RS virus vaccine. Am J Epidemiol 1969; 89(4):405–421.

148. Graham BS, Henderson GS, Tang YW, Lu X, Neuzil KM, Colley DG. Priming immunization determines T helper cytokine mRNA expression patterns in lungs of mice challenged with respiratory syncytial virus. J Immunol 1993; 151(4):2032–2040.

149. Connors M, Giese NA, Kulkarni AB, Firestone CY, Morse HC, III, Murphy BR. Enhanced pulmonary histopathology induced by respiratory syncytial virus (RSV) challenge of formalin-inactivated RSV-immunized BALB/c mice is abrogated by depletion of interleukin-4 (IL-4) and IL-10. J Virol 1994; 68(8):5321–5325.

150. Connors M, Collins PL, Firestone CY, Sotnikov AV, Waitze A, Davis AR, et al. Cotton rats previously immunized with a chimeric RSV FG glycoprotein develop enhanced pulmonary pathology when infected with RSV, a phenomenon not encountered following immunization with vaccinia–RSV recombinants or RSV. Vaccine 1992; 10(7):475–484.

151. Crowe JE, Jr, Collins PL, London WT, Chanock RM, Murphy BR. A comparison in chimpanzees of the immunogenicity and efficacy of live attenuated respiratory syncytial virus (RSV) temperature-sensitive mutant vaccines and vaccinia virus recombinants that express the surface glycoproteins of RSV. Vaccine 1993; 11(14): 1395–1404.

152. Hussell T, Spender LC, Georgiou A, O'Garra A, Openshaw PJ. Th1 and Th2 cytokine induction in pulmonary T cells during infection with respiratory syncytial virus. J Gen Virol 1996; 77(pt 10):2447–2455.

153. Bukreyev A, Whitehead SS, Bukreyeva N, Murphy BR, Collins PL. Interferon gamma expressed by a recombinant respiratory syncytial virus attenuates virus replication in mice without compromising immunogenicity. Proc Natl Acad Sci USA 1999; 96(5):2367–2372.

154. Tripp RA, Jones L, Anderson LJ, Brown MP. CD40 ligand (CD154) enhances the Th1 and antibody responses to respiratory syncitial virus in the BALB/c mouse. J Immunol 2000; 164(11):5913–5921.

9

Use of In Vivo Gene Transfer to Study Pulmonary Fibrosis

THOMAS H. SISSON and RICHARD H. SIMON

University of Michigan
Ann Arbor, Michigan, U.S.A.

I. Introduction

Fibrosis of the lung occurs during many different diseases including idiopathic pulmonary fibrosis, collagen vascular diseases (rheumatoid arthritis, scleroderma, polymyositis, dermatomyositis), sarcoidosis, and hypersensitivity pneumonitis. In addition, lung fibrosis can occur following radiation therapy and as a toxic effect of chemotherapy (e.g., bleomycin, busulfan, 1,3-bis[2-chloroethyl]-1-nitrosourea [BCNU]) and other types of drugs (e.g., amiodarone, nitrofurantoin). Although the factors that initiate the fibrotic process in these diseases are likely different, there may be common downstream steps that are shared. Developing tools to investigate these processes is a high priority. Recent work from a number of research laboratories has shown that in vivo gene transfer can provide a means to manipulate biological cascades that are thought to influence the development of pulmonary fibrosis.

Much of our current understanding of the pathogenesis of human lung fibrosis has come through the use of animal models. Of the various models studied, bleomycin-induced pulmonary fibrosis has received considerable attention. When administered intratracheally, intravenously, or intraperitoneally, bleomycin produces a patchy pulmonary fibrosis that mimics many histological and physiological features of human pulmonary fibrosis (1). In addition, the ability to alter gene expression in mice following bleomycin administration has allowed investigators to uncover important pathogenic mechanisms within the fibrotic pathway. One approach to manipulating gene expression has been accomplished by generating transgenic animals that either overexpress or, as the result of a targeted gene deletion, have no expression of a particular gene. Although the creation of transgenic animal models has been valuable in broadening our understanding of lung fibrosis, they have several disadvantages. First, transgenic animal lines are relatively expensive and time consuming to generate. This limits the number of genetic manipulations that can be feasibly studied. Second, altered gene expression during animal development can potentially have lasting effects on subsequent physiological or pathological events. Furthermore, until recently, alterations in gene expression that result from transgenic manipulation have not been controllable. In vivo gene transfer technology offers an alternative means of manipulating pulmonary gene expression that avoids several of these aforementioned disadvantages.

This chapter will focus on the use of gene transfer technology to study pulmonary fibrosis. To date, gene transfer has been used to investigate whether the overexpression of a particular gene product is sufficient to drive or to ameliorate lung collagen deposition. The first section will review the advantages of a gene transfer approach to study the pathogenesis of fibrosis. The subsequent section will detail studies in which gene transfer techniques have been employed to further our understanding of the pathogenesis of these diseases. The final section of this chapter will outline the current limitations of a gene transfer approach in the study of pulmonary scarring.

II. Advantages of Using a Gene Transfer Approach to Study Lung Fibrosis

Several theoretical advantages exist in the use of a gene transfer approach to study pulmonary fibrosis (Table 1). First, gene transfer makes possible the sustained alteration of gene expression. The ability to maintain altered gene expression for an extended time is important in the study of lung fibrosis, because pathological events take place, at least in the bleomycin model, over a period of several weeks. To obtain the same sustained alteration through exogenous protein administration would require repeat dosing. Such an approach is difficult technically and expensive depending on which protein is being investigated. A prolonged alteration in gene expression is otherwise only achievable through the costly and time-consuming construction of transgenic animal lines. A second advantage to using a gene transfer approach to study the pathogenesis of lung scarring is that the timing of gene expression can be manipulated. In the bleomycin model, the patho-

Table 1 Value of In Vivo Gene Transfer for the Study of Pulmonary Fibrosis

Advantages	Disadvantages
Transgene expression extends for days to weeks	Limited transgene expression beyond several weeks
Transgene expression can be targeted to a desired site	Limited ability to target transgene expression to specific cell types
Ease of generating vectors	Limited ability to transduce cells within inflammatory/fibrotic foci
Constructing vector economical relative to generating transgenic animals	Toxicity of the gene transfer vector; e.g., inflammation

genesis can be divided into an initial inflammatory stage and a subsequent fibroproliferative stage (1). Manipulating gene expression at different points in the pathogenesis of fibrosis can provide clues about how and when a certain gene product may most influence scar formation. Until recently, transgenic animal models only offered the possibility of permanent changes in gene expression. Now with the development of transgenic animal models that possess controllable gene expression (2), the use of gene transfer is not the only means of altering gene expression in a time-dependent manner. Another advantage to employing a gene transfer approach to study lung fibrosis is that, as the vector technology improves, these techniques may be translated directly into therapeutic trials.

Recombinant adenoviruses have been employed most frequently as the vector for transferring genes to the lungs of animals to study pulmonary fibrosis. Adenoviral vectors possess several important features that make them attractive gene transfer tools in the study of lung fibrosis (3). First, these vectors have tropism for alveolar spaces in the lung (4). This tropism allows for very efficient gene transfer to alveolar epithelial cells that ultimately results in an alteration of gene expression at the exact location where the fibrogenic process is taking place. Second, adenoviral vectors are easy to produce at high titers in large quantities. And finally, these vectors have the capacity to accept large constructs of foreign genetic material. On the other hand, the use of adenoviral vectors to study pulmonary fibrosis has uncovered several limitations that prevent them from being ideal gene transfer tools when employed in the study of pulmonary fibrosis. These limitations will be subsequently detailed.

III. Elucidating the Pathogenesis of Pulmonary Fibrosis Through Gene Transfer Technology

Idiopathic pulmonary fibrosis, based on our current understanding, begins with an insult to the capillary-alveolar wall (5). As mentioned above, the particular pathways that lead from lung injury to pulmonary fibrosis are poorly understood. Whether inflammatory cell influx into the lung contributes to the initial injury remains controversial. In the bleomycin model of pulmonary fibrosis, intratracheal or systemic administration of the drug leads to an initial neutrophilic infiltration into the lungs followed by accumulation of mononuclear inflammatory cells. This induced inflammation may contribute to the initial injury of the alveolar-capillary membrane. The recruitment of inflammatory cells into the lung is orchestrated by the expression of various proinflammatory cytokines. In particular, there is an early and sustained production of tumor necrosis factor (TNF-α), interleukin-1β (IL-1β), IL-8, and monocyte chemoattractant protein-1 (MCP-1). Gauldie and colleagues investigated the ability of these early expressed proinflammatory cytokines to initiate lung fibrosis (6,7). Using adenoviral vectors, they transferred the genes for murine TNF-α and human IL-1β into rat lungs to determine if overexpression of these particular cytokines was sufficient to stimulate a fibrotic response. The resultant marked overexpression of both TNF-α and IL-1β resulting from gene transfer persisted for 1 week, and these proinflammatory cytokines predictably attracted a massive influx of lymphocytes, macrophages, and in particular neutrophils into the lungs. With both TNF-α and IL-1β, the inflammatory cell influx reached a peak at day 7 and then began to decline. Despite the observation that both cytokines caused impressive inflammation, only gene transfer of IL-1β caused a significant injury to the alveolar membrane. And, although the upregulated expression of both cytokines did lead to increased lung collagen accumulation, the severity of the resulting fibrosis between the IL-1β– and TNF-α–treated animals was significantly different. TNF-α overexpression produced only patchy areas of scarring, whereas IL-1β initiated a marked fibrotic response. Animals treated with the IL-1β adenoviral vector had increases in lung collagen as measured by hydroxyproline content at the 3-week time point, and fibrosis continued to progress up to 3 months. Although not conclusively linking the cytokine-driven inflammatory cell influx with the subsequent collagen deposition, these experiments do provide evidence suggesting that the overexpression of proinflammatory cytokines can begin a series of pathological changes in the lung that lead to fibrosis. However, the question remains as to why increased TNF-α and IL-1β expression in these particular experiments led to scarring, whereas in other settings (i.e., infection) increased expression of these same cytokines can stimulate inflammation that does not culminate in fibrosis. The authors speculate that an associated increase in transforming growth factor-β (TGF-β) expression may be responsible for the generation of scarring in their studies. They also speculate that the differences in fibrosis that occur following the gene transfer of TNF-α and IL-1β may be related to the amount of TGF-β induced by these two cytokines. IL-1β overexpression was associated with a 2.5-fold increase in TGF-β levels as compared to TNF-α. Why these proinflammatory cytokines are capable of inducing TGF-β expression in this model but not in other situations such as infection remains unclear, but it may be related to the extraordinarily high levels of cytokine expression achieved following adenovirus-mediated gene transfer. Because adenovirus can infect and ultimately injure epithelial cells, the employment of this vector to transfer the IL-1β gene may also have contributed to the final pathology.

The importance of the initial inflammatory insult in the subsequent development of fibrosis is supported by data from experiments involving the transfer of the anti-inflammatory cytokine IL-10 gene (8). In this study, Arai and colleagues transferred the gene for IL-10 using a hemagglutinating virus of Japan (HVJ)–liposomal vector into the peritoneum of mice 3 days prior to the intratracheal administration of bleomycin. The IL-10 gene was selected for transfer because the resultant protein has several anti-inflammatory properties that were hypothesized to be advantageous in mitigating lung fibrosis. Specifically, IL-10 suppresses inflammatory cytokine production. Twenty-four hours after intraperitoneal administration of the IL-10–containing vector, serum IL-10 levels increased significantly. The level of IL-10 then declined so that by 48 hr there was no longer a statistically significant increase in the serum IL-10 levels above that of control animals. The increase in IL-10 production following gene transfer resulted in marked reduction in bleomycin-induced bronchoalveolar lavage (BAL) fluid myeloperoxidase activity, which measures neutrophil accumulation. A day 7 decline in TNF-α messenger RNA from BAL inflammatory cells and in serum TNF-α levels accompanied the decline in BAL fluid myeloperoxidase activity. Ultimately, the intraperitoneal gene transfer of IL-10 also resulted in a significant reduction in lung collagen content as quantified by lung hydroxyproline measured 3 weeks after bleomycin administration. The ability of IL-10 gene transfer to limit the amount of inflammation induced by bleomycin as well as the extent of fibrosis supports a correlation between these two processes. In their report, Arai et al. also demonstrated an IL-10–dependent reduction in fibroblast collagen synthesis in vitro. They proposed this antifibrotic activity of IL-10 as an alternate mechanism by which increased expression of this cytokine might protect against bleomycin-induced collagen accumulation. Although possible, it is notable that, at the time when lung collagen begins to accumulate in the bleomycin model (day 10), the IL-10 expression that resulted from intraperitoneal gene transfer had returned to baseline.

In the pathogenesis of pulmonary fibrosis, the injury to the alveolar membrane is followed by an exudation of serum proteins into the alveolar space that ultimately leads to the formation of a fibrin-rich extracellular matrix. During this initial stage, the activation of plasmin, the enzyme primarily responsible for fibrin degradation, is impaired as the result of an imbalance between urokinase plasminogen activator (uPA) and this latter enzyme's primary inhibitor, plasminogen activator inhibitor-1 (PAI-1) (9,10). In human fibrotic lung disease and in the bleomycin rodent model of pulmonary fibrosis, PAI-1 expression is markedly

increased. The crucial importance of this altered PAI-1 expression in the pathogenesis of pulmonary fibrosis has been demonstrated using PAI-1-deficient and
PAI-1 overexpressing animals in the bleomycin model of pulmonary fibrosis (11).
Transgenic mice lacking PAI-1 are nearly completely protected from bleomycin-
induced fibrosis. On the other hand, mice that overexpress PAI-1 demonstrate
an exuberant response to bleomycin. Through a gene transfer experiment, our
laboratory was able to provide further evidence supporting the role of the plasminogen activator system in the pathogenesis of lung fibrosis. In this experiment,
to correct the imbalance between PAI-1 and uPA, the gene for uPA was transferred via an adenoviral vector into the lungs of mice 21 days following bleomycin injury (12). The extent of lung fibrosis was then assessed 1 week following
intratracheal adenoviral administration. The uPA gene transfer resulted in a 38%
reduction in lung collagen content compared to mice treated with a control vector.
Although this reduction further substantiated the link between the plasminogen
activator system and the development of fibrosis, the magnitude of protection
did not match that obtained through PAI-1 gene deletion. The inability of uPA
gene transfer to completely abrogate fibrosis in this experiment may be related
to the timing of gene transfer. The vector was administered 21 days after bleomycin injury, which is late in the pathogenesis of pulmonary fibrosis. Although the
mechanism by which the imbalance of PAI-1 to uPA leads to fibrosis is unknown,
the correction of this imbalance may need to be achieved earlier in the fibrogenic
process to more efficiently limit collagen accumulation. An alternate explanation
to the limited protection afforded by uPA gene transfer exists, and this alternate
explanation highlights one of the limitations of using a gene transfer approach
to study lung fibrosis. Using immunohistochemistry, a spatial separation between
areas of fibrosis and gene expression was noted. uPA-expressing cells were located almost entirely in areas of normal-appearing airways and alveoli distant
from sites of fibrosis. Thus, intratracheal delivery appears to be a poor method
to deliver a gene of interest to damaged areas of the lung. This separation may
have limited the correction of the imbalance between PAI-1 and uPA at fibrogenic
foci. The addition of dispersing agents such as perfluorochemicals (13) or surfactants (14) may improve the distribution of gene transfer vectors introduced into
the lungs.

Soon after the fibrin-rich matrix has formed, fibroblasts begin to proliferate,
to synthesize collagen, and to migrate from the alveolar interstitium into the alveolar space. These changes in fibroblast behavior require the coordination of many
separate processes. Of critical importance in this alteration of fibroblast behavior
is the increased expression of various growth factors and cytokines. As detailed
earlier, IL-10 may be one cytokine that mitigates fibroblast behavior during the
pathogenesis of fibrosis.

One of several growth factors hypothesized to be of particular importance
in lung scarring is TGF-β (15). In both patients with pulmonary fibrosis as well

as in mice exposed to bleomycin, lung TGF-β levels increase. TGF-β can function as a mitogen and a chemotactic factor for fibroblasts. A temporal relationship exists between the expression of this growth factor and the deposition of extracellular matrix in patients with fibrosing lung disease. Fibroblasts stimulated by TGF-β have been found to change their morphology to that of a myofibroblast, and this conformational change is associated with the synthesis of extracellular matrix proteins in abundant quantities. At the same time, TGF-β is capable of inhibiting fibroblast production of extracellular matrix–degrading enzymes. The increased expression of TGF-β during fibrosing lung processes and its multiple fibrogenic capabilities suggest strongly that this growth factor is an important mediator of pulmonary fibrosis. To substantiate the ability of this protein to orchestrate lung scarring, Yoshida and colleagues overexpressed active TGF-β in rat lungs through HVJ-liposome–mediated gene transfer (16). On day 14, TGF-β expression induced a marked increase in spindle-shaped cells and fibrotic foci located adjacent to alveolar ducts of the treated animals. In a similar experiment, Sime and colleagues transferred a gene expressing the active TGF-β protein into rat lungs (17). The adenovirus-mediated gene transfer resulted in an increased expression of the growth factor for a time period of greater than 14 days. The increased expression of active TGF-β resulted in an early recruitment of mononuclear cells followed by an accumulation of fibroblasts and extensive extracellular matrix deposition. After day 3, a subset of cells making up areas of fibrosis stained positive for a marker of the myofibroblast phenotype. By day 14, lung collagen content was quantitatively increased as measured by hydroxyproline. Collagen accumulation continued through day 64 even though active TGF-β was minimally expressed beyond day 14. Sime et al. hypothesize that this progressive accumulation of collagen occurs as the result of a growth factor–initiated self-perpetuating fibrogenic process. The results of these two experiments demonstrate the capacity of TGF-β to drive lung fibrosis.

The changes in fibroblast behavior following TGF-β exposure occur at least in part through Smad protein signaling (18). Following TGF-β activation of its receptor, Smad2 and Smad3 signaling proteins undergo phosphorylation. Smad2 and Smad3 associate with Smad4, and the entire complex translocates to the nucleus where it then can regulate gene transcription. An additional Smad protein, Smad7, has been found to antagonize TGf-β signaling by binding to its receptor and interfering with Smad2 and Smad3 phosphorylation. Further evidence substantiating the importance of TGF-β in the development of lung fibrosis takes advantage of these recent advances in our understanding of this signaling pathway. Nakao and colleagues developed an adenoviral vector expressing the Smad7 protein to test the hypothesis that blocking TGF-β signaling would lead to a reduction in lung fibrosis (19). This vector was administered intratracheally 12 hr after the initiation of a 7-day subcutaneous bleomycin infusion. Smad7 gene transfer resulted in intrapulmonary expression of the corresponding protein that reached a peak at day 2 and then began to dissipate. Nonetheless, the protein product was detectable for 3 weeks following its initial administration. In accord with their hypothesis, mice treated with the Smad7-containing adenoviral vector developed less fibrosis as measured by both histology and hydroxyproline quantitation. These effects on lung fibrosis occurred independently of lung inflammation and TGF-β expression. The protection from fibrosis afforded by Smad7 gene transfer was incomplete. Nakao et al. theorize that inadequate levels of Smad7 expression in areas of fibrogenesis might explain the partial reduction in lung collagen accumulation. For Smad7 to block TGF-β signaling, the expression of this protein must occur within fibroblasts, cells not easily transduced by adenoviral gene transfer following intratracheal administration. As an alternate explanation for the limited protection against pulmonary fibrosis, the investigators speculate that other growth factors may play a redundant role in the pathogenesis of this disorder.

TGF-β activity can also be modulated by decorin. Decorin is a proteoglycan that possesses two binding sites for all of the TGF-β isotypes and will downregulate TGF-β activity by preventing ligand-receptor binding. Further evidence substantiating the role of TGF-β in the pathogenesis of bleomycin-induced fibrosis is derived from experiments in which the activity of the growth factor is blocked through adenovirus-mediated decorin gene transfer. Kolb and colleagues administered a decorin-containing vector 2 days before intratracheal bleomycin instillation (20). Decorin expression was measured by Northern blot analysis and was found to be detectable for 7 days following adenoviral treatment. The expression of decorin had no influence on bleomycin-induced increases in lung inflammatory cell accumulaton or TGF-β levels. However, decorin expression did significantly reduce lung collagen content as measured by lung hydroxyproline content 21 days following bleomycin administration. The reduction in fibrosis, as was the case with Smad7 gene transfer, was partial.

Because of its ability to serve as a mitogen and chemoattractant for fibroblasts and because of its capacity to stimulate collagen synthesis, platelet-derived growth factor (PDGF) has also been hypothesized to be of critical importance in the pathogenesis of lung fibrosis. Expression of this growth factor in localized fibrotic areas of lung tissue taken from patients with idiopathic pulmonary fibrosis further suggests a role for this growth factor in the pathogenesis of scarring lung disease. To determine if PDGF could stimulate fibrotic foci in rat lungs when overexpressed, Yoshida and colleagues transferred the gene for this growth factor into rat lungs using their HVJ-liposomal vector (16). The resulting pathological changes were similar to those induced by TGF-β overexpression. Specifically, they noted an increase in spindle-shaped cells and an accumulation of mononuclear cells and macrophages. However, the extent of spindle-shaped cell proliferation and collagen accumulation was less impressive than that generated by TGF-β overexpression. To further substantiate the role of PDGF in lung fibrosis, Yoshida and colleagues transferred a gene expressing the extracellular domain of the PDGF beta receptor to the lungs of mice treated with bleomycin (21). The resulting product of this gene transfer was designed to block the cellular effects of PDGF by binding the growth factor and preventing it from interacting with the native receptor. The gene was transferred 3 days following intravenous bleomycin administration by intratracheal instillation of an HVJ-liposomal vector. Using an immunofluorescent technique, Yoshida and colleagues detected gene expression for 2 weeks following vector administration. The administration of their vector reduced both lung wet weight and collagen content as measured by hydroxyproline at a 3-week time point. The reduction in lung collagen content supports the importance of PDGF in the development of bleomycin-induced fibrosis. As in the case with TGF-β inhibition, the protection against fibrosis afforded by this approach was incomplete. Yoshida and colleagues speculate that the dose of gene product generated at the sites of fibrogenesis may have been inadequate to abrogate completely the effects of PDGF. They also suggest that the inhibition of a single growth factor such as PDGF or TGF-β may result in partial protection against fibrosis, because these molecules either work in concert to orchestrate fibrosis or they have redundant activities in the pathogenesis of lung fibrosis.

IV. Limitations of Gene Transfer Technology in the Study of Pulmonary Fibrosis

One of the major limitations of gene transfer in the study of pulmonary fibrosis is the inability to target gene expression directly to the areas of fibrogenesis. As discussed above, this particular difficulty may have prevented a more substantial reduction in lung collagen content following both uPA, Smad7, and PDGF beta receptor gene transfer. The fibrotic areas resulting from bleomycin injury are patchy, and current technology does not allow researchers to direct viral preparations into these regions. In fact, following bleomycin injury, intratracheally delivered gene transfer preparations likely preferentially travel to normal regions of the lung. To test certain hypotheses with gene transfer technology, vectors must not only be targeted to areas of active fibrosis but to specific cells within the areas of fibrosis. Such was the desire of Nakao and colleagues when they administered the Smad7-containing vector to bleomycin-injured mice in hopes of blocking TGF-β effects on fibroblasts (19). To reiterate their results, Nakao et al. were only able to demonstrate partial protection from their experimental approach, and this may have resulted from their inability to target gene transfer to fibroblasts in fibrotic regions.

To avoid the previously described limitation of having gene expression occur in areas spatially separated from fibrotic foci, we administered our adenoviral vector together with the bleomycin in the same inoculum. By so doing, the site of lung injury and site of gene expression would be the same. This approach brought to light a second limitation of using gene transfer to study pulmonary fibrosis. The intratracheal administration of adenoviral vectors produces a predictable inflammatory response (22). As detailed earlier, bleomycin also stimulates an inflammatory cell influx into the lungs of treated animals, and this inflammation may contribute to the initial alveolar membrane injury and the subsequent fibrotic response. When employing gene transfer techniques to study lung fibrosis, the additional inflammation associated with gene transfer can be controlled for through the administration of a second nonexpressing vector. However, in an unpublished experiment, we demonstrated an additive injury when bleomycin and our adenoviral vectors (uPA-containing or control, empty vectors) were administered by intratracheal instillation simultaneously. This additive injury manifested as 70–80% mortality rates in mice treated with both adenovirus and bleomycin versus 0% mortality in those animals treated with either adenovirus or bleomycin alone. Such a high mortality was not reported by Nakao and colleagues (19), although they initiated the bleomycin-induced fibrosis and gene transfer on the same day. However, their bleomycin was administered via an intraperitoneal route over a 1-week period. The separate routes of administration and the slow induction of fibrosis may have averted the synergistic lung injury that we had experienced. However, by using different routes of administration, they may not have achieved an adequate level of gene expression in regions of fibrosis.

The inflammation generated by adenoviral administration to the lung not only causes an additive injury with bleomycin, but this inflammation also ultimately limits the resultant duration of gene expression. In our experience, uPA expression following gene transfer could be detected for approximately 2 weeks (12). In some cases, the expression has persisted for an even shorter duration. Arai and colleagues could detect a significant increase in IL-10 production following intraperitoneal gene transfer for less than 48 hr (8). In other cases, increased gene expression has occurred for up to 3 weeks. The short duration of expression that occurs following gene transfer, particularly when an adenovirus is used as the vector, does not pose a major limitation in the study of bleomycin-induced lung fibrosis. In this model, fibrosis begins to occur at 10–14 days and is well established by 3 weeks. The short duration of gene expression following transfer would, however, limit the prospects of translating these techniques into patient trials. In addition, current gene transfer technology makes it difficult to control not only the duration of gene expression, but also the level of gene expression. Thus, with current technology, using this approach to study the importance of gene's dose response in the pathogenesis of fibrosis would be difficult.

V. Summary

Pulmonary fibrosis is associated with many different diseases. Our current therapy for most of these diseases lacks efficacy and safety. Thus, a desperate need exists for new and more efficacious therapeutic approaches. To develop new therapies requires a better understanding of the pathogenesis of lung fibrosis. Gene transfer techniques have contributed significantly to our understanding of a subset of the important components in the pathway leading to lung collagen accumulation. In particular, gene transfer has demonstrated the importance of the plasminogen activator system and fibroblast growth factors in mitigating fibrosis. In addition, gene transfer has supported the role of early inflammation in the initial alveolar membrane injury. Several limitations prevent gene transfer from being a more powerful tool in the exploration of the pathogenesis of this disease. With the development of new vectors and new techniques to control transgene expression, gene transfer will continue to be an attractive approach to the study of pulmonary fibrosis.

References

1. Adamson IY, Bowden DH. The pathogenesis of bleomycin-induced pulmonary fibrosis in mice. Am J Pathol 1974; 77:185–197.
2. Ray P, Tang W, Wang P, Homer R, Kuhn C III, Flavell RA, Elias JA. Regulated overexpression of interleukin 11 in the lung. Use to dissociate development-dependent and -independent phenotypes. J Clin Invest 1997; 100:2501–2511.
3. Wilson JM. Adenoviruses as gene-delivery vehicles. N Engl J Med 1996; 334:1185–1187.
4. Engelhardt JF, Simon RH, Yang Y, Zepeda M, Weber PS, Doranz B, Grossman M, Wilson JM. Adenovirus-mediated transfer of the CFTR gene to lung of nonhuman primates: biological efficacy study. Hum Gene Ther 1993; 4:759–769.
5. Selman M, King TE, Pardo A. Idiopathic pulmonary fibrosis: prevailing and evolving hypotheses about its pathogenesis and implications for therapy. Ann Intern Med 2001; 134:136–151.
6. Kolb M, Margetts PJ, Anthony DC, Pitossi F, Gauldie J. Transient expression of IL-1beta induces acute lung injury and chronic repair leading to pulmonary fibrosis. J Clin Invest 2001; 107:1529–1536.
7. Sime PJ, Marr RA, Gauldie D, Xing Z, Hewlett BR, Graham FL, Gauldie J. Transfer of tumor necrosis factor-alpha to rat lung induces severe pulmonary inflammation and patchy interstitial fibrogenesis with induction of transforming growth factor-beta1 and myofibroblasts. Am J Pathol 1998; 153:825–832.
8. Arai T, Abe K, Matsuoka H, Yoshida M, Mori M, Goya S, Kida H, Nishino K, Osaki T, Tachibana I, Kaneda Y, Hayashi S. Introduction of the interleukin-10 gene into mice inhibited bleomycin-induced lung injury in vivo. Am J Physiol Lung Cell Mol Physiol 2000; 278:L914–L922.
9. Idell S, James KK, Gillies C, Fair DS. Abnormalities of pathways of fibrin turnover in lung lavage of rats with oleic acid and bleomycin-induced lung injury support alveolar fibrin deposition. Am J Pathol 1989; 137:387–389.
10. Olman MA, Mackman N, Gladson CL, Moser KM, Loskutoff DJ. Changes in procoagulant and fibrinolytic gene expression during bleomycin-induced lung injury in the mouse. J Clin Invest 1995; 96:1621–1630.

11. Eitzman DT, McCoy RD, Zheng X, Fay WP, Shen T, Ginsburg D, Simon RH. Bleomycin-induced pulmonary fibrosis in transgenic mice that either lack or overexpress the murine plasminogen activator inhibitor-1 gene. J Clin Invest 1996; 97:232–237.

12. Sisson TH, Hattori N, Xu Y, Simon RH. Treatment of bleomycin-induced pulmonary fibrosis by transfer of urokinase-type plasminogen activator genes. Hum Gene Ther 1999; 10:2315–2323.

13. Weiss DJ, Bonneau L, Allen JM, Miller AD, Halbert CL. Perfluorochemical liquid enhances adeno-associated virus-mediated transgene expression in lungs. Mol Ther 2000; 2:624–630.

14. Jobe AH, Ueda T, Whitsett JA, Trapnell BC, Ikegami M. Surfactant enhances adenovirus-mediated gene expression in rabbit lungs. Gene Ther 1996; 3:775–779.

15. Brockelmann TJ, Limper AH, Colby TV, McDonald JA. Transforming growth factor beta 1 is present at sites of extracellular matrix gene expression in human pulmonary fibrosis. Proc Natl Acad Sci USA 1991; 88:6642–6646.

16. Yoshida M, Sakuma J, Hayashi S, Abe K, Saito I, Harada S, Sakatani M, Yamamoto S, Matsumoto N, Kaneda Y, Kishimoto T. A histologically distinctive interstitial pneumonia induced by overexpression of the interleukin 6, transforming growth factor beta 1, or platelet-derived growth factor B gene. Proc Natl Acad Sci USA 1995; 92:9570–9574.

17. Sime PJ, Xing Z, Graham FL, Csaky KG, Gauldie J. Adenovector-mediated gene transfer of active transforming growth factor-beta1 induces prolonged severe fibrosis in rat lung. J Clin Invest 1997; 100:768–776.

18. Blobe GC, Schiemann WP, Lodish HF. Role of transforming growth factor beta in human disease. N Engl J Med 2000; 342:1350–1358.

19. Nakao A, Fujii M, Matsumura R, Kumano K, Saito Y, Miyazono K, Iwamoto I. Transient gene transfer and expression of Smad7 prevents bleomycin-induced lung fibrosis in mice. J Clin Invest 1999; 104:5–11.

20. Kolb M, Margetts PJ, Sime PJ, Gauldie J. Proteoglycans decorin and biglycan differentially modulate TGF-beta–mediated fibrotic responses in the lung. Am J Physiol Lung Cell Mol Physiol 2001; 280:L1327–L1334.

21. Yoshida M, Sakuma-Mochizuki J, Abe K, Arai T, Mori M, Goya S, Matsuoka H, Hayashi S, Kaneda Y, Kishimoto T. In vivo gene transfer of an extracellular domain of platelet-derived growth factor beta receptor by the HVJ-liposome method ameliorates bleomycin-induced pulmonary fibrosis. Biochem Biophys Res Commun 1999; 265:503–508.

22. Simon RH, Engelhardt JF, Yang Y, Zepeda M, Weber PS, Grossman M, Wilson JM. Adenovirus-mediated transfer of the CFTR gene to lung of nonhuman primates: toxicity study. Hum Gene Ther 1993; 4:771–780.

Part Three

USE OF GENE THERAPY TO TREAT LUNG DISEASES

10

Gene Therapy for Lung Cancer

RAJ K. BATRA, SHERVEN SHARMA, and STEVEN M. DUBINETT

UCLA School of Medicine
and Veterans Administration Greater Los Angeles Healthcare System
Los Angeles, California, U.S.A.

ROBERT M. STRIETER

UCLA School of Medicine
Los Angeles, California, U.S.A.

I. Introduction

Lung cancer is the leading cause of cancer-related mortality (1), accounting for approximately 30% of all cancer deaths in the United States each year. Nearly half of lung cancers occur in women, and more women die of lung cancer than breast cancer. In fact, lung cancer accounts for more cancer deaths than colo-rectal, breast, and prostate cancers combined (1,2). Using conventional multimo-dality therapy, the 5-year survival rate for all patients with lung cancer is less than 15%, and surgery for early-stage disease remains the only dependable cura-tive option, emphasizing the dire need for new and effective therapies (3–5).

Gene therapy employs the specific transfer of genetic materials to impact a disease process. Thus, gene therapy depends upon understanding the molecular pathogenesis of the disease. As the knowledge underlying the pathogenesis of lung cancer evolves, so too does the ability to test hypothesis-driven strategies that specifically address the molecular and cellular deficits in this disease using gene transfer techniques. Accordingly, over the last several years, investigators have provided experimental proof of concept for the utility of specific strategies that target discrete steps in the pathogenesis of lung cancer. These processes may contribute directly or indirectly to (1) cellular transformation, (2) malignant infiltration, or (3) the systemic progression and metastasis of lung cancer. In this chapter, we will first present an overview of human lung cancer and consider the experimental tools that are used to drive hypotheses from the bench to the clinic. Next, we will describe, in a general fashion, some of the molecular and cellular strategies that appear to hold promise for improving therapy for lung cancer. Rather than catalogue the genetic abnormalities in lung cancer or present the myriad of approaches that have been tested, we will instead focus on themes that underlie the development of rational therapeutics for the treatment of lung cancer.

The development of molecular therapeutics has a rational and predictable course. Because such therapeutics arise from an understanding of molecular mechanisms underlying a disease process, the strategies are hypothesis-driven and targeted toward specific pathways underlying the molecular and cellular pathogenesis. Accordingly, in addition to establishing therapeutic efficacy, the evaluation of molecular therapeutics often confirms the importance of a specific genetic or biological pathway in the *pathogenesis* of a disease process. The evaluation of a molecular therapeutic typically begins by providing a molecular/cellular proof of concept in vitro, followed by an expansion of therapeutic principles and toxicological analyses of the intervention in animal models, and finally a systematic sequence of safety and clinical efficacy trials in human subjects. Logically, gene therapy paradigms can be expected to proceed along this course in order to be considered for the treatment of human disease.

II. Human Lung Cancer

Although susceptibility to environmental carcinogens may be predetermined and, by some reports, may follow a pattern of autosomal dominant Mendelian inheritance (6,7), lung cancer results from an accumulation of acquired genetic mutations (5,8,9). In fact, it is suggested that 10–20 genetic mutations may be necessary for the development of lung cancer (10), although the discrete steps for the progression of a hyperplastic bronchial lesion to metaplasia and anaplasia have not been uncovered. Tobacco use is the strongest epidemiological risk for the development of lung cancer, and it is anticipated that approximately 10% of all smokers will develop lung cancer over their lifetime (11). Current paradigms predict that lung cancer results from the widespread exposure to the carcinogen, leading to a process of "field cancerization" whereby the entire aerodigestive track is exposed to the offending agents and leads to the occurrence of synchronous and metachronous tumors (12,13). The tobacco carcinogens apparently bring about multiple clonal chromosomal abnormalities throughout the airways and alveoli of smokers (14,15). The series of genetic mutations likely results in aberrant signal transduction and cell cycle pathways, eventuating in malignant and metastatic phenotypes (16). The general pattern of genetic chances is characteristic, but not specific, for the various pathological subtypes of lung cancer. Overall, *K-ras* mutations are observed in 20–50% (17), *p53* mutations are present in 50% (18), 60% exhibit reduced expression of *p16-ink4a* (19,20) and 30% show deletion of *Rb*. Small cell lung cancers (SCLCs) display a greater proclivity to c-*myc* amplification and a greater degree of *p53* (80%) and *Rb* mutations (90%). Chromosome 3p deletions, occurring at a chromosomal fragile site that includes the *FHIT* locus, are found in 50% of non–small cell lung cancer (NSCLC) and in 90% of SCLC primary tumors (21). Overexpression of the tyrosine growth factor receptor *erbB2-neu* is seen in 10–30% and overexpression of *bcl-2* (22) in 10–25% of NSCLC tumors (23).

Clinically, lung cancer is categorized as SCLC and NSCLC by histopathology or cytopathology, and by their characteristic clinical presentations and divergent responses to conventional cytoreductive therapies. NSCLC may be further subclassified pathologically into squamous cell (SCCa), adenocarcinoma, bronchoalveolar cell carcinoma (BAC), adenosquamous (mixed pathology), or large cell carcinoma. As noted above, the progression of lung cancer from premalignancy to the clinical/pathological entity that is diagnosed has not yet been fully characterized. Although lung cancer is prevalent, it is typically diagnosed when it is pathologically advanced, and this has hindered full delineation of its molecular pathogenesis. Because of the late stage of diagnosis, there is progressive genetic instability that confers marked genetic and phenotypic heterogeneity within lung cancers even in individual patients. The late stage of diagnosis also results in an absolute lack of premalignant material, making it difficult to assign specific roles for the genetic mutations in the systematic progression of lung cancer. More recently, there has been a concerted effort to identify the early genetic lesions that contribute to the development of lung cancer. Accordingly, some of the characteristic genetic mutations of lung cancer (e.g., loss of heterozygosity [LOH] at chromosome 3p, *p53* mutations), are being identified in microdissected dysplastic epithelium (24). Additionally, screening programs using fluorescence bronchoscopy in individuals at high risk for lung cancer have identified a new lesion, termed angiogenic squamous dysplasia, that is frequently associated with LOH at chromosome 3p (25). Observations in BAC specimens also implicate the characteristic *K-ras* abnormalities in lung cancer as a correlate of mucinous differentiation (26). Similarly, a lesion pathologically termed alveolar atypical hyperplasia (AAH) is being advanced as a precursor to lung adenocarcinoma. AAH is characterized by increased cellular proliferation when compared to adjacent normal parenchyma, by immunohistochemical evidence of *p53* stabilization, *k-ras* mutations, and c-erb-B2 overexpression (27–29). The presence of these mutations in AAH may explain why they may be detectable in sputum cytology specimens that predate the onset of clinical lung cancer (30). Identification of these early events may serve as genetic markers for malignant progression or as targets of specific genetic or chemopreventative approaches.

These early events also may be better modeled in murine models than late-stage lung cancer (see below). Thus, there is an inherent complexity in human lung cancer, and to precisely recapitulate the disease process in animals is not yet possible.

III. Preclinical Murine Models of Human Lung Cancer Utilized in Studies of Gene Therapy

A primary goal of in vivo/animal experimentation is to build on an in vitro proof of concept and to strengthen the rationale for clinical testing of an experimental gene therapy intervention. To justify animal studies, there should be a preexistent pathophysiological rationale and/or in vitro experimental data suggesting that a strategy is likely to be effective. At this juncture, the investigator is faced with the formidable challenge of approximating a human disease in an animal model. Although animal models cannot be exact replicas of the human disease, they should, at the very least, provide useful molecular and cellular similarities to the pathogenesis and clinical manifestations of the target disease (31). For a variety of reasons (low expense for breeding and maintenance, susceptibility to tumorigenesis, well-defined immunosuppressive states, and feasible duration of experimental studies), mice are considered to be the prototypic animal model for experimentation. Ideally, a mouse model used to evaluate lung cancer would mimic the human disease in its etiology, genetics, clinical presentation, and progression. Thus, the ideal mouse model would systematically (in defined pathological stages) develop lung cancer from exposure to cigarette smoke, and the disease could be characterized by sequential gene defects that culminate in the clinical progression that typifies the human disease.

Second, in designing the experimental approach, the pharmacological intervention or drug that is being tested is also important. However, prototypical drugs have reliable delivery/absorption, targeted distribution, a known mechanism of action, and predictable elimination; qualities that are not currently shared by cell or gene-based therapies. Thus, the challenge to aptly test a cell-based therapeutic or gene therapy vector in an animal model is doubly difficult. Consideration must be given to both modeling a complex human disease in vivo and to testing a multifaceted biological compound with ill-defined pharmacokinetic and pharmacodynamic properties that are likely unique to the host and/or the disease state. In order to meet this challenge, perhaps it is safer to adopt an approach that uses a combination of models to overcome specific deficiencies that accompany each individually. Consequently, one may utilize xenogenetic models (engraftment of heterologous tissue derived from donors of a different species, typically into an immunodeficient host) to study the therapeutic-gene effects of vector–target cell interactions. Syngeneic (engraftment of tissue from genetically identical donors) and allogenic (engraftment of tissues from a genetically dissimilar member of the same species) models are used to study host-tumor interactions in terms of immunological parameters and metastasis. To further discern the specific immunological parameters important for tumor rejection in mice, specific knockout (targeted gene disruption) mice are utilized. Finally, transgenic (e.g., referring to the tissue-specific expression of a transforming oncogene) models may be used to study the effects of a molecular therapeutic in the setting of established orthotopic (referring to organ or site-specific) malignancy. Integrating these approaches may allow one to meet the goals of in vivo experimentation for advancing gene therapy.

A. Murine Lung Cancer and Transplantable Allografts

Although murine models of disease are the accepted standards, there are also shortcomings in these models. For example, cigarette smoke, which is a strong epidemiological risk for the development of human lung cancer and is proximally responsible for approximately 85–90% of lung cancer cases in humans (32), is only weakly carcinogenic in most mice (33,34). In addition, although both mouse and human lung adenocarcinomas may share common molecular defects (33), the histopathological repertoire of spontaneous or induced tumors in mice is very limited (35,36), and morphologically, nearly all mouse lung tumors bear structural similarities only to BAC or well-differentiated adenocarcinomas. Consequently, whereas humans typically die from lung cancer of "late-stage" metastatic disease, mice succumb to respiratory failure following the diffuse involvement of their lungs by "early-stage" carcinoma in situ (31).

Spontaneous lung cancer develops in 3% of wild mice (37,38) with strain dependent sensitivity. As noted, murine lung tumors histologically resemble early lesions that originate peripherally (from type 2 alveolar cells or Clara's cells) and simulate papillary or BAC. In contrast, the bulk of human tumors are bronchogenic (arise in the airways) and, as described above, display a broad histopathological variation. In fact, individual human lung cancers may be histologically heterogeneous; often displaying mixed morphologies within the same tumor specimen. These features highlight the difficulty investigators may have in extrapolating interventions from the preclinical setting to the clinic; that is, how does one reconcile the differences between murine lung cancer and human lung cancer, and can one generalize observations and results from one species to another or one individual to another? To overcome deficiencies inherent to individual models of human lung cancer, some investigators may decide to test a therapeutic concept in multiple model systems.

Generally, mice that are sensitive to the development of spontaneous lung tumors are also at the highest risk for chemically induced (including cigarette smoke) tumors (37), and form the basis for the quantitative carcinogenecity bioassays. With respect to induced tumorigenesis, murine A/J and SWR strains are the most sensitive, BALB/c mice are of intermediate sensitivity, and DBA and C57Bl/6 are the most resistant. A variety of agents, including urethane, metals, concentrated components of tobacco smoke such as polyaromatic hydrocarbons, and nitrosoamines (39,40) can induce lung cancer in mice. Although tobacco smoke per se may be weakly carcinogenic (34), strain A/J mice that have been exposed to tobacco smoke reliably have an increased incidence of lung tumors and develop an increased multiplicity of tumors compared to control mice (41). Thus, this model may be the most representative and relevant model to evaluate the effectiveness of putative chemopreventative agents (e.g., genetic or pharmacological blockade of the inducible cyclooxygenase COX-2) for the prevention of human lung cancer (41). The tobacco-induced tumor models may be particularly important, because general chemopreventive methods that have been found to be effective in chemical-induced lung cancer are often ineffective in the tobacco-induced models (41).

Studies of gene therapy efficacy generally utilize transplantable murine tumors for primary analyses (42–47). Although all transplantable allograft systems are artificial, and extrapolating antitumor responses in these mice to humans is not straightforward, these models do provide important insights into the effectiveness of genetic therapies. Isolated clones from spontaneously arising murine tumors have been established as cultures in vitro, and these cultures now serve as a ready source for the generation of transplantable allografts. The best studied of these tumors include line 1 alveolar carcinoma (L1C2), a murine lung cancer cell line that is syngeneic to BALB/c, and 3LL (Lewis lung cancer) that is synergeneic to C57B1/6. Usually, these cell lines are utilized to generate transplantable heterotopic tumors in synegeneic mice, and enable the investigator to study the effectiveness of a therapy without compromising the interplay between the host's immune system and the tumor. Because both L1C2 and 3LL tumors are relatively "nonimmunogenic," as is human lung cancer, immunogenetic strategies that modulate the immune system to generate an antitumor immune response can be investigated in these models.

B. Spontaneously Arising Lung Cancer in Murine Models

Murine models of lung cancer include strains susceptible to chemically induced tumors and transgenic strains that express viral and cellular oncogenes. The simian virus-40 large T-Ag (SV40-TAg) has been commonly used to produce tumors in transgenic mice by promoting its expression in a lung-specific manner (48–51). SV40-TAg binds and incapacitates the cell cycle checkpoint and DNA binding capabilities of the *p53* and *Rb* gene products, resulting in uncontrolled cellular proliferation (52). Animals expressing the SV40-TAg develop multifocal lung adenocarcinomas that have pathological features similar to some human lung adenocarcinomas and succumb to respiratory failure by age 4–5 months. The tumors of these mice vary with respect to the expression of the large TAg, suggesting perhaps that SV40 TAg may contribute to transformation, but continued expression may not be necessary for tumor progression. Within the lungs, tumors consistently involve the bronchiolar and alveolar regions of the lung while sparing the large airways. Likewise, organ-specific expression of SV40-TAg using the Clara's cell–specific MW 10,000 protein (CC-10) also results in the induction of lung tumors (53). CC-10TAg transgenic mice also develop multifocal pulmonary adenocarcinomas and succumb to respiratory failure at 16–20 weeks of age. Pathology is localized to the lungs, and the tumors express the large T-Ag in normal Clara's cells and in transformed tumor cells. Pathological progression is similar to that described above, with the lungs appearing to be pathologically normal at 2 months of age, a number of tumor foci are grossly discernible by 3 months, and the majority of the lung is replaced by coalesced nodules by 4 months of age. As tumor progresses, the expression of endogeneous CC10 expression diminishes, and there is increased nuclear p53 expression, suggesting binding and stabilization of the protein by the large T-Ag (53). The reliable progression of lethal tumors in these transgenic mice enables investigators to test a number of hypotheses, dosing schemes, and dosing routes. Importantly, the effects of immunomodulation by the gene transfer of specific cytokines and chemokines into tumor cells in vivo can be determined. For example, this model has been used to test the immunomodulatory capacity of secondary lymphoid chemokine, or *slc* (45,54), in vivo.

Recently, to better approximate human lung cancer, investigators engineered an oncogenic *K-ras* gene that requires somatic activation in the intact animal (55). Because random recombination events result in the activation of the oncogene, these mice potentially mimic the field effect (56) in the respiratory tract of smokers (57) that is believed to underlie human lung cancer. The sporadic activation of *K-ras* mutations in these mice contributes to the development of lung adenocarcinomas in a staged manner beginning at 1 week of age (55). Immunohistochemistry suggests that the tumor arises from an alveolar type II cell origin, and histopathology, as with other transgenic and spontaneous models, was that of well-differentiated adenocarcinoma or BAC. Undoubtedly, this model will be utilized for a variety of purposes and provide insight into the pathogenesis, prevention, and treatment of lung cancer. Moreover, as other gene families come to be identified that contribute to the malignant phenotype (e.g., *Cox-2*, matrix metalloproteinases and various cytokines/chemokines), the impact of those systems on lung cancer is likely to be carried out in specified transgenic or gene-targeted model systems.

C. Murine Models with Transplantable Xenografts

Xenotransplantation of human tumors into immunocompromised mice began in the late 1960s (58) following the discovery of the node mucosa in 1962 and its characterization as an athymic mutant in 1968 (59). The morphological and karyotypic stability of tumors serially passaged in nude mice was described (60), and it was established that xenotransplanted tumors in nude mice often retained distinctive phenotypic and functional characteristics found in the human host (61). However, the "tumor-take" rate for nude mouse xenotransplants is tumor specific, and, generally, carcinomas are more difficult to establish than melanomas or sarcomas (62). Thus, progressive tumor growth from inoculated primary tumors (i.e., cultured directly from the patient) is observed in only 33% for lung cancers (63). In addition to properties inherent to the tumor, nude mouse–related factors also impact on tumor-take. For example, mice infected with the mouse hepatitis virus do not accept xenotransplants; presumably because of enhanced natural killer (NK) cell activity (64). In this regard, it is important to recall that, although nude mice lack functionally mature T cells, they are capable of mounting normal humoral responses to T-cell–independent antigens (65), and they exhibit high NK cell activity (66). These properties probably impact negatively on the tumor-take rate of xenotransplants. Severe combined immunodeficiency mice (SCID mice) (67) have offered yet another option for hosting human tumor xenografts. The *scid/scid* mice are characterized by the virtual absence of functional T and B lymphocytes due to aberrance in the rearrangement of antigen receptor genes (68). The first successful engraftment of human solid organ tumors into SCID mice began with the subcutaneous inoculation using the A549 lung adenocarcinoma cell line (69). Since that time, a variety of human solid-organ cancers, both from cell lines and primary tumor specimens, have been successfully engrafted. The higher rates of successful engraftment, presumably because of the lack of residual B-cell function in *scid* mice, have led many investigators to prefer *scid/scid* mice over *nu/nu* mice as the host recipients of human xenograft tumors. Furthermore, genetic engineering and gene-targeting technology has helped create murine mutants with exquisitely specific immune defects, including mice in which CD4 or CD8 T cells are deleted (70) and mice which lack β_2-microglobulin and thus do not express transplantation antigens (71).

Xenotransplants have several advantages, including the fact that they provide a replenishable source of human tumor. This enables the genetic characterization and gene discovery of tumor-specific phenotypes, and in rare occasions, the progression toward an advanced or metastatic phenotype of the tumor. Xenotransplants are also useful to assess the mode of delivery and transduction efficiency of gene therapy vectors that are being developed for targeting tumor in vivo (72), and to investigate the scope of polarity of viral attachment receptors in vivo. Indeed, as suggested by in vitro analyses, the histological heterogeneity of lung tumors may be an indicator of differences in adenoviral entry and/or the efficacy of adenoviral gene therapy (73). Extension of this premise in vivo using xenogeneic transplants that represent the various histopathological subtypes of human lung cancer may be useful in the development of disease-specific targeted vectors.

IV. Gene- and Cell-Based Therapies for Lung Cancer

As described, lung cancer results from an accumulation of acquired genetic mutations that eventuate in cellular *transformation* and progressively *invasive/meta-
static* disease (8,9). In this multistep process, transformation is promoted by (1)
growth factors that bind to cell surface receptors and elicit cellular proliferation,
(2) abnormal signaling machinery between the cell surface and the nucleus, and
(3) acceleration of the cell cycle and/or ineffective programmed cell death
(apoptosis) in transformed cells. Once a cell transforms, however, the clinical
manifestations of lung cancer depend on the ability of the malignant cells to form
a tumor mass, to escape immune surveillance, to secure a blood supply, and to
gain the ability to metastasize. These biological features also result from newly
acquired genetic mutations that enable the tumor cells to mediate active immunosuppression, to promote angiogenesis, and to escape into the lymphatic/vascular
tributaries to set up residence in other organ systems. The tumor cells interact
with and often induce stroma formation to advance these aims. Delineating the
molecular mechanisms underlying each step provides an opportunity to intervene
therapeutically, and some of these approaches are described below.

A. Gene-Based Therapies Targeting Molecular Transformation

Abnormalities at the cell surface (e.g., *erB2*), signal transduction (e.g., *ras* oncogene), gene regulation and cell cycle control (e.g., *p53*, *rb*, *myc* oncogene), or
apoptosis (e.g., *p53*, *BCL-2*) are all implicated in the malignant transformation
of pulmonary epithelium. These processes can also serve as targets for rational
therapeutic intervention. For example, the functional loss or the dysregulation of
pathways of the *p53* and *rb* (retinoblastoma) gene products is often critical to
development of lung cancer. Indeed, approximately 50–60% of all human lung
cancers have *p53* mutations that are thought to have significant clinical relevance
(9,74). p53 Is a "tumor suppressor" protein that is critical to maintaining the
integrity of the genome as cells traverse the cell cycle. The majority of *p53* mutations results in the loss of its capacity for DNA binding, and as a result, these
mutations disable the protein's ability to regulate transcription (75). Upon the
loss of p53 function, the mutated cells are left unchecked in replicating damaged
DNA, ultimately resulting in increased genomic instability and neoplastic transformation. In addition to these effects on cell cycle regulation and genomic instability, *p53* mutations may also lead to increased resistance to chemotherapy and
ionizing radiation by interfering with apoptosis (76,77).

To overcome the deficits due to mutated *p53*, one strategy for lung cancer
gene therapy has opted to replace the mutated *p53* gene with a normal copy.
Preclinical studies suggested that replacing mutated *p53* with wild-type decreased
tumorigenicity of human cancer cells in vitro and in animal models (78). Based
on these preliminary studies, clinical gene therapy trials for human NSCLC were

initiated utilizing a *p53* gene transfer strategy (79). In the initial study, nine patients with advanced NSCLC were treated with either bronchoscopic or computed tomography (CT)–guided intratumoral injections of a retroviral *p53* expression vector. Of the seven patients evaluated, three showed evidence of tumor regression at the treatment site and six showed increased apoptosis of tumor cells on posttreatment biopsies. Importantly, there was no significant toxicity associated with the therapy, and in situ gene transfer was achieved (79). However, the mechanism of the tumor regression reported was enigmatic. It was believed that mutated *p53* function would have to be compensated in each and every cell for restoration of the normal apoptosis program. Consequently, how could a significant reduction in tumor volume be explained when only a tiny minority of cells within the tumor mass showed evidence of gene transfer? Because of substantial tumor regression despite poor in situ gene transfer, mechanisms for the observed "bystander effect" were hypothesized (80). The term *bystander effect* refers to the ability of gene-modified (transfected or transduced) tumor cells to mediate killing of neighboring nontransfected cells. One plausible explanation is that wild-type *p53* induces release of inhibitors of angiogenesis (the ability of the tumor to induce the formation of new blood vessels), thus undermining the blood supply to the tumor (81). In addition, the expression of *p53* may also contribute to an immune-mediated response (82,83). These unresolved issues have led to additional mechanism-based bench and animal studies as well as other clinical trials. Because of poor in vivo transduction with retroviral vectors, investigators continued with the theme of *p53* replacement using adenoviral vectors, and commenced trials combining gene therapy with conventional chemotherapy (84–86). Although the study design and objectives varied, both the North American and European studies instilled high doses (7.5 × 10^{12} pfu) of Ad vectors encoding *wt-p53* directly into tumors by endobronchial or transthoracic injections (85,86). Subjects with advanced lung cancer were treated with *p53* gene therapy in combination with platinum-based chemotherapy, and the studies reported the therapy to be generally well tolerated with limited grade 3 toxicity. Again, molecular evidence of in vivo gene transfer and clinical evidence of nonprogressive disease was presented (85,86). However, the investigators interpreted the findings differently, with one group suggesting that there was added benefit of gene therapy with chemotherapy, whereas the second group concluded that there was no advantage of combining *p53* gene therapy to first line chemotherapy. Taken together, these studies may suggest that limited therapeutic efficacy was observed and the mechanisms responsible for the antitumor effects remain unresolved (85,86).

Because of the high frequency of *p53* mutations, another strategy that uses *replication-competent viruses* has been hypothesized to be ideally suited for lung cancer. This approach employs adenoviruses (mutant dl1520, or ONYX-015) that are suggested selectively to replicate in *p53*-mutated (therefore, selectively in cancer) cells (87,88). Consequently, these mutant viruses are promoted as "magic bullets" that kill tumor cells and leave normal tissues intact. This particular approach has generated considerable controversy both in terms of its reputed efficacy as well as its proposed mechanism of action (89–91). Despite mechanistic concerns, the clinical efficacy of this strategy is being tested in a variety of tumors, including advanced lung cancer where the replication-competent vector has been administered intravenously. In this setting, investigators have reportedly injected over 10^{13} particles without observing dose-limiting toxicity and documenting evidence of viral replication in a subset of these subjects (92). In brief, the putative mechanism of action of dl1520 requires additional in vitro and in vivo characterization. Additionally, the safety and effectiveness of conditionally replicative adenoviral (or other candidates; e.g., herpesviruses [93]) remains to be confirmed in ongoing preclinical and clinical trials. Nevertheless, the approach represents a prime example of a "rational therapy" which attempts to exploit the biology of mutant viruses or specific viral proteins to clinical advantage.

Additional strategies that specifically intervene in the various molecular pathways leading to the malignant transformation of pulmonary epithelium are in various stages of development. For example, because mutated *K-ras* contributes to the malignant phenotype by accelerating growth potential, both pharmacological (e.g., farnesyltransferase inhibitors [94]) and gene therapy approaches targeting the *K-ras* oncogene are under investigation. In one such strategy that has reported preclinical efficacy and has been approved for human clinical trials, a vector encoding the "antisense" transcript neutralizes the messenger RNA encoded by *K-ras* oncogene (95,96). An affiliated group has proposed an alternative to this antisense strategy by constructing an adenoviral vector which encodes a hammerhead ribozyme transgene that is specific for the most common (*K-ras* codon 12) mutant found in lung cancer cells. Efficacy using this strategy is cited in vitro and in animal models (97), with further studies pending. Finally, the demonstration that transfection of wild-type *K-ras2* inhibited colony formation and lung tumorigenesis by a murine lung tumor cell line containing an activated *K-ras2* allele implicates a tumor-suppressor role for this proto-oncogene and supports the use of *wt-Kras* in gene therapy (98).

Other investigators have targeted known abnormalities of cell surface receptors in lung cancer. For instance, the *HER-2/neu* (also referred to as *erb-B2*) gene encodes a transmembrane receptor tyrosine kinase that confers an aggressive phenotype and poorer prognosis in lung cancer (23,99). For designing therapy, this cell surface ligand has been used as a cognate receptor for receptor-mediated transfer of genes. Alternatively, the growth-promoting properties of the receptor have been abolished by preventing it from getting sorted to the cell membrane (100) or by using antagonistic antibodies that recognize HER-2/neu (101).

Like *p53,* the tumor-suppressor gene *rb* is mutated or dysregulated in the vast majority of lung cancers. The rb protein is critical to the regulation of cell cycle progression. In this scheme, the status of rb phosphorylation determines its activity as a positive or negative stimulus for cell proliferation (hyperphosphorylation = positive growth, hypophosphorylation = suppression of growth). SCLCs often carry mutations within the *rb* gene per se, whereas NSCLCs inactivate inhibitors of rb kinases (cyclin-dependent kinase inhibitors; e.g., p16-ink-4a), which similarly induce the cell to divide (20). Thus, inhibiting rb phosphorylation by increasing the cellular expression of p16-ink4a is a potential strategy for the treatment of lung cancer, although data reporting the efficacy of molecular therapies targeting the *rb* pathway is generally sparse (102).

Along with the contribution of mutant *p53* to abnormalities in programmed cell death, the antiapoptotic *BCL-2* gene is overexpressed in lung cancer (22,103), and hence is a rational target for intervention (104). Delineating a definitive role for the tumor necrosis factor (TNF)–related apoptosis ligand (TRAIL) in selectively mediating tumor cell death may also yield an effective and safer strategy (105). Similarly, other potential targets that mediate apoptosis resistance have recently been identified. For example, the protein survivin is a putative tumor-specific product (106–108) that suppresses apoptosis, and may be an important gene therapy target. Thus, although fetal tissues express survivin, most normal adult tissues do not (106), and its overexpression is reported to be associated with a poor prognosis in NSCLC (109). Olie et al. (110) and Mesri et al. (111) have recently presented the elemental proof of concept regarding the therapeutic utility of survivin. These investigators induced lung cancer apoptosis by either antisense inhibition of survivin (110) or by using an adenoviral vector that expressed a survivin mutant to induce tumor cell apoptosis and reduce tumor formation in vivo (111).

B. Gene-Based Therapies to Promote Sensitization to Chemotherapy or Radiation

Analogous to inducing cytotoxicity by genetic replacement of *p53*, toxin gene/prodrug or suicide gene therapy has also been used to transfer genes that sensitize the cancer cells to an otherwise nontoxic drug. For lung cancer, the best-studied examples of these toxin gene/prodrug systems include the thymidine kinase/gancyclovir and the cytosine deaminase/5-fluorocytosine combinations. All of such strategies typically aim to effect localized disease, and they all rely on the bystander effect to reduce the overall tumor burden. The bystander response may be specific to the toxin-gene/prodrug system (112,113), or it may attempt to induce an adjuvant or specific antitumor host immune response (42,43,114,115) although selective transcriptional targeting of cancer cells may be hypothetically achieved by regulating the expression of the toxin gene by tumor-specific promoters (116–118), a limitation to the utility of such strategies may well be insufficient transduction to yield a significant bystander response (119). Nevertheless, for lung cancer and malignant mesothelioma, suicide gene therapy paradigms have been tested with some success in preclinical model systems (42,43,72,120–122). Indeed, these experiments have led to Phase I clinical trials targeting malignant mesothelioma with both gene- and cell-based therapy (123), with the initial reports citing low toxicity and molecular evidence for in situ gene transfer (124,125).

Gene therapy strategies may also be used as adjuvants to enhance the efficacy of conventional multimodality (i.e., surgery, radiation, and chemotherapy) approaches for the treatment of lung cancer. For example, a panel of human lung cancer cell lines was systematically tested and demonstrated an additive and/ or synergistic inhibition of growth when *p53* gene transfer was combined with docetaxel and radiation therapy both in vitro and in vivo (126). Similarly, gene therapy may play important synergistic roles in a variety of paradigms, and experimental evidence to validate such synergistic combinations is emerging (127–133). In fact, several approaches highlighted above (e.g., *p53* gene replacement therapy) are already in clinical trials in combination regimens. For many other strategies, there exist a compelling scientific rationale to test them empirically in combination with conventional multimodality therapy. Such rational combinations for synergy may include (inhibitor of nuclear factor kappa B [NF-κB]) IκB gene therapy with radiation or chemotherapy (134–136). IκBα gene transfer can sensitize NSCLC cells to TNF-α–mediated cytoxicity and can induce chemosensitivity (137,138), although the mechanism and generalizability of this effect on lung cancer cells needs further clarification (137,139,140). In addition, a host of other approaches have been described that propose to sensitize the tumor cells to chemotherapy or radiation (e.g., gene transfer of radiosensitizing cytokines IL-1), or, alternatively, to induce the resistance of the normal host tissue to cytoablative or radiation therapy (141) (e.g., myeloprotection: by gene transfer of *thrombopoietin* or other myeloprogenitor growth factors, or prevention of mucositis by *MDR-1, superoxide dismutase,* or *bFGF* gene transfer into the gastrointestinal mucosa).

C. Genetic Immunotherapy

The development of effective immune interventions for lung cancer could have important advantages. In contrast to the other approaches, which rely heavily on gene transfer to the tumor in situ and the accompanying bystander effects for the treatment of local-regional disease, genetic immunotherapy of lung cancer has potential for systemic eradication of disease. The major obstacle for effective immunological intervention for lung cancer has been an incomplete understanding of the immunobiology of this disease. However, basic research focusing on the complex interaction between lung cancer cells and the immune response is providing more direction for fomulating rational therapeutic approaches. In particular, strategies designed to overcome tumor-induced immunosuppression are on the cusp of large-scale clinical experimentation for NSCLC. Autologous or allogeneic tumor cells, genetically modified ex vivo to enhance their immunogenicity by the introduction of cytokine genes or costimulatory molecules, are continuing to undergo preclinical and clinical scrutiny as tumor cell vaccines. Alternatively, in vivo augmentation of the host immune response by attempting direct in situ transduction of target cells with immune stimulatory cytokine genes or by downregulating tumor-mediated immune suppression is being optimized in the preclinical arena. Finally, genetic modification of nontumor host cells ex vivo with specific antigens or cytokines for subsequent in vivo transfer is fast emerging. The target host cells may include lymphocytes, fibroblasts, or antigen-presenting cells such as dendritic cells. Specific examples from each of these approaches (tumor cell vaccines, reversal of immune suppression, and the restoration of antigen-presenting function in lung cancer) are reviewed below.

Methods Used to Identify Specific Tumor Antigens for Use in Lung Cancer Genetic Immunotherapy

Although various methods of immune stimulation have been attempted for the treatment of thoracic malignancies, none has been proven to be reliably effective (142–144). In contrast, immune-based therapies have been proven to be more successful in melanoma and renal cell carcinoma (145,146). This has led to the misconception that thoracic malignancies are nonimmunogenic and will not be amenable to immunological interventions. In groundbreaking studies, however, Boon and colleagues found that protective immunity could be generated against nonimmunogenic murine tumors (147,148). These studies suggested that a tumor's apparent lack of immunogenicity is indicative of a failure to elicit an effective host response rather than a lack of tumor antigen expression (149,150). Accordingly, a new paradigm emerged that focused on generating antitumor responses by therapeutic vaccination (5,151). In this setting, vaccination refers to an intervention that unmasks tumor antigens leading to generation of specific host immune responses against the tumor.

The search for new antigens for use in genetic immunotherapy has involved a variety of techniques. Most investigations have sought to identify antigens capable of eliciting a T-cell–mediated immune response (152). To detect these antigens, genomic DNA or cDNA libraries are typically transfected into cells expressing the appropriate major histocompatibility complex (MHC) phenotype, and antitumor cytotoxic T lymphocytes are then used to identify specificity against the transfectants (153). A second technique to identify tumor antigens includes in vitro sensitization of T cells to candidate antigens. T-cell clones are then assessed for their capacity specifically to release cytokines or for their cytolytic activity against tumor (153). A third (technically difficult) technique is the elutriation of peptides from tumor cells followed by their assessment for the capacity to stimulate CTLs (154). The critical step in all of these techniques is recognition of T-cell responses against antigenic epitopes.

Tumor antigens recognized by T cells can be categorized into four general groups (155). Type I antigens result from somatic mutations in normal gene products. Examples of this type of tumor antigen are the point mutations in connexin 37 discovered in Lewis lung carcinoma by Mandelboim et al. (156). These peptides, termed MUT1 and MUT2, can be used in lung cancer models to immunize and protect mice against tumor challenge as well as to mediate regression of established lung cancer (44,157,158). Type II antigens are those resulting from mutated oncogenes, although it is proposed that the likelihood of a mutation generating an immunodominant epitope is a rare event (159). For example, *p53* has been shown to generate CTL responses in lung cancer (160); however, it is not yet known whether these responses can generate effective, protective immunity. In addition, heterologous antigens expressed by tumors thought to be of viral origin can also be included among the type II antigens. Although the role SV40 proteins play in the pathogenesis of malignant mesothelioma (MM) remains controversial, Waheed et al. (161) showed that antisense to SV40 early gene regions induced growth arrest and apoptosis in SV40 T antigen–positive MM. The significance of these provocative findings awaits further evaluation. Type III antigens are normal gene products that have restricted tissue distribution. These antigens include the MAGE and GAGE antigen families that were initially defined in melanoma, and several of these antigens are expressed in lung cancers (162–164). Type IV antigens have been referred to as "differentiation antigens" and consist of normal tissue-specific gene products. These antigens have been discovered in melanoma and include tyrosinase and MART-1 (162–165).

There is good evidence to suggest that tumor antigens recognized by CTLs play pivotal roles in tumor rejection (166). CTLs have the capacity to discriminate subtle changes in antigens expressed by the MHC class I pathway. Acting in concert with CTLs, CD4$^+$ T cells function to induce and extend the CTL response by producing cytokines requisite for a fully functional cell-mediated response (159). CD4 cells also may be responsible for recognition of MHC class II–dependent epitopes (167). However, not all tumor-*associated* antigens that are recognized by CTLs serve as tumor *rejection* antigens (155). The most prevalent tumor antigens recognized by T cells are actually self-antigens (168), suggesting that tumor immunity may be viewed as a form of autoimmunity (169). The clinical manifestations of the theory linking tumor immunity and autoimmunity are best exemplified in melanoma; patients who develop vitiligo have a better prognosis and are more likely to respond to therapy (170). Similarly, in vivo tumor model systems have shown that immunotherapy directed against tumor antigens can induce autoimmune disease (171,172). However, autoimmunity is not a prerequisite, because effective tumor reduction can be achieved when tumor immunity and autoimmunity are uncoupled (169).

After defining a repertoire of tumor antigens, additional obstacles must be overcome to implement a successful immune-based therapy. First, an immune response to a malignancy may not develop owing to tolerance (173). It has been suggested that the single most important determinant of tumor rejection antigen potency is the avidity of the cognate CTL (174). The tolerogenic response appears to eliminate high-avidity T cells but spare the low-avidity CTL effector populations (175). Thus, the most effective cancer immunotherapies may be those that significantly activate the low-avidity T-cell populations. A second well-documented problem in thoracic malignancies is the active immune suppression induced by the tumor itself (173). Tumor-reactive T cells have been shown to accumulate in lung cancer tissues but fail to respond owing to suppressive tumor cell–derived factors (176). Moreover, tumor cells may also direct surrounding inflammatory cells to release suppressive cytokines in the tumor milieu (177,178). For example, tumor-derived prostaglandin E2 (PGE2) orchestrates an imbalance, favoring the production of suppressive over immune-potentiating cytokines by lymphocytes and macrophages in the tumor environment (177). Importantly, effective antitumor responses can be restored through abrogation of tumor PGE2 production (47).

Tumor Cell Vaccines: Cytokine Gene Therapy for Lung Cancer

A number of models have used the introduction of cytokine genes into tumor cells with the goal of controlling local tumor growth at the primary site while establishing systemic antitumor immunity. In one of the original studies, using retroviral vectors to transduce murine tumors with the interleukin-2 (IL-2) gene, Fearon et al. demonstrated the role of IL-2 in the antitumor response in vivo (179). The investigators speculated that the host's failure to respond to tumor antigens reflected diminished T-cell help for tumor cytolysis by $CD8^+$ lymphocytes. By providing a constant local source of IL-2 via the gene-modified tumor cells, tumors were rejected in vivo primarily by an induced MHC class I–restricted cytotoxic T-lymphocyte response. Subsequently, IL-2 gene therapy also revealed efficacy in lung cancer models. Heike et al. used an adenoviral vector containing IL-2 in the 3LL model (180), and demonstrated a protective effect from tumor rechallenge in 90% of mice following an intrapleural vaccination with irradiated IL-2–transfected 3LL cells. Treatment with subcutaneous injection of irradiated 3LL IL-2 cells, however, had no effect on established pulmonary tumor. Because locally administered recombinant IL-2 has been shown to reduce lung cancer growth in other animal models and preliminary clinical trials, interest in IL-2 gene therapy has persisted (181,182). Other cytokines, however, may be more effective in generating specific antitumor immune responses against lung cancer. In this respect, cytokine gene-modified tumor vaccines have utilized a wide variety of cytokines including interleukins (1–7,10,12,15,18), interferons (γ, α, β), tumor necrosis factor-α (TNF-α), monocyte chemotactic proteins (MCP), granulocyte-macrophage colony-stimulating factor (GM-CSF), granulocyte colony-stimulating factor (G-CSF) in preclinical models (183–210). Although the nature of the inflammatory infiltrates differs depending on the cytokine and model used, most studies indicate that the genetically modified tumors are capable of inducing specific systemic antitumor immunity in vivo. Enhanced immunogenicity has also been documented using tumors transfected with foreign genes (211) or with MHC genes (212,213). Although clinical trials implementing cytokine gene therapy are underway, the clinical setting in which this form of therapy will be efficacious for lung cancer awaits definition. It is speculated that the use of cytokine-producing tumor vaccines may be most applicable in an adjuvant setting in which minimal disease is targeted for elimination (197). In this scenario, cytokine gene transfer stimulates the onset of cytokine cascades in vivo with resultant enhanced tumor immunogenicity, increased cytolytic activity, and further cytokine release by autologous antitumor effector cells. However, it has not yet been determined which cytokines are optimal for lung cancer, especially given the possibility that each primary tumor may have a different immunoregulatory response to a given cytokine. Even so, IL-12, GM-CSF, and IFN-β are of particular interest for cytokine gene therapy of lung cancer.

IL-7, originally described as a growth factor for pre-B cells (214), can also stimulate the growth of mature T cells and is important in promoting T-cell survival by upregulating the antiapoptotic molecules of the bcl-2 family (215). Resting T cells proliferate in direct response to IL-7 as well as through a secondary IL-2–dependent pathway (216). IL-7 modulates peripheral T-cell responses to cognate antigen in vivo (217,218), enhances the generation of CTLs and lymphokine-activated killer (LAK) cells, and induces cytokine secretion and tumoricidal activity in human peripheral blood monocytes (219–221). IL-7 synergizes with IL-12 in the induction of T-cell proliferation, cytotoxicity, and IFN-γ release, a cytokine required for tumor-infiltrating lymphocyte (TIL) antitumor efficacy. IL-7 contributes to this synergy with IL-12 by upregulating IL-12 receptor expression (222). In contrast to IL-2 which upregulates TGF-β, IL-7 down-regulates both macrophage and tumor production of TGF-β, a potent inhibitor of antitumor immuity (223–225). Consistent with these findings, recent studies indicate that IL-7 invokes cell-mediated immune responses characteristic of type 1 cytokines and enhances antigen-specific T-cell cytotoxicity (226,227). Accordingly, IL-7 can mediate significant antitumor responses in vivo in murine models (42,46). Furthermore, IL-7 can directly affect tumor proliferation and cell surface phenotype. For example, when transfected into human NSCLC cells, IL-7 slowed their in vitro proliferation and augmented surface expression of MHC class I and intracellular adhesion molecule-1 (ICAM-1) (228). Thus, IL-7 may enhance the immunogenicity of NSCLC cells, and allogeneic peripheral blood lymphocytes cocultured with IL-7-transduced human tumor cells show enhanced cytolytic and proliferative capacities compared to coculture with parental cells (228). In fact, when used in adoptive transfer, IL-7–generated CTLs reduce metastatic tumor burden as effectively as do CTLs generated in IL-2 (221). IL-7 has also been documented to augment the efficacy of dendritic cell immunotherapy of murine lung cancer (42,46). This compilation of preclinical data has contributed to the translation of IL-7 in multicomponent clinical gene therapy regimes for NSCLC.

Lung cancer cells, and the lymphocytes that infiltrate tumor stroma, both express a predominant immunosuppressive type 2 cytokine pattern (5,229,230). The ability of IL-12 to redirect a type 2 cytokine expression toward an immunostimulatory type 1 cytokine pattern makes its use in gene therapy for lung cancer particularly compelling. IL-12, a 70-kD heterodimer originally identified in supernatants from Epstein-Barr virus (EBV)–transformed B lymphoblastoid cells, is produced by both adherent cells and nonadherent lymphocytes (231,232). The rationale underlying the use of IL-12 in NSCLC is multifaceted. For example, IL-12 (1) induces the proliferation and enhances the cytolytic activity of resting natural killer (NK) and T cells (233); (2) induces the production of IFN-γ and TNF-α from resting and activated NK and T cells (234); (3) synergizes with IL-2 or anti-CD3 in the induction of IFN-γ (235); (4) induces LAK cell activity both directly in the synergy with IL-2 (236,237); (5) acts as a comitogen with anti-CD3 or antigen in the induction of T-cell proliferation (231); and (6) increases specific CTL responses to human tumor in vitro (236). Moreover, IL-12 may augment CTL responses against tumor by one or more mechanisms (236). First, IL-12 may augment the proliferation of a subset of specific CTLs, and/or it may induce the differentiation of precursors into cytolytically active CTLs. IL-12 may also augment MHC antigen or adhesion molecule expression during mixed lymphocyte tumor cell culture, mediating this effect directly or through the increased release of TNF-α or IFN-γ. For example, IL-12 can induce NF-κB–dependent priming for IL-12 production by dendritic cells and can induce an IFN-γ independent induction of MHC class II expression (238). Because IL-12 augments both specific and nonspecific antitumor effector cell populations by inducing the production of TNF-α and IFN-γ, IL-12 may be effective as an adjuvant therapeutic cytokine or for specific cancer immunotherapy/gene therapy (236). Indeed, in experimental models, IL-12 has shown potent antitumor activity when used either as the recombinant protein or in gene therapy strategies (239–241). Preclinical studies have utilized a variety of approaches, including direct intratumoral injection of an adenovirus or vaccinia viral vector expressing IL-12, injections of dendritic cells (DCs) expressing IL-12, or delivery of IL-12 via ex vivo transduced fibroblasts (242–245). Sumimoto et al. (246) found IL-12–transduced murine lung cancer cells were superior to GM-CSF or B7-1 (CD80) transfectants for therapeutic antitumor immunity in syngeneic immunocompetent mice. IL-12 gene transfer also mediated systemic (antimetastatic) effects distant from the site of production (247). The therapeutic effects were attributed to a versatile combination of mechanisms involving CD8$^+$ T cells, NK cells, IFN-γ, and inhibition of angiogenesis (247). In a clinical translation setting, Haku et al. (248) found that IL-12 could induce effective cytotoxicity in peripheral blood mononuclear cells from advanced lung cancer patients.

Initial clinical studies with recombinant IL-12 suggested a significant toxicity profile thought to be associated with elevated levels of IFN-γ (249,250). However, Mazzolini et al. (251) have suggested a possible genetic propensity for this toxicity. The IL-12–mediated heightened IFN-γ production may well be advantageous, eliciting the expression of antiangiogenic IFN-γ–inducible chemokines (e.g., inducible protein-10 [IP-10]). In fact, effective antitumor cell-mediated immunity associated with an enhanced IFN-γ secretion mediated by any cytokine gene transfer has the potential to reduce angiogenesis by way of the induction of antiangiogenic chemokines (54,255,256). Kang et al. undertook a phase I dose-escalation clinical trial in which subjects with disseminated cancer received peritumoral injections of IL-12 (p35 and p40)–transduced autologous fibroblasts. In contrast to earlier reports using systemic administration of IL-12, adverse events were limited to mild to moderate pain at the injection site and clinically significant toxicities were not encountered. Transient reductions of injected tumor were observed in four patients and at noninjected distant sites in one melanoma patient (257). The study demonstrates the potential to reduce toxicity by localizing the administration of gene therapy and raises the prospect of eliciting systemic antitumor immunity by local treatment. Although no patients with lung cancer were treated, the findings may advance the possible use of this strategy in this cohort.

Interferon-β (IFN-β) has potent immunostimulatory, antiproliferative, and antiangiogenic activities. In mice bearing established malignant mesothelioma, Odaka et al. (201) found that a single injection of an adenoviral vector expression murine IFN-β led to long-term survival of more than 90% and long-lasting CD8-dependent antitumor immunity. Consistent with these results, additional studies have demonstrated the efficacy of IFN-β in diverse models (202–209), indicating that this is an attractive candidate cytokine for evaluation in lung cancer gene therapy.

Vaccination with irradiated tumor cells engineered to secrete GM-CSF has been shown to stimulate potent, specific, and long-lasting antitumor immunity (188). Because this cytokine can reverse the downmodulation of T-cell responses induced by pulmonary alveolar macrophages, GM-CSF gene therapy is of particular interest for the treatment of lung cancer (258). The efficacy of GM-CSF gene transfer may result from the induction of DC differentiation and proliferation, and the enhanced tumor antigen presentation induced by this cytokine. When delivered in an adenoviral construct to treat Lewis lung carcinoma by Lee et al. (259),

GM-CSF demonstrated induction of a systemic immune response and regression of established tumor. Consistent with the postulated mechanism, GM-CSF expression induced the accumulation of DCs at the tumor site (259). Clinical studies using GM-CSF transduced tumors have shown encouraging preliminary results in melanoma (260) and renal cell (261,262) and prostate (263) carcinomas, and studies in lung cancer are underway.

Parmiani et al. have recently reviewed the use of gene-modified tumor cells in genetic immunotherapy (197). It was concluded that improvements in gene-modified tumor vaccines could be made by (1) the use of tumor cells that expressed molecularly defined antigens, (2) the introduction of T-cell costimulatory molecules in addition to cytokine genes, (3) the use of vector systems that allow for increased cytokine production by the tumor vaccines, and (4) administration of recombinant cytokines systematically in an effort to expand the T cells activated by the vaccines (197). Further studies will be necessary to determine which of these proposed modifications will be clinically helpful in lung cancer studies. Other possible methods of enhancing immune responses with combinations of cytokine genes or in conjunction with drug-sensitizing (suicide) genes are also being evaluated. The use of suicide gene therapy together with cytokine genes may lead to the release and processing of tumor antigens in the setting of heightened immunity, and understanding the relationship of such gene therapies to induction of immune responses has been the focus of several studies (42,43). The use of gene therapy to create tumor vaccines has also been studied in model systems as an adjuvant to surgery (264). It is quite possible that therein lies the greatest utility of these strategies for clinical translation in the treatment of lung cancer.

Abrogating Lung Cancer–Mediated Suppression of Antitumor Immunity

Current research has intensively focused on understanding the complex mechanisms that comprise the immunosuppressive networks in lung cancer. Lung cancer cells may escape host immune responses via several pathways. Tumors elaborate immunosuppressive cytokines, fail to present antigens, and induce signal transduction defects in host T cells and antigen-presenting cells that can lead to anergy. Gene therapy strategies to overcome these immune inhibitory pathways are being developed, and they potentially represent an opportunity for therapies directed at the major clinical obstacle in lung cancer management—the ability to satisfactorily treat metastatic disease. Importantly, genetic immunotherapies that seek to stimulate specific T-cell–mediated antitumor responses do not require uniform gene transfer into every tumor cell. In this respect, these strategies overcome the dominant obstacle to effective gene therapy: the inability to deliver genes efficiently in vivo. However, although uniform gene transfer may not be required, knowledge of the pathways that prevent specific host T-cell responses against the tumor will aid in the design of clinically relevant therapies.

Lung cancer cells elaborate a number of immune-suppressive mediators including type 2 cytokines, PGE2, and TGF-β that may interfere directly with cell-mediated antitumor responses. In addition to producing their own suppressive factors, tumor cells also induce stromal inflammatory cells to release suppressive cytokines in the milieu. As noted, tumor-derived PGE2 orchestrates a detrimental imbalance of cytokines in the tumor environment. Specifically, PGE2 overproduction by NSCLC cells leads to upregulation of lymphocyte and macrophage IL-10 and downregulation of macrophage IL-12 production (229). Whereas IL-10 inhibits cellular immunity, IL-12 induces type 1 cytokine production and effective cell-mediated immunity. To reinstate a favorable immune environment, inhibiting the tumor cells' production of the cytokine-inducible cyclooxygenase (COX-2) capably restores macrophage IL-12 production and reverses the tumor's capacity to induce lymphocyte IL-10 (265). Expectedly, Stolina et al. found that antisense blockade of COX-2 expression caused significant immune-mediated tumor reduction in the Lewis lung carcinoma model (265). Thus, targeting tumor COX-2 expression (the proximal cause of PGE2 overproduction) may be an important target for gene therapy interventions in NSCLC. Further rational support for specifically targeting tumor COX-2 expression is provided by studies implicating its role in increasing tumor invasiveness (266), apoptosis resistance (267), and angiogenesis (268).

Restoration of Functional Antigen Presentation in Lung Cancer Gene Therapy

Lung cancer cells have defects in antigen processing and diminished MHC expression (269,270), rendering them ineffective as antigen-presenting cells (APCs). Consequently, as determined by Huang et al. (271), professional APCs play a major role in the immune response against cancer. This has led to the recent emphasis on the use of professional APCs as the major source of tumor antigen presentation in vivo in genetic immunotherapies. DCs are highly specialized professional APCs armed with a potent capacity to capture, process, and present antigen to T cells (272). Tumor cells interfere with host DC maturation and function (273,274), nullifying this antigen-presenting capacity. To circumvent the in vivo inhibition of DC maturation and function, protocols have been developed that enable DCs to undergo cytokine-stimulated maturation ex vivo. These cells can then be utilized to generate antigen-specific CTL responses, as demonstrated in a variety of models as well as in clinical trials (42,43,158,275–279).

Pulsed or transfected DCs may also be useful in presenting tumor antigens to mount a specific antitumor response in vivo. Currently, although specific tumor antigens may be identified, specific tumor antigen–based therapies are difficult to achieve for human lung cancer (5). To optimize such therapy, however, several points need to be considered. For example, delivery of tumor antigens by ex vivo stimulated DCs may be superior to a single purified peptide in avoiding CTL tolerization (280), and vaccination with multiple tumor antigens may be superior to the use of a single epitope (280,281). Indeed, immunization with individual peptides may contribute to tolerance (280) and consequently an inability of animals to reject antigen-expressing tumors (280). Second, there is strong evidence for immunoselection of antigen-loss variants in human cancer (146,282). One may overcome these limitations by administering competent DCs intratumorally, where the tumor provides an array of immunogenic epitopes in situ. Introducing immune-potentiating cytokine genes (which serve to augment antigen uptake and/or presentation or enhance trafficking to regional and systemic lymph nodes) into these DCs may further boost the antitumor response with resultant systemic antitumor responses and long-term immunity (46). To date, intratumoral therapy with cytokine gene-modified DCs has yielded systemic antitumor effects comparable to those achieved with specific tumor antigen–pulsed DCs. The effect use of DC administered in this manner (i.e., without antigen pulsing ex vivo) implies that cross presentation (the MHC class I–restricted presentation of exogeneous antigens leading to CD8$^+$ T-cell responses [282]) is operative. In fact, DCs may represent the APCs that are predominantly effective in cross presentation (284). Accordingly, tumor antigen delivery systems utilizing cytokine gene-transduced tumor cells and DCs (42,43) or fusion of tumor cells with DCs can induce antitumor immunity (285,286). In a recent clinical study, tumor cell–dendritic cell hybrids administered to 17 patients with metastatic renal cell carcinoma resulted in seven antitumor responses, including four complete antitumor responses (145). These and other results (200,287) suggest that intratumoral DC genetic immunotherapy may be a highly effective alternative to specific tumor antigen immunization strategies. An additional advantage to this approach is that it does not exclude patients on the basis of HLA phenotype or degree or expression of a particular tumor antigen. As such, this therapy could be available to all patients with lung cancer in the appropriate clinical setting and could be utilized alone or in conjunction with other therapeutic modalities. However, additional questions regarding the effective dose, appropriate cytokines, and optimal parameters for monitoring immune responses with this mode of therapy will require ongoing assessment in preclinical models as well as clinical trials.

Another method to colocalize potent APCs with tumor antigens and T cells is to use genes that encode the chemoattractants for these cells. For example, secondary lymphoid chemokine (SLC), normally expressed in high endothelial venules and in T-cell zones of spleen and lymph nodes, strongly attracts naive T cells and DCs, colocalizing these early immune response constituents and culminating in cognate T-cell activation (288–295). The capacity of SLC to chemo-attract DCs (296) is a property shared with other chemokines (297–299). However, SLC may be distinctly advantageous because of its added ability to elicit a TH1 cytokine response in vivo (45) and participate in generating antiangiogenic responses (300). Sharma et al. (45) demonstrated that intratumoral injection of recombinant SLC led to significant CD4 and CD8 lymphocyte-dependent tumor reduction in weakly immunogenic syngeneic murine lung cancer models. More recent studies indicate that SLC is also effective in mediating significant tumor reduction following intra-axillary lymph node (LN) injection in mice bearing spontaneously occurring bronchoalveolar carcinoma (54). In mediating tumor regression, SLC induced extensive CD4 and CD8 lymphocytic infiltration of the pulmonary tumors and marked DC and lymphocyte infiltration of the injected LN sites. The cellular infiltrates were accompanied by the enhanced elongation of TH1 cytokines and increased production of the antiangiogenic chemokines, IFN–IP-10 and monokine induced by IFN-γ (MIG). Consistent with the induction of specific immunity, spleen-derived cells from SLC-treated mice secreted enhanced concentrations of IFN-γ and GM-CSF in response to the autologous tumor (54). These findings provide a strong rationale for further evaluation of SLC in tumor immunity and its use in lung cancer genetic immunotherapy.

D. Targeting Angiogenesis and Metastasis

Thirty years ago, Folkman proposed that tumors have an absolute prerequisite for securing a blood supply to acquire the malignant phenotype (301). That hypothesis has gained wide acceptance, and the complex process of angiogenesis is being gradually unraveled. As such, experimental paradigms suggest somewhat contrasting views on the acquisition of tumor-associated vasculature. One hypothesis is that tumors, and metastases, arise as small avascular entities, existing in a state of equilibrium between proliferation and apoptosis until a "switch" confers to the tumor an angiogenic phenotype (302–304). This concept supports the observation that the transformation from a preneoplastic to the neoplastic state is correlated with the switch to a proangiogenic microenvironment. In this scenario, inhibitors of angiogenesis may function to induce and retain a balance between proliferation and cell death (305). A competing hypothesis suggests that tumor cells select vascular beds for metastatic seeding and grow there by usurping host vessels (306,307); that is, tumors emerge endowed with a vascular supply. In this schema, there is generally a constant pathological cycling of neovascularization and vascular regression that results from disequilibrium between angiogenic and angiostatic factors in the tumor microenvironment. Both models predict that certain pathways are indispensable for the tumor to grow and metastasize. Our purpose in this section is to provide an overview of tumor-associated angiogenesis so that the reader understands the rationale for specific interventions.

Several detailed reviews on the topic of angiogenesis and therapeutic options have recently been published to gain a broader perspective (303,304,308–312).

Angiogenesis, defined as the growth of new capillaries from preexisting vessels, is a pervasive biological phenomenon that is at the core of both physiological and pathological processes. It is distinct from vasculogenesis, or the primordial process for the de novo development of the heart and great vessels. In contrast, further organ development (e.g., brain, lung, kidney) and tumorigenesis occurs by angiogenesis (313), a process whereby new vessels are formed by sprouting from preexisting vessels. Unlike physiological processes (e.g., physiological growth, wound repair, and menstruation), chronic inflammatory fibroproliferative disorders and tumorigenesis are associated with aberrant angiogenesis (311). In this respect, angiogenesis is a prerequisite for successful tumorigenesis and metastatic potential.

Several molecular and cellular mechanisms have been identified as being important for *physiological* angiogenesis, although their role in pathological states is less well defined. First, quiescent endothelial cells are activated or induced to degrade their basement membrane and extracellular matrix, migrate directionally, divide, and organize into functioning capillaries invested by a new basal lamina (314,315). The signal(s) that initiates angiogenesis likely varies with the conditions and may be organ specific (316). Under some conditions, these processes occur rapidly in response to tissue injury, and they do not require new protein synthesis. For instance, during the wound response, angiogenic factors may be released through platelet degranulation (317) or proteolytic digestion of extracellular matrix (318). Inhibitors of angiogenesis, including platelet factor-4, thrombospondins, and proteinases that cause the proteolytic conversion of plasminogen to angiostatin and collagen XVIII to endostatin, may also be released into the wound by cellular components of blood.

Alternatively, *pathological* angiogenic signals may arise from various cellular sources, including tumor cells (319), fibroblasts (320), epithelial cells (321), activated macrophages (322), or endothelial cells themselves (323,324). These signals prompt the detachment of endothelial cells from tight junctions (comprising specific vascular endothelial cadherin molecules, termed VE-Cad), with their neighbors. This dissolution of tight junctions leads to increased pericellular permeability, and the endothelial cells begin to digest and migrate through their basement membrane (325,326). Endothelial cell proliferation is mandatory for effective neovascularization, and most angiogenic factors are also endothelial cell mitogens (327). For initiating sprouting angiogenesis, vascular endothelial growth factor (VEGF), signaling through VEGF receptor 2 (VEGF-R2 or Flk-1) prompts endothelial cell proliferation, vascular dilatation, and leakage (306,310). Proteinase activity is necessary to digest the basement membrane, and inhibitors of matrix metalloproteinases are capable of inhibiting the earliest stages of angiogenesis (328). As the endothelium proliferates, remodeling, maturation, and stabilization of this early vasculature requires the reestablishment of cell-cell tight junctions, mediated by VE-Cad and platelet endothelial cell adhesion molecule (PECAM-1) (329–331), as well as membranes of the angiopoietin family (primarily Ang 1). Ang 2, as well as matrix metalloproteinases (MMPs), facilitate the migration of tumor and endothelial cells through the extracellular matrix (ECM) (332). The ECM is composed of diverse components, including fibrin, fibronectin, vitronectin, and hyaluronan as well as other glycosaminoglycans (333), and migration of cells through this matrix is mediated by a host of surface adhesion receptors that signal cellular motility. For example, $\alpha_v\beta_3$ integrins may be selectively expressed on cells comprising neovasculature but not on quiescent vasculature (334). These integrins mediate promiscuous interactions with a variety of ECM components, and moreover, they bind activated MMP-2 onto the surface of migrating cells, thus facilitating their journey through the ECM (335). In fact, specific inhibition of integrin binding in angiogenic endothelium leads to apoptosis of the endothelial cells (336). Thus, integrin binding and subsequent signaling not only facilitate adhesive and locomotive functions, but also inhibit endothelial cell death (336). If $\alpha_v\beta_3$ integrins are indeed selectively expressed on tumor neovasculature, they may provide a specific molecular target to ablate tumor-associated angiogenesis. Following endothelial cell migration, modeling, and canalization, the neovasculature is fortified with a vessel wall and basement membrane. Members of the platelet-derived growth factor family (PDGF-BB) and transforming growth factor-$\beta1$ (TGF-$\beta1$) mediate important interactions in recruiting smooth muscle cells into the vessel walls (310,337,338). Finally, basement membrane is deposited, and inhibition of collagen biosynthesis can impair basement membrane formation and angiogenesis (339).

After neovascularization is complete, its maintenance requires the *persistence* of a proangiogenic environment; that is, a paracrine imbalance with local angiogenic factors outweighing the expression of angiostatic factors. The specific events and the number of factors capable of regulating this imbalance have not been fully defined. However, it is recognized that once this imbalance favors angiostasis, the angiogenic vessels regress by cellular apoptosis (340), and tissue homeostasis resumes (341). In contrast, tumor-associated neovascularization favors a persistent imbalance of angiogenic over angiostatic factors, with resultant unregulated and aberrant angiogenesis.

The process of angiogenesis and metastasis utilize similar pathways, which are emerging as a frequent target for biological discovery and for developing therapies of lung cancer. The divergent genetic profiles of metastatic versus nonmetastatic lung tumors are being studied by cDNA microarray screening in xenograft lung cancer models (342). Clinically, the expression of VEGF and its receptors has been investigated in lung tumors (343,344). Early reverse transcriptase–polymerase chain reaction (RT-PCR) analyses of VEGF mRNAs revealed transcripts for the secretory forms of VEGF (VEGF121 and VEGF165) in resected lung cancer, and the investigators correlated the VEGF121 mRNA expression with poor prognosis (344). Tsao et al. similarly confirmed VEGF to be a major angiogenic factor in NSCLC (345), and angiogenesis was suspected to be an independent poor prognostic factor in NSCLC. More recently, however, VEGF transcription was again studied in a panel of non–small cell lung cancers using RT-PCR and correlated to tumor angiogenesis using immunohistochemical staining. By multivariate analysis, the VEGF189 mRNA isoform expression ratio was associated with a high intratumoral microvessel count, short survival, and early postoperative relapse. In contrast to earlier reports, VEGF165 and VEGF 206 mRNA showed no statistical correlation with tumor angiogenesis, postoperative relapse time, or survival (346). VEGF expression has additionally been implicated in disorders of serosal permeability associated with malignancy. For example, Zebrowski et al. observed that VEGF could induce permeability and accumulation of malignant pleural effusions in a xenograft nude mouse model (347). Yano et al. extended this observation by demonstrating that pharmacological inhibition of VEGF receptor tyrosine kinase phosphorylation diminished the accumulation of effusions, although this blockade had no effect on the tumor burden per se in this model (348). Therapeutic targeting of the VEGF signaling cascade has also been directed at VEGF receptors. As noted, VEGFR2 (KDR/Flk-1) is believed to mediate endothelial cell mitogenesis and permeability increases. Monoclonal antibody blockade of VEGFR2 inhibited the growth of established human tumor xenografts in mice (349) and potentiated radiation-induced tumor cell death (350). Another strategy utilized an adenoviral vector that encoded a soluble form of VEGFR1 (flt-1) (351) to serve as a soluble decoy. The soluble receptor secreted from AdVEGF-R1–infected cells bound VEGF, with resultant diminished angiogenesis and tumor growth in a variety of xenogeneic lung cancer transplants.

In parallel with the growing list of factors that promote angiogenesis (308,352), there is a matching list of angiogenesis inhibitors (337,353,354). For instance, thrombospondin-1 (TSP-1) is a naturally occurring inhibitor of angiogenesis that limits vessel density in normal tissues and curtails tumor growth, apparently inducing receptor-mediated apoptosis in activated microvascular endothelial cells through signaling mediated through CD36 and the stress-activated MAP kinases (355). Perhaps the most studied angiogenesis inhibitors are angiostatin and endostatin. O'Reilly et al. initially demonstrated that a Lewis lung carcinoma (LLC-LM) primary tumor could suppress the growth of its metastases by generating an inhibitor of angiogenesis (337). Angiostatin, a 38-kD internal fragment of plasminogen, was purified from the serum and urine of mice bearing LLC-LM, and its systemic administration induced regression in a wide variety of malignant tumors in vivo. However, because the tumor cells were not found to express angiostatin or other fragments of plasminogen, the source of this inhibitor remained unclear until it was determined that ECM degradation mediated by tumor MMP-2 resulted in the production of angiostatin (356). In a like manner, Dong et al. demonstrated that melanoma cells that were genetically modified to express GM-CSF upregulate angiostatin production and suppress growth of metastases (357). Interestingly, angiostatin expression by immunohistochemistry has been investigated in non–small cell lung cancer (358). Patients with angiostatin-positive tumors reportedly survived longer than patients with angiostatin-negative tumors in this study population.

In a mechanically similar strategy, gene therapy using recombinant adenovirus expressing murine endostatin resulted in diminished growth of primary tumor and prevented the formation of pulmonary micrometastases by Lewis lung carcinoma (359). In a different model, stable transfectants of RenCa mouse renal carcinoma cells and SW620 human colon carcinoma cells, engineered to secrete constitutively mouse endostatin, demonstrated suppressed growth and impaired metastasis compared to parental controls (360). More recently, however, although inhibition of lung metastasis was observed, mice developed an acute severe toxicity after receiving intravenous delivery of rAds encoding human endostatin. The toxicity appeared to be due to the transgene product rather than due to immunogenicity against the recombinant human protein (361). These observations emphasize the stance that the safety and efficacy profiles of such therapies need to be established in multiple models before they are considered for human clinical trials.

Modulating factors that have been delineated as having a role in angiogenesis and metastasis may engender several rational gene and cell-based therapies for lung cancer. As described, a number of strategies are envisioned to disrupt the angiogenic phenotype (303). In general, trials are underway that employ pharmacological or biological compounds that interfere with angiogenic ligands, their receptors, or their intracellular signaling. Strategies to deliver angiogenic inhibitors (synthetic or by gene delivery) or to destroy selectively the tumor vasculature have had some success in animal models (362,363) and are in early clinical trials. Similarly, compounds that interfere with the response of endothelial cells to angiogenic peptides and/or inhibit the actions of the MMPs have demonstrated utility in animal models (364–366) are also in clinical trials (304,310).

Chemokines in Angiogenesis

An important, yet relatively underappreciated, regulator of angiogenesis is the balance between chemokines in the tumor environment. CXC chemokines are heparin binding proteins that have four highly conserved cysteine amino acid residues in their primary structure, with the first two cysteines being separated by one nonconserved amino acid residue (367–369). Members of this family have dissimilar roles in regulating angiogenesis by virtue of a glutamic acid–leucine-arginine (ELR) motif in their amino terminus that precedes the first cysteine amino acid residue of the primary structure of these cytokines (370). The family members that contain the ELR motif (ELR$^+$) are potent promoters of angiogenesis in physiological concentrations of 1–100 nM (370). In contrast, members of the family that lack the ELR motif (ELR$^-$) and, in general, are interferon inducible, are potent inhibitors of angiogenesis in physiological concentrations of 500 pM to 100 nM (371–373). The angiogenic (ELR$^+$) CXC chemokines include IL-8, epithelial neutrophil-activating protein-78 (ENA-78), and the growth-related genes (GRO-α, -β, and -γ). These molecules possess both endothelial cell chemotactic and proliferative activity, and these effects are distinct from their ability to induce inflammation. Furthermore, ELR$^+$ CXC chemokines induce the expression of the metalloproteinases MMP-2 and MMP-9 by tumor cells, promoting tumorigenesis and metastasis (374,375). All ELR$^+$ CXC chemokines mediate angiogenesis, and the common receptor mediating this effect has been putatively identified as CXCR2 (376–378). In contrast, IFN-inducible (ELR$^-$) CXC chemokines are inhibitors of angiogenesis. These angiostatic members include PF4, monokine induced by INF-γ (MIG), and INF-γ–IP-10 (379–382). Recently, a new ELR$^-$ member of the CXC chemokine family, IFN-inducible T-cell alpha chemoattractant (I-TAC), has been cloned and its expression appears to be induced primarily by IFN-γ (383). I-TAC, similar to IP-10 and MIG, inhibits neovascularization in a rabbit corneal micropocket (CMP) assay in response to either ELR$^+$ CXC chemokines or VEGF, suggesting that all these IFN-inducible ELR-CXC chemokines are potent inhibitors of angiogenesis. In fact, the ability of molecules such as IL-18 and IL-12 that stimulate the expression of IFN may indirectly contribute to angiostasis through the inducible expression of ELR-CXC chemokines. The receptor(s) mediating these angiostatic effects has yet to be characterized, and although ELR-CXC chemokines may have similar mechanisms to mediate the inhibition of bFGF, VEGF, EGF, and ELR$^+$ CXC chemokine-induced angiogenesis, this hypothesis requires additional empirical proof.

The relative importance of angiogenic factors may be variable and tumor specific; however, the ELR$^+$ CXC chemokines unequivocally contribute to tumorigenesis by their angiogenic properties. For instance, IL-8 directly increases angiogenesis and indirectly induces MMP-2 to promote the invasion of tumor cells through the host stroma to enhance metastasis concomitantly (375). In fact, in an ovarian cancer model, the expression of IL-8 was directly correlated with neovascularization and inversely correlated with survival, whereas VEGF expression was only correlated with production of ascites, and no correlation was founded for bFGF with either tumor neovascularization or survival (384). Similarly, IL-8 is markedly elevated and contributes to the overall angiogenic activity of NSCLC (385–387). Tumor-derived IL-8 directly correlates with tumorigenesis, and animals depleted of IL-8 demonstrated a >40% reduction in tumor growth and a reduction in spontaneous metastasis (386). Although IL-8 is important, ENA-78 may be more predictive of NSCLC-derived angiogenesis (388). Analogous to IL8, in a SCID mouse model of human NSCLC tumorigenesis, ENA-78 expression directly correlates with tumor growth, and both tumor growth and spontaneous metastases are markedly attenuated in tumor-bearing animals depleted of ENA-78 (388). There is a reduction of angiogenesis accompanied by an increase in tumor cell apoptosis, whereas proliferation of NSCLC cells is unaffected by the presence of ENA-78 in vitro. However, despite reductions in angiogenesis, tumor growth, and metastases, ENA-78 depletion does not completely inhibit tumor growth. This reflects that the angiogenic activity of NSCLC tumors is related to many overlapping and potentially redundant factors acting in a parallel or serial manner.

Conversely, to test the pathophysiological role of ELR$^-$-CXC angiostatic chemokines, Addison et al. hypothesized that the monokine induced by interferon-γ (MIG) might be an endogeneous inhibitor of NSCLC growth. As expected, the overexpression of MIG by three different strategies, including gene transfer, resulted in a decrease in tumor-derived vessel density and an inhibition of NSCLC tumor growth and metastasis. The findings support the importance of MIG in inhibiting NSCLC tumor growth by attenuation of tumor-derived angiogenesis and demonstrate that gene therapy may be a viable means to deliver and overexpress a potent angiostatic CXC chemokine (389). Similarly, the concentration of another ELR$^-$-CXC angiostatic chemokine, IP-10, was examined in human surgical NSCLC tumor specimens (390). There was an increase in IP-10 from squamous cell carcinoma (SCCA) as compared to lung adenocarcinoma. The difference in the local concentration and bioactivity of IP-10 in the different NSCLC subtypes may be clincally relevant, and may represent a possible mechanism for variations in phenotype exhibited by these subtypes. For example, patient survival is lower, metastatic potential is higher, and evidence of angiogenesis is greater for adenocarcinoma than for SCCA of the lung (391). In an analogous manner, the production of IP-10 from NSCLC subtypes inversely correlated with tumor growth, angiogenesis, and metastatic potential in a SCID mouse model (390).

V. Gene Delivery for Lung Cancer Therapy

In general, efficient gene transfer is requisite for effective gene therapy. There are a number of barriers that intervene in the process of achieving efficient gene transfer/expression. First, the ability of any vector to approach the target cell is contingent on the vector mode of delivery and the anatomical (e.g., endothelium for intravascular delivery) (392,393) and biochemical (e.g., neutralizing antibodies, glycocalyx) (394,395) barriers that must be overcome. Subsequent transduction of target cells is mediated by vector–target cell interactions that utilize vector-specific attachment, internalization, and intracellular transport processes to effect gene delivery to the nucleus (396–399). The transferred gene, as an episome or integrated provirus, must conform to structural requirements that allows it to be appropriately engaged by the transcriptional machinery and be expressed. Efficacious (i.e., therapeutic) gene transfer may be limited in a myriad of ways through this process. For instance, the gene transfer vector may be seized by innate (e.g., macrophages) reticuloendothelial cells (400) or be neutralized by a preexisting or an induced humoral immune response. Upon reaching its target, a vector may not be recognized by its attachment receptor, because the cell has an absolute paucity of such receptors or because the receptor is expressed in a polarized fashion (73,401). Upon entry, a vector may not be capable of escaping the endosomal compartment. And upon gaining entry to the nucleus, gene transcription may be acutely silenced by paracrine or autocrine factors or the cellular immune response (402,403). The resultant inability to achieve efficient transduction in vivo is considered by many to be the major barrier to successful gene therapy.

Although both viral and nonviral vectors (404) continue to be developed, to date, various viral vectors (adenoviral, retroviral, adeno-associated virus [AAV], and herpes simplex virus [HSV]) have demonstrated the best gene transfer efficiency in experimental trials, and this discussion will focus on those viral vectors employed in human trials for lung cancer gene therapy. Retroviral vectors are single-stranded RNA vectors capable of stable integration into the target cell genome, and until recently were the most commonly used vector in human cancer gene therapy trials (405,406). The earlier retroviral vectors were based on the murine Moloney leukemia virus and were capable of transducing only replicating cells. However, newer human lentiviral vectors have also shown the capacity to transduce nondividing cells in vivo (407,408). In addition, modifications of the original amphotropic and ecotropic envelope glycoproteins by the introduction of novel binding (cell attachment) domains have enabled selective targeting of cells in vitro (409,410). Although retroviral vectors have been utilized for in vivo gene delivery in a human NSCLC trial (79), they have shown a limited capacity for in vivo transduction. There are a number of reasons that likely play a role in this regard. For example, these vectors are targets for complement-mediated lysis in vivo (411), and a variety of newer modifications are being made to avoid inactivation by human complement (412). In addition, connective tissue or cell-derived chondroitin sulfate proteoglycans and glycosaminoglycans have been implicated as inhibitors of transduction mediated by amphotropic and vesicular stomatitis virus G-protein (VSV-G)–enveloped retroviral vectors (395). Moreover, most gene therapy strategies that target malignant disease do not require stable transduction and/or long-lasting transgene expression. Thus, for in situ delivery of genes to lung cancer cells, these vectors have generally fallen out of favor. However, these vectors may continue to have utility in ex vivo transduction of tumor or immune cells for the creation of antitumor vaccines or adoptive immunotherapy strategies or for testing a proof of concept in preclinical studies.

Adenoviral (Ad) vectors are double-stranded DNA viruses that function as transiently expressing episomes (413). Ad vectors are advantageous in that they can be concentrated to high titer and have demonstrated the capacity to transfer genes to a variety of cell types in vitro and in vivo. However, both in animal models and in human trials for gene replacement therapy of genetic diseases, the systemic use of Ad vectors has been accomplished by deleterious immune responses (403,414) and, in at least one case, lethal multiorgan failure (415). Although there is no consensus on the exact pathogenesis of the multiorgan failure, an acute cytokine syndrome mediating a systemic inflammatory response appears to be likely. Thus, though it has been suggested that an adjuvant immune response induced by the low-level expression of viral antigens may be of benefit for gene therapy of lung cancer, most investigators believe that noninflammatory vectors are desirable. To this end, "gutted" Ad vectors with all or most of their viral genes removed are being developed (416). In fact, such gutted vectors have enabled prolonged transgene expression with an apparent lack of inflammation in animal models (417). Coadministration of immunosuppressive agents to limit the acute host inflammatory response has been considered, although it is unclear whether this measure serves to augment gene transfer (125). The success of these approaches to ablate Ad-induced inflammation may depend upon the inflammatory capacity of the Ad capsid per se. Early studies by McCoy et al. suggested that inactivated Ad particles were inflammatory at high doses irrespective of whether their genes were expressed (418). More recently, the acute cytokine response to the systemic administration of Ad vectors has been attributed to uptake of the vector by reticuloendothelial cells before viral gene expression takes place (419,420). In addition, a recent report cites that the Ad capsid independently activates NF-κB in renal epithelial cells, also suggesting that overcoming the host response to the Ad vector may not be overcome by deleting viral gene expression (421). It is noteworthy, however, that cationic lipid-DNA complexes also evoke an acute activation of innate immune responses, suggesting that physiochemical characteristics of gene delivery vectors rather than elements specific to the Ad capsid may be responsible (422). Finally, if the Ad capsid is indeed capable of mediating systemic inflammation, perhaps altering the capsid may attenuate this response. In an effort to "hide" the capsid, investigators have conjugated the Ad to polyethylene glycols. Although the impact of this process on the immediate release of cytokines is not known, diminished CTL and antibody responses against the virus were documented (423).

Ad gene transfer into lung cancer cells is heterogeneous and is correlated (in vitro) with the cellular expression of the high-affinity Ad attachment receptor (73). The distribution and "polarity" of these receptors in situ have not been determined for lung cancer. However, the limited clinical trials that have been performed using replication-deficient Ad vectors have been informative in terms of the expected in vivo transduction efficiency. Tursz et al. injected 10^7 or 10^8 plaque-forming units (PFUs) of recombinant Ad (AdRSVLacZ: E1-deleted Ad vector encoding the marker gene β-galactosidase driven by the Rous sarcoma virus promoter) suspension into endobronchial tumors via fiberoptic bronchoscopy (424). Of the six patients with stage IIIB or stage IV NSCLC who received the vector, β-gal expression was seen in three. PCR for Ad genes was positive at day 8 in five of six patients and at 3 months in two patients. In another study, Gahery-Segard et al. assessed the immune response to a single injection of 10^9 PFUs of recombinant Ad expressing Lacz in four patients (425). Vector DNA was detected in three or four patients at 30 and 60 days, and strong antivirus and anti–β-galactosidase–specific CTL responses were observed. The investigators concluded that the transgene is appropriately expressed and that the immunogenecity of the vector does not prohibit specific cellular immune responses against the transgene product (425). Indeed, transgenic-specific responses were long-lived; persisting for over 2 years following vector administration (426). Because evidence of "tumor regression" was noted in these studies using "control" adenoviruses, caution against overinterpreting any transgene-specific "therapeutic response" is warranted. As with all experimental therapeutics, appropriately controlled studies are needed to reach any conclusions that guide therapy.

More recently, larger studies have been undertaken using Ad vectors in combination with conventional chemotherapy (84–86). These studies instilled high doses of Ad directly into the tumors by bronchoscopy or transthoracic computed tomography (CT)–guided injection. Whereas Swisher and Nemunaitis injected doses of up to 10^{11} viral particles, Schuler et al. injected up to 7.5×10^{12} particles (84–86). Although the exact multiplicity of infectious units per cell (Ad-MOI) cannot be determined, assuming that Schuler et al. injected a 3-cm^3 tumor mass, an estimate of the MOI would be 250 viral particles/cell. Using intratumoral transgene mRNA (by RT-PCR of vector-specific sequences) as a marker of transduction efficiency, Swisher and Nemunaitis both reported less than 40–50% expression in a dose-dependent manner, and Schuler et al. reported transgene expression in 68% of subjects after multiple biopsies. Since it may require an MOI greater than 1000 particles/cell to achieve uniform transduction of certain lung cancer subtypes in vitro (73), the dose or delivery scheme of the Ad vectors will need to be changed for more efficient gene delivery in vivo. Alternatively, investigators may continue to attempt to target lung cancer transductionally using retargeted vectors that are specific for ligands on lung cancer cells, or transcriptionally target the expression of the transgene to these cells by incorporating lung cancer–specific promoter or enhancer sequences. Unfortunately, such specific cell surface ligands or regulatory sequences have yet to be identified or validated.

VI. Summary

This chapter has focused on the developing field of genetic therapies for lung cancer. Although the field is still in its infancy, investigators in gene therapy have made notable achievements in enabling gene transfer and expression. However, there are significant shortcomings that are due, in part, to an incomplete understanding of the molecular pathogenesis of lung cancer. In addition, the implementation of genetic therapies continues to be limited by the lack of efficient and specific gene delivery systems. To overcome these limitations, investigators have tailored the therapeutic approaches to minimize the limitations of current gene delivery vectors. For example, many strategies are emerging that employ ex vivo cellular gene modification. Because there persists a strong belief that gene therapy has the versatility to respond quickly to discoveries underlying molecular pathogenesis, the paradigms in which gene transfer is utilized to achieve a therapeutic aim continue to expand. Improvements in gene transfer technologies and identification of relevant hurdles to effective gene therapy in translational studies will bring many of these strategies to the clinical arena.

References

1. Landis SH, Murray T, Bolden S, Wingo PA. Cancer statistics. CA Cancer J Clin 1999; 49:8–31.
2. Jett J. Screening for lung cancer in high risk groups. Semin Respir Crit Care Med 2000; 21:385–392.
3. Greenlee RT, Murray T, Bolden S, Wingo PA. Cancer statistics, 2000. CA Cancer J Clin 2000; 50:7–33.
4. Haura EB. Treatment of advanced non–small-cell lung cancer: a review of current randomized clinical trials and an examination of emerging therapies. Cancer Control 2001; 8:326–336.
5. Dubinett SM, Miller PW, Sharma S, Batra RK. Gene therapy for lung cancer. Hematol Oncol Clin North Am 1998; 12:569–594.
6. Seller TA, Bailey-Wilson JE, Elston RC, et al. Evidence for Mendelian inheritance in the pathogenesis of lung cancer. J Natl Cancer Inst 1990; 82:1272–1279.
7. Schwartz AG, Yang P, Swanson GM. Familial risk of lung cancer among nonsmokers and their relatives. Am J Epidemiol 1996; 144:554–562.
8. Carbone D. The biology of lung cancer. Semin Oncol 1997; 24:388–401.
9. Salgia R, Skarin AT. Molecular abnormalities in lung cancer. J Clin Oncol 1998; 16:1207–1217.
10. Sethi T. Science, medicine, and the future. Lung cancer. BMJ 1997; 314:652–655.
11. Shopland DR, Eyre JH, Pechacek TF. Smoking-attributable cancer mortality in 1991: is lung cancer now the leading cause of death among smokers in the United States? J Natl Cancer Inst 1991; 83:1142–1148.

12. Sozzi G, Miozzo M, Pastorino U, et al. Genetic evidence for an independent origin of multiple preneoplastic and neoplastic lung lesions. Cancer Res 1995; 55:135–140.

13. Franklin WA, Gazdar AF, Haney J, et al. Widely dispersed *p53* mutation in respiratory epithelium. A novel mechanism for field carcinogenesis. J Clin Invest 1997; 100:2133–2137.

14. Mao L, Lee JS, Kurie JM, et al. Clonal genetic alterations in the lungs of current former smokers. J Natl Cancer Inst 1997; 89:857–862.

15. Wistuba I II, Lam S, Behrens C, et al. Molecular damage in the bronchial epithelium of current and former smokers. J Natl Cancer Inst 1997; 89:1366–1373.

16. Batra R, Sharma S, Dubinett S. New gene and cell-based therapies for lung cancer. Semin Respir Med 2000; 21:463–473.

17. Slebos R, Kibbelaar R, Dalesio O, et al. K-ras oncogene activation as a prognostic marker in adenocarcinoma of the lung. N Engl J of Med 1990: 323:561–565.

18. Mitsudomi T, Steinberg SM, Nau MM, et al. *p53* Gene mutations in non–small-cell lung cancer cell lines and their correlation with the presence of ras mutations and clinical features. Oncogene 1992; 7:171–180.

19. Kamb A, Shattuck-Eidens D, Eeles R, et al. Analysis of the *p16* gene (CDKN2) as a candidate for the chromosome 9p melanoma susceptibility locus. Nat Genet 1994; 8:23–26.

20. Shapiro GI, Edwards CD, Kobzik L, et al. Reciprocal Rb in activation and p16INK4 expression in primary lung cancers and cell lines. Cancer Res 1995; 55:505–509.

21. Sozzi G, Veronese ML, Negrini M, et al. The *FHIT* gene 3p14.2 is abnormal in lung cancer. Cell 1996; 85:17–26.

22. Pezzella F, Turley H, Kuzu I, et al. bcl-2 Protein in non–small cell lung carcinoma. N Engl J Med 1993; 329:690–694.

23. Kern JA, Schwartz DA, Norberg JE, et al. p185neu Expression in human lung adenocarcinomas predicts shortened survival. Cancer Res 1990; 50:5184–5187.

24. Sundaresan V, Ganly P, Hasleton P, et al. p53 And chromosome 3 abnormalities, characteristic of malignant lung tumours, are detectable in preinvasive lesions of the bronchus. Oncogene 1992; 7:1989–1997.

25. Keith RL, Miller YE, Gemmill RM, et al. Angiogenic squamous dysplasia in bronchi of individuals at high risk for lung cancer. Clin Cancer Res 2000; 6:1616–1625.

26. Marchetti A, Pellegrini S, Bertacca G, et al. *FHIT* and *p53* gene abnormalities in bronchioloalveolar carcinomas. Correlations with clinicopathological data and K-ras mutations. J Pathol 1998; 184:240–246.

27. Kerr KM, Carey FA, King G, Lamb D. Atypical alveolar hyperplasia: relationship with pulmonary adenocarcinoma, p53, and c-erB-2 expression. J Pathol 1994; 174: 249–256.

28. Westra WH, Baas IO, Hruban RH, et al. K-ras oncogene activation in atypical alveolar hyperplasias of the human lung. Cancer Res 1996; 56:2224–2228.

29. Cooper CA, Carby FA, Bubb VJ, Lamb D, Kerr KM, Wyllie AH. The pattern of K-ras mutation in pulmonary adenocarcinoma defines a new pathway of tumour development in the human lung. J Pathol 1997; 181:401–404.

30. Mao L, Hruban RH, Boyle JO, Tockman M, Sidransky D. Detection of oncogene

mutations in sputum precedes diagnosis of lung cancer. Cancer Res 1994; 54:1634–1637.

31. Malkinson AM. Molecular comparison of human and mouse pulmonary adenocarcinomas. Exp Lung Res 1998; 24:541–555.

32. Yesner R. Pathogenesis and pathology. Clin Chest Med 1993; 14:17–30.

33. Tuveson DA, Jacks T. Modeling human lung cancer in mice: similarities and shortcomings. Oncogene 1999; 18:5318–5324.

34. Witschi H. Tobacco smoke as a mouse lung carcinogen. Exp Lung Res 1998; 24:385–394.

35. Malkinson A, Belinsky S. The use of animal models in preclinical studies. In: Pass H, Mitchell J, Johnson D, Turrisi A, eds. Lung Cancer: Principles and Practice. Philadelphia: Lippincott-Raven, 1996:273–284.

36. Stoner GD. Introduction to mouse lung tumorigenesis. Exp Lung Res 1998; 24:375–383.

37. Shimkin MB, Stoner GD. Lung tumors in mice: application to carcinogenesis bioassay. Adv Cancer Res 1975; 21:1–58.

38. Malkinson AM. Primary lung tumors in mice: an experimentally manipulable model of human adenocarcinoma. Cancer Res 1992; 52:2670s–2676s.

39. Hecht SS, Morse MA, Amin S, et al. Rapid single-dose model for lung tumor induction in A/J mice by 4-(methylnitrosamino)-1-(3-pyridyl)-1-butanone and the effect of diet. Carcinogenesis 1989; 10:1901–1904.

40. Kim SH, Lee CS. Induction of benign and malignant pulmonary tumours in mice with benzo(a)pyrene. Anticancer Res 1996; 16:465–470.

41. Witschi H. Successful and not so successful chemoprevention of tobacco smoke-induced lung tumors. Exp Lung Res 2000; 26:743–755.

42. Sharma S, Miller P, Stolina M, et al. Multi-component gene therapy vaccines for lung cancer: effective eradication of established murine tumors in vivo with interleukin 7/herpes simplex thymidine kinase–transduced autologous tumor and ex vivo–activated dendritic cells. Gene Ther 1997; 4:1361–1370.

43. Miller PW, Sharma S, Stolina M, et al. Dendritic cells augment granulocyte-macrophage colony-stimulating factor (GM-CSF)/herpes simplex virus thymidine kinase–mediated gene therapy of lung cancer. Cancer Gene Ther 1998; 5:380–389.

44. Sharma S, Stolina M, Lin Y, et al. T cell–derived IL-10 promotes lung cancer growth by suppressing both T cell and APC function. J Immunol 1999; 163:5020–5028.

45. Sharma S, Stolina M, Luo J, et al. Secondary lymphoid tissue chemokine mediates T cell–dependent antitumor responses in vivo. J Immunol 2000; 164:4558–4563.

46. Miller PW, Sharma S, Stolina M, et al. Intratumoral administration of adenoviral interleukin 7 gene-modified dendritic cells augments specific antitumor immunity and achieves tumor eradication. Hum Gene Ther 2000; 11:53–65.

47. Stolina M, Sharma S, Lin Y, et al. Specific inhibition of cyclooxygenase 2 restores antitumor immunity by altering the balance of IL-10 and IL-12 synthesis. J Immunol 2000; 164:361–370.

48. Compere SJ, Baldacci P, Jaenisch R. Oncogenes in transgenic mice. Biochim Biophys Acta 1988; 948:129–149.

49. Kao C, Huang J, Wu SQ, Hauser P, Reznikoff CA. Role of SV40 antigen binding

to pRB and p53 in multistep transformation in vitro of human uroepithelial cells. Carcinogenesis 1993; 14:2297–2302.

50. Wikenheiser K, Clark J, Linnoila R, Stahlman M, Whitsett J. Simian virus 40 large T antigen directed by transcriptional elements of the human surfactant protein C gene produces pulmonary adenocarcinomas in transgenic mice. Cancer Res 1992; 52:5342–5352.

51. Wikenheiser K, Whitsett J. Tumor progression and cellular differentiation of pulmonary adenocarcinomas in SV40 large T antigen transgenic mice. Am J Respir Cell Mol Biol 1997; 16:713–723.

52. Levine AJ, Momand J. Tumor suppressor genes: the p53 and retinoblastoma sensitivity genes and gene products. Biochim Biophys Acta 1990; 1032:119–136.

53. Magdaleno S, Wang G, Mireles V, Ray M, Finegold M, Demayo F. Cyclin-dependent kinase inhibitor expression in pulmonary clara cells transformed with SV40 large t antigen in transgenic mice. Cell Growth Diff 1997; 8:145–155.

54. Sharma S, Stolina M, Zhu L, et al. Secondary lymphoid organ chemokine reduces pulmonary tumor burden in spontaneous murine bronchoalveolar cell carcinoma. Cancer Res 2001; 61:6406–6412.

55. Johnson L, Mercer K, Greenbaum D, et al. Somatic activation of the K-ras oncogene causes early onset lung cancer in mice. Nature 2001; 410:1111–1116.

56. Garcia SB, Park HS, Novelli M, Wright NA. Field cancerization, clonality, and epithelial stem cells: the spread of mutatee clones in epithelial sheets. J Pathol 1999; 187:61–81.

57. Berns A. Cancer: improved mouse models. Nature 2001; 410:1043–1044.

58. Rygaard J, Povlsen CO. Heterotransplantation of a human malignant tumour to "nude" mice. Acta Pathol Microbiol Scand 1969; 77:758–760.

59. Pantelouris EM. Absence of thymus in a mouse mutant. Nature 1968; 217:370–371.

60. Povlsen CO, Visfeldt J, Rygaard J, Jensen G. Growth patterns and chromosome constitutions of human malignant tumours after long-term serial transplantation in nude mice. Acta Pathol Microbiol Scand [A] 1975; 83:709–716.

61. Shimosata Y, Kameya T, Hirohashi S. Growth, morphology, and function of xeno-transplanted human tumors. Pathol Annu 1979; 14 Pt 2:215–257.

62. Fidler IJ. Rationale and methods for the use of nude mice to study the biology and therapy of human cancer metastasis. Cancer Metatasis Rev 1986; 5:29–49.

63. Bepler G, Neumann K. Nude mouse xenografts as in vivo models for lung carcinomas. In Vivo 1990; 4:309–315.

64. Kyriazis AP, DiPersio L, Michael JG, Pesce AJ. Influence of the mouse hepatitis virus (MHV) infection on the growth of human tumors in the athymic mouse. Int J Cancer 1979; 23:402–409.

65. Reed ND, Manning JK, Baker PJ, Ulrich JT. Analysis of 'thymus-independent' immune responses using nude mice. In: Rygaard J, Povlsen CO, eds. Proceedings of the First International Workshop on Nude Mice. Stuttgart: Verlag 1974: 19:19.

66. Hann N. Role of natural killer cells in control of cancer metastasis. Cancer Metastasis Rev 1982; 1:45–64.

67. Bosma GC, Custer RP, Bosma MJ. A severe combined immunodeficiency mutation in the mouse. Nature 1983; 301:527–530.

68. Bosma MJ, Carroll AM. The SCID mouse mutant: definition, characterization, and potential uses. Annu Rev Immunol 1991; 9:323–350.

69. Reddy S, Piccione D, Takita H, Bankert RB. Human lung tumor growth established in the lung and subcutaneous tissue of mice with severe combined immunodeficiency. Cancer Res 1987; 47:2456–2460.

70. Mak TW, Rahemtulla A, Schilham M, Koh DR, Fung-Leung WP. Generation of mutant mice lacking surface expression of CD4 or CD8 by gene targeting. J Autoimmun 1992; 5(Suppl A):55–59.

71. Koller BH, Smithies O. Altering genes in animals by gene targeting. Annu Rev Immunol 1992; 10:705–730.

72. Hoganson D, Matsui H, Batra R, Boucher R. Toxin gene-mediated growth inhibition of lung adenocarcinoma in an animal model of pleural malignancy. Hum Gene Ther 1998; 9:1143–1156.

73. Batra R, Olsen J, Pickles R, Hoganson S, Boucher R. Transduction of non–small cell lung cancer cells by adeniviral and retroviral vectors. Am J Cell Mol Biol 1998; 18:402–410.

74. Nishio M, Koshikawa T, Kuroishi T, et al. Prognostic significance of abnormal p53 accumulation in primary, resected non–small-cell lung cancers. J Clin Oncol 1996; 14:497–502.

75. Kern S, Pietenpol J, Thiagalingam S, Seymour A, Kinzler K, Vogelstein B. Oncogenic forms of p53 inhibit p53-regulated gene expression. Science 1992; 256:827–830.

76. Joseph B, Lewensohn R, Zhivotovsky B. Role of apoptosis in the response of lung carcinomas to anti-cancer treatment. Ann NY Acad Sci 2000; 926:204–216.

77. McGill G, Fisher DE. p53 and cancer therapy: a double-edged sword. J Clin Invest 1999; 104:223–225.

78. Fujiwara T, Cai D, Georges R, Mukhopadhyay T, Grimm E, Roth J. Therapeutic effect of a retroviral wild-type p53 expression vector in an orthotopic lung cancer model. J Natl Cancer Inst 1994; 86:1458–1462.

79. Roth JA, Nguyen D, Lawrence DD, et al. Retrovirus-mediated wild-type p53 gene transfer to tumors of patients with lung cancer. Nat Med 1996; 2:985–991.

80. Freeman SM, Abboud CN, Whartenby KA, et al. The "bystander effect": tumor regression when a fraction of the tumor mass is genetically modified. Cancer Res 1993; 53:5274–5283.

81. Nishizaki M, Fujiwara T, Tanida T, et al. Recombinant advenovirus expressing wild-type p53 is antiangiogenic: a proposed mechanism for bystander effect. Clin Cancer Res 1999; 5:1015–1023.

82. Chen H, Carbone D. p53 As a target for anti-cancer immunotherapy. Mol Med Today 1997; 3:160–167.

83. Vierboom MP, Nijman HW, Offringa R, et al. Tumor eradication by wild-type p53-specific cytotoxic T lymphocytes. J Exp Med 1997; 186:695–704.

84. Swisher SG, Roth JA, Nemunaitis J, et al. Adenivirus-mediated p53 gene transfer in advanced non–small-cell lung cancer. J Natl Cancer Inst 1999; 91:763–771.

85. Nemunaitis J, Swisher SG, Timmons T, et al. Adenovirus-mediated p53 gene transfer in sequence with cisplatin to tumors of patients with non–small-cell lung cancer. J Clin Oncol 2000; 18:609.

86. Schuler M, Herrmann R, De Greve J, et al. Adenovirus-mediated wild-type p53 gene transfer in patients receiving chemotherapy for advanced non–small-cell lung cancer: results of a multicenter phase II study. J Clin Oncol 2001; 19:1750–1758.

87. Bischoff JR, Kirn DH, Williams A, et al. An adenovirus mutant that replicates selectively in p53-deficient human tumor cells. Science 1996; 274:373–376.

88. Heise C, Sampson-Johannes A, Williams A, McCormick F, Von Hoff D, Kirn D. ONYX-015, an E1B gene-attenuated adenovirus, causes tumor-specific cytolysis and antitumoral efficacy that can be augmented by standard chemotherapeutic agents. Nat Med 1997; 3:639–645.

89. Hall AR, Dix BR, O'Carroll SJ, Braithwaite AW. p53-Dependent cell death/apoptosis is required for a productive adenovirus infection. Nat Med 1998; 4:1068–1072.

90. Harada JN, Berk AJ. p53-Independent and -dependent requirements for E1B-55K in adenovirus type 5 replication. J Virol 1999; 73:5333–5344.

91. Rothmann T, Hengstermann A, Whitaker NJ, Scheffner M, zur Hausen H. Replication of ONYX-015, a potential anticancer adenovirus, is independent of p53 status in tumor cells. J Virol 1998; 72:9470–9478.

92. Nemunaitis J, Cunningham C, Buchanan A, et al. Intravenous infusion of a replication-selective adenovirus (ONYX-015) in cancer patients: safety, feasibility and biological activity. Gene Ther 2001; 8:746–759.

93. Lambright E, Kang E, Force S, et al. Effect of preexisting anti-herpes immunity on efficacy of herpes simplex viral therapy in a murine intraperitoneal tumor model. Mol Ther 2000; 2:387–393.

94. Gibbs JB, Oliff A, Kohl NE. Farnesyltransferase inhibitors: Ras research yields a potential cancer therapeutic. Cell 1994; 77:175–178.

95. Mukhopadhyay T, Tainsky M, Cavender A, et al. Specific inhibition of K-ras expression and tumorigenicity of lung cancer cells by antisense RNA. Cancer Res 1991; 51:1744–1748.

96. Roth J. Modification of tumor suppressor gene expression and induction of apoptosis in non–small cell lung cancer (NSCLC) with an adenovirus vector expressing wildtype p53 and cisplatin. Hum Gene Ther 1996; 7:1013–1030.

97. Zhang Y, Nemunaitis J, Tong A. Generation of a ribozyme-adenoviral vector against K-ras mutant human lung cancer cells. Mol Biotechnol 2000; 15:39–49.

98. Zhang Z, Wang Y, Vikis HG, et al. Wildtype Kras2 can inhibit lung carcinogenesis in mice. Nat Genet 2001; 29:25–33.

99. Yamamoto T, Ikawa S, Akiyama T, et al. Similarity of protein encoded by the human c-erbB-2 gene to the epidermal growth factor receptor. Nature 1986; 319:230–234.

100. Deshane J, Siegal G, Alvarez R, et al. Targeted tumor killing via an intracellular antibody against erbB-2. J Clin Invest 1995; 96:2980–2989.

101. Agus D, Bunn PJ, Franklin W, Garcia M, Ozols R. HER-2/neu as a theraeutic target in non-small cell lung cancer, prostate cancer, and ovarian cancer. Semin Oncol 2000; 27:53–63.

102. Craig C, Kim M, Ohri E, et al. Effects of adenovirus-mediated p16INK4A expres-

sion on cell cycle arrest are determined by endogenous p16 and Rb status in human cancer cells. Oncogene 1998; 16:265–272.

103. Brambilla E, Gazzeri S, Lantuejoul S, et al. p53 mutant immunophenotype and deregulation of p53 transcription pathway (Bcl2, Bax, and Waf1) in precursor bronchial lesions of lung cancer. Clin Cancer Res 1998; 4:1609–1618.

104. Ziegler A, Luedke GH, Fabbro D, Altmann KH, Stahel RA, Zangemeister-Wittke U. Induction of apoptosis in small-cell lung cancer by an antisense oligodeoxynucleotide targeting the Bcl-2 coding sequence. J Natl Cancer Inst 1997; 89:1027–1036.

105. Kagawa S, He C, Gu J, et al. Antitumor activity and bystander effects of the tumor necrosis factor-related apoptosis-inducing ligand (TRAIL) gene. Cancer Res 2001; 61:3330–3338.

106. Reed JC. The survivin saga goes in vivo. J Clin Invest 2001; 108:965–969.

107. Altieri DC, Marchisio PC, Marchisio C. Survivin apoptosis: an interloper between cell death and cell proliferation in cancer. Lab Invest 1999; 79:1327–1333.

108. Ambrosini G, Adida C, Altieri DC. A novel anti-apoptosis gene, survivin, expressed in cancer and lymphoma. Nat Med 1997; 3:917–921.

109. Monzo M, Rosell R, Felip E, et al. A novel anti-apoptosis gene: re-expression of survivin messenger RNA as a prognosis marker in non–small-cell lung cancers. J Clin Oncol 1999; 17:2100–2104.

110. Olie RA, Simoes-Wust AP, Baumann B, et al. A novel antisense oligonucleotide targeting survivin expression induces apoptosis and sensitizes lung cancer cells to chemotherapy. Cancer Res 2000; 60:2805–2809.

111. Mesri M, Wall NR, Li J, Kim RW, Altieri DC. Cancer gene therapy using a surviving mutant adenovirus. J Clin Invest 2001; 108:981–990.

112. Hoganson D, Bantra R, Olsen J, Boucher R. Comparison of the effects of three different toxin genes and their levels of expression on cell growth and bystander effect in lung carcinoma. Cancer Res 1996; 56:1315–1323.

113. Imaizumi K, Hasegawa Y, Kawabe T, et al. Bystander tumoricidal effect and gap junctional communication in lung cancer cell lines. Am J Respir Cell Mol Biol 1998; 18:205–212.

114. Nanni P, De Giovanni C, Nicoletti G, et al. The immune response elicited by mammary adenocarcinoma cells transduced with interferon-γ and cytosine deaminase genes cures lung metastases by parental cells. Hum Gene Ther 1998; 9:217–224.

115. Consalvo M, Mullen CA, Modesti A, et al. 5-fluorocytosine-induced eradication of murine adenocarcinomas engineered to express the cytosine deaminase suicide gene requires host immune competence and leaves an efficient memory. J Immunol 1995; 154:5302–5312.

116. Tanaka M, Inase N, Miyake S, Yoshizawa Y. Neuron specific enolase promoter for suicide gene therapy in small cell lung carcinoma. Anticancer Res 2001; 21: 291–294.

117. Osaki T, Tanio Y, Tachibana I, et al. Gene therapy for carcinoembryonic antigen-producing human lung cancer cells by cell type–specific expression of herpes simplex virus thymidine kinase gene. Cancer Res 1994; 54:5258–5261.

118. Inase N, Horita K, Tanaka M, Miyake S, Ichioka M, Yoshizawa Y. Use of gastrin-

releasing peptide promoter for specific expression of thymidine kinase gene in small-cell lung carcinoma cells. Int J Cancer 2000; 85:716–719.

119. Zhang L, Wikenheiser K, Whitsett J. Limitations of retrovirus-mediated HSV-tk gene transfer to pulmonary adenocarcinoma cells in vitro and in vivo. Hum Gene Ther 1997; 8:563–574.

120. Hwang HC, Smythe WR, Elshami AA, et al. Gene therapy using adenivorus carrying the herpes simplex–thymidine kinase gene to treat in vivo models of human malignant mesothelioma and lung cancer. Am J Respir Cell Mol Biol 1995; 13: 7–16.

121. Smythe WR, Hwang HC, Amin KM, et al. Use of recombinant adenovirus to transfer the herpes simplex virus thymidine kinase (HSVtk) gene to thoracic neoplasms: an effective in vitro drug sensitization system. Cancer Res 1994; 54:2055–2059.

122. Schwarzenberger P, Lei D, Freeman S, et al. Antitumor activity with the HSV-tk-gene–modified cell line PA-1-STK in malignant mesothelioma. Am J Respir Cell Mol Biol 1998; 19:333–337.

123. Schwarzenberger P, Harrison L, Weinacker A, et al. The treatment of malignant mesothelioma with a gene modified cancer cell line: a phase I study. Hum Gene Ther 1998; 9:2641–2649.

124. Sterman D, Treat J, Litzky L, et al. Adenovirus-mediated herpes simplex virus thymidine kinase/ganciclovir gene therapy in patient with localized malignancy: results of a phase I clinical trial in malignant mesothelioma. Hum Gene Ther 1998; 9:1083–1092.

125. Sterman D, Molnar-Kimber K, Iyengar T, et al. A pilot study for systemic corticosteroid administration in conjunction with intrapleural adenoviral vector administration in patients with malignant pleural mesothelioma. Cancer Gene Ther 2000; 7:1511–1518.

126. Nishizaki M, Meyn RE, Levy LB, et al. Synergistic inhibition of human lung cancer cell growth by adenovirus-mediated wild-type p53 gene transfer in combination with docetaxel and radiation therapeutics in vitro and in vivo. Clin Cancer Res 2001; 7:2887–2897.

127. Kim JH, Kim SH, Brown SL, Freytag SO. Selective enhancement by an antiviral agent of the radiation-induced cell killing of human glioma cells transduced with HSV-tk gene. Cancer Res 1994; 54:6053–6056.

128. Anello R, Cohen S, Atkinson G, Hall S. Adenovirus mediated cytosine deaminase gene transduction and 5-fluorocytosine therapy sensitizes mouse prostate cancer cells to irradiation. J Urol 2000; 164:2173–2177.

129. Wildner O, Blaese R, Morris J. Synergy between the herpes complex virus tk/ganiciclovir prodrug suicide system and the topoisomerase I inhibitor topotecan. Human Gene Ther 1999; 10:2679–2687.

130. Sutherland R. Managing cancer through synergy. Radiation and molecular medicine. Adm Radiol j 1996; 15:21–27.

131. Nielsen L, Lipari P, Dell J, Gurnani M, Hajian G. Adenovirus-mediated p53 gene therapy and paclitaxel have synergistic efficacy in models of human head and neck, ovarian, prostate, and breast cancer. Clin Cancer Res 1998; 4:835–846.

132. McBride W, Dougherty G. Radiotherapy for genes that cause cancer. Nat Med 1995; 1:1215–1217.

133. McIlwrath A, Vasey P, Ross G, Brown R. Cell cycle arrests and radiosensitivity of human tumor cell lines: dependence on wild-type p53 for radiosensitivity. Cancer Res 1994; 54:3718–3722.

134. Wang C-Y, Mayo MW, Baldwin ASJ. TNF- and cancer therapy-induced apoptosis: potentiation by inhibition of NF-κB. Science 1996; 274:784–787.

135. Baldwin A. Control of oncogenesis and cancer therapy resistance by the transcription factor NF-κB. J Clin Invest 2001; 107:241–246.

136. Wang C, Cusack JJ, Liu R, Baldwin AJ. Control of inducible chemoresistance: enhanced anti-tumor therapy through increased apoptosis by inhibition of NF-κB. Nat Med 1999; 5:412–417.

137. Batra RK, Guttridge DC, Bennner DA, Dubinett SM, Baldwin AS, Boucher RC. IkappaBalpha gene transfer is cytotoxic to squamous-cell lung cancer cells and sensitizes them to tumor necrosis factor-alpha-mediated cell death. Am J Respir Cell Mol Biol 1999; 21:238–245.

138. Jones D, Broad R, Madrid L, Baldwin AJ, Mayo M. Inhibition of NF-kappaB sensitizes non-small cell lung cancer cells to chemotherapy-induced apoptosis. Ann Thorac Surg 2000; 70:930–936.

139. Tabata M, Tabata R, Grabowski D, Bukowski R, Ranapathi M, Ganapathi R. Roles of NF-kappaB and 26 S proteasome in apoptotic cell death induced by topoisomerase I and II poisons in human nonsmall cell lung carcinoma. J Biol Chem 2001; 276:8029–8036.

140. Jiang Y, Cui L, Yie T, Rom W, Cheng H, Tchou-Wong K. Inhibition of anchorage-independent growth and lung metastasis of A549 lung carcinoma cells by IκBβ. Oncogene 2001; 20:2254–2263.

141. Stickle RL, Epperly MW, Klein E, Bray JA, Greenberger JS. Prevention of irradiation-induced esophagitis by plasmid/liposome delivery of the human manganese superoxide dismutase transgene. Radiat Oncol Invest 1999; 7:204–217.

142. O'Reilly EM, Ilson DH, Saltz LB, Heelan R, Martin L, Kelsen DP. A phase II trial of interferon alpha-2a and carboplatin in patients with advanced malignant mesothelioma. Cancer Invest 1999; 17:195–200.

143. Sterman DH, Kaiser LR, Albelda SM. Advances in the treatment of malignant pleural mesothelioma. Chest 1999; 116:504–520.

144. Dubinett S. The immune response of lung tumors and the effects of cytokine administration on pulmonary immune cells. In: Kradin R, Robinson B, eds. Immunopathology of Lung Disease. Boston: Butterworth-Heinemann, 1996:469–490.

145. Kugler A, Stuhler G, Walden P, et al. Regression of human metastatic renal cell carcinoma after vaccination with tumor cell-dendritic cell hybrids. Nat Med 2000; 6:332–336.

146. Thurner B, Haendle I, Roder C, et al. Vaccination with mage-3A1 peptide-pulsed mature, monocyte-derived dendritic cells expand specific cytotoxic T cells and induces regression of some metastases in advanced stage IV melanoma. J Exp Med 19099; 190:1669–1678.

147. Van Pel A, Boon T. Protection against a nonimmunogenic mouse leukemia by an immunogenic variant obtained by mutagenesis. Proc Natl Acad Sci USA 1982; 79:4718–4722.

148. Boon T, Old L. Cancer tumor antigens. Curr Opin Immunol 1997; 9:681–683.

149. Boon T, Gajewski TF, Coulie PG. From defined human tumor antigens to effective immunization? Immunol Today 1995; 16:334–336.

150. Boon T, van der Bruggen P. Human tumor antigens recognized by T lymphocytes. J Exp Med 1996; 183:725–729.

151. Pardoll D. Cancer vaccines. Nat Med 1998; 4 (5 Suppl):525–531.

152. Rosenberg SA. A new era for cancer immunotherapy based on the genes that encode cancer antigens. Immunity 1999; 10:281–287.

153. De Plaen E, Lurquin C, Lethe B, et al. Identification of genes coding for tumor antigens recognized by cytolytic T lymphocytes. Methods 1997; 12:125–142.

154. Cox AL, Skipper J, Chen Y, et al. Identification of a peptide recognized by five melanoma-specific human cytotoxic T cell lines. Science 1994; 264:716–719.

155. Gilboa E. The makings of a tumor rejection antigen. Immunity 1999; 11:263–270.

156. Mandelboim O, Berke G, Fridkin M, Feldman M, Eisenstein M, Eisenbach L. CTL induction by a tumor-associated antigen octapeptide derived from a murine lung carcinoma. Nature 1994; 369:67–71.

157. Mandelboim O, Vaidai E, Fridkin M, et al. Regression of established murine carcinoma metastases following vaccination with tumour-associated antigen peptides. Nat Med 1995; 1:1179–1183.

158. Mayordomo JI, Zorina T, Storkus WJ, et al. Bone marrow-derived dendritic cells pulsed with synthetic tumor peptides elicit protective and therapeutic antitumor immunity. Nat Med 1995; 1:1297–1302.

159. Yewdell JW, Bennink JR. Immunodominance in major histocompatibility complex class I-restricted T lymphocyte responses. Annu Rev Immunol 1999; 17:51–88.

160. Ciernik IF, Berzofsky JA, Carbone DP. Human lung cancer cells endogenously expressing mutant p53 process and present the mutant epitope and are lysed by mutant-specific cytotoxic T lymphocytes. Clin Cancer Res 1996; 2:877–882.

161. Waheed I, Guo ZS, Chen GA, Weiser TS, Nguyen DM, Schrump DS. Antisense to SV40 early gene region induces growth arrest and apoptosis in T-antigen-positive human pleural mesothelioma cells. Cancer Res 1999; 59:6068–6073.

162. Nakao M, Schichijo S, Imaizumi T, et al. Identification of a gene coding for a new squamous cell carcinoma antigen recognized by the CTL. J Immunol 2000; 164:2565–2574.

163. Iwamoto O, Nagao Y, Schichijo S, Eura M, Kameyama T, Itoh K. Detection of MAGE-4 protein in sera of patients with head-and-neck squamous-cell carcinoma. Int J Cancer 1997; 70:287–290.

164. Shichijo S, Nakao M, Imai Y, et al. A gene coding antigenic peptides of human squamous cell carcinoma recognized by cytotoxic T lymphocytes. J Exp Med 1998; 187:277–288.

165. Takaki T, Hiraki A, Uenaka A, et al. Variable expression on lung cancer cell lines of HLA-A2–binding MAGE-3 peptide recognized by cytotoxic T lymphocytes. Int J Oncol 1998; 12:1103–1109.

166. Townsend A, Bodmer H. Antigen recognition by class I-restricted T lymphocytes. Annu Rev Immunol 1989; 7:601–624.

167. Jager E, Jager D, Karbach J, et al. Identification of NY-ESO-1 epitopes presented by human histocompatibility antigen (HLA)-DRB4*0101–0103 and recognized by

CD4(+) T lymphocytes of patients with NY-ESO-1-expressing melanoma. J Exp Med 2000; 191:625–630.

168. Houghton AN. Cancer antigens: immune recognition of self and altered self. J Exp Med 1994; 180:1–4.

169. Bowne WB, Srinivasan R, Wolchok JD, et al. Coupling and uncoupling of tumor immunity and autoimmunity. J Exp Med 1999; 190:1717–1722.

170. Rosenberg SA, White DE. Vitiligo in patients with melanoma: normal tissue antigens can be targets for cancer immunotherapy. J Immunother Emphasis Tumor Immunol 1996; 19:81–84.

171. Ludewig B, Ochsenbein AF, Odermatt B, Paulin D, Hengartner H, Zinkernagel RM. Immunotherapy with dendritic cells directed against tumor antigens shared with normal host cells results in severe autoimmune disease. J Exp Med 2000; 191: 795–804.

172. Overwijk WW, Lee DS, Surman DR, et al. Vaccination with a recombinant vaccinia virus encoding a "self" antigen induces autoimmune vitiligo and tumor cell destruction in mice: requirement for CD4(+) T lymphocytes. Proc Natl Acad Sci USA 1999; 96:2982–2987.

173. Sogn JA. Tumor immunology: the glass is half full. Immunity 1998; 9:757–763.

174. Zeh HJ, 3rd, Perry-Lalley D, Dudley ME, Rosenberg SA, Yang JC. High avidity CTLs for two self-antigens demonstrate superior in vitro and in vivo antitumor efficacy. J Immunol 1999; 162:989–994.

175. Poplonski L, Vukusic B, Prawling J, et al. Tolerance is overcome in beef insulin-transgenic mice by activation of low-affinity autoreactive T cells. Eur J Immunol 1996; 26:601–609.

176. Yoshino I, Yano T, Murata M, et al. Tumor-reactive T-cells accumulate in lung cancer tissues but fail to respond due to tumor cell-derived factor. Cancer Res 1992; 52:775–781.

177. Huang M, Sharma S, Mao JT, Dubinett SM. Non-small cell lung cancer-derived soluble mediators and prostaglandin E_2 enhance peripheral blood lymphocyte IL-10 transcription and protein production. J Immunol 1996; 157:5512–5520.

178. Alleva DG, Burger CJ, Elgert KD. Tumor-induced regulation of suppressor macrophage nitric oxide and TNF-alpha production: role of tumor-derived IL-10, TGF-beta and prostaglandin E2. J Immunol 1994; 153:1674.

179. Fearon E, Pardoll D, Itaya T, et al. Interleukin-2 production by tumor cells bypasses T helper function in the generation of an antitumor response. Cell 1990; 60:397–403.

180. Heike Y, Takahashi M, Ohira T, et al. Genetic immunotherapy by intrapleural, intraperitoneal and subcutaneous injection of IL-2 gene-modified lewis lung carcinoma cells. Int J Cancer 1997; 73:844–849.

181. Dubinett SM, Patrone L, Tobias J, Cochran A, Ren DR, McBride WH. Intratumoral interleukin 2 immunotherapy: activation of tumor-infiltrating and splenic lymphocytes in vivo. Cancer Immunol Immunother 1993; 36:156–162.

182. Scudeletti M, Filaci G, Imro MA, et al. Immunotherapy with intralesional and systemic interleukin-2 of patients with non-small-cell lung cancer. Cancer Immunol Immunother 1993; 37:119–124.

183. Allione A, Consalvo M, Nanni P, et al. Immunizing and curative potential of repli-

cating and nonreplicating murine mammary adenocarcinoma cells engineered with interleukin (IL)-2, IL-4, IL-6, IL-7, IL-10, tumor necrosis factor alpha, granulocyte-macrophage colony-stimulating factor, and gamma-interferon gene or admixed with conventional adjuvants. Cancer Res 1994; 54:6022–6026.

184. Asher AL, Mule JJ, Kasid A, et al. Murine tumor cells transduced with the gene for tumor necrosis factor-α. J Immunol 1991; 146:3227–3234.

185. Bottazzi B, Walter S, Govoni D, Colotta F, Mantovani A. Monocyte chemotactic cytokine gene transfer modulates macrophage infiltration, growth, and susceptibility to IL-2 therapy of a murine melanoma. J Immunol 1992; 148:1280–1285.

186. Colombo MP, Ferrari G, Stoppacciaro A, et al. Granulocyte colony-stimulation factor (G-CSF) gene transfer suppress tumorigenicity of a murine adenocarcinoma in vivo. J Exp Med 1991; 173:889–897.

187. Douvdevani A, Huleihel M, Zoller M, Segal S, Apte RN. Reduced tumorigenicity of fibrosarcomas which constitutively generate IL-1 alpha either spontaneously or following IL-1 alpha gene transfer. Int J Cancer 1992; 51:822–830.

188. Dranoff G, Jaffe E, Lazenby A, et al. Vaccination with irradiated tumor cells engineered to secrete murine granulocyte-macrophage colony-stimulating factor stimulates potent, specific, and long-lasting anti-tumor immunity. Proc Natl Acad Sci USA 1993; 90:3539–3543.

189. Gansbacher B, Bannerji R, Daniels B, Zier K, Cronin K, Gilboa E. Retroviral vector-mediated gamma-interferon gene transfer into tumor cells generates potent and long lasting antitumor immunity. Cancer Res 1990; 50:7820–7825.

190. Gansbacher B, Zier K, Daniels B, Cronin L, Bannerji R, Gilboa E. Interleukin 2 gene transfer into tumor cells abrogates tumorigenicity and induces protective immunity. J Exp Med 1990; 172:1217–1224.

191. Mastrangeli A, Danel C, Rosenfeld M, et al. Diversity of airway epithelial cell targets for in vivo recombinant adenovirus-mediated gene transfer. J Clin Invest 1993; 91:225–234.

192. McBride WH, Thacker JD, Comora S, et al. Genetic modification of a murine fibrosarcoma to produce IL-7 stimulates host cell infiltration and tumor immunity. Cancer Res 1992; 52:3931–3937.

193. Porgador A, Tzehoval E, Katz A, et al. Interleukin 6 gene transfection into Lewis lung carcinoma tumor cells suppresses the malignant phenotype and confers immunotherapeutic competence against parental metastic cells. Cancer Res 1992; 52: 3679–3686.

194. Tepper R, Pattengale P, Leder P. Murine interleukin-4 displays potent antitumor activity in vivo. Cell 1989; 57:503–512.

195. Suzuki K, Nakazato H, Matsui H, et al. NK cell–mediated anti-tumor immune response to human prostate cancer cell, PC-3: immunogene therapy using a highly secretable form of interleukin-15 gene transfer. J Leukoc Biol 2001; 69:531–537.

196. Hazama S, Noma T, Wang F, et al. Tumour cells engineered to secrete interleukin-15 augment anti-tumor immune responses in vivo. Br J Cancer 1999; 80:1420–1426.

197. Parmiani G, Rodolfo M, Melani C. Immunological gene therapy with ex vivo gene-modified tumor cells: a critique and a reappraisal. Hum Gene Ther 2000; 11:1269–1275.

198. Hara S, Nagai H, Miyake H, et al. Secreted type of modified interleukin-18 gene transduced into mouse renal cell carcinoma cells induces systemic tumor immunity. J Urol 2001; 165:2039–2043.

199. Usuda J, Okunaka T, Furukawa K, et al. Increased cytotoxic effects of photodynamic therapy in IL-6 gene transfected cells via enhanced apoptosis. Int J Cancer 2001; 93:475–480.

200. Nishioka Y, Hirao M, Robbins PD, Lotze Mt, Tahara H. Induction of systemic and therapeutic antitumor immunity using intratumoral injection of dendritic cells genetically modified to express interleukin 12. Cancer Res 1999; 59:4035–4041.

201. Odaka M, Sterman DH, Wiewrodt R, et al. Eradication of intraperitoneal and distant tumor by adenovirus-mediated interferon-beta gene therapy is attributable to induction of systemic immunity. Cancer Res 2001; 61:6201–6212.

202. Cao G, Su J, Lu W, et al. Adenovirus-mediated interferon-beta therapy suppresses growth and metastasis of human prostate cancer in nude mice. Cancer Gene Ther 2001; 8:497–505.

203. Kageshita T, Mizuno M, Ono T, Matsumoto K, Saida T, Yoshida J. Growth inhibition of human malignant melanoma transfected with the human interferon-beta gene by means of cationic liposomes. Melanoma Res 2001; 11:337–342.

204. Tada H, Maron DJ, Choi EA, et al. Systemic IFN-beta gene therapy results in long-term survival in mice with established colorectal liver metastases. J Clin Invest 2001; 108:83–95.

205. Eck SL, Alavi JB, Judy K, et al. Treatment of recurrent or progressive malignant glioma with a recombinant adenovirus expressing human interferon-beta (H5.010CMVhIFN-beta): a phase I trial. Hum Gene Ther 2001; 12:97–113.

206. Natsume A, Tsujimura K, Mizuno M, Takahashi T, Yoshida J. IFN-beta gene therapy induces systemic antitumor immunity against malignant glioma. J Neurooncol 2000; 47:117–124.

207. Lu W, Fidle IJ, Dong Z. Eradication of primary murine fibrosarcomas and induction of systemic immunity by adenovirus-mediated interferon beta gene therapy. Cancer Res 1999; 59:5202–5208.

208. Natsume A, Mizuno M, Ryuke Y, Yoshida J. Antitumor effect and cellular immunity activation by murine interferon-beta gene transfer against intracerebral glioma in mouse. Gene Ther 1999; 6:1626–1633.

209. Dong Z, Greene G, Pettaway C, et al. Suppression of angiogenesis, tumorigenicity, and metastasis by human prostate cancer cells engineered to produce interferon-beta. Cancer Res 1999; 59:872–879.

210. Toda M, Martuza RL, Rabkin SD. Tumor growth inhibition by intratumoral inoculation of defective herpes simplex virus vectors expressing granulocyte-macrophage colony-stimulating factor. Mol Ther 2000; 2:324–329.

211. Fearon E, Itaya T, Hunt Barbara H, Vogelstein B, Frost P. Induction in a murine tumor of immunogenic tumor variants by transfection with a foreign gene. Cancer Res 1988; 48:2975–2980.

212. Nabel GJ, Nabel EG, Yang Z-Y, et al. Direct gene transfer with DNA-liposome complexes in melanoma: expression, biologic activity, and lack of toxicity in humans. Proc Natl Acad Sci USA 1993; 90:11307–11311.

213. Ostrand-Rosenberg S, Thakur A, Clements V. Rejection of mouse sarcoma cells after transfection of MHC class II genes. J Immunol 1990; 144:4068–4071.

214. Namen AE, Lupton S, Hjerrild K, et al. Stimulation of B-cell progenitors by cloned murine interleukin-7. Nature 1988; 333:571–573.

215. Vella A, Teague TK, Ihle J, Kappler J, Marrack P. Interleukin 4 (Il-4) or IL-7 prevents the death of resting T cells: stat6 is probably not required for the effect of IL-4. J Exp Med 1997; 186:325–330.

216. Chazen GD, Pereira GMB, Le Gros G, Gillis S, Shevach EM. Interleukin 7 is a T cell growth factor. Proc Natl Acad Sci USA 1989; 86:5923–5927.

217. Fry TJ, Connick E, Falloon J, et al. A potential role for interleukin-7 in T-cell homeostasis. Blood 2001; 97:2983–2990.

218. Fry TJ, Mackall CL. Interleukin-7: master regulator of peripheral T-cell homeostasis? Trends Immunol 2001; 22:564–571.

219. Alderson MR, Tough TW, Ziegler SF, Grabstein KH. Interleukin 7 induces cytokine secretion and tumoricidal activity by human peripheral blood monocytes. J Exp Med 1991; 173:923–930.

220. Stotter H, Custer MC, Bolton ES, Guedez L, Lotze MT. IL-7 induces human lymphokine-activated killer cell activity and is regulated by IL-4. J Immunol 1991; 146:150–155.

221. Jicha DL, Mule JJ, Rosenberg SA. Interleukin 7 generates antitumor cytotoxic T lymphocytes against murine sarcomas with efficacy in cellular adoptive immunotherapy. J Exp Med 1991; 174:1511–1515.

222. Mehrotra PT, Grant AJ, Siegel JP. Synergistic effects of IL-7 and IL-12 on human T cell activation. J Immunol 1995; 154:5093–5102.

223. Dubinett S, Huang M, Dhanani S, et al. Down-regulation of murine fibrosarcoma transforming growth factor-b1 expression by interleukin 7. J Natl Cancer Inst 1995; 87:593–597.

224. Dubinett SM, Huang M, Dhanani S, Wang J, Beroiza T. Down-regulation of macrophage transforming growth factor-b messenger RNA expression by interleukin-7. J Immunol 1993; 151:6670–6680.

225. Miller AR, McBride WH, Dubinett SM, et al. Transduction of human melanoma cell lines with the human interleukin-7 gene using retroviral-mediated gene transfer: comparison of immunological properties with IL-2. Blood 1993; 82:3686–3694.

226. Sieling PA, Sakimura L, Uyemura K, et al. IL-7 in the cell-mediated immune response to a human pathogen. J Immunol 1995; 154:2775–2783.

227. Kos FJ, Mullbacher A. IL-2-independent activity of IL-7 in the generation of secondary antigen-specific cytotoxic T cell responses in vivo. J Immunol 1993; 150: 387–393.

228. Sharma S, Wang J, Huang M, et al. Interleukin-7 gene transfer in non–small cell lung cancer decreases tumor proliferation, modifies cell surface molecule expression, and enhances antitumor reactivity. Can Gene Ther 1996; 3:302–313.

229. Huang M, Stolina M, Sharma S, et al. Non–small cell lung cancer cyclooxygenase-2–dependent regulation of cytokine balance in lymphocytes and macrophages: upregulation of interleukin 10 and down-regulation of interleukin 12 production. Cancer Res 1998; 58:1208–1216.

230. Huang M, Wang J, Lee P, et al. Human non-small cell lung cancer cells express a type 2 cytokine pattern. Cancer Res 1995; 55:3847–3853.

231. D'Andrea A, Rengaraju M, Valiante NM, et al. Production of natural killer cell stimulatory factor (interleukin 12) by peripheral blood mononuclear cells. J Exp Med 1992; 176:1387–1398.

232. Kobayashi M, Fitz L, Ryan M, et al. Identification and purification of natural killer cell stimulatory factor (NKSF), a cytokine with multiple biologic effects on human lymphocytes. J Exp Med 1989; 170:827.

233. Chehimi J, Starr S, Frank I, et al. Natural killer (NK) cell stimulatory factor increases the cytotoxic activity of NK cells from both healthy donors and human immunodeficiency virus-infected patients. J Exp Med 1992; 175:789.

234. Chan SH, Perussia B, Gupta JW, et al. Induction of interferon γ production by natural killer cell stimulatory factor: characterization of the responder cells and synergy with other inducers. J Exp Med 1991; 173:869.

235. Chan SH, Kobayashi M, Santoli D, Perussia B, Trinchieri G. Mechanisms of IFN-γ induction by natural killer cell stimulatory factor (NKSF/IL-12): role of transcription and mRNA stability in the synergistic interaction between NKSF and IL-2. J Immunol 1992; 148:92.

236. Gately MK, Wolitzky AG, Quinn PM, Chizzonite R. Regulation of human cytolytic lymphocyte responses by interleukin-12. Cell Immunol 1992; 143:127–142.

237. Naume B, Gately M, Espevik T. A comparative study of IL-12 (cytotoxic lymphocyte maturation factor)–, IL-2–, and IL-7–induced effects on immunomagnetically purified CD56+ NK cells. J Immunol 1992; 148:2429–2436.

238. Grohamm U, Belladonna ML, Bianchi R, et al. IL-12 acts directly on DC to promote nuclear localization of NF-kappaB and primes DC for IL-12 production. Immunity 1998; 9:315–323.

239. Brunda MJ, Luistro L, Warrier RR, et al. Antitumor and antimetastatic activity of interleukin 12 against murine tumors. J Exp Med 1993; 178:1223–1230.

240. Nastala CL, Edington HD, McKinney TG, et al. Recombinant IL-12 administration induces tumor regression in association with IFN-gamma production. J Immunol 1994; 153:1697–1706.

241. Tahara H, Zeh III HJ, Storkus WJ, et al. Fibrosis genetically engineered to secrete interleukin 12 can suppress tumor growth and induce antitumor immunity to a murine melanoma in vivo. Cancer Res 1994; 54:182–189.

242. Zitvogel L, Tahara H, Robbins P, et al. Cancer immunotherapy of established tumors with IL-12: effective delivery by genetically engineered fibroblasts. J Immunol 1995; 155:1393–1403.

243. Bramson J, Hitt M, Addison C, Muller W, Gauldie J, Graham F. Direct intratumoral injection of an adenovirus expressing interleukin-12 induces regression and long-lasting immunity that is associated with highly localized expression of interleukin-12. Hum Gene Ther 1996; 7:1995–2002.

244. Meko J, Yim J, Tsung K, Norton J. High cytokine production and effective antitumor activity of a recombinant vaccinia virus encoding murine interleukin 12. Cancer Res 1995; 55:4765–4770.

245. Kang W, Park C, Yoon H, et al. Interleukin 12 gene therapy of cancer by peritu-

moral injection of transduced autologous fibroblasts: outcome of a phase I study. Hum Gene Ther 2001; 12:671–684.

246. Sumimoto H, Tani K, Nakazaki Y, et al. Superiority of interleukin-12-transduced murine lung cancer cells to GM-CSF or B7-1 (CD80) transfectants for therapeutic antitumor immunity in syngeneic immunocompetent mice. Cancer Gene Ther 1998; 5:29–37.

247. Oshikawa K, Rakhmilevich AL, Shi F, Sondel PM, Yang N, Mahvi DM. Interleukin 12 gene transfer into skin distant from the tumor site elicits antimetastatic effects equivalent to local gene transfer. Hum Gene Ther 2001; 12:149–160.

248. Haku T, Yanagawa H, Nabioullin R, Takeuchi E, Sone S. Interleukin-12–mediated killer activity in lung cancer patients. Cytokine 1997; 9:846–852.

249. Jenks S. Genes to order: regulators struggle against future abuses. J Natl Cancer Inst 1997; 89:1478–1479.

250. Coughlin CM, Wysocka M, Trinchieri G, Lee WM. The effect of interleukin 12 desensitization on the antitumor efficacy of recombinant interleukin 12. Cancer Res 1997; 57:2460–2467.

251. Mazzolini G, Narvaiza I, Perez-Diez A, et al. Genetic heterogeneity in the toxicity to systemic adenoviral gene transfer of interleukin-12. Gene Ther 2001; 8:259–267.

252. Coughlin CM, Salhany KE, Gee MS, et al. Tumor cell responses to IFNgamma affect tumorigenicity and response to IL-12 therapy and antiangiogenesis. Immunity 1998; 9:25–34.

253. Duda DG, Sunamura M, Lozonschi L, et al. Direct in vitro evidence and in vivo analysis of the antiangiogenesis effects of interleukin 12. Cancer Res 2000; 60: 1111–1116.

254. Pertl U, Luster AD, Varki NM, et al. IFN-gamma–inducible protein-10 is essential for the generation of a protective tumor-specific CD8 T cell response induced by single-chain IL-12 gene therapy. J Immunol 2001; 166:6944–6951.

255. Bukowski RM, Rayman P, Molto L, et al. Interferon-gamma and CXC chemokine induction by interleukin 12 in renal cell carcinoma. Clin Cancer Res 1999; 5:2780–2789.

256. Kahn ML, Nakanishi-Matsui M, Shapiro MJ, Ishihara H, Coughlin SR. Protease-activated receptors 1 and 4 mediate activation of human platelets by thrombin. J Clin Invest 1999; 103:879–887.

257. Kang WK, Park C, Yoon HL, et al. Interleukin 12 gene therapy of cancer by peritumoral injection of transduced autologous fibroblasts: outcome of a phase I study. Hum Gene Ther 2001; 12:671–684.

258. Bilyk N, Holt PG. Inhibition of the immunosuppressive activity of resident pulmoary alveolar macrophages by granulocyte/macrophage colony-stimulating factor. J Exp Med 1993; 177:1773–1777.

259. Lee C-T, Wu S, Ciernik F, et al. Genetic immunotherapy of established tumors with adenovirus-murine granulocyte-macrophage colony-stimulating factor. Hum Gene Ther 1997; 8:187–193.

260. Chang AE, Li Q, Bishop DK, Normolle DP, Redman BD, Nickoloff BJ. Immunogenetic therapy of human melanoma utilizing autologous tumor cells transduced to

secrete granulocyte-macrophage colony-stimulating factor. Hum Gene Ther 2000; 11:839–850.

261. Berns AJ, Clift S, Cohen LK, et al. Phase I study of non-replicating autologous tumor cell injections using cells prepared with or without GM-CSF gene transduction in patients with metastatic renal cell carcinoma. Gene Ther 1995; 6:347–368.

262. Tani K, Nakazaki Y, Hase H, et al. Progress reports on immune gene therapy for stage IV renal cell cancer using lethally irradiated granulocyte-macrophage colony-stimulating factor-transduced autologous renal cancer cells. Cancer Chemother Pharmacol 2000; 46 Suppl:S73–76.

263. Simons JW, Mikhak B, Chang JF, et al. Induction of immunity to prostate cancer antigens: results of a clinical trial of vaccination with irradiated autologous prostate tumor cells engineered to secrete granulocyte-macrophage colony-stimulating factor using ex vivo gene transfer. Cancer Res 1999; 59:5160–5168.

264. Mukherjee S, Nelson D, Loh S, et al. The immune anti-tumor effects of GM-CSF and B7-1 gene transfection are enhanced by surgical debulking of tumor. Cancer Gene Ther 2001; 8:580–588.

265. Stolina M, Sharma S, Lin Y, et al. Specific inhibition of cyclooxygenase 2 restores antitumor reactivity by altering the balance of IL-10 and IL-12 synthesis. J Immunol 2000; 164:361–370.

266. Dohadwala M, Luo J, Zhu L, et al. Non small cell lung cancer cylooxygenase-2–dependent invasion is mediated by CD44. J Biol Chem 2001; 276(24):20809–20812.

267. Tsujii M, Dubois R. Alterations in cellular adhesion and apoptosis in epithelial cells overexpressing prostaglandin endoperoxide synthase-2. Cell 1995; 83:493–501.

268. Masferrer JL, Leahy KM, Koki AT, et al. Antiangiogenic and antitumor activities of cyclooxygenase-2 inhibitors. Cancer Res 2000; 60:1306–1311.

269. Restifo NP, Esquivel F, Kawakami Y, et al. Identification of human cancers deficient in antigen processing. J Exp Med 1993; 177:265–272.

270. Hiraki A, Kaneshige T, Kiura K, et al. Loss of HLA haplotype in lung cancer cell lines: implications for immunosurveillance of altered HLA class I/II phenotypes in lung cancer. Clin Cancer Res 1999; 5:933–936.

271. Huang AYC, Golumbek P, Ahmadzadeh M, Jaffee E, Pardoll D, Levitsky H. Role of bone marrow-derived cells in presenting MHC class I-restricted tumor antigens. Science 1994; 264:961–965.

272. Banchereau J, Steinman RM. Dendritic cells and the control of immunity. Nature 1998; 392:245–252.

273. Gabrilovich DI, Chen HL, Girgis KR, et al. Production of vascular endothelial growth factor by human tumors inhibiting the functional maturation of dendritic cells. Nature Med 1996; 2:1096–1103.

274. Kiertscher SM, Luo J, Dubinett SM, Roth MD. Tumors promote altered maturation and early apoptosis of monocyte-derived dendritic cells. J Immunol 2000; 164: 1269–1276.

275. Nestle F, Alijagic S, Gilliet M, et al. Vaccination of melanoma patients with peptide- or tumor lysate-pulsed dendritic cells. Nat Med 1998; 4:328–332.

276. Ribas A, Butterfield L, McBride W, et al. Genetic immunization for the melanoma

antigen MART-1/Melan-A using recombinant adenovirus-transduced murine dendritic cells. Cancer Res 1997; 57:2865–2869.

277. Zitvogel L, Mayordomo JI, Tjandrawan T, et al. Therapy of murine tumors with tumor peptide-pulsed dendritic cells: dependence on T cells, B7 costimulation, and T helper cell 1–associated cytokines. J Exp Med 1996; 183:87–97.

278. Boczkowski D, Nair SK, Snyder D, Gilboa E. Dendritic cells pulsed with RNA are potent antigen-presenting cells in vitro and in vivo. J Exp Med 1996; 184:465–472.

279. Celluzzi CM, Mayordomo JI, Storkus WJ, Lotze MT, Falo Jr. LD. Peptide-pulsed dendritic cells induce antigen-specific, CTL-mediated protective tumor immunity. J Exp Med 1996; 183:283–287.

280. Toes R, van der Voort E, Schoenberger S, et al. Enhancement of tumor outgrowth through CTL tolerization after peptide vaccination is avoided by peptide presentation on dendritic cells. J Immunol 1998; 160:4449–4456.

281. Fields RC, Shimizu K, Mule JJ. Murine dendritic cells pulsed with whole tumor lysates mediate potent antitumor immune responses in vitro and in vivo. Proc Natl Acad Sci USA 1998; 95:9482–9487.

282. Jager E, Ringhoffer M, Karbach J, Arand M, Oesch F, Knuth A. Inverse relationship of melanocyte differentiation antigen expression in melanoma tissues and CD8+ cytotoxic-T-cell responses: evidence for immunoselection of antigen-loss variants in vivo. Int J Cancer 1996; 66:470–476.

283. Bevan MJ. Antigen presentation to cytotoxic T lymphocytes in vivo. J Exp Med 1995; 182:639–641.

284. Waldrop S, Pitcher C, Peterson D, Maino V, Picker L. Determination of antigen-specific memory/effector CD4+ T cell frequencies by flow cytometry. J Clin Invest 1997; 99:1739–1750.

285. Gong J, Chen D, Kashiwara M, Kufe D. Induction of antitumor activity by immunization with fusions of dendritic and carcinoma cells. Nat Med 1997; 3:558–561.

286. Celluzzi C, Falo LJ. Cutting edge: Physical interaction between dendritic cells and tumor cells result in an immunogen that induces protective and therapeutic tumor rejection. J Immunol 1998; 160:3081–3085.

287. Kirk CJ, Hartigan-O'Connor D, Nickoloff BJ, et al. T cell-dependent antitumor immunity mediated by secondary lymphoid tissue chemokine: augmentation of dendritic cell–based immunotherapy. Cancer Res 2001; 61:2062–2070.

288. Cyster JG. Chemokines and the homing of dendritic cells to the T cell areas of lymphoid organs. J Exp Med 1999; 189:447–450.

289. Ogata M, Zhang Y, Wang Y, et al. Chemotactic response toward chemokines and its regulation by transforming growth factor-beta1 of murine bone marrow hematopoietic progenitor cell–derived different subset of dendritic cells. Blood 1999; 93: 3225–3232.

290. Chan VW, Kothakota S, Rohan MC, et al. Secondary lymphoid-tissue chemokine (SLC) is chemotactic for mature dendritic cells. Blood 1999; 93:3610–3616.

291. Hedrick JA, Zlotnik A. Identification and characterization of a novel beta chemokine containing six conserved cysteines. J Immunol 1997; 159:1589–1593.

292. Hromas R, Kim CH, Klemsz M, et al. Isolation and characterization of Exodus-2,

a novel C-C chemokine with a unique 37-amino acid carboxyl-terminal extension. J Immunol 1997; 159:2554–2558.

293. Nagira M, Imai T, Hieshima K, et al. Molecular cloning of a novel human CC chemokine secondary lymphoid-tissue chemokine that is a potent chemoattractant for lymphocytes and mapped to chromosome 9p13. J Biol Chem 1997; 272:19518–19524.

294. Tanabe S, Lu Z, Luo Y, et al. Identification of a new mouse beta-chemokine, thymus-derived chemotactic agent 4, with activity on T lymphocytes and mesangial cells. J Immunol 1997; 159:5671–5679.

295. Willimann K, Legler DF, Loetscher M, et al. The chemokine SLC is expressed in T cell areas of lymph nodes and mucosal lymphoid tissues and attracts activated T cells via CCR7. Eur J Immunol 1998; 28:2025–2034.

296. Kellermann SA, Hudak S, Oldham ER, Liu YJ, McEvoy LM. The CC chemokine receptor-7 ligands 6Ckine and macrophage inflammatory protein-3 beta are potent chemoattractants for in vitro– and in vivo–derived dendritic cells. J Immunol 1999; 162:3859–3864.

297. Sallusto F, Schaerli P, Loetscher P, et al. Rapid and coordinated switch in chemokine receptor expression during dendritic cell maturation. Eur J Immunol 1998; 28:2760–2769.

298. Sozzani S, Allavena P, D'Amico G, et al. Differential regulation of chemokine receptors during dendritic cell maturation: a model for their trafficking properties. J Immunol 1998; 161:1083–1086.

299. Dieu MC, Vanbervliet B, Vicari A, et al. Selective recruitment of immature and mature dendritic cells by distinct chemokines expressed in different anatomic sites. J Exp Med 1998; 188:373–386.

300. Arenberg DA, Zlotnick A, Strom SRB, Burdick MD, Strieter RM. The murine CC chemokine, 6Ckine, inhibits tumor growth and angiogenesis in a human lung cancer SCID mouse model. Cancer Immunol Immunother 2000; 49:587–592.

301. Folkman J. Tumor angiogenesis: therapeutic implications. N Engl J Med 1971; 285:1182–1186.

302. Holmgren L, O'Reilly MS, Folkman J. Dormancy of micrometastases: balanced proliferation and apoptosis in the presence of angiogenesis suppression (see comments). Nat Med 1995; 1:149–153.

303. Folkman J. Tumor angiogenesis. In: Mendelsohn J, Howley P, Israel M, eds. The Molecular Basis of Cancer. Philadelphia: Saunders, 1995:206–232.

304. Pluda JM. Tumor-associated angiogenesis: mechanisms, clinical implications, and therapeutic strategies. Semin Oncol 1997; 24:203–218.

305. O'Reilly MS, Holmgren L, Chen C, Folkman J. Angiostatin induces and sustains dormancy of human primary tumors in mice. Nat Med 1996; 2:689–692.

306. Yancopoulos GD, Davis S, Gale NW, Rudge JS, Wiegand SJ, Holash J. Vascular-specific growth factors and blood vessel formation. Nature 2000; 407:242–248.

307. Holash J, Maisonpierre PC, Compton D, et al. Vessel cooption, regression, and growth in tumors mediated by angiopoietins and VEGF. Science 1999; 284:1994–1998.

308. Risau W. Mechanisms of angiogenesis. Nature 1997; 386:671–674.

309. Carmeliet P. Mechanisms of angiogenesis and arteriogenesis. Nat Med 2000; 6: 389–395.

310. Carmeliet P, Jain RK. Angiogenesis in cancer and other diseases. Nature 2000; 407:249–257.

311. Strieter R, Belperio J. CXC chemokines in angiogenesis. In: Ransohoff R, ed. Universes in Delicate Balance: Chemokines and the Nervous System. Amsterdam: Elsevier Science. In press.

312. Ferrara N, Alitalo K. Clinical applications of angiogenic growth factors and their inhibitors. Nat Med 1999; 5:1359–1364.

313. Risau W. Vasculogenesis, angiogenesis and endothelial cell differentiation during embryonic development. In: Feinberg RN, Sherer GK, Auerbach R, eds. The Development of the Vascular System. Basel: K. Karger, 1991:58–68.

314. Engerman R, Pfaffenenbach D, Davis M. Cell turnover of capillaries. Lab Invest 1967; 17:738–743.

315. Tannock I, Hayashi H. The proliferation of capillary and endothelial cells. Cancer Res 1972; 32:77–82.

316. Auerbach R, Auerbach W, Polakowski I. Assays for angiogenesis: a review. Pharmacol Ther 1991; 51:1–11.

317. Sato N, Beitz JG, Kato J, et al. Platelet-derived growth factor indirectly stimulates angiogenesis in vitro. Am J Pathol 1993; 142:1119–1130.

318. Vlodavsky I, Fuks Z, Ishai-Michaeli R, et al. Extracellular matrix-resident basic fibroblast growth factor: implication for the control of angiogenesis. J Cell Biochem 1991; 45:167–176.

319. Gimbrone MA, Leapman SB, Cotran RS, Folkman J. Tumor dormancy in vivo by prevention of neovascularization. J Exp Med 1972; 136:261–276.

320. Keane MP, Arenberg DA, Lynch JP, 3rd, et al. The CXC chemokines, IL-8 and IP-10, regulate angiogenic activity in idiopathic pulmonary fibrosis. J Immunol 1997; 159:1437–1443.

321. Nickoloff BJ, Karabin GD, Barker JWCN, et al. Cellular localization of interleukin-8 and its inducer, tumor necrosis factor-alpha in psoriasis. Am J Pathol 1991; 138: 129–140.

322. Leibovich SJ, Wiseman DM. Macrophages, wound repair and angiogenesis. Prog Clin Biol Res 1988; 266:131–145.

323. Vlodavski I, Folkman J, Sullivan R, et al. Endothelial cell–derived basic fibroblast growth factor: synthesis and deposition into subendothelial extracellular matrix. Proc Natl Acad Sci USA 1987; 84:2292–2296.

324. Strieter RM, Kunkel SL, Showell HJ, Marks RM. Monokine-induced gene expression of human endothelial cell–derived neutrophil chemotactic factor. Biochem Biophys Res Commun 1998; 156:1340–1345.

325. Dejana E. Endothelial adherens junctions: implications in the control of vascular permeability and angiogenesis. J Clin Invest 1997; 100:S7–10.

326. Pepper MS, Vassaui JD, Orci L, Montesano R. Proteolytic balance and capillary morphogenesis in vitro. In: Steiner R, Weisz PB, Langer R, eds. Angiogenesis: Key Principles. Basel: Birkhauser Verlag, 1992:137–145.

327. Sunderkotter C, Goebeler M, Schulze-Osthoff K, Bhardwaj R, Sorg C, Macrophage-derived angiogenesis factors. Pharmacol Ther 1991; 51:195–216.

328. Takigawa M, Nishida Y, Suzuki F, Kishi J, Yamashita K, Hayakawa T. Induction of angiogenesis in chick yolk-sac membrane by polyamines and its inhibition by tissue inhibitors of metalloproteinases (TIMP and TIMP-2). Biochem Biophys Res Commun 1990; 171:1264–1271.

329. Matsumura T, Wolff K, Petzelbauer P. Endothelial cell tube formation depends on cadherin 5 and CD31 interactions with filamentous actin. J Immunol 1997; 158: 3408–3416.

330. DeLisser HM, Newman PJ, Albelda SM. Platelet endothelial cell adhesion molecule (CD31). Curr Top Microbiol Immunol 1993; 184:37–45.

331. DeLisser HM, Christofidou-Solomidou M, Strieter RM, et al. Involvement of endothelial PECAM-1/CD31 in angiogenesis. Am J Pathol 1997; 151:671–677.

332. Ray JM, Stetler-Stevenson WG. The role of matrix metalloproteases and their inhibitors in tumour invasion, metastasis and angiogenesis. Eur Respir J 1994; 7: 2062–2072.

333. Arnold F, West DC. Angiogenesis in wound healing. Pharmacol Ther 1991; 52: 407–422.

334. Brooks P, Clark R, Cheresh D. Requirements of vascular integrin $\alpha_v\beta_3$ for angiogenesis. Science 1994; 264:569–571.

335. Brooks PC, Stromblad S, Sanders LC, et al. Localization of matrix metalloproteinase MMP-2 to the surface of invasive cells by interaction with integrin alpha v beta 3. Cell 1996; 85:683–693.

336. Brooks P, Montgomery A, Rosenfeld M, et al. Integrin $\alpha_v\beta_3$ antagonist promote tumor regression by inducing apoptosis of angiogenic blood vessels. Cell 1994; 79:1157–1164.

337. O'Reilly MS, Holmgren L, Shing Y, et al. Angiostatin: a novel angiogenesis inhibitor that mediates the suppression of metastases by a Lewis lung carcinoma. Cell 1994; 79:315–328.

338. O'Reilly MS, Boehm T, Shing Y, et al. Endostatin: an endogenous inhibitor of angiogenesis and tumor growth. Cell 1997; 88:277–285.

339. Haralabopoulos GC, Grant DS, Kleinman HK, Lelkes PI, Papaioannou SP, Maragoudakis ME. Inhibitors of basement membrane collagen synthesis prevent endothelial cell alignment in matrigel in vitro and angiogenesis in vivo. Lab Invest 1994; 71:575–582.

340. Robaye B, Mosselmans R, Fiers W, Dumont JE, Galand P. Tumor necrosis factor induces apoptosis (programmed cell death) in normal endothelial cells in vitro. Am J Pathol 1991; 138:447–453.

341. Ausprunk DH, Folkman J. The sequence of events in the regression of corneal capaillaries. Lab Invest 1978; 38:284–296.

342. Chen JJ, Peck K, Hong TM, et al. Global analysis of gene expression in invasion by a lung cancer model. Cancer Res 2001; 61:5223–5230.

343. Mattern J, Koomagi R, Volm M. Association of vascular endothelial growth factor expression with intratumoral microvessel density and tumour cell proliferation in human epidermoid lung carcinoma. Br J Cancer 1996; 73:931–934.

344. Ohta Y, Endo Y, Tanaka M, et al. Significance of vascular endothelial growth factor messenger RNA expression in primary lung cancer. Clin Cancer Res 1996; 2:1411–1416.

345. Tsao MS, Liu N, Nicklee T, Shepherd F, Viallet J. Angiogenesis correlates with vascular endothelial growth factor expression but not with Ki-ras oncogene activation in non–small cell lung carcinoma. Clin Cancer Res 1997; 3:1807–1814.

346. Yuan A, Yu CJ, Kuo SH, et al. Vascular endothelial growth factor 189 mRNA isoform expression specifically correlates with tumor angiogenesis, patient survival, and postoperative relapse in non–small-cell lung cancer. J Clin Oncol 2001; 19: 432–441.

347. Zebrowski BK, Yano S, Liu W, et al. Vascular endothelial growth factor levels and induction of permeability in malignant pleural effusions. Clin Cancer Res 1999; 5:3364–3368.

348. Yano S, Herbst RS, Shinohara H, et al. Treatment for malignant pleural effusion of human lung adenocarcinoma by inhibition of vascular endothelial growth factor receptor tyrosine kinase phosphorylation. Clin Cancer Res 2000; 6:957–965.

349. Brekken RA, Overholser JP, Stastny VA, Waltenberger J, Minna JD, Thorpe PE. Selective inhibition of vascular endothelial growth factor (VEGF) receptor 2 (KDRE/Flk-1) activity by a monoclonal anti-VEGF antibody blocks tumor growth in mice. Cancer Res 2000; 60:5117–5124.

350. Kozin SV, Boucher Y, Hicklin DJ, Bohlen P, Jain RK, Suit HD. Vascular endothelial growth factor receptor-2-blocking antibody potentiates radiation-induced long-term control of human tumor xenografts. Cancer Res 2001; 61:39–44.

351. Takayama K, Ueno H, Nakanishi Y, et al. Suppression of tumor angiogenesis and growth by gene transfer of a soluble form of vascular endothelial growth factor receptor into a remote organ. Cancer Res 2000; 60:2169–2177.

352. Hotfidler M, Nowak-Gottl U, Wolff JE. Tumorangiogenesis: a network of cytokines. Klin Padiatr 1997; 209:265–270.

353. Pike Se, Yao L, Jones KD, et la. Vasostatin, a calreticulin fragment, inhibits angiogenesis and suppresses tumor growth. J Exp Med 1998; 188:2349–2356.

354. Vazquez F, Hastings G, Ortega MA, et al. METH-1, a human ortholog of ADAMTS-1, and METH-2 are members of a new family of proteins with angioinhibitory activity. J Biol Chem 1999; 274:23349–23357.

355. Jimenez B, Volpert OV, Crawford SE, Febbraio M, Silverstein RL, Bouck N. Signals leading to apoptosis-dependent inhibition of neovascularization by thrombospondin-1. Nat Med 2000; 6:41–48.

356. O'Reilly MS, Wiederschain D, Stetler-Stevenson WG, Folkman J, Moses MA. Regulation of angiostatin production by matrix metalloproteinase-2 in a model of concomitant resistance. J Biol Chem 1999; 274:29568–29571.

357. Dong Z, Yoneda J, Kumar R, Fidler IJ. Angiostatin-mediated suppression of cancer metastases by primary neoplasms engineered to produce granulocyte/macrophage colony-stimulating factor. J Exp Med 1998; 188:755–763.

358. Volm M, Mattern J, Koomagi R. Angiostatin expression in non–small cell lung cancer. Clin Cancer Res 2000; 6:3236–3240.

359. Sauter BV, Martinet O, Zhang WJ, Mandeli J, Woo SL. Adenovirus-mediated gene transfer of endostatin in vivo results in high level of transgene expression and inhibition of tumor growth and metastases. Proc Natl Acad Sci USA 2000; 97:4802–4807.

360. Yoon SS, Eto H, Lin CM, et al. Mouse endostatin inhibits the formation of lung and liver metastases. Cancer Res 1999; 59:6251–6256.

361. Wen XY, Bai Y, Stewart AK. Adenovirus-mediated human endostatin gene delivery demonstrates strain-specific antitumor activity and acute dose-dependent toxicity in mice. Hum Gene Ther 2001; 12:347–358.

362. Kumar CC, Malkowski M, Yin Z, et al. Inhibition of angiogenesis and tumor growth by SCH221153, a dual alpha(v)beta3 and alha(v)beta5 integrin receptor antagonist. Cancer Res 2001; 61:2232–2338.

363. Silletti S, Kessler T, Goldberg J, Boger DL, Cheresh DA. Disruption of matrix metalloproteinase 2 binding to integrin alpha vbeta 3 by an organic molecule inhibits angiogenesis and tumor growth in vivo. Proc Natl Acad Sci USA 2001; 98: 119–124.

364. Shalinsky DR, Brekken J, Zou H, et al. Marked antiangiogenic and antitumor efficacy of AG3340 in chemoresistant human non-small cell lung cancer tumors: single agent and combination chemotherapy studies. Clin Cancer Res 1999; 5:1905–1917.

365. Li H, Lindenmeyer F, Grenet C, et al. AdTIMP-2 inhibits tumor growth, angiogenesis, and metastasis, and prolongs survival in mice. Hum Gene Ther 2001; 12:515–526.

366. Liao F, Li Y, O'Connor W, et al. Monoclonal antibody to vascular endothelial-cadherin is a potent inhibitor of angiogenesis, tumor growth, and metastasis. Cancer Res 2000; 60:6805–6810.

367. Luster AD. Chemokines—chemotactic cytokines that mediate inflammation. N Engl J Med 1998; 338:436–445.

368. Baggiolini M, Dewald B, Moser B. Human chemokines: an update. Annu Rev Immunol 1997; 15:675–705.

369. Strieter RM, Kunkel SL, Shanafelt AB, Arenberg DA, Koch AE, Polverini PJ. CXC chemokines in regulation of angiogenesis. In: Koch AE, Strieter RM, eds. Chemokines in Disease. Austin, TX: Landes, 1996:195–210.

370. Strieter R, Polverini P, Kunkel S, et al. The functional role of the 'ELR' motif in CXC chemokine-mediated angiogenesis. J Biol Chem 1995; 270:27348–27357.

371. Angiolillo AL, Sgadari C, Taub DD, et al. Human interferon inducible protein 10 is a potent inhibitor of angiogenesis in vivo. J Exp Med 1995; 182:155.

372. Luster AD, Greenberg SM, Leder P. The IP-10 chemokine binds to a specific cell surface heparan sulfate site shared with platelet factor 4 and inhibits endothelial cell proliferation. J Exp Med 1995; 182:219.

373. Sgadari C, Farber JM, Angiolillo AL, et al. Mig, the monokine induced by interferon-gamma, promotes tumor necrosis in vivo. Blood 1997; 89:2635–2643.

374. Inoue K, Slaton J, Eve B, Kim S, Perrotte P, Balbay M. Interleukin 8 expression regulates tumorigenicity and metastases in androgen-independent prostate cancer. Clin Cancer Res 2000; 6:2104–2119.

375. Bar-Eli M. Role of interleukin-8 in tumor growth and metastasis of human melanoma. Pathobiology 1999; 67:12–18.

376. Arenberg DA, Polverini PJ, Kunkel SL, Shanafelt A, Strieter RM. In vitro and in vivo systems to assess role of C-X-C chemokines in regulation of angiogenesis. Methods Enzymol 1997; 288:190–220.

377. Addison C, Daniel T, Burdick M, Liu H, Ehlert J, Xue Y. The CXC chemokine

receptor 2, CXCR2, is the putative receptor for ELR(+) CXC chemokine-induced angiogenic activity. J Immunol 2000; 165:5269–5277.

378. Devalarja R, Nanney L, Qian Q, Du J, Yu Y, Devalarja M. Delayed wound healing in CXCR2 knockout mice. J Invest Dermatol 2000; 115:234–244.

379. Farber JM. HuMIG: a new member of the chemokine family of cytokines. Biochem Biophys Res Commun 1993; 192:223–230.

380. Farber JM. A macrophage mRNA selectively induced by gamma-interferon encodes a member of the platelet factor 4 family of cytokines. Proc Natl Acad Sci USA 1990; 87:5238–5242.

381. Luster AD, Unkeless JC, Ravetch JV. Gamma-interferon transcriptionally regulates an early-response gene containing homology to platelet proteins. Nature 1985; 315: 672–676.

382. Luster AD, Ravetch JV. Biochemical characterization of a gamma interferon-inducible cytokine (IP-10). J Exp Med 1987; 166:1084–1097.

383. Cole KE, Strict CA, Paradis TJ, et al. Interferon-inducible T cell alpha chemoattractant (I-TAC): a novel non-ELR CXC chemokine with potent activity on activated T cells through selective high affinity binding to CXCR3. J Exp Med 1998; 187: 2009–2021.

384. Yoneda J, Kuniyasu H, Crispens MA, Price JE, Bucana CD, Fidler IJ. Expression of angiogenesis-related genes and progression of human ovarian carcinomas in nude mice. J Natl Cancer Inst 1998; 90:447–454.

385. Smith DR, Polverini PJ, Kunkel SL, et al. Inhibition of interleukin 8 attenuates angiogenesis in bronchogenic carcinoma. J Exp Med 1994; 179:1409–1415.

386. Arenberg D, Kunkel S, Polverini P, Glass M, Burdick M, Strieter R. Inhibition of interleukin-8 reduces tumorigenesis of human non–small cell lung cancer in SCID mice. J Clin Invest 1996; 97:2792–2802.

387. Yatsunami J, Tsuruta N, Ogata K, et al. Interleukin-8 participates in angiogenesis in non–small cell, but not small cell carcinoma of the lung. Cancer Lett 1997; 120: 101–108.

388. Arenberg DA, Keane MP, DiGiovine B, et al. Epithelial-neutrophil activating peptide (ENA-78) is an important angiogenic factor in non–small cell lung cancer. J Clin Invest 1998; 102:465–472.

389. Addison C, Arenberg D, Morris S, et al. The CXC chemokine, monokine induced by interferon gamma, inhibits non-small cell lung carcinoma tumor growth and metastasis. Hum Gene Ther 2000; 11:247–261.

390. Arenberg DA, Kunkel SL, Polverini PJ, et al. Interferon-gamma-inducible protein 10 (IP-10) is an angiostatic factor that inhibits human non–small cell lung cancer (NSCLC) tumorigenesis and spontaneous metastases. J Exp Med 1996; 184:981–992.

391. Yuan A, Yang PC, Yu CJ, et al. Tumor angiogenesis correlates with histologic type and metastasis in non–small-cell lung cancer. Am J Respir Crit Care Med 1995; 152:2157–2162.

392. Jain RK. Delivery of molecular medicine to solid tumors. Science 1996; 271:1079–1080.

393. Jain RK. The next frontier of molecular medicine: delivery of therapeutics. Nat Med 1998; 4:655–657.

394. Molnar-Kimber KL, Sterman DH, Chang M, et al. Impact of preexisting and induced humoral and cellular immune responses in an adenovirus-based gene therapy phase I clinical trial for localized mesothelioma. Hum Gene Ther 1998; 9:2121–2133.

395. Batra R, Olsen J, Hoganson D, Caterson B, Boucher R. Retroviral gene transfer is inhibited by chondroitin sulfate proteoglycans/glycosaminoglycans in malignant pleural effusions. J Biol Chem 1997; 18:11736–11743.

396. Bergelson JM, Cunningham JA, Droguett G, et al. Isolation of a common receptor for coxsackie B viruses and adenoviruses 2 and 5. Science 1997; 275:1320–1323.

397. Wickham TJ, Mathias P, Cheresh DA, Nemerow GR. Integrins alpha v beta 3 and alpha v beta 5 promote adenovirus internalization but not virus attachment. Cell 1993; 73:309–319.

398. Seth P. Adenovirus-dependent release of choline from plasma membrane vesicles at an acidic pH is mediated by the penton base protein. J Virol 1994; 68:1204–1206.

399. Greber UF, Willetts M, Webster P, Helenius A. Stepwise dismantling of adenovirus 2 during entry into cells. Cell 1993; 75:477–486.

400. Wolff G, Worgall S, van Rooijen N, Song WR, Harvey BG, Crystal BG, Crystal RG. Enhancement of in vivo adenovirus-mediated gene transfer and expression by prior depletion of tissue macrophages in the target organ. J Virol 1997; 71:624–629.

401. Walters RW, Grunst T, Bergelson JM, Finberg RW, Welsh MJ, Zabner J. Basolateral localization of fiber receptors limits adenovirus infection from the apical surface of airway epithelia. J Biol Chem 1999; 274:10219–10226.

402. Sung RS, Qin L, Bromberg JS. TNFalpha and IFNgamma induced by innate anti-adenoviral immune responses inhibit adenovirus-mediated transgene expression. Mol Ther 2001; 3:757–767.

403. Yang Y, Li Q, Ertl H, Wilson J. Cellular and humoral immune responses to viral antigens create barriers to lung-directed gene therapy with recombinant adenoviruses. J Virol 1995; 69:2004–2015.

404. Ramesh R, Saeki T, Templeton NS, et al. Successful treatment of primary and disseminated human lung cancers by systemic delivery of tumor suppressor genes using an improved liposome vector. Mol Ther 2001; 3:337–350.

405. Kay M, Liu D, Hoogerbrugge P. Gene Therapy. Proc Natl Acad Sci USA 1997; 94:12744–12746.

406. Boris-Lawrie K, Temin HM. The retroviral vector. Replication cycle and safety considerations for retrovirus-mediated gene therapy. Ann NY Acad Sci 1994; 716:59–70; discussion 71.

407. Naldini L, Blomer U, Gallay P, et al. In vivo gene delivery and stable transduction of nondividing cells by a lentiviral vector. Science 1996; 272:263–267.

408. Naldini L, Blomer U, Gage F, Trono D, Verma I. Efficient transfer, integration, and sustained long-term expression of the transgene in adult rat brains injected with a lentiviral vector. Proc Natl Acad Sci USA 1996; 93:11382–11388.

409. Kasahara N, Dozy A, Kan Y. Tissue-specific targeting of retroviral vectors through ligand-receptor interactions. Science 1994; 266:1373–1376.

410. Valsesia-Wittmann S, Drynda A, Deleage G, et al. Modifications in the binding

domain of avian retrovirus envelope protein to redirect the host range of retroviral vectors. J Virol 1994; 68:4609–4619.

411. Miller N, Whelan J. Progress in transcriptionally targeted and regulatable vectors for genetic therapy. Hum Gene Ther 1997; 8:803–815.

412. Cosset FL, Takeuchi Y, Battini JL, Weiss RA, Collins MK. High-titer packaging cells producing recombinant retroviruses resistant to human serum. J Virol 1995; 69:7430–7436.

413. Imler J. Adenovirus vectors as recombinant viral vaccines. Vaccine 1995; 13:1143–1151.

414. Crystal R, McElkvaney N, Rosenfeld M, et al. Administration of an adenovirus containing the human CFTR cDNA to the respiratory tract of individuals with cystic fibrosis. Nature Genet 1994; 8:42–51.

415. Lehrman S. Virus treatment questioned after gene therapy death (news). Nature 1999; 401:517–518.

416. Mitani K, Graham F, Caskey C, Kochanek, S. Rescue, propagation, and partial purification of a helper virus–dependent adenovirus vector. Proc Natl Acad Sci USA 1995; 92:3854–3858.

417. Morsy MA, Gu M, Motzel S, et al. An adenoviral vector deleted for all viral coding sequences results in enhanced safety and extended expression of a leptin transgene. Proc Natl Acad Sci USA 1998; 95:7866–7871.

418. McCoy RD, Davidson BL, Roessler BJ, et al. Pulmonary inflammation induced by incomplete or inactivated adenoviral particles. Hum Gene Ther 1995; 6:1553–1560.

419. Zhang Y, Chirmule N, Gao GP, et al. Acute cytokine response to systemic adenoviral vectors in mice is mediated by dendritic cells and macrophages. Mol Ther 2001; 3:697–707.

420. Schnell MA, Zhang Y, Tazelaar J, et al. Activation of innate immunity in nonhuman primates following intraportal administration of adenoviral vectors. Mol Ther 2001; 3:708–722.

421. Borgland SL, Bowen GP, Wong NC, Libermann TA, Muruve DA. Adenovirus vector-induced expression of the C-X-C chemokine IP-10 is mediated through capsid-dependent activation of NF-kappaB. J Virol 2000; 74:3941–3947.

422. Dow SW, Fradkin LG, Liggitt DH, Willson AP, Heath TD, Potter TA. Lipid-DNA complexes induce potent activation of innate immune responses and antitumor activity when administered intravenously. J Immunol 1999; 163:1552–1561.

423. Croyle MA, Chirmule N, Zhang Y, Wilson JM. Stealth adenoviruses blunt cell-mediated and humoral immune responses against the virus and allow for significant gene expression upon readministration in the lung. J Virol 2001; 75:4792–4801.

424. Tursz T, Cesne A, Baldeyrou P, et al. Phase I study of a recombinant adenovirus-mediated gene transfer in lung cancer patients. J Natl Cancer Inst 1996; 88:1857–1863.

425. Gahery-Segard H, Molinier-Frenkel V, Le Boulaire C, et al. Phase I trial of recombinant adenovirus gene transfer in lung cancer: longitudinal study of the immune responses to transgene and viral products. J Clin Invest 1997; 100:2218–2226.

426. Molinier-Frenkel V, Le Boulaire C, Le Gal FA, et al. Longitudinal follow-up of

cellular and humoral immunity induced by recombinant adenovirus-mediated gene therapy in cancer patients. Hum Gen Ther 2000; 11:1911–1920.

427. Douglas JT, Rogers BE, Rosenfeld ME, Michael SI, Feng M, Curiel DT. Targeted gene delivery by tropism-modified adenoviral vectors. Nat Biotechnol 1996; 14: 1574–1578.

428. Wickham T, Roelvink P, Brough D, Kovesdi I. Adenovirus targeted to heparan-containing receptors increases its gene delivery efficiency to multiple cell types. Nature Biotechnol 1996; 14:1570–1573.

11

Gene Therapy for Malignant Mesothelioma

DANIEL H. STERMAN

University of Pennsylvania Medical Center
Philadelphia, Pennsylvania, U.S.A.

I. Introduction

Mesotheliomas are neoplasms of the serosal membranes of the body cavities, arising from the pleura, peritoneum, pericardium, ovarian epithelium, tunica vaginalis, and testis. Eighty percent of mesotheliomas originate in the pleural space, and they represent the most common primary tumor of the pleural cavity. Malignant pleural mesothelioma is minimally responsive to most chemotherapy and radiotherapy regimens, and it is almost uniformly fatal. New chemotherapy drugs may provide symptomatic relief and perhaps transitory clinical/radiographic responses to patients with advanced mesothelioma, but they have not been shown to prolong survival. Radiation therapy is primarily useful for palliation of localized chest wall invasion or implantation. Even radical surgical resection of all involved pleural surfaces, ipsilateral lung, pericardium, and diaphragm has not been demonstrated to prolong survival except in highly selected groups of patients as part of multimodality treatment involving surgery, chemotherapy, and radiation therapy (1–5).

As the incidence of pleural mesothelioma peaks in the United States and Europe over the next 10–20 years, new therapeutic approaches are imperative.

The genetic revolution in cancer medicine over the past 30 years facilitated the development of gene therapy trials in which therapeutic genes were inserted via various vectors into tumor cells to induce apoptosis, necrosis, and antitumor immune responses. Malignant mesothelioma has several characteristics that make it an attractive target for gene therapy: (1) absence of standard, effective therapy; (2) accessibility in the pleural space for biopsy, vector delivery, and analysis of treatment effects; and (3) morbidity and mortality related to local extension of disease rather than distant metastases. Therefore, unlike other tumors that metastasize earlier in their course, small increments of improvement in local control in mesothelioma could result in significant benefit in survival. In addition, experimental gene therapy for malignant pleural mesothelioma could serve as a paradigm for treatment of other localized malignancies such as bladder and ovarian carcinoma.

Several different cancer gene therapy approaches are currently being explored for malignant pleural mesothelioma including the use of so-called "suicide genes," delivery of tumor-suppressor genes, and transfer of immunomodulatory genes. Several of these have been applied in Phase I clinical trials of malignant pleural mesothelioma utilizing a variety of vector systems including recombinant adenovirus, vaccinia virus, and modified ovarian carcinoma cells (6–8). Others remain in the preclinical stage, but with plans for clinical trials in the near future (Table 1). This chapter will discuss these aspects of gene therapy for mesothelioma, as well as possible future approaches.

II. Suicide Gene Therapy

One prominent approach in cancer gene therapeutics is so-called suicide gene therapy. This method involves the transduction of a neoplasm with cDNA encoding for an enzyme rendering tumor cells sensitive to a "benign" agent by converting the "prodrug" to a toxic metabolite (9). The enzymes encoded by the suicide gene are often of nonhuman origin, that is, the *Escherichia coli* cytosine deaminase (CDA) gene (10) or the herpes simplex virus-1 thymidine kinase (HSV*tk*) gene (11). HSV*tk* differs significantly from mammalian thymidine kinases in that, once incorporated by malignant cells, it renders them sensitive to the nucleoside analog ganciclovir (GCV).

GCV (9-[1,3 dihydroxy-2-propoxy)methyl]-guanine) is an acyclic nucleoside that is poorly metabolized by mammalian cells and is therefore generally nontoxic. However, after enzymatic conversion to GCV *mono*phosphate (GCV-MP) by HSV*tk*, it is rapidly metabolized to GCV *tri*phosphate (GCV-TP) by endogenous mammalian kinases. GCV-TP is a potent inhibitor of viral DNA polymerase and competes with normal *mammalian* nucleosides for DNA replication (12). In addition, incorporation of GCV-MP into the DNA template can

Table 1 Gene Therapy Approaches for Mesothelioma

Strategy	Vector	Therapeutic gene	Molecular mechanism	Location
Suicide gene	Recombinant, replication-deficient adenovirus	Herpes simplex thymidine kinase	Delivery of enzyme capable of generating toxic metabolite after exposure to ganciclovir	University of Pennsylvania Medical Center, Philadelphia
Genetic immuno-potentiation	Replication-restricted vaccinia virus	Human IL-2	Augmentation of immune response to tumor	Queen Elizabeth II Medical Center, Perth, Australia
	Vaccinia virus	Modified SV40 T antigen	Stimulation of immune response against SV40(+) mesothelioma cells	Wayne State University Medical Center, Detroit
	Replication-deficient adenovirus	Interferon-β	Induction of antitumor immune response	University of Pennsylvania Medical Center (pending)
	Cationic liposome	Prokaryotic DNA	Nonspecific induction of innate and acquired immunity	Protocol pending
Combination suicide gene/tumor vaccine	Irradiated, allogeneic ovarian carcinoma cells	Herpes simplex thymidine kinase	Generation of toxic metabolite and antitumor immune responses	LSU Medical Center, New Orleans
Mutation compensation	Oligonucleotides	Anti-sense SV40 TAG	Inhibition of dominant oncogenes	Protocol pending
	Adenovirus	Wild-type p14(ARF)/p16	Restoration of tumor suppressors	Protocols pending
	Adenovirus	Wild-type p53/Bak	Induction of apoptosis	Protocols pending
Replication-competent viral lytic therapy	HSV-1 mutants (HSV-1716)	Herpes simplex thymidine kinase	Tumor-restricted viral replication and cytotoxicity	Protocol pending
	Replication-restricted adenovirus: ONYX-015	None	Tumor-restricted viral replication and cytotoxicity	Protocol pending

itself induce significant cytotoxicity (13). Intracellular production of these GCV metabolites engenders a "suicidal" path to tumor cell death (9,12). A "bystander" effect, whereby neighboring tumor cells also perish, appears to be important in achieving maximal tumor response (14).

A. Bystander Effects of HSV*tk* Suicide Gene Therapy

Given the limited gene transfer efficiency of current vector systems, the primary reason for the success of in vivo HSV*tk* experiments appeared to be the finding that transgene expression in every cell was *not* required for complete tumor regression. This so-called bystander effect was demonstrated in in vitro mixing experiments using retrovirally infected tumor cells, as well as in vivo experiments involving tumors with only 10–20% HSV*tk* expression. Complete tumor regression was noted in animals after ganciclovir treatment (15–19). The nature of this bystander effect is complex and appears to involve passage of toxic GCV metabolites from transduced to nontransduced cells via gap junctions or apoptotic vesicles (20,21) and induction of antitumor immune responses capable of killing tumor cells not expressing the HSV*tk* transgene (14).

B. Adenoviral Delivery Systems

The transfer of HSV*tk* DNA to target tumor cells can be accomplished in a variety of ways including the use of viral vectors, lipsomes, cellular delivery systems, and naked DNA electrocorporation (22).

Early in vitro and in vivo studies utilized retroviral vectors to facilitate HSV*tk* DNA transfer into tumors including the injection of "producer" cell lines that secrete retrovirus expressing the suicide gene (23,24). These retrovirus-based approaches have been used successfully in animal models of brain tumor, ovarian cancer, and hepatocellular carcinoma (25).

Adenoviruses have since become the vector of choice for delivery of the HSV*tk* gene, as well as other therapeutic genes, in many cancer gene therapy experimental models. Adenoviral vectors are preferred, because they infect both dividing and nondividing cells, do not carry the theoretical risk of insertional mutagenesis (they deliver their DNA episomally), and are much easier to produce in lots large enough for use in clinical studies (26). Based on these factors, our group and others have produced recombinant, replication-deficient adenoviral vectors encoding the HSV*tk* gene (AdHSV*tk*). We and others have shown that this AdHSV*tk* vector, in combination with GCV, could eradicate tumor cells in vitro and in in vivo models of malignant mesothelioma, as well as in lung cancer, brain tumors, colon carcinoma, hepatocellular carcinoma, glioma, and melanoma (27–31).

C. Malignant Mesothelioma: Paradigm for HSV*tk*/GCV Gene Therapy

Preclinical Data: Animal and Toxicity Studies

Initial experiments demonstrated that replication-deficient adenoviral HSV*tk* vectors efficiently transduced mesothelioma cells both in tissue culture and in animal models and facilitated HSV*tk*-mediated killing of human mesothelioma cells in the presence of low concentrations of GCV (32,33). Subsequently, AdHSV*tk*/GCV gene therapy was used to treat established, intraperitoneal human mesothelioma and lung cancer xenografts in immunodeficient mice (27,29) resulting in significant tumor reduction and prolongation of survival (30). The in vitro and in vivo sensitivities of human mesothelioma cells to HSV*tk*/GCV gene therapy have been confirmed by other independent investigators (34).

Based on this efficacy data in animals, we conducted preclinical toxicity studies designed to simulate human clinical trials. Rats were given high doses of virus intrapleurally followed by intraperitoneal administration of GCV at the same dose proposed for initial use in the clinical trial (10 mg/kg/day). Toxicity was limited to localized inflammation of the pleural and pericardial surfaces. Formal toxicology studies were also done in three nonhuman primates given high doses of AdHSV*tk* (10^{12} pfu) and GCV (35). There were no adverse clinical effects documented nor any hematological or biochemical abnormalities. Necropsy findings were limited to inflammatory changes in the chest wall and intrathoracic serosa.

Initial Phase I Clinical Trial

A Phase I clinical trial for patients with pleural mesothelioma began in November 1995 at the University of Pennsylvania Medical Center in conjunction with Penn's Institute for Human Gene Therapy. In this dose-escalation protocol, mesothelioma patients who met strict inclusion criteria (including patent pleural cavities) underwent intrapleural administration of a single dose of AdHSV*tk* vector followed by 2 weeks of intravenous GCV (36,37). The initial adenoviral vector used was a so-called "first-generation" replication-incompetent virus deleted in the early genes E1 and E3 with the HSV*tk* gene inserted in the E1 region. The overall goals of this trial were to determine the toxicity, gene transfer efficacy, and immune responses generated in response to the intrapleural instillation of AdHSV*tk*. The protocol was designed as a dose-escalation study that started with a vector dose of 1×10^9 plaque-forming units (pfu) and increased in half-log increments to the maximal dose level of 1×10^{12} pfu. Throughout the study, participants were carefully evaluated for evidence of toxicity, viral shedding, immune responses to the virus, and radiographic evidence of tumor response.

Twenty-six patients (21 male, 5 female), ranging in age from 37 to 81, were enrolled in the study between November 1995 and November 1997 (Table 2) (37). Intratumoral HSV*tk* gene transfer was documented in 17 of 25 evaluable patients in a dose-related fashion by DNA polymerase chain reaction (PCR), reverse transcription PCR, in situ hybridization, and immunohistochemistry (IHC) utilizing a murine monoclonal antibody directed against HSV*tk*. All patients treated at dose levels of 3.2×10^{11} pfu or greater demonstrated evidence of intratumoral HSV*tk* expression via IHC (37). Clinical toxicities of the Ad*tk*/ GCV gene therapy were well tolerated, and a maximum-tolerated dose (MTD) was not achieved. Toxicities included reversible liver function test abnormalities, anemia, fever, and bullous exanthem at the instillation site. At the highest dose level of 1×10^{12} pfu, two of three patients developed transitory hypotension and hypoxemia within hours after vector instillation that resolved with supplemental oxygen and intravenous fluids (37).

Strong antiadenoviral humoral and cellular immune responses were noted, including generation of high serum and pleural fluid titers of antiadenoviral neutralizing antibodies, generation of serum antibodies against adenoviral structural proteins, and increased peripheral blood mononuclear cell proliferative responses to adenoviral proteins (38).

In a small, pilot study, five patients (patients 19–23) received intravenous corticosteroids around the time of vector instillation. This trial was designed preliminarily to assess the effects of immunosuppression upon the degree of intratumoral gene transfer and antiadenoviral immune responses. Decreased fever and hypoxemia was noted in the corticosteroid-treated cohort, but there was also an increased incidence of reversible mental status changes (39). No diminution in antiadenoviral immune responses was demonstrated in the group receiving corticosteroids, nor were there any appreciable differences in the degree of intratumoral gene transfer.

Of the 26 patients enrolled in the initial Phase I trial, 25 have since died, with a median posttreatment survival of approximately 11 months (see Table 2). One patient (20) in the corticosteroid pilot study who had stage IV mesothelioma at the time of enrollment died 2 weeks after completion of the protocol from rapid progression of his mesothelioma with malignant involvement of the contralateral hemithorax.

Several patients with stage IA/IB epithelioid mesothelioma had posttreatment survivals of greater than 3 years, with one patient surviving over 4 years. The initial patient enrolled in the trial (patient 1) is now surviving 6 years after completion of the AdHSV*tk*/GCV protocol. He did have evidence of minimal disease progression approximately 3 years after enrollment, and he subsequently underwent pleurectomy/decortication followed by intraoperative photodynamic therapy. Of the trial participants who are deceased, all had progressive mesothelioma as their primary cause of death, typically with invasion of mediastinum,

Table 2 Results of University of Pennsylvania Phase I Clinical Trials of Ad.*tk*/GCV Gene Therapy for Mesothelioma

Patient age/sex	Stage/ cell type	Vector dose (pfu)	Post-Rx survival (months)	Gene transfer	Tumor response
1 62/M	IA/E[a]	1×10^9	72	−	SD[e] × 2 yrs
2 56/M	III/E	1×10^9	8[c]	−	−
3 69/M	III/B[b]	1×10^9	20[c]	+	−
4 66/M	II/E	3.2×10^9	11[c]	−	−
5 71/M	IA/E	3.2×10^9	58[c]	−	SD × 3 yrs
6 71/M	II/B	1×10^{10}	4[c]	+	−
7 70/M	II/E	1×10^{10}	6[c]	−	−
8 60/M	II/E	1×10^{10}	27[c]	+	−
9 74/M	II/B	3.2×10^{10}	2[c]	NP[d]	−
10 60/M	III/E	3.2×10^{10}	9[c]	−	−
11 37/F	IV/E	1×10^{11}	16[c]	−	−
12 37/M	III	1×10^{11}	2[c]	−	−
13 65/F	III/E	1×10^{11}	10[c]	+	−
14 66/F	IA/E	3.2×10^{11}	50[c]	+	SD × 2 yrs
15 60/M	IV/B	3.2×10^{11}	5[c]	+	−
16 69/M	IB/E	3.2×10^{11}	8[c]	+	−
17 70/F	IB/E	3.2×10^{11}	15[c]	+	−
18 69/F	IB/E	3.2×10^{11}	14[c]	+	−
19 75/M[f]	II/E	3.2×10^{11}	8[c]	+	−
20 68/M[f]	IV/B	3.2×10^{11}	1[c]	+	−
21 71/M[f]	IB/E	3.2×10^{11}	41[c]	+	−
22 76/M[f]	IB/E	3.2×10^{11}	33[c]	+	−
23 81/M[f]	II/E	3.2×10^{11}	25[c]	+	−
24 71/M	II/E	1×10^{12}	21[c]	+	−
25 65/M	II/E	1×10^{12}	5[c]	+	−
26 67/M	IA/E	1×10^{12}	22[c]	+	PR (CT)
27 67/M[g]	III/B	1×10^{11}	7[c]	+	−
28 53/M[g]	III/E	1×10^{11}	13[c]	+	−
29 30/F[g]	I/E	5×10^{11}	37	+	SD
30 56/F[g]	IA/E	5×10^{11}	37	+	SD
31 66/M[g]	II/E	5×10^{11}	9[c]	+	−
32 74/M[g,h]	I/E	5×10^{11}	19[c]	+	PR (PET)
33 64/M[g,h]	I/E	5×10^{11}	10[c]	+	−
34 69/M[g,h]	II/E	5×10^{11}	26	NP	−

[a] Epithelioid.
[b] Biphasic.
[c] Deceased (11/1/01). Received third-generation E1/E4–deleted adenoviral vector.
[d] Test not performed.
[e] Stable disease (CT ± PET).
[f] Received adjuvant corticosteroids.
[g] Received third-generation E1/E4–deleted adenoviral vector.
[h] Received 15 mg/kg/day of GCV × 14 days.

contralateral hemithorax, and transdiaphragmatic extension, as well as with widespread metastatic disease, which is a fairly common finding in advanced mesothelioma. Only one of the 26 patients (patient 26) had radiographic evidence of intrathoracic tumor regression post–Ad*tk*/GCV on follow-up chest computed tomographic (CT) scan. This patient eventually died from intraperitoneal disease progression. At autopsy there was extensive intraabdominal tumor but scant disease in the treated thoracic cavity.

Additional Phase I Trials of AdHSV*t*k Gene Therapy for Mesothelioma

We demonstrated in our first Phase I trial that intrapleural AdHSV*tk* gene therapy had minimal toxicity, could effectively deliver transgene to superficial areas of mesothelioma tumor nodule, and induced significant humoral and cellular responses to the Ad vector (37,38). Nevertheless, we felt that improved intratumoral gene transfer was necessary. We decided to achieve this goal initially by increasing the vector dose, but doing so with the "first-generation" vector became problematic because of high levels of replication-competent adenovirus in the vector lots.

For these reasons, in June 1998, we initiated a Phase I clinical trial employing an advanced-generation adenoviral vector containing deletions in the E1 and E4 regions with preservation of the E3 region. The presence of an intact E4 region, unlike E3, is critical to the late phase of the viral life cycle: E4 deletions decrease viral DNA synthesis and late gene expression. Adenoviral vectors with lethal deletions in E1 and E4 offered theoretical advantages over first-generation vectors for diminished cytopathic effects and reduced cellular immune responses (40). In addition, since two replication-necessary genes are deleted, simple recombination could not produce replication-competent virus in the vector production process.

The primary goals of the second Phase I clinical trial were to determine the toxicity, gene transfer efficiency, and immune responses associated with the intrapleural injection of high titers of the E1/E4–deleted AdRSV*tk* vector combined with systemic ganciclovir. Five patients were treated under this protocol, starting at a dose 1 log lower than the highest dose used with the E1/E3–deleted Ad vector (1.5×10^{13} viral particles). At this lower dose, we saw minimal toxicity, primarily transitory fever (grade 1). The next three patients were treated with a dose of 5×10^{13} viral particles with evidence of increased but non–dose-limiting toxicity. All three patients experienced acute febrile responses (grade 1) after vector instillation with rapid defervescence. One patient (29) developed hypotension and hypoxemia (grade 2) within hours after vector administration that resolved with supplemental oxygen and intravenous fluids. Patient 29 also developed elevated serum transaminases to levels approximately two to three times normal (grade 2) after vector delivery, peaking during the first week of ganciclovir therapy, but returning to normal levels by the completion of the protocol. The patient had no associated elevations in serum bilirubin or prothrombin time and no clinical evidence of hepatic dysfunction. The third patient treated at the higher dose level (patient 31) developed low-grade fever (grade 1) post–intrapleural vector instillation, as well as a contralateral pleural inflammation. Overall, there appeared to be a trend toward lower hepatoxicity in the patients treated with the E1/E4–deleted vector compared to patients treated with equivalent doses of the E1/E3–deleted adenovirus but a similar pattern of increased systemic side effects at higher dose levels (41).

Dose-related gene transfer was detected in all patients at both dose levels via immunohistochemistry using an anti-HSV*tk* monoclonal antibody. As in the initial Phase I trial, significant humoral responses to the recombinant adenoviral vector were seen in all five patients, with the development of high serum titers of total and neutralizing antiadenoviral antibodies within 15–20 days of vector instillation (41).

Of the five patients treated in this second Phase I trial, there are two surviving (patients 29 and 30), both of whom were treated at the higher dose level of 5.0×10^{13} particles of AdHSV*tk* (Table 2). Each of the patients had stage I epithelioid mesothelioma at diagnosis. Both have had clinically and radiographically stable disease without other antitumor therapy for 36 months after treatment. Patient 29, a 34-year-old female, has demonstrated diminished tumor metabolic activity on serial follow-up 18-fluordeoxyglucose positron emission tomography (18-FDG PET) scans (Fig. 1). This delayed decrease in tumor metabolic activity

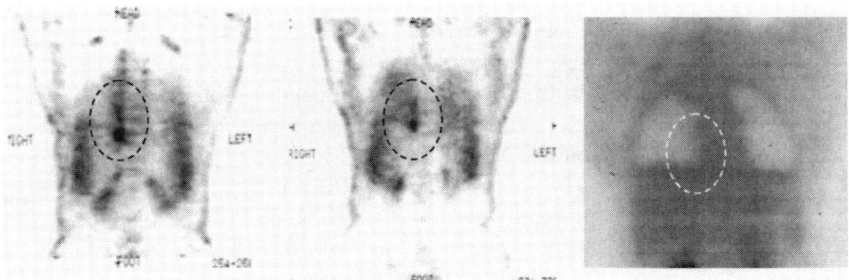

Figure 1 One of the eight patients enrolled in E1/E4–deleted vector protocols, patient 29, had objective evidence of tumor response before and after gene therapy 18-fluorodeoxyglucose (FDG) PET imaging, with near-complete absence of FDG uptake on an 18-FDG PET scan performed 18 months after completion of the protocol (see text). This objective metabolic response correlated with the patient's excellent clinical status and stability on serial chest CT scans. She has had no other antineoplastic therapy other than our gene therapy protocol.

several months after completion of the gene therapy protocol suggests the induction of a secondary immune bystander effect induced by AdRSV*tk*/GCV (41).

Based upon in vitro and animal experiments in mesothelioma models demonstrating a direct correlation between GCV dose and cytotoxic response after tumor transduction with HSV*tk*, we initiated another Phase I clinical trial involving gradual dose escalation of the nucleoside analog in combination with intrapleural delivery of the E1/E4–deleted Ad vector (29,31,37,42,43). We completed the first cohort of three patients each of whom were treated with 3×10^{13} particles of AdRSV*tk* (E1/E4–deleted) and 7.5 mg/kg ganciclovir IV twice a day (15 mg/kg/day). All three patients tolerated the treatment well. Toxicities were non–dose limiting and included fever, lymphopenia, liver function test abnormalities, hyponatremia, and hypokalemia. One of three patients is still alive, albeit with evidence of significant tumor progression, now 26 months after treatment (see Table 1). No durable clinical responses were noted in any of the three patients treated in this protocol, although the initial patient (101) treated demonstrated reduced 18-FDG uptake in the mediastinal and parietal pleural regions on his posttreatment scan. Subsequent 18-FDG PET scanning at day 170, however, showed a significant increase in tracer uptake consistent with increased tumor metabolic activity. This correlated with the patient's increasing clinical symptoms and progressive pleural thickening and nodularity on repeat chest CT scan. Patients 102 and 103 both demonstrated increased 18-FDG uptake on their follow-up day 80 PET studies, and they also had clear evidence of progression on chest CT.

Challenges and Future Directions

Based upon our clinical trial experiences of limited toxicity, successful gene transfer, and anecdotal tumor responses, the AdHSV*tk*/GCV suicide gene therapy approach has potential for the treatment of malignant mesothelioma, as well as other localized malignancies. Unfortunately, these Phase I trials were halted in midstream because of the death of a participant in a gene therapy trial for ornithine transcarbamylase (OTC) deficiency at the University of Pennsylvania Medical Center utilizing a similar adenoviral vector backbone (44). Nonetheless, one of the most valuable aspects of our trial has been the identification of specific challenges that need to be addressed, such as gene transfer efficiency.

Using the current strategy, therapeutic efficacy could only be expected in patients with relatively small tumor burdens (small nodules or diffuse, "thin" tumors). An alternative treatment schema maximizing the vector:tumor cell ratio would involve surgical "debulking" to minimize tumor mass followed by adjuvant administration of AdHSV*tk*/GCV. Another method of improving intratumoral gene transfer would be repeated administration of vector and GCV (i.e., three doses over a 3-week period). Recently completed studies in immunocompetent mice with established peritoneal tumors by our group (45) and others (46) showed marked increases in efficacy after multiple intraperitoneal injections of AdHSV*tk*, each followed by a course of GCV. Importantly, data from our initial clinical trials suggest that gene transfer is possible even in patients with titers of anti-Ad neutralizing antibodies of up to 1:500, as would be expected with repeated administration of Ad vector.

Another approach to the gene transfer problem is to maximize the efficacy of the expressed HSV*tk* enzyme. The underlying principal of our suicide gene approach is that the herpes simplex thymidine kinase-1 enzyme has a relaxed specificity (in comparison to mammalian thymidine kinase) that allows it to phosphorylate not only thymidine but other nucleoside analogs such as ganciclovir (GCV) and acyclovir (ACV). Unfortunately, HSV*tk* has a high affinity for thymidine ($K_m = 0.5$ μM), whereas the affinities for GCV ($K_m = 45$ μM) and ACV ($K_m \geq 400$ μM) are much lower (47). "Molecular remodeling" of the HSV*tk* enzyme has allowed increasing specificity for GCV and ACV and concomitantly decreased thymidine utilization (47). These HSV*tk* mutants show increased ACV- and GCV-mediated cytotoxicity and enhanced bystander effects in mixing experiments (48,49). We have produced adenoviral vectors containing the mutated HSV*tk*s and demonstrated enhanced cell killing and augmented bystander effect in in vitro and in vivo models of mesothelioma. (S.M. Albelda, personal communication).

An additional mechanism of maximizing intratumoral gene transfer would be to produce adenoviral vectors capable of selective replication in mesothelioma cells. In this system, tumor killing could occur via two mechanisms: direct tumor lysis due to viral replication and by HSV*tk*-mediated killing after administration of GCV. Widespread dissemination will be precluded by the intact host immune response (50). We are developing tumor-selective replicating AdHSV*tk* vectors by substituting the adenoviral E1 promoter with promoters for tumor-related proteins such as manganese superoxide dismutase (MnSOD), calretinin, and mesothelin. Recent work by the Kinnula group in Finland has shown that MnSOD is very highly expressed in human malignant mesothelioma tissues and cell lines (51). Calretinin is a 29-kD calcium-binding protein that is expressed primarily in the nervous system, but high levels of expression have also been noted in cells of mesothelial origin (52,53). Mesothelin is 40-kD surface protein of unknown function that is expressed only on the tissues forming the pleural, pericardial, and peritoneal membranes (54). Other more general tumor-selective promoters, such as promoters responsive to the transcription factor E2F (55) or the survivin gene (56) would also be candidates.

III. Suicide Gene Vaccines

A growing body of evidence supports the hypothesis that in most models tested, treatment with HSV*tk*/GCV results in an immunological bystander effect that enhances antitumor cytotoxicity both at the site of vector delivery as well as at distant, nontransduced tumor site (14,19,57–59). We believe that we have seen evidence of this immune bystander effect in our mesothelioma Phase I clinical trials with the progressive decline in tumor metabolic activity seen on PET scan in patient 29 over 36 months posttreatment. This putative antitumor immune reaction may result from *non*apoptotic HSV*tk*/GCV–mediated tumor necrosis, a type of cell death that releases so-called "danger signals" that then activate significant cellular immune responses (59,60). Generation of these danger signals may be enhanced by transduction of tumor cells with the HSV*tk* gene *plus* a cytokine gene such as the gene for interleukin-2 (IL-2). Augmented tumor cytotoxicity has been reported with HSV*tk* plus IL-2 in mouse liver metastasis from colon carcinoma (61), a mouse squamous cell carcinoma model (62), a murine melanoma model (63), and a rat intraperitoneal colon cancer model (64). Animal studies are underway in mouse models of mesothelioma to determine the best combination of cytokines with HSV*tk*, as well as the best way to combine these therapies (i.e., direct injection of cytokine versus delivery of cytokine using gene therapy). This method of causing mesothelioma tumor destruction via the immunological bystander effects of HSV*tk*/GCV gene therapy, a presumptive "suicide gene vaccine," was studied in a Phase I clinical trial conducted by Schwarzenberger and colleagues at the Louisiana State University (LSU) Medical Center in New Orleans (see Table 1) (7). The protocol designed by the LSU investigators consisted of the intrapleural instillation via an indwelling pleural catheter of an irradiated ovarian carcinoma cell line retrovirally transfected with HSV*tk* (PA1-STK cells) followed by systemic administration of GCV (7). Schwarzenberger and colleagues hypothesized that the PA1-STK cells would migrate to areas of intrapleural tumor after instillation, undergo necrotic cell death after exposure to GCV, and generate immune responses that would facilitate killing of adjacent mesothelioma cells. The LSU group performed in vitro mixing experiments showing that PA1-STK cells, in combination with GCV, killed both mouse and human mesothelioma cells in a dose-dependent manner. In syngeneic murine models of mesothelioma, PA1-STK cells administration (with GCV) prolonged survival when the percentage of transduced tumor cells was high (70%), but there was no survival benefit when the percentage of PA1-STK cells was low (30%) (65).

Anti-mesothelioma immune responses in this system are related to the local generation of proinflammatory cytokines which, in turn, summon an influx of cytotoxic lymphocytes to the area producing hemorrhagic tumor necrosis (7,66). In patients treated to date, minimal side effects have been seen, whereas preliminary findings showed significant posttreatment increases in the percentage of CD8 T lymphocytes in pleural fluid (66).

The LSU investigators have also demonstrated that PA1-STK cells home to mesothelioma deposits in patients after intrapleural instillation. They performed a substudy in which the gene-modified ovarian cancer cells expressing the thymidine kinase gene (PA1-STK) were radiolabeled with ^{99}technecium and infused into the pleural space of four patients with malignant pleural mesothelioma. The patients were then scanned to determine the distribution of the cells. PA1-STK cells recognized and adhered preferentially to mesothelioma lining the chest wall, confirming the feasibility of this treatment concept (67).

IV. Cytokine Gene Therapy for Mesothelioma

There has been significant interest at many centers in the delivery of genes encoding for proinflammatory cytokines to the pleural space of patients with malignant mesothelioma. The hypothesis behind this approach is that the expression of cytokine genes by tumor cells generates a high level of intratumoral cytokines in a paracrine fashion, inducing powerful local cytokine effects without significant systemic toxicity. Prolonged local cytokine expression can induce activation of tumor-infiltrating dendritic cells (DCs) to express major histocompatibility complex (MHC)–tumor antigen complexes in conjunction with costimulatory molecules. These activated DCs can then migrate to regional lymph nodes where they stimulate proliferation of tumor specific CD8 and CD4 lymphocytes, inducing antitumor cytotoxicity at distant sites of tumor. In addition, some proinflammatory cytokines such as IL-2 have the capability of direct intratumoral activation of CD8$^+$ tumor-infiltrating lymphocytes, overcoming tolerance signals to produce tumor specific cytotoxic lymphocytes (CTLs). Increased intratumoral IL-2 may also activate natural killer (NK) cells and lymphokine-activated killer cells (LAKs). Animal experiments have shown that injection of IL-2–transduced tumor cells increases specific antitumor activity, generates systemic responses to the parental tumor, augments the immune response against autologous tumor, and causes rejection of rechallenged tumor cells (68,69).

One of the rationales for the use of cytokine gene therapy in mesothelioma is that exogenous cytokines are known to have direct antiproliferative effects upon mesothelioma cells, as well as the ability to activate intrapleural and intratumoral immune effector cells in vivo. Several published Phase I and Phase II clinical trials have documented mesothelioma tumor responses to intrapleural infusion of interleukin-2 (IL-2), interferon-β (IFN-β), and interferon-γ (IFN-γ) (70–76). In particular, Boutin and colleagues at the Hôpital de la Conçeption in Marseille, France, demonstrated significant response rates in pleural mesothelioma after intrapleural instillation of IFN-γ, including several complete pathological responses in patients with stage IA disease (tumor limited to the parietal and diaphragmatic pleural surfaces) (73,74).

In the first human clinical trial of direct intratumoral delivery of cytokine genes in malignant pleural mesothelioma, this method of in vivo genetic immunotherapy was conducted by investigators at Queen Elizabeth II Hospital in Perth, Australia, using a recombinant vaccinia virus (VV) expressing the human IL-2 gene (see Table 1). A vaccinia vector was chosen because of its large genome, proven safety in human vaccines, and availability of anti-VV antibodies for evaluation of vector-induced immune responses. In addition, insertion of the IL-2 gene into the thymidine kinase region of the VV rendered it partially replication restricted, allowing for relatively more expression in tumor cells. The VV–IL-2 vector at a dose of 1×10^7 pfu was serially injected into palpable chest wall lesions of six patients with advanced malignant mesothelioma. Toxicities were minimal, and there was no clinical or serological evidence of spread of VV to patient contacts. No significant tumor regression was seen in any of the patients, and only modest intratumoral T-cell infiltration was detected. VV–IL-2 mRNA was detected by reverse transcriptase PCR in serial tumor biopsies for up to 6 days after injection, but it declined to low levels by day 8. The prolonged nature of IL-2 gene expression in this trial was remarkable considering the fact that significant serum titers of anti-VV neutralizing antibodies were generated in all patients (77).

The use of cellular vectors to deliver the IL-2 gene in patients with pleural mesothelioma is currently being studied in a Phase II European clinical trial sponsored by Transgene, Inc. (Strasburg, France). Mertelsmann and colleagues in Freiburg, Germany, are conducting a Phase II randomized study of nonspecific immunotherapy of malignant mesothelioma by repeated intratumoral injection of "Vero cells" engineered to produce human IL-2 (Vero-IL2). Vero cells are immortalized monkey fibroblasts capable of constitutive expression of therapeutic human proteins such as inflammatory cytokines. Vero cells can be grown in culture, packaged in vials, tested for quality, stored, and administered to the patient like a standard medicinal product. Transgene, Inc. has engineered Vero cells to secrete very high levels of either human IL-2 or other cytokines including IFN-γ. The first two mesothelioma patients in this study were enrolled in March 1999 with the plan to enroll 20 patients in total. This Phase II trial is based upon earlier animal studies demonstrating efficacy of Vero-IL2 therapy in the treatment of spontaneously occurring tumors, as well as two Phase I clinical trials completed in France and Switzerland documenting safety of this product in human subjects and preliminary evidence of antitumor activity (78).

A. Future of Genetic Immunotherapy for Mesothelioma

Several other candidate cytokine genes are being evaluated for therapeutic effectiveness in animal models of mesothelioma. Caminschi and colleagues at Queen Elizabeth II Medical Center in Perth have investigated genetic alteration of murine mesothelioma cell lines with the gene for IL-12, one of the most active immunomodulatory cytokines. This same group previously demonstrated that systemic administration of exogenous IL-12 induced strong antitumor immune responses in mice bearing syngeneic mesothelioma tumors (79). The Perth group showed that injection of murine mesothelioma cells transfected with the IL-12 gene (AB1–IL-12) did not produce tumors in immune-competent mice, but did so in athymic nude mice, implicating a T-cell–dependent mechanism of IL-12 activity. Immune competent mice challenged with AB1–IL-12 were protected from subsequent challenge with parental tumor not expressing IL-12, demonstrating induction of long-term immunity. In addition, AB1–IL-12 injection reduced the incidence of tumor development from parental cell challenge at a distant site (80).

B. Nonspecific Immune Stimulation

Innate and adaptive antitumor immune responses can also be elicited by delivery of nonspecific immunostimulatory genes. As an example of this paradigm, Lukacs and colleagues transferred mycobacterial heat shock protein gene (HSP-65) via a cationic liposome into the abdominal cavities of mice bearing intraperitoneal sarcomas resulting in a significant antitumor response (81). The rationale for the in vivo efficacy of HSP gene transfer was that HSPs, expressed in tumor cells, could serve as "molecular chaperones," facilitating more efficient tumor antigen presentation via MHC molecules. Interestingly, Lanuti and colleagues in our laboratory found that the antitumor effects of HSP gene transfer via cationic liposomes could be reproduced in a syngeneic murine model of mesothelioma, but appeared to be related to nonspecific effects of lipid-pDNA complexes. Significant survival advantages compared with saline control were observed with plasmid delivery of HSP-65, the *E. coli* β-galactosidase marker gene *lacZ*, as well as with a null vector (82). Surprisingly, there did not appear to be a survival benefit for heat shock gene transfer compared with the null vector alone. Lanuti and colleague therefore postulated that the unmethylated CpG motifs of the prokaryotic DNA in the null vector were sufficient to activate danger signals and initiate innate and adaptive antitumor immune responses (82).

These findings were similar to those of Lukacs and colleagues in their study of intraperitoneal delivery of the β-gal gene into immunocompetent mice bearing intraperitoneal mesotheliomas. Transfection of tumor cells with plasmid-liposome complexes or replication-incompetent retroviruses (with and without liposomes) encoding for β-gal engendered significant reduction in intraperitoneal mesothelioma burden in immunocompetent but not immunodeficient mice. Although the retrovirus-liposome constructs provided the greatest β-gal expression, there was no correlation to superior antitumor response. Lukacs' group demonstrated as well the generation of tumor-specific CTLs in mice treated with intraperitoneal β-gal–plasmid/liposome complexes. Therefore, the antitumor effect induced by the expression of bacterial antigen in tumor cells is likely mediated via a T-cell mechanism (83).

Rudginsky and colleagues at Genzyme Corporation (Framingham, MA) further explored the potential of prokaryotic DNA induction in mesothelioma cells. They conducted a series of experiments confirming antitumor responses and increased survival with liposomal delivery of fragments of bacterial plasmid DNA, genomic *E. coli* DNA, and synthetic CpG oligonucleotides. No increased survival or tumor reductions were seen with liposomal delivery of eukaryotic DNA or with methylated bacterial DNA. Therefore, the unmethylated CpG motifs of prokaryotic DNA play a crucial role in the development of innate and adaptive antitumor immune responses. Intraperitoneal lavage after liposomal delivery revealed elevations in the proinflammatory cytokines tumor necrosis factor-α (TNF-α) and IL-12 only with those complexes inducing antitumor immunity (84). Based upon the Lanuti, Lukacs, and Rudginsky experiences, therefore, a case could then be made for a straightforward clinical trial of intrapleural delivery of nonspecific lipid-pDNA in patients with mesothelioma (see Table 1).

C. INF-β Gene Therapy

As previously mentioned, the type I (α, β) and type II (γ) interferons have been shown to have clinical antitumor activity when administered exogenously to patients with pleural mesothelioma. IFN-β, for example, has potent antiproliferative in vitro effects on mesothelioma cells and strong immunostimulatory actions in animal models, but it is limited in clinical use by toxicity of systemic administration (85). Odaka and colleagues at the University of Pennsylvania Medical Center therefore investigated the effects of IFN-β gene therapy in murine models of mesothelioma. The Penn investigators showed that a single intraperitoneal (i.p.) injection of a recombinant adenovirus engineered to express the murine INF-β gene (AdmuIFN-β) can eradicate syngeneic murine mesothelioma in >90% of animals tested. Intraperitoneal AdmuIFN-β gene therapy resulted as well in significant reduction of subcutaneous tumors at a distant site. These effects of AdmuIFN-β were clearly shown in several experiments to be mediated by CD8+ T lymphocytes. The Penn investigators hope to develop human clinical trials of intrapleural delivery of AdmuIFN-β for the treatment of mesothelioma (see Table 1) (86).

V. Induction of Apoptosis

One of the primary approaches to cancer gene therapy research over the past decade has been mutation compensation—the replacement of absent or mutated tumor-suppressor genes responsible, at least in part, for the malignant phenotype of the cancer cell. Intratumoral delivery of the wild-type p53 gene, for example, has been the most frequent method of experimental gene therapy of solid tumors, as mutations in the p53 tumor-suppressor gene account for the majority of genetic abnormalities in solid tumors. Most mesotheliomas, however, contain wild-type p53 and a normal copy of the cell cycle regulator pRB. The most common molecular abnormality found in pleural mesotheliomas is absent expression of the cyclin-dependent kinase (cdk) inhibitor, p16^{INK4a}. This mutation can lead to unmitigated progression through the cell cycle despite the presence of normal pRB expression and wild-type p53, and therefore the development of a neoplastic phenotype (87).

Kratzke and colleagues at the University of Minnesota School of Medicine have demonstrated that reexpression of p16^{INK4a} in mesothelioma cells in vitro and in vivo results in cell cycle arrest, cell growth inhibition, apoptosis, and tumor reduction (88). In addition, the Minnesota investigators have recently shown that repeated administration of an adenoviral vector expressing wild-type p16^{INK4a} into established human mesothelioma xenografts in athymic nude mice resulted in prolongation of survival compared with controls receiving saline or an Ad vector expressing the marker gene *lacZ* (87). Successful application of this technology to human clinical trials is dependent upon the development of more efficient means of tumor cell transduction.

Investigators at the Thoracic Oncology Laboratory, University of California, San Francisco (UCSF) Cancer Center are targeting another common mutation in mesotheliomas for mutation compensation gene therapeutic approaches. Jablons and colleagues at UCSF have demonstrated that homozygous deletion of the INK4a/ARF locus is common in human mesotheliomas. The p14(ARF) protein encoded by the INK4a/ARF locus promotes degradation of the MDM2 protein and thus prevents the MDM2-mediated inhibition of p53. Deletion of the INK4a/ARF locus, therefore, may abrogate p14(ARF) protein expression, thereby inactivating p53 (via MDM2), and leading to unchecked progression through the cell cycle. The UCSF transfected human mesothelioma cell lines with an adenoviral vector encoding for human p14(ARF) complementary DNA (Adp14). Overexpression of p14(ARF) within the mesothelioma cells led to increased amounts of p53 and p21 and dephosphorylation of pRb. In addition, Adp14 inhibited mesothelioma cell growth via induction G1 phase cell cycle arrest and apoptotic cell death. To date, this approach has not yet been tested in human clinical trials (89).

Interestingly, Jablons and colleagues have also investigated the efficacy of the ONYX-015 adenovirus in mesothelioma cells, and they found that the cytolytic effect of this agent in mesothelioma is dependent upon absence of p14(ARF) expression. ONYX-015 is a conditionally replication-competent adenovirus lacking the E1b–55-kD gene, and therefore can only replicate in tumor cells lacking functional p53. (One of the functions of E1b–55-kD is to bind and inactivate wild-type p53.) Clinical trials of ONYX-015 in patients with cancers of the head and neck and lung have shown evidence of tumor reduction with minimal toxicity. As described above, in mesothelioma, unlike many other solid tumors, genetic alterations in p53 are uncommon, but functional inhibition of p53 can be achieved via deletions in the INK4a/ARF locus. The UCSF group demonstrated in vitro cytotoxicity of ONYX-015 on mesothelioma cell lines lacking p14(ARF), and increased resistance of these same cell lines to ONYX-015 after transfection of the tumor cells with Adp14 (90).

Despite the fact that most mesotheliomas have wild-type p53 (wt-p53), the function of p53 in mesothelioma cells may be abnormal secondary to binding of p53 by inhibitor proteins such as mdm2 and simian virus 40 (SV40) large T antigen. Therefore, there may be a rationale for gene therapy of mesothelioma via overexpression of wt-p53 within the cell. Giuliano and colleagues in Chieti, Italy, performed a series of experiments in which they transfected human mesothelioma cells with a replication-deficient adenoviral vector carrying the wt-p53 gene (91). They demonstrated greater than 80% inhibition of tumor cell growth in vitro at a multiplicity of infection (MOI) of 25 with documentation of induction of apoptosis in the dying tumor cells. In addition, Giuliano and colleagues showed that ex vivo transfer of the wt-p53 gene to mesothelioma cells inhibited growth of tumor implants in nude mice. In immunodeficient mice with established human mesothelioma xenografts, intratumoral injection of the wt-p53 gene inhibited tumor growth and prolonged survival (91). It is not inconceivable, therefore, to consider human clinical trials of Adwt-p53 gene therapy in mesothelioma akin to those conducted in lung cancer, head and neck cancer, and metastatic colon cancer (see Table 1).

An alternate method of inhibiting mesothelioma cells is the introduction of "downstream" promoters of apoptosis such as the proapoptotic Bcl-2 family member Bak. Pataer and colleagues at M.D. Anderson Cancer Center in Houston codelivered binary adenoviral-Bak/GV-16 vectors into wt-p53–positive and mutated p53 mesothelioma cell lines in vitro, along with binary Ad*lacZ*/GV-16 control vectors (92). The M.D. Anderson group demonstrated marked induction of apoptosis and decreased cellular viability in *both* p53 "sensitive" and "resistant" cell lines with *Bak* gene transfer but not with *lacZ* delivery. Thus, gene transfer in vivo with proapoptotic Bcl-2 family members would be a reasonable strategy for future mesothelioma gene therapy clinical trials.

VI. SV40: Is There a Role in Therapy for Mesothelioma?

One of the most remarkable developments in mesothelioma research over the past several years has been the discovery of SV sequences in mesothelioma tumor specimens from the United States and several European countries. SV40, a nonhuman polyomavirus which was a contaminant of some polio vaccines in the 1950s and 1960s, carries the ability to transform normal cells via the oncogenic properties of its large T antigen (Tag), and can induce the formation of mesotheliomas in hamsters after injection into the pleural space or peritoneal cavity (93). Laboratory analysis of a subset of human mesotheliomas has demonstrated coimmunoprecipitation of SV40 Tag with tumor-suppressor gene products such as the p53 and pRB proteins (94). The presence of SV40 Tag within tumor cells binding and inactivating wt-p53 and pRB may explain the unusually high rate of wt-p53 and pRb within mesotheliomas, unlike most other solid tumors.

The potential role for SV40 as a causative factor in mesothelioma oncogenesis and proliferation has inspired several new experimental gene therapy approaches. Schrump and colleagues at the Thoracic Oncology branch of the National Cancer Institute have shown that antisense oligonucleotides designed to abrogate SV40 Tag expression induce apoptosis and enhance sensitivity to chemotherapeutic agents in SV40(+) mesothelioma cells in vitro (95). Another strategy has been advocated by Imperiale and colleagues at the University of Michigan and Wayne State University Medical Centers who are developing a genetically engineered vaccine to SV40 Tag. SV40 is an excellent candidate for antigen-specific immunotherapy, because Tag is a viral antigen which should not induce immune tolerance unlike most other tumor antigens. The Michigan group has created a recombinant, truncated version of Tag (mTag) modified to exclude the domains involved in oncogenic function: the J domain and the p53 and pRB binding domains. They have cloned the mTag gene into a vaccinia vector (vac-mTag), and have demonstrated significant antitumor immune responses in Balb/c mice carrying Tag(+) tumors. A Phase I dose-escalation safety and toxicity trial in patients with Tag-expressing mesotheliomas is planned (see Table 1) (96).

VII. Conclusions

Gene therapy for mesothelioma is in its infancy, yet the results of recent Phase I clinical trials and ongoing preclinical studies offer significant promise for the future. Intrapleural and intratumoral injections of viral and vectors encoding therapeutic genes have proved to be safe in humans with evidence of intratumoral gene transfer and expression of therapeutic proteins. Anecdotal tumor responses have been seen in suicide gene therapy trials either as a resultant of direct cytotoxicity or via induction of bystander immunological phenomena. Expanding knowledge of the cellular and molecular abnormalities responsible for the carcinogenesis of mesothelioma has led to the development of gene therapy approaches targeting oncoproteins and mutant tumor-suppressor genes. Implementation of these experimental modalities on a routine basis for mesothelioma patients remains several years in the future. Nevertheless, the lack of significant benefit from standard anticancer treatments in the disease argues strongly for patient enrollment in clinical studies of various gene therapy approaches to determine safety, toxicity, and efficacy, as well as to guide future laboratory investigation.

Acknowledgments

The HSV*tk* studies were supported by Grant No. P01 CA66726 from the National Cancer Institute and Grant MO1-RR00040 to the General Clinical Research Center of the University of Pennsylvania Medical Center from the National Gene Vector Laboratories, the Nicolette Asbestos Trust, the Benjamin Shein Foundation for Humanity, and the Samuel H. Lunenfeld Charitable Foundation. Institutional support was provided by the University of Pennsylvania Cancer Center.

References

1. Sterman D, Kaiser L, Albelda S. Advances in the treatment of malignant pleural mesothelioma. Chest 1999; 116:504–520.
2. Rusch V. Trials in malignant mesothelioma. LCSG 851 and 882. Chest 1994; 106: 359S–362S.
3. Rusch V. Pleurectomy/decortication and adjuvant therapy for malignant mesothelioma. Chest 1993; 103:382S–384S.
4. Martini N, McCormack PM, Bains MS, Kaiser LR, Burt ME, Hilaris BS. Pleural mesothelioma. Ann Thorac Surg 1987; 43:113–120.
5. Rusch VW, Figlin R, Godwin D, Piantadosi S. Intrapleural cisplatin and cytarabine in the management of malignant pleural effusions: a Lung Cancer Study Group trial. J Clin Oncol 1991; 9:313–319.
6. Treat J, Kaiser LR, Sterman DH, Litzky L, Davis A, Wilson JM, Albelda SM. Treatment of advanced mesothelioma with the recombinant adenovirus H5.010RSVTK: a phase 1 trial (BB-IND 6274). Hum Gene Ther 1996; 7:2047–2057.
7. Schwarzenberger P, Harrison L, Weinacker A, Gaumer R, Theodossiou C, Summer W, Ye P, Marrogi AJ, Ramesh R, Freeman S, Kolls J. Gene therapy for malignant mesothelioma: a novel approach for an incurable cancer with increased incidence in Louisiana. J La State Med Soc 1998; 150:168–174.
8. Robinson BW, Mukherjee SA, Davidson A, Morey S, Musk AW, Ramshaw I, Smith D, Lake R, Haenel T, Garlepp M, Marley J, Leong C, Caminischi I, Scott B. Cytokine gene therapy or infusion as treatment for solid human cancer. J Immunother 1998; 21:211–217.
9. Tiberghien P. Use of suicide genes in gene therapy. J Leukoc Biol 1994; 56:203–209.
10. Huber BE, Austin EA, Richards CA, Davis ST, Good SS. Metabolism of 5-fluorocytosine to 5-fluorouracil in human colorectal tumor cells transduced with the cytosine

deaminase gene: significant antitumor effects when only a small percentage of tumor cells express cytosine deaminase. Proc Natl Acad Sci USA 1994; 91:8302–8306.

11. Hoganson DK, Batra RK, Olsen JC, Boucher RC. Comparison of the effects of three different toxin genes and their levels of expression on cell growth and bystander effect in lung adenocarcinoma. Cancer Res 1996; 56:1315–1323.

12. Matthews T, Boehme R. Antiviral activity and mechanism of action of ganciclovir. Rev Infect Dis 1988; 10:S490–S494.

13. Rubsam LZ, Davidson BL, Shewach DS. Superior cytotoxicity with ganciclovir compared with acyclovir and 1-β-D-arabinofuranosylthymine in herpes simplex virus–thymidine kinase expressing cells: a novel paradigm for cell killing. Cancer Res 1998; 58:3873–3882.

14. Pope IM, Poston GJ, Kinsella AR. The role of the bystander effect in suicide gene therapy. Eur J Cancer 1997; 33:1005–1016.

15. Moolten FL, Wells JM, Mroz PJ. Multiple transduction as a means of preserving ganciclovir chemosensitivity in sarcoma cells carrying retrovirally transduced herpes thymidine kinase genes. Cancer Lett 1992; 64:257–263.

16. Ram Z, Culver KW, Walbridge B, Blaese RM, Oldfield EH. In situ retroviral-mediated gene transfer for the treatment of brain tumors in rats. Cancer Res 1993; 53:83–88.

17. Freeman SM, Abboud CN, Whartenby KA, Packman CH, Koeplin DS, Moolten FL, Abraham GN. The "bystander effect": tumor regression when a fraction of the tumor mass is genetically modified. Cancer Res 1993; 53:5274–5283.

18. Hasegawa Y, Emi N, Shimokata K, Abe A, Kawabe T, Hasegawa T, Kirioka T, Saito H. Gene transfer of herpes simplex virus type I thymidine kinase gene as a drug sensitivity gene into human lung cancer lines using retroviral vectors. Am J Respir Cell Mol Biol 1993; 8:655–661.

19. Caruso M, Panis Y, Gagandeep S, Houssin D, Salzmann JL, Klatzmann D. Regression of established macroscopic liver metastases after in situ transduction of a suicide gene. Proc Natl Acad Sci USA 1993; 90:7024–7028.

20. Elshami AA, Saavedra A, Zhang HB, Kucharczuk JC, Spray DC, Fishman GI, Kaiser LR, Albelda SM. Gap junctions play a role in the bystander effect of the herpes simplex virus thymidine kinase/ganciclovir system in vitro. Gene Ther 1996; 3:85–92.

21. Mesnil M, Yamasaki H. Bystander effect in herpes simplex virus–thymidine kinase/ganciclovir cancer gene therapy: role of gap-junctional intercellular communication. Cancer Res 2000; 60:3989–3999.

22. Vile RG, Hart IR. Use of tissue-specific expression of the herpes simplex virus thymidine kinase gene to inhibit growth of established murine melanomas following direct intratumoral injection of DNA. Cancer Res 1993; 53:3860–3864.

23. Culver KW, Ram Z, Wallbridge S, Ishii I, Oldfield EH, Blaese RM. In vivo gene transfer with retroviral vector-producer cells for treatment of experimental brain tumors. Science 1992; 256:1550–1552.

24. Vile RG, Nelson JA, Castleden S, Chong H, Hart IR. Systemic gene therapy of murine melanoma using tissue specific expression of the HSV*tk* gene involves an immune component. Cancer Res 1994; 54:6228–6234.

25. Moolten FL. Drug sensitivity ("suicide") genes for selective cancer therapy. Cancer Gene Ther 1994; 1:279–287.
26. Kozarsky K, Wilson JM. Gene Therapy: Adenovirus vectors. Curr Opin Genet Dev 1993; 3:499–503.
27. Smythe WR, Hwang HC, Elshami AA, Amin K, Eck S, Davidson B, Wilson J, Kaiser LR, Albelda SM. Successful treatment of experimental human mesothelioma using adenovirus transfer of the herpes simplex–thymidine kinase gene. Ann Surg 1995; 222:78–86.
28. Chen SH, Shine HD, Goodman JC, Grossman R, Woo SLC. Gene therapy for brain tumors: regression of experimental gliomas by adenovirus-mediated gene transfer in vivo. Proc Natl Acad Sci USA 1994; 91:3054–3057.
29. Hwang HC, Smythe WR, Elshami AA, Kucharczuk JC, Amin K, Williams JP, Litzky LA, Kaiser LR, Albelda SM. Gene therapy using adenovirus carrying the herpes simplex thymidine kinase gene to treat in vitro models of human malignant mesothelioma and lung cancer. Am J Respir Cell Mol Biol 1995; 13:7–16.
30. Elshami A, Kucharczuk J, Zhang H, Smythe W, Huang H, Amin K, Litzky L, Kaiser LR, Albelda SM. Treatment of pleural mesothelioma in an immunocompetent rat model utilizing adenoviral transfer of the HSV–thymidine kinase gene. Hum Gene Ther 1996; 7:141–148.
31. Perez-Cruet MJ, Trask TW, Chen SH, Goodman JC, Woo SLC, Grossman RG, Shine HD. Adenovirus-mediated gene therapy of experimental gliomas. J Neurosci Res 1994; 39:506–511.
32. Smythe WR, Hwang HC, Amin KM, Eck S, Wilson J, Kaiser LR, Albelda SM. Use of recombinant adenovirus to transfer the herpes simplex virus thymidine kinase (HSV*tk*) gene to thoracic neoplasms: an effective in vitro drug sensitization system. Cancer Res 1994; 54:2055–2059.
33. Smythe WR, Kaiser LR, Amin KM, Pilewski J, Eck S, Wilson J, Albelda SM. Successful adenovirus-mediated gene transfer in an in vivo model of human malignant mesothelioma. Ann Thor Surg 1994; 57:1395–1401.
34. Esandi MC, van Someren GD, Vincent AJ, van Bekkum DW, Valerio D, Bout A, Noteboom JL. Gene therapy of experimental malignant mesothelioma using adenovirus vectors encoding the HSV*tk* gene. Gene Ther 1997; 4:280–287.
35. Kucharczuk JC, Raper S, Elshami AA, Amin K, Sterman DH, Litzky LA, Kaiser LR, Albelda SM. Safety of adenoviral-mediated transfer of the herpes simplex thymidine kinase cDNA to the pleural cavity of rats and non-human primates. Hum Gene Ther 1996; 7:2225–2233.
36. Treat J, Kaiser LR, Sterman DH, Litzky LA, Davis A, Wilson JM, Albelda SM. Treatment of advanced mesothelioma with the recombinant adenovirus H5.010RSV*TK*: a phase 1 trial (BB-IND 6274). Hum Gene Ther 1996; 7:2047–2057.
37. Sterman DH, Treat J, Litzky LA, Amin K, Molnar-Kimber K, Wilson J, Albelda SM, Kaiser LR. Adenovirus-mediated herpes simplex virus thymidine kinase gene delivery in patients with localized malignancy: results of a phase 1 clinical trial in malignant mesothelioma. Hum Gene Ther 1998; 9:1083–1092.
38. Molnar-Kimber KL, Sterman DH, Chang M, Elbash M, Elshami A, Roberts JR, Treat J, Wilson JM, Kaiser LR, Albelda SM. Humoral and cellular immune re-

sponses induced by adenoviral-based gene therapy for localized malignancy: results of a phase 1 clinical trial for malignant mesothelioma. Hum Gene Ther 1998; 9: 2121–2133.

39. Sterman DH, Molnar-Kimber K, Iyengar T, Chang M, Lanuti M, Amin KM, Pierce BK, Kang E, Treat J, Recio A, Litzky LA, Wilson JM, Kaiser LR, Albelda SM. A pilot study of systemic corticosteroid administration in conjunction with intrapleural adenoviral vector administration in patients with malignant pleural mesothelioma. Cancer Gene Therapy 2000; 7(12):1511–1518.

40. Gao GP, Yang Y, Wilson JM. Biology of adenovirus vectors with E1 and E4 deletions for liver-directed gene therapy. J Virol 1996; 70:8934–8943.

41. Sterman DH, Recio A, Molnar-Kimber K, Knox L, Hughes J, Alavi A, Lanuti M, Litzky LA, Albelda SM, Kaiser LR. Herpes simplex virus thymidine kinase (HSV*tk*) gene therapy utilizing an E1/E4-deleted adenoviral vector: preliminary results of a phase I clinical trial for pleural mesothelioma. Am J Respir Crit Care Med 1999; 159:A237.

42. Alavi JB, Eck SL. Gene therapy for malignant gliomas. Hematol Oncol Clin North Am 1998; 12:617–629.

43. Morris JC, Ramsey WJ, Wildner O, Muslow HA, Aguilar-Cordova E, Blaese RM. A phase I study of intralesional administration of an adenovirus vector expressing the HSV-1 thymidine kinase gene (AdV.RSV-*TK*) in combination with escalating doses of ganciclovir in patients with cutaneous metastatic melanoma. Hum Gene Ther 2000; 11:487–503.

44. Carmen IH. A death in the laboratory: the politics of the Gelsinger aftermath. Mol Ther: J Am Soc Gen Ther 2001; 3(4):425–428.

45. Lambright ES, Force SD, Lanuti M, Wasfi DS, Amin K, Albelda SM, Kaiser LR. Efficacy of repeated adenoviral suicide gene therapy in a localized murine tumor model. Ann Thor Surg 2000. In press.

46. Al-Hendry A, Magliocco AM, Al-Tweigeri T, Braileanu G, Crellin N, Li H, Strong T, Curiel D, Chedrese PJ. Ovarian cancer gene therapy: repeated treatment with thymidine kinase in an adenovirus vector and ganciclovir improves survival in a novel immunocompetent murine model. Am J Obstet Gynecol 2000; 182:553–559.

47. Black ME, Newcomb TG, Wilson HMP, Loeb LA. Creation of drug-specific herpes simplex virus type 1 thymidine kinase mutants for gene therapy. Proc Natl Acad Sci USA 1996; 93:3525–3529.

48. Qiao HJ, Black ME, Caruso M. Enhanced ganciclovir killing and bystander effect of human tumor cells transduced with retroviral vector carrying a herpes simplex thymidine kinase gene mutant. Hum Gene Ther 2000; 11:1569–1576.

49. Black ME, Kokoris MS, Sabo P. Herpes simplex virus-1 thymidine kinase mutants created by semi-random sequence mutagenesis improve prodrug-mediated tumor cell killing. Cancer Res 2001; 61(7):3022–3026.

50. Alemany R, Balague Curiel C. Replicative adenoviruses for cancer therapy. Nat Biotechnol 2000; 18:723–727.

51. Kahlos K, Anttila S, Asikainen T, Kinnula K, Raivio KO, Mattson K, Linnainmaa K, Kinnula VL. Manganese superoxide dismutase in healthy human pleural mesothelium and in malignant pleural mesothelioma. Am J Respir Cell Mol Biol 1998; 18: 579–580.

52. Doglioni C, Dei Tos AP, Laurino L, Iuzzolino P, Chiarelli C, Celio MR, Viale G. Calretinin: a novel immunocytochemical marker for mesothelioma. Am J Surg Pathol 1996; 20:1037–1046.

53. Gotzos V, Vogt P, Celio M. The calcium binding protein calretinin is a selective marker for malignant pleural mesotheliomas of the epithelial type. Pathol Res Pract 1996; 192:137–147.

54. Chang K, Pastan I. Molecular cloning of mesothelin, a differentiation antigen present on mesothelium, mesotheliomas, and ovarian cancers. Proc Natl Acad Sci USA 1996; 93:136–140.

55. Amin KM, Tsukuda K, Odaka M, Molnar-Kimber K, Kaiser LR, Albelda SM. The development and characterization of a mutant oncolytic adenovirus that replicates selectivity in ovarian and lung cancer cells over-expressing E2F-1 protein (abst). American Association for Cancer Research Annual Meeting, Philadelphia, 2001: 3716.

56. Ambrosini G, Adid C, Altieri DC. A novel anti-apoptosis gene, surviving, expressed in cancer and lymphoma. Nat Med 1997; 3:917–921.

57. Hall SJ, Sanford MA, Atkinson G, Chen SH. Induction of potent antitumor natural killer cell activity by herpes simplex virus–thymidine kinase and ganciclovir therapy in an orthotopic mouse model of prostate cancer. Cancer Res 1998; 58:3221–3225.

58. Freeman SM, Ramesh R, Marogi AJ. Immune system in suicide gene therapy. Lancet 1997; 349:2–3.

59. Vile RG, Castleden S, Marshall J, Camplejohn R, Upton C, Chong H. Generation of an anti-tumor immune response in a non-immunogenic tumour: HSV*tk* killing in vivo stimulates a mononuclear cell infiltrate and a Th1-like profile of intratumoural cytokine expression. Int J Cancer 1997; 71:267–274.

60. Melcher A, Todryk S, Hardwick N, Ford M, Jacobson M, Vile R. Tumor immunogenicity is determined by the mechanism of cell death via induction of heat shock protein expression. Nat Med 1998; 4:581–587.

61. Chen SH, Li Chen XH, Wang Y, Kosai KI, Finegold MJ, Rich SS, Woo SC. Combination gene therapy for liver metastasis of colon carcinoma in vivo. Proc Natl Acad Sci USA 1995; 92:2577–2581.

62. O'Malley B, Jr Cope KA, Chen SH, Li D, Schwartz M, Woo SLC. Combination gene therapy for oral cancer in a murine model. Cancer Res 1996; 56:1737–1741.

63. Castleden SA, Chong H, Garcia-Ribas I, Melcher AA, Hutchinson G, Roberts B, Hart IR, Vile RG. A family of bicistronic vectors to enhance both local and systemic antitumor effects of HSV*tk* or cytokine expression in a murine melanoma model. Hum Gene Ther 1997; 8:2087–2102.

64. Coll J, Mesnil M, Lefebvre M, Lancon A, Favrot M. Long-term survival of immunocompetent rats with intraperitoneal colon carcinoma tumors using herpes simplex thymidine kinase/ganciclovir and IL-2 treatments. Gene Ther 1997; 4:1160–1166.

65. Schwarzenberger P, Lei D, Freeman SM, Ye P, Weinacker A, Theodossiou C, Summer W, Kolls JK. Antitumor activity with the HSV-*tk*-gene cell line PA-1-STK in malignant mesothelioma. Am J Respir Cell Mol Biol 1998; 19(2):333–337.

66. Kolls J, Freeman S, Ramesh R, Marroqi A, Weinacker A, Summer W, Schwarzenberger P. The treatment of malignant pleural mesothelioma with gene modified cancer cells: a Phase I study. Am J Respir Crit Care Med 1998; 157:A563.

67. Harrison LH Jr, Schwarzenberger PO, Byrne PS, Marrogi AJ, Kolls JK, McCarthy KE. Gene-modified PA1-STK cells home to tumor sites in patients with malignant pleural mesothelioma. Ann Thorac Surg 2000; 70(2):407–411.

68. Leong CC, Marley JV, Loh S, Robinson BWS, Garlepp MJ. The induction of immune responses to murine mesothelioma by IL-2 gene transfer. Immunol Cell Biol 1997; 75:356–359.

69. Fakharai H, Shawler D, Gjerset R, Naviaux RK, Koziol J, Royston I, Sobol RE. Cytokine gene therapy with interleukin-2–transduced fibroblasts: effects of IL-2 dose on anti-tumor immunity. Hum Gen Ther 1995; 6:591–601.

70. Christmas T, Manning LS, Garlepp MJ, Mush AW, Robinson BW. Effect of interferon-alpha 2a on malignant mesothelioma. Interferon Res 1993; 13:9–12.

71. Astoul P, Viallat JR, Laurent JC, Brandley M, Boutin C. Intrapleural IL-2 in passive immunotherapy for malignant pleural effusion. Chest 1993; 103(1):209–213.

72. Astoul P, Picat-Joossen D, Viallat J, Boutin C. Intrapleural administration of interleukin-2 for the treatment of patients with malignant pleural mesothelioma: a Phase II study. Cancer 1998; 83:2099–2104.

73. Boutin C, Viallat J, VanZandwijk N, Douillard JT, Paillard JC, Guerin JC, Mignot P, Migueres J, Varlet F, Jehan A. Activity of intrapleural recombinant gamma-interferon in malignant mesothelioma. Cancer 1991; 67:2033–2037.

74. Boutin C, Nussbaum E, Monnet I, Bignon J, Vanderscheuren R, Guerin JC, Menard O, Mignot P, Dabouis G, Douillard JT. Intrapleural treatment with recombinant gamma-interferon in early stage malignant pleural mesothelioma. Cancer 1994; 74: 2460–2467.

75. Robinson B, Bowman R, Manning L, Musk A, Van Hazel G. Interleukin-2 and lymphokine-activated killer cells in malignant mesothelioma. Eur Respir Rev 1993; 3:220–222.

76. Goey SH, Eggermont AM, Punt CJ, Slingerland R, Gratama JW, Oosterom R, Oskam R, Bolhuis RL, Stoter G. Intrapleural administration of interleukin-2 in pleural mesothelioma: a Phase I-II study. Br J Cancer 1995; 72:1283–1288.

77. Mukherjee S, Haenel T, Himbeck R, Scott B, Ramshaw I, Lake RA, Harnett G, Phillips P, Morey S, Smith D, Davidson JA, Musk AW, Robinson B. Replication-restricted vaccinia as a cytokine gene therapy vector in cancer: persistent transgene expression despite antibody generation. Cancer Gen Ther 2000; 7(5):663–670.

78. Rochlitz C, Jantscheff P, Bongartz G, Dietrich PY, Quiquerez AL, Schatz C, Mehtali M, Courtney M, Tartour E, Dorval T, Fridman WH, Herrmann R. Gene therapy study of cytokine-transfected xenogeneic cells (Vero–interleukin-2) in patients with metastatic solid tumors. Cancer Gene Ther 1999; 6(3):271–278.

79. Caminschi I, Venetsanakos E, Leong CC, Garlepp MJ, Scott B, Robinson BWS. Interleukin-12 induces an effective antitumor response in malignant mesothelioma. Am J Respir Cell Mol Biol 1998; 19:738–746.

80. Caminschi I, Venetsanakos E, Leong CC, Garlepp MJ, Robinson BW, Scott B. Cytokine gene therapy of mesothelioma. Immune and antitumor effects of transfected interleukin-12. Am J Respir Cell Mol Biol 1999; 21:347–356.

81. Lukacs KV, Nakakes A, Atkins CJ, Lowrie DB, Colston MJ. In vivo gene therapy of malignant tumors with heat shock protein-65 gene. Gen Ther 1997; 4:345–350.

82. Lanuti M, Rudginsky S, Force S, Lambright ES, Chang MY, Amin K, Kaiser LR,

Scheule RK, Albelda SM. Cationic lipid: bacterial DNA complexes elicit anti-tumor effects and adaptive immunity in murine intraperitoneal tumor models. Cancer Res 2000; 60:2955–2963.

83. Lukacs KV, Porter CD, Pardo OE, Oakley RE, Steel RM, Judd DV, Browning JE, Geddes DM, Alton EW. In vivo transfer of bacterial marker genes results in differing levels of gene expression and tumor progression in immunocompetent and immuno-deficient mice. Hum Gene Ther 1999; 10(14):2373–2379.

84. Rudginsky S, Siders W, Ingram L, Marshall J, Scheule R, Kaplan J. Antitumor activity of cationic lipid complexed with immunostimulatory DNA. Mol Med 2001; 4(4): 347–355.

85. Rosso R, Rimoldi R, Salvati F, DePalma M, Cinquegrana A, Nicolo G, Ardizzoni A, Fusco U, Capaccio A, Centofanti R, Neri M, Cruciani AR, Maisto L. Intrapleural natural beta interferon in the treatment of malignant pleural effusions. Oncology 1988; 45:253–256.

86. Odaka M, Sterman DH, Wiewrodt R, Zhang Y, Kiefer M, Amin KM, Gao GP, Wilson JM, Barsoum J, Kaiser LR, Albelda SM. Eradication of intraperitoneal and distant tumor by adenovirus-mediated interferon-β gene therapy is attributable to induction of systemic immunity. Cancer Res 2001; 61:6201–6212.

87. Frizelle SP, Rubins JB, Zhou JX, Curiel DT, Kratzke RA. Gene therapy of established mesothelioma xenografts with recombinant p16[INK4a] adenovirus. Cancer Gene Ther 2000; 7:1421–1425.

88. Frizelle SP, Grim J, Zhou JX, Gupta P, Curiel DT, Geradts J, Kratzke RA. Reexpression of p16[INK4a] in mesothelioma cells results in cell cycle arrest, cell death, tumor suppression, and tumor regression. Oncogene 1998; 16:3087–3095.

89. Yang C, You L, Yeh C, Chang J, Chang F, McCormick F, Jablons DM. Cell cycle arrest and induction of apoptotic death in mesothelioma cells by the adenovirus-mediated p14[ARF] expression. J Natl Cancer Instit 2000; 92(8):636–641.

90. Yang C, You L, Yeh C, Uematsu K, Yeh C, McCormick F, Jablons DM. p14[ARF] Modulates the cytolytic effect of ONYX-015 in mesothelioma cells with wild-type p53. Cancer Res 2001; 61:5959–5963.

91. Giuliano M, Catalano A, Strizzi L, Vianale G, Capogrossi M, Procopio A. Adenovirus-mediated wild-type p53 overexpression reverts tumourigenicity of human mesothelioma cells. Int J Mol Med 2000; 5(6):591–596.

92. Pataer A, Smythe WR, Yu R, Fang B, McDonnell T, Roth JA, Swisher SG. Adenovirus-mediated Bak gene transfer induces apoptosis in mesothelioma cell lines. J Thorac Cardiovasc Surg 2001; 121(1):61–67.

93. Cicala C, Pompetti F, Carbone M. SV40 induces mesothelioma in hamsters. Am J Pathol 1993; 142(5):1524–1533.

94. Carbone M, Rizzo P, Grimley PM, Procopio A, Mew DJ, Shridhar V, de Bartolomeis A, Esposito V, Giuliano MT, Steinberg SM, Levine AS, Giordano A, Pass HI. Simian virus-40 large-T antigen binds p53 in human mesotheliomas. (comments). Nat Med 1997; 3(8):908–912.

95. Schrump DS, Waheed I. Strategies to circumvent SV40 oncoprotein expression in malignant pleural mesothelioma. Semin Cancer Biol 2001; 11:73.

96. Imperiale MJ, Pass HI, Sanda MG. Prospects for an SV40 vaccine. Semin Cancer Biol 2001; 11:81–85.

12

Strategies for Gene Therapy of Cystic Fibrosis

LARRY G. JOHNSON and RICHARD C. BOUCHER

Cystic Fibrosis Pulmonary Research and Treatment Center
University of North Carolina at Chapel Hill
Chapel Hill, North Carolina, U.S.A.

I. Introduction

Cystic fibrosis (CF) is a common inherited disorder affecting a variety of epithelial tissues. The disease is caused by mutations in the cystic fibrosis transmembrane conductance regulator gene (CFTR) that lead to abnormal secretions, recurrent infection and inflammation, bronchiectasis, and premature death. Because lung disease is the major cause of morbidity and mortality in this disorder, gene therapy efforts have focused on treatment of CF lung disease. Since CF is an autosomal recessive disorder in which heterozygotes exhibit a normal phenotype, introduction of a single wild-type (normal) copy of the gene into a defective CF cell should restore the normal phenotype. Transfer of wild-type *CFTR* into CF airway epithelial cells by retroviral, vaccinia viral, adenoviral, or nonviral vectors has been shown to restore CFTR-mediated Cl⁻ transport function, which is consistent with this concept (1–5). These studies demonstrating restoration of normal Cl⁻ transport by in vitro gene transfer of wild-type (i.e., normal) CFTR have established the feasibility of gene therapy for CF.

The in vivo cellular targets for CF gene therapy in humans have not been clearly elucidated. The site where CF lung disease begins remains controversial with both the superficial columnar epithelial cells lining the lumen of the small airways and the serous cells of submucosal glands having been identified as potential sites. Clinical data tend to support the theory that the disease begins in the small airways (6,7), whereas the submucosal glands are the predominant site of CFTR expression (8). Where the disease begins is relevant, since luminal (airway) delivery of gene transfer vectors primarily targets the superficial columnar airway epithelium, whereas intravenous (blood) delivery may be required to target the submucosal glands and basal cells in the airway.

Recent studies have suggested that stem cell niches may also exist within the lung that may ultimately be the targets for airway gene transfer. These stem cell niches appear to consist of subpopulations of submucosal gland duct cells in the proximal airways and subpopulations of Clara cell and/or Clara cell secretory protein-expressing cells in the distal airway (9,10). The ability of bone marrow–derived and mesenchymal stem cells to traffick to multiple organs following intravenous injection have also raised hopes for ex vivo approaches to gene therapy of CF lung disease (11,12). However, current strategies focus on delivery of gene transfer vectors to the airway lumen.

Following initial in vitro complementation studies, investigators rapidly moved to clinical safety and efficacy trials of gene transfer vectors delivered by luminal application to the airways of CF patients. Although some evidence for gene transfer was detected, the efficiency and efficacy of gene transfer failed to meet expectations and did not fully correct the known functional defects ascribed to this disorder (13–26). This failure forced exploration of potential barriers to gene transfer in airways and stimulated efforts to develop strategies to overcome these barriers. In this chapter, we review current vectors for airway gene transfer, discuss the barriers that have become apparent from preclinical and human studies, and explore current strategies to overcome these barriers to luminal airway gene transfer.

II. Vectors for Lung Gene Transfer

Naturally occurring viruses known to cause human disease introduce their own viral nucleic acid (DNA or RNA) into the host cell nucleus leading to expression of viral genes that promote viral replication. This property of naturally occurring viruses led to the development of viral vectors that introduce and express therapeutic genes (cDNAs) in lieu of their viral structural genes, which have been deleted. Adenoviruses (Ads), adeno-associated viruses (AAVs), and retroviruses each have been altered to introduce therapeutic cDNAs. Ad and AAV have already been evaluated in clinical trials in CF patients (13,15–18,21,22,27), and retroviral vectors have undergone substantial improvements in recent years that may permit their application to CF patients (see retroviral sections below). Of the nonviral methods, only cationic liposomes have been tested in Phase I clinical

Table 1 Vectors for Airway Gene Transfer

Gene transfer vectors	cDNA insert size (kbp)	Duration of expression	Transduction of nondividing cells	Risk of insertional mutagenesis
Adenovirus				
First- and second-generation	7–8	Transient	Yes	Minimal
Helper-dependent	>30	Transient[c]	Yes	Minimal
Adeno-associated virus	4.5	Long-term	Yes	Yes
Retrovirus				
MLV[a]	7	Long-term	No	Yes
Lentivirus[b]	>7	Long-term	Yes	Yes
Cationic liposomes	>10	Transient	Yes	No
Molecular conjugates	>10	Transient	Yes	No

[a] Derived from murine leukemia virus.
[b] Derived from human immunodeficiency virus, equine infectious anemia virus, or feline leukemia virus. Experience with helper-dependent adenoviral vectors is limited.
[c] Transient expression from helper-dependent Ad vectors can be prolonged.

gene transfer safety and efficacy trials in the lung (14,19,20,23–26), although two molecular conjugate vectors appear promising, the serpin enzyme complex (SEC) receptor-targeted poly-L-lysine complexes and lactosylated poly-L-lysine complexes (28–30). The characteristics of the different vector systems have been outlined in Table 1 and are discussed in more detail with regard to vector-specific barriers to transduction below.

III. Barriers to Airway Gene Transfer

Multiple barriers to airway gene transfer have been identified in the lung. Nonspecific barriers include airway mucus, cell surface glycoconjugates, and the inflammatory milieu, whereas vector-specific barriers include factors affecting cell binding and entry, nuclear translocation, and factors limiting transgene expression post nuclear entry. These barriers combine to make in vivo gene transfer to human airways inefficient.

A. Nonspecific Barriers to Gene Transfer

Luminal Contents

In cystic fibrosis, mutant CFTR mediates defective ion transport that reduces airway surface liquid (ASL) height and volume with resultant abnormal secretions, ineffective mucociliary clearance, bacterial proliferation with multiresistant organisms and chronic inflammation, bronchiectasis, and ultimately death (31–34). The inflammatory response is characterized by a massive influx of neutrophils, which release oxidants and proteolytic enzymes promoting tissue injury and bronchiectasis. The influx of neutrophils also increases the load of DNA and actin in the airway secretions of the CF lung, leading to a markedly increased sputum viscosity with markedly elevated levels of the proinflammatory cytokines tumor necrosis factor-α (TNF-α), interleukin-1β (IL-1β), IL-6, and IL-8 that perpetuate the inflammatory response (35). Abnormal secretions, inflammation, and *Pseudomonas* colonization is established early in life, often in the first year (36–39). Because current therapies do not eradicate the chronic pulmonary infection and inflammation of the CF lung, luminal gene transfer approaches targeting the superficial airway epithelium will have to overcome the inflammatory response in order to gain vector access to the airway epithelium.

Stern et al. investigated the effect of fresh sputum obtained from CF patients on gene transfer to primary airway cells and to CF cell lines in vitro (40). A dose-dependent inhibition of gene transfer to COS-7, 16HBE14o⁻, and 2-CFSMEO cells mediated by the cationic liposome DC-Chol/DOPE and an Ad-*lacZ* vector was detected in the presence of ultraviolet light-sterilized CF sputum. The effects of CF sputum on liposomal gene transfer were partially reversible with recombinant DNAse (rDNAse) pretreatment and completely reversible when rDNAse pretreatment preceded Ad gene transfer. Pretreatment with other mucolytic agents, including nacystelyn, lysine, n-acetylysteine, and ralginase, failed to increase liposomal or Ad gene transfer efficiency. Application of genomic DNA to cultures prior to transduction with DC-Chol/DOPE or an Ad-*lacZ* vector simulated the inhibitory effects of sputum on gene transfer. Thus, excessive DNA appears to be a major contributor to the inhibitory effects of noninfectious sputum components on gene transfer mediated by cationic liposomes and adenoviruses.

In a similar experiment, Perricone et al. evaluated the effect of the CF sputum on Ad vector infectivity (41). Sputum was collected from CF patients with acute exacerbations receiving antibiotics and rDNAse and was separated into aqueous (sol) and gel components by ultracentrifugation. Pooled CF sol samples inhibited Ad gene transfer to fetal rat tracheal and normal human bronchial epithelial cells. Subsequent studies demonstrated that Ad-specific antibodies in the sol of CF sputum inhibited Ad gene transfer, since removal of antibodies with a heat inactivated irrelevant Ad vector eliminated the inhibitory effect of CF sol on Ad gene transfer. Although neutrophil elastase (NE) was also detected in the CF sol, pretreatment of CF sol with proteinase inhibitors did not prevent CF sol-induced inhibition of Ad gene transfer.

The technique of bronchoalveolar lavage (BAL) harvests luminal contents from the airways and the alveolar region of the lung. It may also harvest soluble components from the airway and alveolar surfaces. BAL fluid from CF patients has been shown to inhibit AAV gene transfer to IB3-1 cells and C12 cells in vitro (42). This inhibitory effect was reversible when CF BAL fluid was incubated with α_1-antitrypsin (α_1AT) and correlated with markedly elevated levels of NE and human neutrophil peptide (HNP) in BAL fluid from CF subjects. However, studies with purified HNP and NE demonstrated that HNP, rather than NE, mediated the major inhibitory effect on AAV gene transfer. Thus, HNP in BAL fluid from CF patients may have inhibitory effects on AAV gene transfer.

Pseudomonas aeruginosa–induced bronchopulmonary inflammation may also inhibit Ad-mediated gene transfer (43). In an animal model of chronic bronchopulmonary infection, in which mice inoculated with *P. aeruginosa*–laden agarose beads develop bronchitis, bronchopneumonia, bronchiectasis, mucous plugging, and alveolar exudate with acute and chronic inflammatory cells, a greater than twofold reduction in gene transfer efficiency was detected following nasal instillation of an Ad-*lacZ* vector as compared to mice that had sterile beads or Ad vector alone instilled. Similarly, the efficiency of Ad-*lacZ* gene transfer to nasal airways of *Pseudomonas* (PAO1 strain)–infected mice was reduced by 10-fold as compared to noninfected nasal airways (44). Thus, the inflammatory milieu induced by *Pseudomonas* is a formidable barrier to transduction.

Airway and alveolar macrophages may also serve as barriers. Worgall et al. (45) used Ad-specific probes and Southern analysis to demonstrate a 70% loss of Ad-*lacZ* genomes within 24 hr in both immunocompetent and immunodeficient mice 24 hr following transtracheal administration of an Ad-*lacZ* vector. Pretreatment of murine lungs with liposomes containing dichloromethylene biphosphonate to eliminate macrophages followed by administration of an Ad-*lacZ* vector resulted in a significant increase in lung DNA and subsequent β-galactosidase expression. In vitro studies in cultured human alveolar macrophages demonstrated rapid loss of Ad vector genomes consistent with the in vivo data.

Alveolar macrophages have also been shown to inhibit retrovirus-mediated gene transfer to airway epithelia (46). Transduction of human airway epithelial cells by an amphotropic enveloped retroviral vector was inhibited ~40% by alveolar macrophages and by more than 60% by lipopolysaccharide (LPS)–activated alveolar macrophages (39). Incubation of macrophages with dexamethasone (1 μM) partially reversed this inhibition of retroviral transduction. Rapid uptake of labeled vector into vesicles of macrophages was associated with loss of DNA within 24 hr, which is consistent with rapid degradation rather than rapid transduction, of alveolar macrophages. These data suggest that macrophages can play a significant role in inhibiting in vivo gene transfer to lung epithelia.

Cell Surface Components

Components of the airway surface liquid and the glycocalyx may also have inhibitory effects on airway gene transfer. The effect of airway surface liquid on airway gene transfer has not been extensively evaluated. McCray and coworkers (46) demonstrated that airway surface liquid from well-differentiated (WD) human airway epithelial (HAE) cell cultures harvested in a small volume of distilled water failed to inhibit retroviral transduction to naïve airway cells in vitro. Airway surface fluid, obtained by washing the surfaces of WD airway cell cultures and bronchial xenografts also had no effect on transduction mediated by AAV vectors (47). Although the samples of the airway surface fluid used in these studies were dilute, these data would suggest that insignificant levels of vector-inhibitory substances are present within the soluble components of airway surface fluid.

The glycocalyx is a complex structure on the apical surfaces of airways consisting of complex carbohydrate moieties (sugars), glycolipids, and glycoproteins. At least three mucin glycoproteins have been localized to airway surfaces: MUC1 and MUC4, which are tethered mucins, and MUC5ac, which is thought to adhere to the cell surface (48–52). Arcasoy and colleagues (51,53) demonstrated that overexpression of the mucin MUC1 reduced Ad-mediated gene transfer to MDCK and bronchial epithelial cells that could be overcome by removal of sialic acid residues from the apical surface by neuraminidase pretreatment (51,53). Two groups have recently taken advantage of glycosylphosphatidyl inositol (GPI)–linked coxsackie and adenovirus 2/5 receptor (CAR) to evaluate more carefully the role of the glycocalyx as a barrier to gene transfer. GPI-linked CAR when overexpressed in MDCK cells and HAE cells localizes primarily to the apical membrane of polarized cells (54,55). Pickles et al. demonstrated that an Ad-5 vector failed to transduce efficiently MDCK cells overexpressing GPI-linked CAR following apical application, an effect that was reversible with removal of sialic residues by neuraminidase (54). In contrast, Walters et al. demonstrated that luminal application of an Ad-2 vector efficiently transduced HAE cells overexpressing GPI-linked CAR on the apical membrane and that neuraminidase had no effect on gene transfer efficiency (55). Since Ad-2 and Ad-5 target the same region of CAR, it is unlikely that this incongruity results from differences in vector serotype. Rather it may reflect differences in the levels of expression of glycocalyeal components between the different culture systems.

B. Vector-Specific Barriers to Luminal Airway Gene Transfer

Coincident with the initiation of clinical gene transfer efficacy and safety trials, in vitro and in vivo preclinical studies revealed that gene transfer to airway epithelial cells was inefficient when vector was delivered to the luminal surface. In this section, we review data identifying the barriers to gene transfer for vectors that have been evaluated in clinical trials and for vectors that exhibit potential for use in clinical trials.

Ad Vectors

Adenoviruses are double-stranded DNA viruses, of which human serotypes 2 and 5 (90% homology) provide the backbone for current Ad vectors (56–59). Wild-type adenoviruses have a 36-kbp genome consisting of a series of early genes that are responsible for viral replication, antigen presentation and surveillance, and a series of late genes that encode viral structural proteins (56–59). Several generations of Ad vectors have been developed based on Ad serotypes 2 (Ad-2) and 5 (Ad-5) (Fig. 1). First-generation vectors have had the early region 1 (E1) genes deleted to make the vector replication defective (60). Deletion of the E3 region creates sufficient room to insert therapeutic cDNAs with a suitable promoter.

E1-deleted second-generation vectors have been developed in which the E2a region has also been mutated to form a temperature-sensitive mutant virus

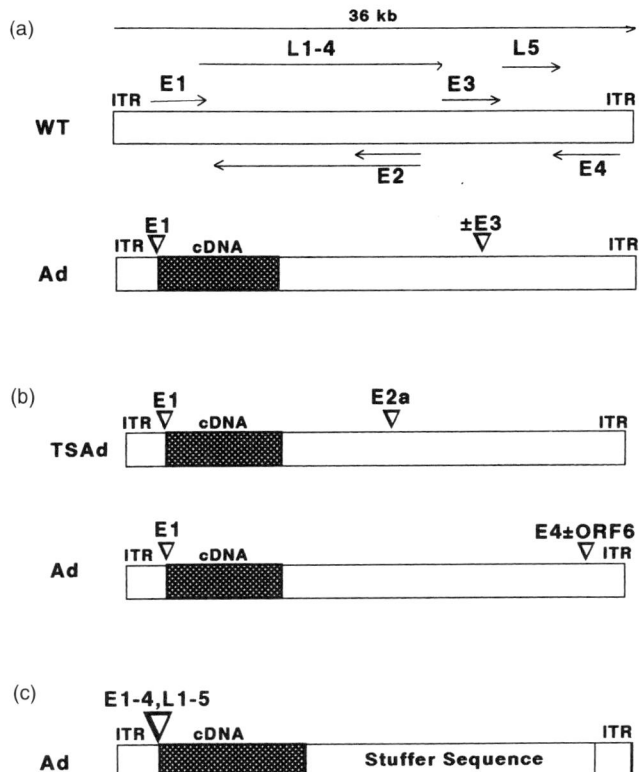

Figure 1 Map of adenoviral vectors derived from wild-type adenovirus. (a) First-generation vectors. (b) Second-generation vectors. (c) Third-generation vectors. Abbreviations: Ad, adenovirus vector; E, early region viral genes; ITR, inverted terminal repeat; L, late region viral genes; WT, wild-type; TS, temperature-sensitive; ∇, deletion of an early or late region gene; ±, with or without.

(Fig. 1b). This mutant replicates in 293 cells at 32°C, but not at 39°C, potentially bringing an additional safety feature to this vector (61–64). E1-deleted second-generation vectors have also been developed with deletions in most (except for open reading frame six, ORF6) or all of the E4 region (Fig. 1b) in an attempt to limit late viral gene expression (65–67).

All viral genes have been deleted from third-generation Ad vectors (Fig. 1c), retaining only a small packaging signal and the inverted terminal repeats (68–74). These vectors are attractive, because they can accept insert cDNAs or even genomic DNA in excess of 30 kb (58). For adequate packaging of vector constructs containing smaller cDNAs, these vectors often require a stuffer sequence (72,74). The absence of viral proteins also decreases the immune response to these vectors. However, these completely deleted vectors require coinfection of producer cells with an Ad helper virus for production of viral structural proteins, which may contaminate vector production stocks. The advent of Cre-lox recombination techniques has led to a reduction in the amount of Ad helper contamination to as low as 0.5–1.0%. Thus, Ad vectors that have complete deletions of the Ad genome are often referred to as gutless, high-capacity, or helper-dependent (HD) Ad vectors.

Ad enters cells by receptor-mediated endocytosis (75). It binds to a high-affinity coxsackie and adenoviral 2/5 receptor (CAR) (76) and is internalized through an $\alpha_v\beta_{3/5}$ integrin-mediated vesicular (endocytic) process (77). As a result of endosomolytic properties mediated by the Ad penton base, Ad avoids lysosomal degradation and efficiently translocates to the nucleus where it exists as an episome (extrachromosomal DNA) mediating expression of therapeutic genes (cDNAs). Because Ad vectors do not integrate at high frequencies, transient expression occurs, so repetitive administration will be required for CF gene therapy.

Clinical trials and preclinical studies have established that luminal Ad gene transfer to airways is inefficient. Grubb et al. demonstrated that luminal application of an Ad-*lacZ* vector efficiently transduced basal cells, the predominant cell type at the site of mechanical injury in human and mouse tracheal explants, whereas uninjured lumen-facing columnar cells were resistant to gene transfer (27). Pickles et al. confirmed this observation in model systems of WD rat and human airway epithelia and extended it to human intrapulmonary (bronchial) airways (78). Parallel experiments in excised human airway specimens demonstrated preferential transduction of undifferentiated regenerating or wound repairing cells by Ad vectors, as compared to WD pseudostratified columnar epithelia (79).

The reasons for the inefficiency of Ad gene transfer to WD airway epithelial cells following luminal application were delineated in subsequent studies. An early observation was that $\alpha_v\beta_{3/5}$ integrins, which mediate uptake of Ad vectors (77), were localized to the basolateral membrane, rather than the apical membrane, of columnar cells limiting vector entry and, hence, efficient gene transfer

(80). Subsequent experiments with radio- and fluorescent-labeled Ad vectors revealed evidence for decreased binding to the apical membrane of these polarized airway epithelial cells as compared to poorly differentiated airway cells, and a low rate of vector internalization out of proportion to the reduction in binding (78,81,82). Preferential transduction of polarized WD airway epithelia following basolateral application of vector as compared to the apical application was consistent with the binding and uptake studies (78,81,82). Immunofluorescent antibody studies ultimately localized CAR to the basolateral membrane (54).

While the resistance of the epithelium to Ad-mediated gene transfer may be partially overcome by increasing the duration of Ad vector incubation with the epithelium (83,84), direct measurements of nonspecific (fluid phase) endocytosis with radiolabeled markers demonstrated a markedly reduced rate of endocytic uptake in WD airway epithelia as compared to poorly differentiated airway epithelia (85). These data suggest that minimal enhancement of gene transfer would result from increasing nonspecific binding of Ad vectors to WD airway epithelia. Thus, vector-specific barriers to Ad-mediated gene transfer present on the apical membrane of WD airways lead to decreased uptake and decreased entry of vector. Strategies to improve vector access with luminal application must address these considerations.

AAV Vectors

AAV vectors are attractive for gene therapy, because they offer the possibility of long-term expression with a high degree of safety. They are derived from the naturally defective and nonpathogenic wild-type human parvoviruses, AAV-2 and AAV-3 (86–90). An AAV requires the presence of a helper virus, for example, Ad or herpes simplex virus, to replicate or to cause a lytic infection. In the absence of a helper virus, the AAV integrates into the host cell genome and becomes latent. Upon a subsequent wild-type Ad or wild-type herpes virus infection, the AAV genome can be rescued (excised) from the chromosome to generate a lytic infection (86–90).

The small AAV genome ($\sim$4.7 kbp) consists of the following: (1) inverted terminal repeats at the 5' and 3' ends of the molecule (86–89), which play a role in replication and are important for integration into the host cell genome, and (2) the viral genes *rep* and *cap* which mediate viral replication and nucleocapsid formation. Deletion of *rep* and *cap* creates an AAV vector with an insert size of $\sim$4.5 kb, which is at the upper size limit for insertion of full-length wild-type CFTR (coding region of $\sim$4.5 kb) driven by an exogenous promoter. Thus, the small insert size of AAV vectors may serve as a barrier to gene transfer of human CFTR.

Inefficient transduction of WD airway epithelia by luminal application of AAV vectors may also be limiting for CFTR gene transfer. A membrane-associated heparan sulfate proteoglycan has been identified as a receptor for AAV-2, the most common serotype developed into gene transfer vectors (91). Fibroblast growth factor-1 (FGF-1) and $\alpha_v \beta_5$ integrins act as coreceptors for AAV-2 (92,93). Heparan sulfate proteoglycans and the coreceptors have been localized predominantly to the basolateral surface of WD HAE cells (47), which correlates with preferential transduction of these cells when vector is applied to the basolateral membrane relative to the apical membrane. However, binding studies of radiolabeled AAV-2 have shown only a four- to sevenfold reduction in binding to the apical membrane of WD HAE in culture as compared to the basal membrane. Because gene transfer efficiency was 200-fold greater following basal application than for luminal application, the existence of apical membrane receptors for AAV-2 that are not functional for vector expression have been proposed (47,94).

A postentry barrier to transduction is the persistence of AAV-2 genomes as single-stranded episomes (ssDNA), which are inefficiently converted to double-stranded DNA (dsDNA), a requirement for transgene expression (95,96). This limitation leads to a delay in the onset of transgene expression which may be overcome by waiting long enough for maximal transgene expression to occur (~4 wk) or by the use of DNA-damaging agents, topoisomerase inhibitors, and Ad early gene products (97–99). Thus, barriers to AAV-mediated transduction of CFTR into CF airways include small insert size, decreased binding and uptake of vector due to absent or decreased functional receptor expression on the apical membrane, and inefficient single-strand to double-strand conversion of AAV genomes.

Retroviral Vectors

Retroviruses are members of a large group of viruses known as the Retroviridae that infect vertebrates (100,101), which consists of seven genera. Several members of the mammalian C-type genus, which includes a variety of oncogenic retroviruses, and the lentivirus genus, which is associated with slowly progressive immunodeficiency states, have been developed into gene transfer vectors. Many of the commonly used C-type retroviral vectors are based on murine leukemia virus (MLV). The best-known and perhaps most actively studied lentiviruses are the human immunodeficiency viruses (HIV-1 and HIV-2) and simian immunodeficiency viruses (SIVs). Feline immunodeficiency virus (FIV) and equine infectious anemia virus (EIAV) have also been developed as gene transfer vectors for CF.

Retroviruses have been extensively tested in the laboratory for stable expression of therapeutic cDNAs. Simple C-type retroviruses are RNA viruses whose genomes consist of two viral long terminal repeats (LTRs) that are important for cellular integration, but also contain promoter elements, a packaging signal, and a series of structural genes, *gag*, *pol*, and *env* (Fig. 2A). These structural genes encode the capsid protein, reverse transcriptase, protease, an integrase,

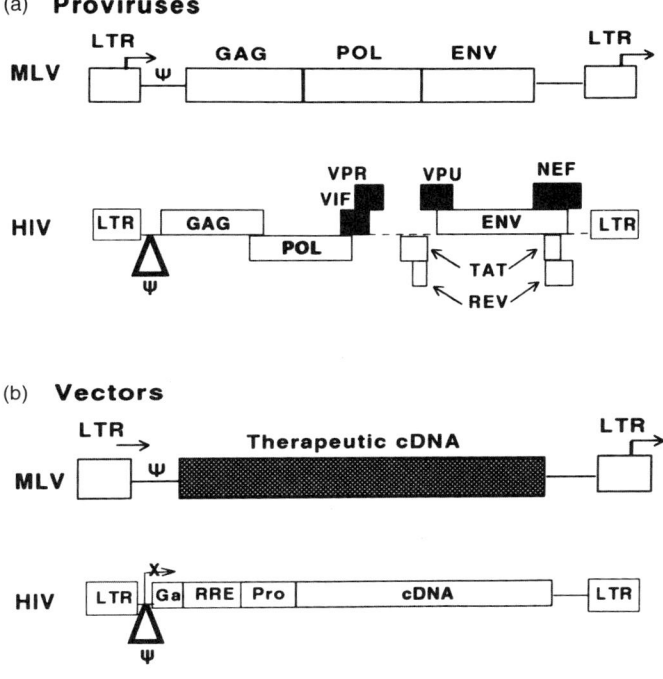

Figure 2 Maps of murine leukemia virus (MLV)–derived retroviral and human lentiviral (HIV-derived) vectors. (a) Proviruses of wild-type MLV and HIV. Note the more complex genome of HIV, which contains a number of accessory genes not present in MLV including *vif*, *vpr*, *vpu*, *nef*, *rev*, and *tat*. (b) MLV- and HIV-based derived vectors. Vectors are produced by providing the envelope and viral genes deleted from the vector in *trans* with stably transfected producer cell lines or by transient transfection. Abbreviations: LTR, long terminal repeat; Ψ, viral packaging signal; pro, promoter; Ga, gag; RRE, rev response element.

and the envelope glycoprotein. Deletion of *gag*, *pol*, and *env* creates room for insertion of therapeutic cDNAs (genes) into the retroviral genome forming a replication defective retroviral vector (102). Production of the vector is performed by supplying the deleted functions in *trans* with stable cell lines overexpressing helper proteins or by transient transfection.

The genomes of lentiviruses (Fig. 2B) are more complex, encoding a variety of regulatory accessory proteins and pathogenesis factors that are not present in the genomes of simple retroviruses (103–106). Furthermore, genes encoding proteins that utilize the cellular nuclear import machinery, for example, MA, IN, and Vpr of HIV-1, to target the preintegration complex to the nucleus are also encoded within this complex genome. Major deletions in these accessory and pathogenetic factor genes have enabled the development of lentiviral vectors for gene transfer (103–106). Exogenous (internal) promoters have also been included within the sequences of the inserted gene cassette, since transcription from the viral LTR may constitute a safety hazard. Deletions in the LTR to prevent transcription (self-inactivating or SIN vectors) have been introduced as a safety feature of retroviral vectors based on MLV and HIV (107,108).

The envelope glycoproteins of wild-type retroviruses and lentiviruses bind to cell surface receptors to facilitate entry of the virus into the cytoplasm where the viral RNA is reverse transcribed to form a cDNA, the provirus. This provirus is translocated to the nucleus where it integrates into the host cell chromosomes and through the normal process of DNA transcription encodes new viral proteins and new viral RNA, which are assembled at the cell surface into new viral particles. Replication-defective retroviral and lentiviral vectors infect cells by similar mechanisms, but unlike wild-type viruses, the integrated provirus from these vectors encodes the therapeutic gene and viral particles are not produced.

The lack of cell proliferation in WD airway epithelia in vivo (109) and low titers have traditionally served as major barriers to application of the C-type retroviral vectors derived from MLV to in vivo airway gene transfer efforts. The development of HIV, EIAV, and FIV vectors (103,104,106,108,110,111), which can transduce nondividing airway cells, may overcome the requirement for cell proliferation by oncogenic retroviruses (112). Advances in retroviral production techniques and pseudotyping of vectors to create stable envelopes that permit concentration of vector stocks may also soon overcome the limitations of titer (113). However, titers of retroviruses remain ~1–2 logs lower than that of Ad vectors.

Current data suggest that apical membrane barriers to efficient transduction of WD airway cells are also limiting for retroviruses. Wang et al. demonstrated efficient transduction of polarized WD airway cells stimulated to proliferate with keratinocyte growth factor (KGF) when amphotropic enveloped MLV vectors were applied to the basolateral surface as compared to minimal to no gene transfer when vector was applied to the apical surface (114). The data are consistent with localization of the amphotropic receptor (RAM-1 or Pit-2) to the basolateral surface of polarized WD airway cells. Western blot data from this study suggested that receptor levels were extremely low in the absence of KGF. In vivo studies have confirmed low levels of expression of RAM-1 or Pit-2 in murine lung (115). However, recently, Wang and colleagues have suggested that nonfunctional amphotropic receptors may be present on the apical membrane (116).

Similar findings have been observed with retroviral vectors bearing different envelopes. Wild-type vesicular stomatitis virus (VSV) preferentially infects polarized MDCK cells, a model for polarized airway epithelia, across the basolateral membrane (117). Since MLV and lentiviral vectors derived from HIV, EIAV, and FIV have each been pseudotyped with the envelope glycoprotein (G) of VSV, these vectors would be expected preferentially to transduce polarized MDCK cells from the basolateral surface. In vitro and in vivo studies of transduction have confirmed this notion in MDCK cells, polarized WD HAE cells, and murine, rat, and rabbit tracheas in vivo (110,111,114,118,119).

Nonviral Vectors

Cationic Liposomes

Cationic liposomes and naked plasmid DNA have been the principal nonviral vectors evaluated in clinical trials. Cationic liposomes are composed of cationic lipids mixed in varying molar ratios with cholesterol and dioleylphosphatidylethanolamine (DOPE), a neutral phospholipid (120,121). Commonly used cationic lipids for gene transfer include N[1-(2,3-dioleoxy)propyl] N,N,N trimethylammonium (DOTMA), 1,2-dimyristyloxypropyl-3-dimethylhydroxyethylammonium bromide (DMRIE), or 3β[N-N',N'-dimethylamino ethanecarbamoyl] cholesterol (DC-Chol), N[1-(2,3-dioleoxy)propyl] N,N,N trimethylammonium methyl sulfate (DOTAP), p-ethyl dimyristoyl phosphatidyl choline (EDMPC) cholesterol, and N⁴-sperminine cholesteryl carbamate (GL-67). Cationic liposomes bind to negatively charged plasmid DNA to form DNA-liposome complexes which may, under conditions of excess molar DNA, have a net negative charge. DNA-liposome complexes (also known as lipoplexes) enter cells primarily by endocytosis (122,123), although the mechanism and specificity of binding to the cell surface has not been clearly delineated. Cationic liposomes also promote the release of plasmid DNA from the endosome into the cytoplasm (123). Like adenoviruses, cationic liposomes do not integrate into the host cell genome, so that expression may be lost with cell division. Thus, repetitive administration of lipoplexes will be required for CF gene therapy.

Naked DNA

Naked or plasmid DNA has also been shown to mediate gene transfer to lung epithelia in vitro and in vivo. In a clinical trial of lipid GL-67 in the nasal epithelium of CF patients, plasmid DNA alone was as effective as GL-67/CFTR plasmid DNA lipoplexes, although the restoration of chloride secretion was small in both cases (25).

DNA-Ligand-Polymer Complexes

When plasmid DNA is linked to a polymer, for example, poly-L-lysine, and a receptor ligand, this forms a DNA-ligand-polymer complex (molecular conjugate or polyplex). This complex may then bind to a specific cell surface receptor and enter the cell by receptor-mediated endocytosis. Ferkol and colleagues have shown that molecular conjugates that use a Fab fragment of IgG against human secretory component can deliver reporter genes to the airway epithelia in vitro and in vivo following intravenous administration (124,125). These complexes appeared preferentially to target the larger cartilaginous airways where expression of the polymeric IgA receptor predominates, but they were immunogenic.

Poly-L-lysine has been linked to specific peptides that bind the serpin enzyme complex receptor in an attempt to increase luminal airway epithelial gene transfer efficiency (28). The poly-L-lysine polymer has also been modified to enhance gene transfer efficiency. Kollen et al. (29,30) have demonstrated that lactosylated poly-L-lysine can significantly enhance gene DNA transfer to cultured CF cells in vitro.

Two barriers to liposome-mediated gene transfer have been identified. Nuclear entry has been identified as the rate-limiting factor for efficient liposome-mediated gene transfer into cell lines resistant to transfection (126), whereas gene transfer to WD airway epithelial cells may be limited by both inefficient nuclear entry and failure of DNA-liposome complexes to enter the cell (85). Matsui et al. used rat and human airway cells grown as islands on permeable collagen substrates in which poorly differentiated cells form on the edges of the islands and polarized (well-differentiated) cells form in the central portions to investigate the relative efficiency of liposome mediated gene transfer (85). Matsui et al. demonstrated loss of phagocytic entry mechanisms, decreased cell surface binding, and decreased uptake in differentiated airway epithelial cells (central cells) as compared to poorly differentiated cells (edge cells) as the reason for inefficient transduction. A subsequent study confirmed these observations by demonstrating decreased amounts of cell-associated lipoplexes in differentiated airway epithelia as compared to poorly differentiated epithelia (127). Liposome-mediated gene transfer into proliferating cells was also enhanced relative to quiescent cells, raising the possibility of enhanced nuclear transport of DNA during mitosis due to breakdown of the nuclear envelope. The choice of lipid used in these two studies did not affect the low efficiency of gene transfer to differentiated epithelia. Thus, barriers to efficient transduction of WD airway cells by lipoplexes include decreased binding and uptake of lipoplexes and poor nuclear translocation of DNA.

Molecular conjugates are typically designed to target specific receptors on cell surfaces to improve binding and uptake. However, poor nuclear translocation with trafficking of significant portions of vector to lysosomal compartments for degradation remains a concern for molecular conjugates.

C. Inflammatory and Immune Barriers to Airway Epithelial Gene Transfer

The induction of immune and inflammatory responses by gene transfer vectors may serve as a significant barrier to the use of gene transfer vectors clinically. To date, the responses induced by Ad vectors have been the most pronounced

(57,128–136). However, humoral immune responses have also been noted with AAV vectors and inflammatory conditions have been detected following delivery of nonviral vectors (26,137–141).

Ad Vectors

The immunogenic responses induced by Ad vectors are a major concern for gene therapy. The death of a subject in an adenoviral gene transfer trial for ornithine transcarbamylase deficiency has heightened these concerns (142,143). Ad vectors induce an acute nonspecific mixed cellular inflammatory response and a late specific dose-related, lymphocyte-predominant, cell-mediated immune response (57,128–136). The acute response is nonspecific and likely induced by cytokines. The later specific immune response is mediated by cytotoxic (CD8) T lymphocytes directed against viral gene products and transgene proteins, leading to destruction of transduced cells with resultant decreased persistence. Despite the E1 deletion, first-generation vectors have been shown to express late gene products. Second-generation E2a-defective vectors reduce late gene expression and inflammation, extending the duration of transgene expression in nonhuman primates and in rodents. However, the duration of the cellular inflammation is also extended (61–64,140).

Second-generation E1-deleted Ad-2 vectors with deletions of the E4 region, except for ORF6 (Fig. 1B), have also been associated with cellular inflammation. Studies in nonhuman primates examining toxicity with repetitive administration (every 3 weeks for up to 11 doses) of these vectors suggest that histopathological changes of inflammation are minimal at doses of up to 3×10^9 IU delivered to a single lobe of the lung (132). However, doses of vector greater than 3×10^9 IU generated the expected histological changes of inflammation. Subsequent studies of Ad-d2 vectors with wild-type E4 regions, partial deletions of E4 retaining only ORF6, and complete deletions of E4 displayed a complex relationship between promoters and the persistence of gene transfer. Sustained expression of the *lacZ* transgene occurred when driven by a CMV promoter in nude mice in the presence of wild-type E4 *cis* elements, whereas transgene expression from vectors with deletions of E4 did not persist (66,144). Surprisingly, other promoters did not mediate persistent *lacZ* expression.

Helper-dependent vectors that have had all of the viral genes deleted (ΔrAd) have not been extensively evaluated in the lung, but may have an improved safety profile (73,74,145). Complete removal of helper virus (E1-deleted virus used to produce ΔrAd) from ΔrAd vector is a current limitation to the widespread application of completely deleted vectors.

Humoral immune responses to Ad vectors include the development of mucosal and neutralizing antibodies (129,131,136,146–149). This immune response arises from helper (CD4$^+$) T-lymphocyte response directed against the adenoviral capsid proteins. The major limitation of these antibodies is the inhibition of Ad infection upon subsequent readministration of vector.

Neurogenic inflammation and dose dependent increases in apoptosis are additional limitations of Ad vectors for airway gene transfer (150,151). Intra-airway administration of E1, E3-deleted Ad vectors induced a dose-dependent potentiation in capsaicin-stimulated vascular permeability in rat airways consistent with neurogenic inflammation (150,151). This dose-dependent effect was reduced by UV-psoralen inactivation of the Ad vector, consistent with inhibition of viral gene expression, and by administration of a selective substance P (NK1) receptor antagonist. Dose-dependent induction of apoptosis and cell cycle alterations occurring after Ad infection of airway cells may be harmful to the reparative responses in the lung (151).

AAV Vectors

Cell-mediated immune responses have not been reported with AAV vectors. However, contradictory results have been published regarding the generation of a humoral immune response. Halbert et al. demonstrated transduction of ~5–6% of rabbit airway cells by an AAV-2 alkaline phosphatase and *lacZ* vectors following balloon treatment of rabbit airway (138). However, AAV failed to transduce the balloon-treated right lower lobe (RLL) airway epithelia of rabbits that had received administration of an AAV vector to the left lower lobe (LLL) 14 days previously. This failure to transduce rabbit airways upon readministration of vector correlated with an increase in neutralizing antibody that could be overcome by transient immunosuppression. Beck reported increased levels of neutralizing antibody to AAV in rabbits following nasal and bronchoscopic administration (137). However, no inhibition of AAV gene transfer was detected despite the increased levels of neutralizing antibody. Potential reasons for the differences between these studies include differences in delivery technique, with perhaps greater injury in the balloon catheter model leading to greater antigen exposure and wild-type. Ad contamination of AAV vector stocks. The results from these animal studies are consistent with the low frequency with which antibodies obtained from the sera of normal and CF subjects inhibited AAV transduction in vitro (32%) relative to the high prevalence of seropositivity (96%) for AAV-2 in the sera (152). Further studies of AAV produced from helper virus–free systems are required to answer fully the role of neutralizing antibody–mediated inhibition of gene transfer following repetitive administration.

Cationic Liposomes

Liposomes may also elicit lung inflammation. GL-67 has been shown to induce an acute dose-dependent neutrophil-predominant inflammatory response following intratracheal administration to murine lung, which tends to be less severe following aerosol administration (141,153). In a clinical trial, bronchoscopic, but not nasal, administration, of $CFTR/GL-67/DOPE/DMPE-PEG_{5000}$ complexes induced an influenza-like syndrome characterized by fever, myalgias, and headache with negative chest x-rays and blood cultures (26). The etiology of this inflammatory response was unclear, although unmethylated CpG dinucleotide sequences of bacterial origin within the plasmid DNA and the lipid have both been implicated. However, the inflammation per se did not demonstrate a clear effect on either efficiency or persistence of gene transfer.

In summary, a variety of barriers to efficient transduction of airways in vivo by luminal application of vector exist. Decreased binding and uptake of vector due to lack of apical membrane receptors and internalization pathways appears to be a common barrier to all vectors tested in clinical trials to date. Other barriers such as second-strand synthesis and nuclear entry are more vector specific. Thus, strategies that permit better apical membrane entry or that allow access of vector to the basolateral surface are likely to be generally useful. Circumventing the immune response will be necessary to alleviate safety concerns and to facilitate repetitive administration of transient expression vectors.

IV. Strategies to Overcome Apical Membrane Barriers to Efficient Transduction

Since the apical membrane of WD airway cells is a major barrier to efficient transduction by all the current gene transfer vectors, strategies to overcome apical membrane barriers are crucial. Intravenous approaches have been considered (124,125), but the multiple barriers that must be crossed, for example, endothelium, endothelial basement membrane, interstitium, and epithelial basement membrane, have made luminal delivery of vectors more attractive. Current strategies have not fully addressed the problem with luminal contents, that is, neutrophils, bacteria, excess DNA, and inflammation, focusing instead on improving apical membrane binding and entry. The hope is that pretreatment with $\alpha_1 AT$, rDNase, or antibiotic therapy will limit the effects of luminal contents on gene transfer.

Two strategies have been proposed for overcoming barriers to airway epithelial gene transfer following luminal application of vector. One strategy focuses on modification of the host airway to enhance gene transfer and the other strategy modifies vectors to target receptors expressed on the apical membrane of airways in vivo that have the capacity to internalize. We elaborate on these two strategies in more detail below.

A. Host Modification

Modulating Paracellular Permeability

A number of agents have been proposed for modification of paracellular permeability as a means to enhance drug absorption (154,155). These agents can generally be grouped into those that have relatively nonspecific effects and those that target specific components of the intercellular junction. The application of methods modulating paracellular permeability to enhance gene transfer has also been recently established. Inhalation of the oxidant gas sulfur dioxide promotes denuding of the surface epithelium in a dose-dependent manner while also increasing paracellular permeability in less severely injured regions (118,119,156). Johnson and colleagues demonstrated that this oxidant model could be used to stimulate epithelial cell proliferation and enable relatively efficient gene transfer to the airways of mice by VSV-G pseudotyped retroviral and lentiviral vectors (118, 119). Subsequently, Parsons and colleagues demonstrated that low doses of the surface active detergent polidocanol increased airway permeability of polidocanol-treated murine airways, but not that of control animals without inducing frank morphological injury (44). Pretreatment of nasal airways with polidocanol enhanced gene transfer mediated by an Ad-*lacZ* vector and facilitated partial correction of the Cl$^-$ transport defect in the nasal epithelium of CF mice following a single dose of vector. The single dose of Ad-CFTR vector used following pretreatment with the surface agent polidocanol generated the same degree of CFTR correction previously reported by Grubb (27) in which four doses of an Ad vector were required to generate a 40–50% correction of Cl$^-$ transport.

Agents that more specifically alter paracellular permeability of airways to enhance gene transfer have also been tested. Wang et al. demonstrated enhanced retroviral gene transfer mediated by an amphotropic enveloped vector applied to the apical membrane of WD airway epithelia following pretreatment with the calcium chelator ethylene glycol bis-(β-aminoethyl ether)-N,N,N',N'-tetraacetic acid (EGTA) and hypotonic solutions (114). A 7- to 10-fold increase in transduction of WD primary HAE cells cultures by an AAV-GFP vector and transient permeabilization with EGTA/hypotonic solution has also been reported (47). EGTA/hypotonic solution treatment has enabled investigators to correct the Cl$^-$ transport defect in WD CF HAE cells stimulated to proliferate with keratinocyte growth factor (KGF) when vector was applied to the luminal surface (114) and has enhanced FIV-based lentiviral gene transfer to rabbit airways in vivo (111), Ad gene transfer in vitro, and Ad gene transfer to murine airways in vivo (157). Recently, Chu et al. demonstrated that high concentrations of EGTA (0.1–0.4 M) were optimal for enhancement of Ad gene transfer to nasal and lower airway epithelia of mice in vivo (158). Medium chain fatty acids have also been shown to enhance airway gene transfer in vitro (159) and in preliminary studies in vivo (160). These studies established the feasibility of transient permeabilization of the paracellular path to enhance airway gene transfer in vivo mediated by vectors that bind to receptors that are localized on the basolateral membrane.

Enhancing Endosomal Processing

Duan et al. have suggested that receptors for AAV-2 may exist on the apical membrane of polarized WD HAE cells that can bind and mediate AAV-2 entry, but fail to mediate transgene expression (47,94). The rationale for their hypothesis was an observation in which rAAV-2 transduction of WD HAE was 200-fold more efficient following basolateral application of 10^4 rAAV particles/cell as compared to apical application of an equal number of particles (47). This observation was incongruent with binding studies which demonstrated only a four- to sevenfold difference in binding between the apical or basolateral membranes. To evaluate their observation further, these investigators explored differences in the molecular state of rAAV 50 days after apical or basolateral transduction by Southern blot analysis of Hirt DNA (47). Following apical application of vector, rAAV genomes were detected consistent with cellular entry, but remained as ssDNA. In contrast, rAAV genomes that had been converted to dsDNA forms were detected after basolateral application of vector. DNA-damaging agents did not increase gene transfer following apical infection, but the proteasome inhibitors z-LLL and LLnL, which prevent ubiquitination of molecules targeted for degradation, increased gene transfer efficiency to levels that were one-eighth of those observed following basolateral transduction. These data are consistent with a lumen-specific block to AAV endosomal processing and trafficking. Agents inhibiting proteasomal degradation also enhanced luminal rAAV-2-mediated airway gene transfer in vivo. These findings have not yet been verified by others in airways, although barriers to endosomal processing of AAV-2 have been identified in undifferentiated cell lines (161,162).

B. Vector Modification

Modifications to specific gene transfer vectors is an alternative approach to enhancing gene transfer efficiency. Targeting the vector to receptors that are endogenously expressed on the apical membrane of WD HAE cells is the goal of this approach. The concept of targeting gene transfer vectors to known alternative (non–wild-type) receptors is well established in the literature for adenoviral, retroviral, and nonviral vectors (163–174).

Ad Vectors

Three general approaches have been described for retargeting of Ad vectors: (1) genetic engineering of peptide ligand sequences or single chain antibody fragments (scFv) into the fiber knob domain of Ad (164,173); (2) the use of scFv-fusion proteins with specificities for an Ad epitope while bearing a ligand binding domain for a specific cell surface receptor, the adenobody approach (171); and (3) the use of bispecific antibodies composed of two antibodies—one directed against the Ad vector and the other against the specific cell surface receptor—that have been cross linked (172).

Although each of these methods has been successful at increasing binding, successful vector specific transduction has been more difficult. Genetic incorporation of ligands into Ad vectors is limited by size of the peptide sequence and the ability to incorporate the chimeras into viral particles, whereas bispecific antibodies and adenobodies must fold properly to bind specifically and enter with the target receptor (163,175). A membrane or endosomolytic fusion event must also occur for the vector to gain access to the cytoplasm and henceforth the nucleus. Nevertheless, the aforementioned approaches have been successfully used in vitro to target a variety of receptors including α_v-integrins (77), the epidermal growth factor receptor (171), stem cell factor receptor (170,174), and T-cell receptors such as CD3 (172).

Major concerns are which receptors are expressed on the apical membrane and whether the levels of expression are sufficient to promote successful gene transfer. P2Y$_2$-R, a seven-transmembrane purinoceptor that normally mediates acute airway epithelial cell responses to the luminal environment, the serpin enzyme complex receptor (SEC-R), and the urokinase plasminogen activator receptor (uPA-R) have been proposed as potential targets on the apical membrane (28,176–179). Studies in polarized cells have documented that bispecific monoclonal antibody-Ad vector complexes directed toward epitope-tagged external domains of P2Y$_2$-R can promote enhanced gene transfer efficiency (180) and targeted transduction of wild-type P2Y$_2$-R–expressing cell lines mediated by vector conjugates composed of Ad complexed to chemically modified ligands such as biotin-UTP has also been demonstrated (181). A uPA-polyethylene glycol (PEG)–coated Ad vector has also been shown to enhance Ad gene transfer to polarized airway epithelia (178,182).

Alternatively, chimeric Ad vectors that target apical membrane of airway cells have been proposed. Zabner et al. screened 12 adenoviral serotypes from Ad subgroups A–F for their ability to bind and infect the apical surface of polarized WD HAE cells in culture (183). Wild-type Ad-17 bound to WD HAE cells more efficiently than wild-type Ad-2. Subsequently chimeric Ad-2 vectors with Ad-17 fiber transduced WD HAE cells ∼100 fold more efficiently than the original Ad-2 vector. These data suggested that it may be possible to generate chimeric Ad vectors that more efficiently transduce HAE cells following luminal application.

AAV Vectors

Although retargeting of AAV-2 vectors with single-chain antibodies may be feasible (184), efforts to improve apical membrane targeting of AAV vectors have focused on identifying wild-type AAV vectors of other serotypes. Once identified, the alternative serotypes can be developed into new gene transfer vectors, or alternatively their cap genes can serve as pseudotypes for AAV-2 vectors. At least six serotypes of AAV vectors have been cloned (185–187).

Halbert et al. developed AAV-2 vectors pseudotyped with an AAV-6 capsid generated by transient transfection techniques (188). These AAV-6 pseudotypes bound heparin columns weakly as compared to AAV-2 and were not inhibited by soluble heparin sulfate, but luminally applied vector transduced polarized primary CF HAE cells up to 100-fold more efficiently than AAV-2. AAV-6 pseudotypes also transduced a high percentage (up to 80%) of cells in some mouse airways in vivo that was 100- to 1000-fold higher than detected following AAV-2 gene transfer. Of note, AAV-6–pseudotyped AAV-2 vectors were produced in much higher titers than AAV-6 vectors, suggesting that pseudotyping may offer advantages for vector production.

Zabner and colleagues evaluated the molecular characteristics of different AAV serotypes focusing on AAV-4 and AAV-5, which appeared to differ from AAV-2 genetically (189). Recombinant vector stocks generated in the presence of Ad helper virus were used to infect the apical membrane of WD HAE cells. Although significantly more AAV-4 and AAV-5 bound to the apical membrane than AAV-2, only AAV-5 efficiently transduced airway cells following apical application, an effect that was not affected by pretreatment with soluble heparin. AAV-5 vector-transduced lungs exhibited a fivefold increase in the number of transduced cells/microscopic field for airways and 20- to 30-fold increase for alveoli as compared to AAV-2-transduced lungs. Recent data suggest that 2,3-linked sialic acid residues may serve as the receptor for AAV-5 (190). Thus, AAV-5 and AAV-6 may be candidates for enhancing AAV gene transfer following luminal delivery. However, confirmatory studies of gene transfer efficiency, CFTR transduction, and safety will be required. Large-scale production techniques must also be developed.

An additional barrier to AAV-mediated CFTR gene transfer has been the restriction on insert size that limits efficient packaging of wild-type CFTR with a suitable promoter. Expression from AAV-CFTR vectors in clinical trials has been driven by endogenous promoter elements within the viral terminal repeats due to limits on insert size (21,191,192). Because AAV vectors undergo intermolecular circular concatermerization and recombination, a trans-splicing strategy has been proposed for full-length cDNAs in excess of the packaging size limits (193). In this strategy (Fig. 3), rAAV vectors encoding either the 5′ or 3′ portions of a therapeutic transgene with splice donor sites intact would be delivered into the same cell where circular concatamers arising from intermolecular recombination permit functional transsplicing of the component portions of the molecule into full-length therapeutic cDNAs (193). This strategy has been successfully applied to the human erythropoietin (Epo) gene in vitro and to animal models of renal failure–induced anemia (193). A similar strategy has been proposed to restore CFTR chloride channel function to CF epithelia, but the feasibility of this approach will depend on efficient delivery of the vector encoding each half of CFTR, or alternatively a CFTR transgene in one vector and a promoter with a superenhancer in another to the same cell with a high frequency of trans-splicing (194).

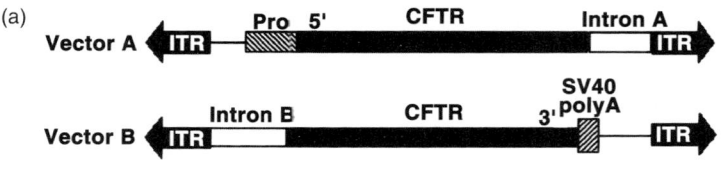

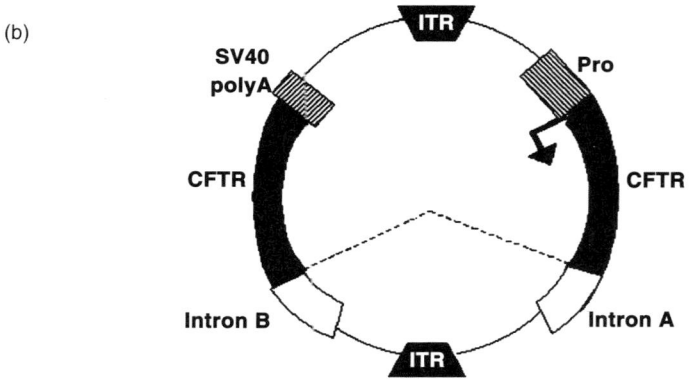

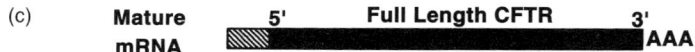

Figure 3 Schematic representation of a proposed trans-splicing strategy for expression of CFTR. Two AAV vectors are shown in (a). Vector A contains an exogenous promoter (pro) and the 5′ portion of CFTR. Vector B contains the remaining 3′ portion of CFTR. Following successful coinfection of an airway cell with both vectors, circular concatamers form (b), which ultimately undergo functional transsplicing to yield a mature full length CFTR mRNA (c). An alternative strategy would include the promoter and enhancer elements in one vector and only CFTR in the other (see Ref. 193).

Retroviral Vectors

Strategies to overcome in vivo barriers to retroviral transduction must address issues of titer, cell proliferation, and receptor localization. Retroviral vectors based on MLV have generally been produced by the generation and selection of stable cell lines, which then allow continuous production of vector over many passages. These cell lines are derived from fibroblast and human embryonic kidney 293 cells stably transfected with envelope, helper, and vector, with propagation of clones producing the highest titers. These titers have traditionally been in the range of 10^5–10^6 infectious units (IU)/mL, with further increases in titer limited in part by the stability of the envelope protein. Envelope proteins from a variety of viruses can be incorporated into the viral membrane of retroviral vectors, a process known as pseudotyping, which is common to most retroviruses including lentiviruses.

VSV-G–pseudotyped MLV and lentiviral vectors have been developed that can be concentrated to high titer by ultracentrifugation without significant loss of infectivity (103–106,110,111,113,118,195). Following concentration, retroviral titers approach titers within a log of AAV and Ad vectors and high titer VSV-G–pseudotyped MLV and lentiviral vectors have been shown to correct Cl⁻ permeability defect in poorly differentiated dividing (subconfluent) and WD primary CF HAE cells without selection (111,118). The toxicity of VSV-G envelope protein and some lentiviral accessory proteins initially limited the ability to develop stable packaging cells lines for vector production, but regulated expression of helper and envelope components with tetracycline-inducible promoters has permitted the development of stable VSV-G–pseudotyped MLV and lentiviral vector producer lines (196–198).

Oncogenic retroviral vectors based on MLV require cell proliferation for nuclear entry, integration, and subsequent transgene expression. Studies in freshly excised human airways from CF and non-CF individuals suggest that the rates of airway epithelial cell proliferation in the chronically inflamed CF lung may be as high as 18% in regions as compared to 0.1–2.0% in non-CF individuals (109). Areas of increased proliferation were patchy and perhaps more frequent in regions of severe injury. One strategy to overcome low rates of epithelial cell proliferation was to deliver gene transfer vectors in utero where rates of epithelial proliferation were presumed to be higher. Pitt et al. demonstrated successful retrovirus-mediated gene transfer to fetal lamb airways in utero (199). Although the efficiency of transduction was not quantified, this study established the feasibility of retroviral gene transfer to proliferating airways in vivo. However, techniques that stimulate epithelial cell proliferation are required for successful retroviral gene transfer to airway epithelia in the postnatal lung. Two models were developed to stimulate epithelial cell proliferation in vivo. (1) oxidant gas injury models and (2) growth factors (114,115,118,119,200).

Johnson and coworkers developed a sulfur dioxide (SO_2) inhalational injury model to stimulate airway epithelial cell proliferation in vivo (118). Mice exposed to SO_2 (500 ppm for 3 hr) demonstrated an increase in the number of proliferating tracheal epithelial cells to ≥50% of cells that peaked at 24 hr after SO_2 inhalation, with a rapid decline in the number of proliferating cells over the ensuing 48 hr. Importantly, no significant cell proliferation was detected in the first 12 hr after SO_2 exposure. Subsequently, vector was instilled into the tracheas of anesthetized mice through a proximal tracheostomy while the mice breathed through a distal tracheostomy, limiting vector to the region between the two ostomies for up to 2 hr. This technique produced relatively efficient gene transfer to murine tracheas (~6% of cells) with a MLV (VSV-G) *lacZ* vector construct as compared to <0.1% of cells in air exposed tracheas, which were not different from vehicle controls. The known toxicity of oxidant gas injury will likely prevent the use of this method for enhancing MLV-based retroviral gene transfer to airways in humans.

Wang et al. demonstrated that polarized WD HAE cells treated with keratinocyte growth factor (KGF) to stimulate epithelial cell proliferation could be transduced with amphotropic enveloped MLV vectors following apical application of vector, but only if airways were either pretreated with or vector was coadministered with EGTA and hypotonic solutions (114). However, because no significant gene transfer occurred in the absence of EGTA and hypotonic solutions, factors other than proliferation were limiting. Similarly, intratracheal administration of KGF in vivo stimulated bronchiolar and alveolar type II cell proliferation in murine lung which increased transduction by amphotropic and 10A1-enveloped vectors in murine lung in vivo (115,200). Despite the increased rate of epithelial cell proliferation, retrovirus-mediated gene transfer was inefficient. Subsequent immunohistochemical and molecular studies demonstrated minimal levels of amphotropic receptor expression (RAM-1 or Pit-2) in murine lung. Thus, MLV-based retroviral vectors must not only overcome the limitations of cell proliferation, but must also circumvent the lack of apical membrane receptors to transduce airway epithelial cells in vivo.

Lentiviral vectors have been shown to transduce a variety of nondividing cell types in vitro and in vivo, and thus offer the possibility to overcome the limitation of cell proliferation typical of oncogenic retroviruses (103–106, 108,110,111,119,195). Goldman and colleagues demonstrated that HIV (VSV-G) vectors failed to transduce WD primary human airway epithelia cells in bronchial xenografts (201). Subsequently, Johnson et al. evaluated whether HIV (VSV-G) vectors could transduce nondividing airway epithelial cells (119). An amphotropic enveloped vector (MLV [ampho]), a HIV (VSV-G) vector, and a MLV (VSV-G) vector each efficiently transduced growing or dividing CF tracheal epithelia cells (CFT1), whereas only the HIV (VSV-G) vector efficiently transduced aphidicolin-treated (growth-arrested) airway epithelial cells. However, because luminal application of pseudotyped lentiviral vectors failed to transduced WD primary human airway epithelia in vitro and murine airways in vivo, strategies to circumvent the lack of apical membrane receptors will still be required.

To evaluate the polarity of lentiviral transduction, VSV-G pseudotyped vectors derived from HIV, EIAV, and FIV were applied to either the apical or the basolateral surfaces of polarized WD HAE cells. A 30-fold greater transduction efficiency was observed in vitro when HIV (VSV-G) vectors were applied to the basolateral surface as compared to apical application of vector. Similar data have evolved for EIAV and FIV vectors pseudotyped with VSV-G in vitro and in vivo. These data suggest that although lentiviral vectors can transduce nondividing cells, the receptors for uptake and entry of amphotropic and VSV-G pseudotyped MLV and lentiviral vectors are predominantly localized to the basolateral membrane. Two strategies have been proposed to overcome the lack of apical membrane receptor expression: (1) host modification with injury models and agents that permeabilize tight junctions to increase vector access to basolateral membrane receptors and basal cells (110,111,114,118,119) and (2) targeting the apical membrane of polarized airway epithelia by pseudotyping retroviruses with envelope proteins from other viruses that bind and enter across the apical membrane of polarized airway epithelial cells. Modification of host cells to increase access to the basolateral receptors has been discussed above. We focus here on targeting retroviral vectors to receptors on the apical membrane as an alternative strategy to increase airway gene transfer.

The usual paradigm for retroviral targeting is the generation of pseudotypes from envelope proteins of other viruses that target specific cell types. Toward this goal, investigators have initiated screening studies of enveloped viruses for their ability to infect WD HAE cells from the apical surface. Although some efforts have focused on common respiratory viruses, several investigators have broadened their search to include other enveloped viruses. Of the respiratory viruses considered as candidates for pseudotyping, influenzavirus, respiratory syncytial virus (RSV), and human coronavirus have received the most attention. Influenza A virus subtype H2N2/Japan/305/57 has been shown preferentially to infect the apical rather than the basolateral membrane of polarized WD HAE cells, whereas apical infection of HAE cells with subtypes H1N1 and H3N2 was inefficient (202). The binding of the H2N2 subtype appeared to be specific for sialic acid $\alpha2,3$-gal residues, suggesting that these sialic acid residues may serve as an apical membrane receptor for targeting of retroviral pseudotypes. In preliminary studies, wild-type RSV has been shown to infect or enter cells from the apical membrane of WD HAE cells (203,204). Human coronavirus 229E (HcoV229E) has also been shown to bind and enter across the apical membrane of WD HAE cells (205). No successful retroviral pseudotypes derived from the Env proteins of these respiratory viruses have been reported.

A variety of nonrespiratory enveloped viruses have also been evaluated as candidates to increase targeting of retroviruses to the apical surfaces of HAE cells. Rai et al. identified a type D simple retrovirus, jaagsiekte sheep retrovirus (JSRV), which is the causative agent for the contagious lung cancer of sheep known as ovine pulmonary carcinoma (206). These investigators have successfully pseudotyped MLV vectors with the Env glycoprotein of JSRV and demonstrated that the vectors can infect human airway cells in vitro. However, the ability of this pseudotyped vector efficiently to target the apical membrane of

WD HAE from either the large or small airways has not been demonstrated. In a preliminary study, MLV- and FIV-based vectors were pseudotyped with amphotropic, xenotropic, VSV-G, RD-114, 10A1, ecotropic, GALV, Marburg, and Ebola envelope glycoproteins by transient transfection techniques. Application of these pseudotyped vectors to the apical surface of WD HAE cells demonstrated efficient transduction only with FIV vectors pseudotyped with the Marburg virus envelope glycoprotein (207).

Kobinger and colleagues have also explored the potential of a family of viruses known as the Filoviridae to target the apical membrane of airway epithelia (208). Filoviridae are enveloped nonsegmented negative sense RNA viruses, which include Ebola virus and Marburg virus among its members. To identify viral envelopes capable of mediating apical transduction of polarized air-liquid interface cultures, HIV vectors were pseudotyped with MLV, influenza-hemagglutinin, RSV F and G proteins, Mokola, Ebola Reston (Ebo-R), or Ebola Zaire (EboZ) envelopes. Concentrated stocks of EboZ, but not EboR or other pseudotypes, efficiently transduced polarized HAE cells following apical application with gene transfer in up to 70% of cells as compared to up to 40% of cells following basolateral transduction. EboZ-pseudotyped HIV vectors also transduced WD HAE cells in xenografts and in freshly excised human tracheal explants. Thus, lentiviral vectors may overcome the limitations of low rates of cellular proliferation and pseudotyping lentiviral vectors with specific envelope proteins may overcome barriers to titer and lack of apical membrane receptors.

Nonviral Vectors

Barriers to nonviral vectors include poor apical membrane binding and entry and inefficient nuclear transport. Cationic lipids and naked DNA have been the only nonviral vectors evaluated in CF clinical trials to date, but newer nonviral gene transfer vectors have been developed based on polymers that may have advantages over cationic lipids. These polymers are inherently more flexible, since they can readily be linked to ligands preferentially targeting the apical membrane. The localization of the serpin enzyme complex receptor to the apical membrane of WD HAE cells has stimulated the production of polymer complexes (polyplexes) of SEC-R–targeted peptide ligand-poly-L-lysine-DNA (28,179). In preliminary studies, these polyplexes efficiently targeted the apical membranes of murine nasal epithelia in vivo and partially corrected the functional chloride permeability defect in CF mouse nasal epithelia (28,179). Lactosylated poly-L-lysine has also been suggested as a nonviral polymer that may promote binding to the apical membrane of airways (29,30,209). Although this vector has shown promise in vitro, the ability to mediate efficient transduction of polarized WD HAE cells in vitro or in vivo has not been demonstrated.

To overcome inefficient nuclear transport of nonviral vectors, fusogenic peptides, weak bases such as chloroquine, and glycerol, which presumably has an osmotic effect on intracellular vesicles, have been proposed as agents promoting endolysosomal escape (210). None of these agents have been verified in WD HAE cells or in vivo. Polyethylenimine polymers may also promote endosomal release (211), but appear to lack specific targeting moieties. Recent studies have suggested that polyplexes of lactosylated poly-L-lysine and SEC-R targeted poly-L-lysine with condensed DNA may be more efficiently translocated DNA to the nucleus (210,212). Lactosylated poly-L-lysine-DNA complexes appear to enter undifferentiated CF primary and immortalized cells by a receptor-mediated process. Confocal micrographs of labeled complexes demonstrated rapid perinuclear accumulation of lactosylated poly-L-lysine polyplexes with a small amount of nuclear entry. However, agents that inhibit lysosomal trafficking markedly increased nuclear delivery, suggesting that the majority of the lactosylated polyplexes trafficked to the endolysosomal pathway (210).

SEC-R–targeted polyplexes may be more efficiently translocated to the nucleus than lactosylated polyplexes. In preliminary studies of human hepatoma cells (HuH7), fluorescently labeled complexes, which enter the cell by receptor mediated endocytosis, were delivered to the perinuclear region within 5 min of binding with some free DNA, but no poly-L-lysine, appearing in the nucleus (212). In contrast to studies with lactosylated poly-L-lysine, chloroquine did not increase gene transfer mediated by SEC-R–targeted polyplexes, consistent with nuclear translocation with efficient escape from the endolysosomal pathway (212). Targeting of these polyplexes has not been verified in airway cells.

New Vector Systems

Recently, the paramyxoviruses have shown promise for gene transfer (213,214). Sendai virus (SeV) is an enveloped single-stranded nonsegmented negative-strand RNA virus that mediates cell attachment and entry via the envelope glycoproteins hemagglutinin-neuraminidase (HN) and fusion protein (F). The ability of the ribonucleoprotein (RNP) of this virus—and Paramyxoviridae family members in general—to mediate transcription and replication independent of nuclear functions or a DNA phase permits infection of nondividing cells. Reverse genetics has permitted the development of replication-competent SeV vectors, and recently a nontransmissable SeV vector has been developed (214). Replication-competent SeV vectors have been shown to mediate efficient reporter gene transfer to murine lung throughout the conducting airways with expression present in ciliated columnar, nonciliated secretory cells, and submucosal gland cells but not basal cells (213). Similar results were obtained following delivery to ferret lung in vivo and to freshly excised human airways ex vivo. Importantly, only a modest inhibition (50%) of SeV-mediated gene transfer has been reported in the presence of mucus. Dose-dependent inflammatory responses, which were detected in third-generation and smaller airways, and the loss of SeV-mediated expression with cell division are potential limitations of this vector.

Respiratory syncytial virus is another member of the Paramyxoviridae family of viruses that has been considered for new vector development. RSV mediates cell entry through its glycoproteins G and F (215). Like SeV, transcription and replication are cystoplasmic events. In preliminary studies, a replication-competent RSV-GFP virus efficiently transduced WD HAE cells following apical, but not basolateral, application of vector (203). RSV will likely have similar limitations as SeV for vector development. However, SeV and RSV offer exciting promise for future human airway gene transfer efforts.

C. Circumventing the Immune Response

This strategy primarily addresses cell-mediated and humoral immune responses to Ad vectors and humoral responses mediated by AAV (130,139,216). Two major approaches have been developed to blunt the cell-mediated responses: (1) elimination of specific genes that initiate or amplify the cell-mediated immune responses from the vector and (2) reinsertion of vector genes that have evolved to subvert antiviral mechanisms in host cells into completely or partially deleted Ad vectors to modulate host-cell defense responses (144,217). With regard to the former, the removal of specific viral gene products (e.g., E2A, E4) and complete deletions of all genes in the vectors that express viral proteins (e.g., helper-dependent Ad vectors) are examples (61–63,68–74,144). Reinsertion of 19-kD glycoprotein encoded in the Ad E3 region to reduce cytotoxicity to viral infected host cells by inhibiting MHC class I transport to the cell surface is an example of the latter (217). An Ad vector in which high-level E3 expression was ensured by promoter selection has been demonstrated to improve transgene persistence in an animal model, and some investigators have demonstrated increased persistence of transgene expression by retention of the E4 region (144,217,218).

Serotype switching (146,147) and transient immunosuppression (139, 219,220) have been proposed as methods to overcome the humoral immune response that leads to inhibition of repetitive viral vector administration. With regard to serotype switching, alternate dosing with Ad vectors from different subgroups and even different serotypes has been proposed as an approach to circumvent the anti-Ad humoral response, limiting gene transfer with repetitive administration (146,147). Intratracheal administration of wild-type Ad-5 (subgroup C), but not wild-type Ad-4 (subgroup E) or wild-type Ad-30 (subgroup D), has been reported to prevent subsequent gene transfer mediated by intratracheal administration of an Ad-5–*CAT* or Ad-5–*lacZ* vector (subgroup C) 7 days later (147).

Transient immunosuppression may also prevent inhibition of Ad gene transfer by neutralizing antibody production with readministration of vector. Intratracheal and/or intraperitoneal delivery of interleukin-12 (IL-12) and interferon-γ (IFN-γ) has been shown markedly to reduce (60-fold) production of vector-specific neutralizing and IgA antibodies in bronchoalveolar lavage (BAL) fluid of mice infected with an Ad-5 vector (149). Furthermore, coadministration of IL-12 and IFN-γ with an Ad-*lacZ* vector permitted successful gene transfer 28 days after previous intratracheal dosing with an Ad-*ALP* (alkaline phosphatase) vector. Blockade of T-cell costimulatory pathways with antibodies against CD40 ligand and CTLA4 and the use of pharmacological agents such as corticosteroids and cyclophosphamide at the time of vector administration could also inhibit the development of neutralizing antibodies to Ad vectors (139,219,220). Successful repetitive AAV gene transfer has also been reported following blockade of costimulatory pathways at the time of initial AAV administration to inhibit formation of neutralizing antibody to AAV (139).

Coating of Ad vector capsids by covalent linkage of polyethylene glycol (PEG) and related compounds has been suggested as another approach by which Ad vectors might escape antibody neutralization (182,221). This approach increased the duration of Ad-mediated gene expression and facilitated successful readministration of Ad vectors in vivo, although more than two repeat doses of vector were not feasible. Surprisingly, pegylation also reduced CTL responses. This approach, although promising, may be limited by the deleterious effects of PEG and related compounds on vector titer and aggregation (182). Even with the strategies discussed here, overcoming the numerous immune and inflammatory concerns raised by Ad vectors remains a formidable task.

D. Other Approaches

Polycations have been used to enhance airway gene transfer. A variety of polycations including poly-L-lysine, DEAE-dextran, polybrene, and protamine sulfate have been shown to enhance Ad-mediated gene transfer to airway epithelia in vitro and in vivo (218,222). Polycations may increase nonspecific Ad and AAV vector binding and uptake in cell lines and undifferentiated primary airway epithelial cell cultures (222). However, a role for changes in epithelial permeability as a mechanism of gene transfer enhancement has not been excluded. Further safety studies of polycations are required, although toxicity appears to be limited with current concentrations of polycations used.

Calcium phosphate coprecipitation creates aggregates of Ad that lead to enhanced non–CAR-dependent binding and uptake of Ad vectors in NIH 3T3 cells (223). These coprecipitates have been reported to increase Ad- and AAV-mediated gene transfer to airway epithelia in vitro and in vivo (223,224). Whether enhanced nonspecific binding and uptake is operative in vivo where the rate of

Table 2   Strategies for Overcoming Barriers to Airway Gene Transfer

	Barrier	Strategy
Nonspecific Barriers		
Luminal contents	Mucus, neutrophils, excess DNA, cytokines, proteases	Antibiotics, rDNAse, $\alpha_1 AT$
Cell-associated	Glycocalyx	Neuraminidase, new vector design; e.g., paramyxoviruses
Adenovirus		
Inefficient binding/entry	Absence of apical membrane receptors and coreceptors	Retargeting with chimeric Ad vectors, bispecific antibodies, adenobodies, host modification
Immune response	Cell-mediated response	HD Ad vectors, PEGylation
	Humoral response	Transient immunosuppression with CTLA4, CD40 ligand; seroswitching, stealth Ad vectors (PEGylation); IL-12 and IFN_γ
Adeno-Associated Virus		
Binding/entry	Absence of apical membrane receptors and coreceptors	Alternative serotypes, retargeting Host modification
Small insert size	4.5-kb insert limitation	Transsplicing
Postnuclear entry	SsDNA $\pm$ dsDNA conversion	Time, DNA topoisomerase inhibitors, Ad E4 gene products
Immune response	Neutralizing antibody[a]	Transient immunosuppression
Retroviruses		
MLV	Titer	Pseudotyping, vector concentration
	Cell proliferation	Lentiviruses, KGF, host modification
	Absence of apical receptors	Pseudotyping
Lentivirus	Absence of apical receptors	Pseudotyping
Nonviral Vectors		
Cationic liposomes	Inefficient binding and entry	New formulations, host modification
	Poor nuclear translocation	Fusogenic peptides, alternative formulations, weak bases
Molecular conjugates (polymers)	Inefficient binding and entry	Targeting with specific ligands
	Poor nuclear translocation	Targeting, lactosylated polymers, fusogenic peptides, weak bases, osmotic agents

[a] Whether or not neutralizing antibodies to AAV-2 act as a barrier to gene transfer is controversial.

endocytosis across the apical membrane by nonspecific mechanisms is low has not been delineated. Possible effects on cellular and paracellular permeability have not been investigated.

V. Conclusions

Significant advances have been made in the design and production of vectors for lung gene transfer. However, the lung remains a formidable target for gene transfer approaches owing to its complex anatomy, large surface area, protective immune functions, and the presence of specific barriers that limit entry of foreign particles. Progress has been made and a number of strategies have evolved to address the barriers (Table 2). Efforts to improve the ability of vectors to target the apical membrane of airway epithelia in vivo and methods that modify the host to increase vector access to cell targets offer hope, but more basic research is needed to achieve successful gene therapy of cystic fibrosis lung disease.

Acknowledgments

The authors thank Miriam Kelly and Carolyn Coyne for their assistance with figures and Marguerite Applin for clerical assistance. This work was supported by HL58342 (LGJ) and HL51818 (RCB) from the National Heart Lung and Blood Institute, National Institutes of the Health and a grant (S880) from the Cystic Fibrosis Foundation.

References

1. Olsen JC, Johnson LG, Stutts MJ, Sarkadi B, Yankaskas JR, Swanstrom R, Boucher RC. Correction of the apical membrane chloride permeability defect in polarized cystic fibrosis airway epithelia following retroviral-mediated gene transfer. Hum Gene Ther 1992; 3:253–266.
2. Drumm ML, Pope HA, Cliff WH, Rommens JM, Marvin SA, Tsui LC, Collins FS, Frizzell RA, Wilson JM. Correction of the cystic fibrosis defect in vitro by retrovirus-mediated gene transfer. Cell 1990; 62:1227–1233.
3. Egan M, Flotte T, Afione S, Solow R, Zeitlin PL, Carter BJ, Guggino WB. Defective regulation of outwardly rectifying Cl^- channels by protein kinase A corrected by insertion of CFTR. Nature 1992; 358:581–584.
4. Rich DP, Anderson MP, Gregory RJ, Cheng SH, Paul S, Jefferson DM, McCann JD, Klinger KW, Smith AE, Welsh MJ. Expression of cystic fibrosis transmembrane conductance regulator corrects defective chloride channel regulation in cystic fibrosis airway epithelial cells. Nature 1990; 347:358–363.
5. Rosenfeld MA, Yoshimura K, Trapnell BC, Yoneyama K, Rosenthal ER, Dalemans

W, Fukayama M, Bargon J, Stier LE, Stratford-Perricaudet L, et al. In vivo transfer of the human cystic fibrosis transmembrane conductance regulator gene to the airway epithelium. Cell 1992; 68:143–55.

6. Brasfield D, Hicks G, Soong S, Peters J, Tiller R. Evaluation of scoring system of the chest radiograph in cystic fibrosis: a collaborative study. AJR Am J Roentgenol 1980; 134:1195–1198.

7. Tepper RS, Montgomery GL, Ackerman V, Eigen H. Longitudinal evaluation of pulmonary function in infants and very young children with cystic fibrosis. Pediatr Pulmonol 1993; 16:96–100.

8. Engelhardt JF, Yankaskas JR, Ernst SA, Yang Y, Marino CR, Boucher RC, Cohn JA, Wilson JM. Submucosal glands are the predominant site of CFTR expression in the human bronchus. Nat Genet 1992; 2:240–248.

9. Borthwick DW, Shahbazian M, Krantz QT, Dorin JR, Randell SH. Evidence for stem-cell niches in the tracheal epithelium. Am J Respir Cell Mol Biol 2001; 24: 662–670.

10. Hong KU, Reynolds SD, Giangreco A, Hurley CM, Stripp BR. Clara cell secretory protein-expressing cells of the airway neuroepithelial body microenvironment include a label-retaining subset and are critical for epithelial renewal after progenitor cell depletion. Am J Respir Cell Mol Biol 2001; 24:671–681.

11. Deng W, Obrocka M, Fischer I, Prockop DJ. In vitro differentiation of human marrow stromal cells into early progenitors of neural cells by conditions that increase intracellular cyclic AMP. Biochem Biophys Res Commun 2001; 282:148–152.

12. Krause DS, Theise ND, Collector MI, Henegariu O, Hwang S, Gardner R, Neutzel S, Sharkis SJ. Multi-organ, multi-lineage engraftment by a single bone marrow–derived stem cell. Cell 2001; 105:369–377.

13. Zabner J, Petersen DM, Puga AP, Graham SM, Couture LA, Keyes LD, Lukason MJ, St George JA, Gregory RJ, Smith AE, et al. Safety and efficacy of repetitive adenovirus-mediated transfer of CFTR cDNA to airway epithelia of primates and cotton rats. Nat Genet 1994; 6:75–83.

14. Caplen NJ, Alton EW, Middleton PG, Dorin JR, Stevenson BJ, Gao X, Durham SR, Jeffery PK, Hodson ME, Coutelle C, et al. Liposome-mediated CFTR gene transfer to the nasal epithelium of patients with cystic fibrosis. Nat Med 1995; 1: 39–46.

15. Knowles MR, Hohneker KW, Zhou Z, Olsen JC, Noah TL, Hu PC, Leigh MW, Engelhardt JF, Edwards LJ, Jones KR, et al. A controlled study of adenoviral-vector–mediated gene transfer in the nasal epithelium of patients with cystic fibrosis. N Engl J Med 1995; 333:823–831.

16. Bellon G, Michel-Calemard L, Thouvenot D, Jagneaux V, Poitevin F, Malcus C, Accart N, Layani MP, Aymard M, Bernon H, Bienvenu J, Courtney M, Doring G, Gilly B, Gilly R, Lamy D, Levrey H, Morel Y, Paulin C, Perraud F, Rodillon L, Sene C, So S, Touraine-Moulin F, Pavirani A, et al. Aerosol administration of a recombinant adenovirus expressing CFTR to cystic fibrosis patients: a phase I clinical trial. Hum Gene Ther 1997; 8:15–25.

17. Crystal RG, McElvaney NG, Rosenfeld MA, Chu CS, Mastrangeli A, Hay JG,

Brody SL, Jaffe HA, Eissa NT, Danel C. Administration of an adenovirus containing the human CFTR cDNA to the respiratory tract of individuals with cystic fibrosis. Nat Genet 1994; 8:42–51.

18. Hay JG, McElvaney NG, Herena J, Crystal RG. Modification of nasal epithelial potential differences of individuals with cystic fibrosis consequent to local administration of a normal CFTR cDNA adenovirus gene transfer vector. Hum Gene Ther 1995; 6:1487–96.

19. Hyde SC, Southern KW, Gileadi U, Fitzjohn EM, Mofford KA, Waddell BE, Gooi HC, Goddard CA, Hannavy K, Smyth SE, Egan JJ, Sorgi FL, Huang L, Cuthbert AW, Evans MJ, Colledge WH, Higgins CF, Webb AK, Gill DR. Repeat administration of DNA/liposomes to the nasal epithelium of patients with cystic fibrosis. Gene Ther 2000; 7:1156–1165.

20. Noone PG, Hohneker KW, Zhou Z, Johnson LG, Foy C, Gipson C, Jones K, Noah TL, Leigh MW, Schwartzbach C, Efthimiou J, Pearlman R, Boucher RC, Knowles MR. Safety and biological efficacy of a lipid-CFTR complex for gene transfer in the nasal epithelium of adult patients with cystic fibrosis. Mol Ther 2000; 1:105–114.

21. Wagner JA, Messner AH, Moran ML, Daifuku R, Kouyama K, Desch JK, Manley S, Norbash AM, Conrad CK, Friborg S, Reynolds T, Guggino WB, Moss RB, Carter BJ, Wine JJ, Flotte TR, Gardner P. Safety and biological efficacy of an adeno-associated virus vector–cystic fibrosis transmembrane regulator (AAV-CFTR) in the cystic fibrosis maxillary sinus. Laryngoscope 1999; 109:266–274.

22. Zabner J, Ramsey BW, Meeker DP, Aitken ML, Balfour RP, Gibson RL, Launspach J, Moscicki RA, Richards SM, Standaert TA, et al. Repeat administration of an adenovirus vector encoding cystic fibrosis transmembrane conductance regulator to the nasal epithelium of patients with cystic fibrosis. J Clin Invest 1996; 97:1504–1511.

23. Gill DR, Southern KW, Mofford KA, Seddon T, Huang L, Sorgi F, Thomson A, MacVinish LJ, Ratcliff R, Bilton D, Lane DJ, Littlewood JM, Webb AK, Middleton PG, Colledge WH, Cuthbert AW, Evans MJ, Higgins CF, Hyde SC. A placebo-controlled study of liposome-mediated gene transfer to the nasal epithelium of patients with cystic fibrosis. Gene Ther 1997; 4:199–200.

24. Porteous DJ, Dorin JR, McLachlan G, Davidson-Smith H, Davidson H, Stevenson BJ, Carothers AD, Wallace WA, Moralee S, Hoenes C, Kallmeyer G, Michaelis U, Naujoks K, Ho LP, Samways JM, Imrie M, Greening AP, Innes JA. Evidence for safety and efficacy of DOTAP cationic liposome mediated CFTR gene transfer to the nasal epithelium of patients with cystic fibrosis. Gene Ther 1997; 4:210–218.

25. Zabner J, Cheng SH, Meeker D, Launspach J, Balfour R, Perricone MA, Morris JE, Marshall J, Fasbender A, Smith AE, Welsh MJ. Comparison of DNA-lipid complexes and DNA alone for gene transfer to cystic fibrosis airway epithelia in vivo. J Clin Invest 1997; 100:1529–1537.

26. Alton EW, Stern M, Farley R, Jaffe A, Chadwick SL, Phillips J, Davies J, Smith SN, Browning J, Davies MG, Hodson ME, Durham SR, Li D, Jeffery PK, Scallan M, Balfour R, Eastman SJ, Cheng SH, Smith AE, Meeker D, Geddes DM. Cationic

lipid-mediated CFTR gene transfer to the lungs and nose of patients with cystic fibrosis: a double-blind placebo-controlled trial. Lancet 1999; 353:947–954.

27. Grubb BR, Pickles RJ, Ye H, Yankaskas JR, Vick RN, Engelhardt JF, Wilson JM, Johnson LG, Boucher RC. Inefficient gene transfer by adenovirus vector to cystic fibrosis airway epithelia of mice and humans. Nature 1994; 371:802–807.

28. Ziady AG, Keefer R, Ferkol T, Davis PB. Serpin enzyme complex receptor targeted DNA complexes deliver genes to airway epithelia. Pediatr Pulmonol 1999; (Suppl): 233.

29. Kollen WJ, Schembri FM, Gerwig GJ, Vliegenthart JF, Glick MC, Scanlin TF. Enhanced efficiency of lactosylated poly-L-lysine–mediated gene transfer into cystic fibrosis airway epithelial cells. Am J Respir Cell Mol Biol 1999; 20:1081–1086.

30. Kollen WJ, Mulberg AE, Wei X, Sugita M, Raghuram V, Wang J, Foskett JK, Glick MC, Scanlin TF. High-efficiency transfer of cystic fibrosis transmembrane conductance regulator cDNA into cystic fibrosis airway cells in culture using lactosylated polylysine as a vector. Hum Gene Ther 1999; 10:615–622.

31. Matsui H, Grubb BR, Tarran R, Randell SH, Gatzy JT, Davis CW, Boucher RC. Evidence for periciliary liquid layer depletion, not abnormal ion composition, in the pathogenesis of cystic fibrosis airways disease. Cell 1998; 95:1005–1015.

32. Matsui H, Randell SH, Peretti SW, Davis CW, Boucher RC. Coordinated clearance of periciliary liquid and mucus from airway surfaces. J Clin Invest 1998; 102:1125–1131.

33. Tarran R, Grubb BR, Parsons D, Picher M, Hirsh AJ, Davis CW, Boucher RC. The cf salt controversy in vivo observations and therapeutic approaches. Mol Cell 2001; 8:149–158.

34. Boucher RC. Pathogenesis of cystic fibrosis airways disease. Trans Am Clin Climatol Assoc 2001; 112:99–107.

35. Bonfil TL. Inflammatory cytokines in cystic fibrosis lungs. Am J Respir Crit Care Med 1995; 152:2111–2118.

36. Black HR, Yankaskas JR, Johnson LG, Noah TL. Interleukin-8 production by cystic fibrosis nasal epithelial cells after tumor necrosis factor-alpha and respiratory syncytial virus stimulation. Am J Respir Cell Mol Biol 1998; 19:210–215.

37. Khan TZ, Wagener JS, Bost T, Martinez J, Accurso FJ, Riches DW. Early pulmonary inflammation in infants with cystic fibrosis. Am J Respir Crit Care Med 1995; 151:1075–1082.

38. Kirchner KK, Wagener JS, Khan TZ, Copenhaver SC, Accurso FJ. Increased DNA levels in bronchoalveolar lavage fluid obtained from infants with cystic fibrosis. Am J Respir Crit Care Med 1996; 154:1426–1429.

39. Davis PB. Clinical pathophysiology and manifestations of lung disease. In: Yankaskas JR, Knowles MR, eds. Cystic Fibrosis in Adults. Philadelphia: Lippincott-Raven, 1999.

40. Stern M, Caplen NJ, Browning JE, Griesenbach U, Sorgi F, Huang L, Gruenert DC, Marriot C, Crystal RG, Geddes DM, Alton EW. The effect of mucolytic agents on gene transfer across a CF sputum barrier in vitro. Gene Ther 1998; 5:91–98.

41. Perricone MA, Rees DD, Sacks CR, Smith KA, Kaplan JM, St George JA. Inhibi-

tory effect of cystic fibrosis sputum on adenovirus-mediated gene transfer in cultured epithelial cells. Hum Gene Ther 2000; 11:1997–2008.

42. Virella-Lowell I, Poirier A, Chesnut KA, Brantly M, Flotte TR. Inhibition of recombinant adeno-associated virus (rAAV) transduction by bronchial secretions from cystic fibrosis patients. Gene Ther 2000; 7:1783–1789.

43. van Heeckeren A, Ferkol T, Tosi M. Effects of bronchopulmonary inflammation induced by pseudomonas aeruginosa on adenovirus-mediated gene transfer to airway epithelial cells in mice. Gene Ther 1998; 5:345–351.

44. Parsons DW, Grubb BR, Johnson LG, Boucher RC. Enhanced in vivo airway gene transfer via transient modification of host barrier properties with a surface-active agent. Hum Gene Ther 1998; 9:2661–2672.

45. Worgall S, Leopold PL, Wolff G, Ferris B, Van Roijen N, Crystal RG. Role of alveolar macrophages in rapid elimination of adenovirus vectors administered to the epithelial surface of the respiratory tract. Hum Gene Ther 1997; 8:1675–1684.

46. McCray PB, Jr., Wang G, Kline JN, Zabner J, Chada S, Jolly DJ, Chang SM, Davidson BL. Alveolar macrophages inhibit retrovirus-mediated gene transfer to airway epithelia. Hum Gene Ther 1997; 8:1087–1093.

47. Duan D, Yue Y, Yan Z, McCray PB, Jr., Engelhardt JF. Polarity influences the efficiency of recombinant adenoassociated virus infection in differentiated airway epithelia. Hum Gene Ther 1998; 9:2761–2776.

48. Bernacki SH, Nelson AL, Abdullah L, Sheehan JK, Harris A, William Davis C, Randell SH. Mucin gene expression during differentiation of human airway epithelia in vitro. Muc4 and muc5b are strongly induced. Am J Respir Cell Mol Biol 1999; 20:595–604.

49. Gray T, Nettesheim P, Basbaum C, Koo J. Regulation of mucin gene expression in human tracheobronchial epithelial cells by thyroid hormone. Biochem J 2001; 353:727–734.

50. Gray T, Koo JS, Nettesheim P. Regulation of mucous differentiation and mucin gene expression in the tracheobronchial epithelium. Toxicology 2001; 160:35–46.

51. Arcasoy SM, Latoche J, Gondor M, Henderson RA, Hughey R, Finn OJ, Pilewski JM. The effects of sialoglycoconjugates on adenovirus-mediated gene transfer to epithelial cells in vitro and in human airway xenografts. Chest 1997; 111:142S–143S.

52. Meerzaman D, Shapiro PS, Kim KC. Involvement of the MAP kinase ERK2 in MUC1 mucin signaling. Am J Physiol Lung Cell Mol Physiol 2001; 281:L86–91.

53. Arcasoy SM, Latoche J, Gondor M, Watkins SC, Henderson RA, Hughey R, Finn OJ, Pilewski JM. MUC1 and other sialoglycoconjugates inhibit adenovirus-mediated gene transfer to epithelial cells. Am J Respir Cell Mol Biol 1997; 17:422–435.

54. Pickles RJ, Fahrner JA, Petrella JM, Boucher RC, Bergelson JM. Retargeting the coxsackievirus and adenovirus receptor to the apical surface of polarized epithelial cells reveals the glycocalyx as a barrier to adenovirus-mediated gene transfer. J Virol 2000; 74:6050–6057.

55. Walters RW, van't Hof W, Yi SM, Schroth MK, Zabner J, Crystal RG, Welsh MJ. Apical localization of the coxsackie-adenovirus receptor by glycosyl-phosphatidyl-

inositol modification is sufficient for adenovirus-mediated gene transfer through the apical surface of human airway epithelia. J Virol 2001; 75:7703–7711.

56. Berkner K. Development of adenovirus vectors from the expression of heterologous genes. Biotechniques 1998; 6:616–629.

57. Ginsberg HS, Lundholm-Beauchamp U, Horswood RL, Pernis B, Wold WS, Chanock RM, Prince GA. Role of early region 3 (E3) in pathogenesis of adenovirus disease. Proc Natl Acad Sci USA 1989; 86:3823–3827.

58. Kovesdi I, Brough DE, Bruder JT, Wickham TJ. Adenoviral vectors for gene transfer. Curr Opin Biotechnol 1997; 8:583–589.

59. Rich DP, Couture LA, Cardoza LM, Guiggio VM, Armentano D, Espino PC, Hehir K, Welsh MJ, Smith AE, Gregory RJ. Development and analysis of recombinant adenoviruses for gene therapy of cystic fibrosis. Hum Gene Ther 1993; 4:461–476.

60. Engelhardt JF, Yang Y, Stratford-Perricaudet LD, Allen ED, Kozarsky K, Perricaudet M, Yankaskas JR, Wilson JM. Direct gene transfer of human CFTR into human bronchial epithelia of xenografts with E1-deleted adenoviruses. Nat Genet 1993; 4:27–34.

61. Engelhardt JF, Litzky L, Wilson JM. Prolonged transgene expression in cotton rat lung with recombinant adenoviruses defective in E2a. Hum Gene Ther 1994; 5: 1217–1229.

62. Engelhardt JF, Ye X, Doranz B, Wilson JM. Ablation of E2A in recombinant adenoviruses improves transgene persistence and decreases inflammatory response in mouse liver. Proc Natl Acad Sci USA 1994; 91:6196–6200.

63. Goldman MJ, Litzky LA, Engelhardt JF, Wilson JM. Transfer of the CFTR gene to the lung of nonhuman primates with E1-deleted, E2a-defective recombinant adenoviruses: a preclinical toxicology study. Hum Gene Ther 1995; 6:839–851.

64. Yang Y, Nunes FA, Berencsi K, Gonczol E, Engelhardt JF, Wilson JM. Inactivation of E2a in recombinant adenoviruses improves the prospect for gene therapy in cystic fibrosis. Nat Genet 1994; 7:362–369.

65. Wang Q, Jia XC, Finer MH. A packaging cell line for propagation of recombinant adenovirus vectors containing two lethal gene-region deletions. Gene Ther 1995; 2:775–783.

66. Kaplan JM, Armentano D, Sparer TE, Wynn SG, Peterson PA, Wadsworth SC, Couture KK, Pennington SE, St George JA, Gooding LR, Smith AE. Characterization of factors involved in modulating persistence of transgene expression from recombinant adenovirus in the mouse lung. Hum Gene Ther 1997; 8:45–56.

67. Armentano D, Sookdeo CC, Hehir KM, Gregory RJ, St George JA, Prince GA, Wadsworth SC, Smith AE. Characterization of an adenovirus gene transfer vector containing an E4 deletion. Hum Gene Ther 1995; 6:1343–1353.

68. Parks RJ, Chen L, Anton M, Sankar U, Rudnicki MA, Graham FL. A helper-dependent adenovirus vector system: removal of helper virus by Cre-mediated excision of the viral packaging signal. Proc Natl Acad Sci USA 1996; 93:13565–13570.

69. Fisher KJ, Choi H, Burda J, Chen SJ, Wilson JM. Recombinant adenovirus deleted of all viral genes for gene therapy of cystic fibrosis. Virology 1996; 217:11–22.

70. Hardy S, Kitamura M, Harris-Stansil T, Dai Y, Phipps ML. Construction of adenovirus vectors through Cre-lox recombination. J Virol 1997; 71:1842–1849.

71. Hartigan-O'Connor D, Amalfitano A, Chamberlain JS. Improved production of gut-

ted adenovirus in cells expressing adenovirus preterminal protein and DNA polymerase. J Virol 1999; 73:7835–7841.

72. Kochanek S, Clemens PR, Mitani K, Chen HH, Chan S, Caskey CT. A new adenoviral vector: replacement of all viral coding sequences with 28 kb of DNA independently expressing both full-length dystrophin and beta-galactosidase. Proc Natl Acad Sci USA 1996; 93:5731–5736.

73. Lieber A, He CY, Kirillova I, Kay MA. Recombinant adenoviruses with large deletions generated by Cre-mediated excision exhibit different biological properties compared with first-generation vectors in vitro and in vivo. J Virol 1996; 70:8944–8960.

74. Morsy MA, Gu M, Motzel S, Zhao J, Lin J, Su Q, Allen H, Franlin L, Parks RJ, Graham FL, Kochanek S, Bett AJ, Caskey CT. An adenoviral vector deleted for all viral coding sequences results in enhanced safety and extended expression of a leptin transgene. Proc Natl Acad Sci USA 1998; 95:7866–7871.

75. FitzGerald DJ, Padmanabhan R, Pastan I, Willingham MC. Adenovirus-induced release of epidermal growth factor and pseudomonas toxin into the cytosol of KB cells during receptor-mediated endocytosis. Cell 1983; 32:607–617.

76. Bergelson JM, Cunningham JA, Droguett G, Kurt-Jones EA, Krithivas A, Hong JS, Horwitz MS, Crowell RL, Finberg RW. Isolation of a common receptor for coxsackie B viruses and adenoviruses 2 and 5. Science 1997; 275:1320–1323.

77. Wickham TJ, Mathias P, Cheresh DA, Nemerow GR. Integrins alpha v beta 3 and alpha v beta 5 promote adenovirus internalization but not virus attachment. Cell 1993; 73:309–319.

78. Pickles RJ, Barker PM, Ye H, Boucher RC. Efficient adenovirus-mediated gene transfer to basal but not columnar cells of cartilaginous airway epithelia. Hum Gene Ther 1996; 7:921–931.

79. Dupuit F, Zahm JM, Pierrot D, Brezillon S, Bonnet N, Imler JL, Pavirani A, Puchelle E. Regenerating cells in human airway surface epithelium represent preferential targets for recombinant adenovirus. Hum Gene Ther 1995; 6:1185–1193.

80. Goldman MJ, Wilson JM. Expression of alpha v beta 5 integrin is necessary for efficient adenovirus-mediated gene transfer in the human airway. J Virol 1995; 69:5951–5958.

81. Zabner J, Freimuth P, Puga A, Fabrega A, Welsh MJ. Lack of high affinity fiber receptor activity explains the resistance of ciliated airway epithelia to adenovirus infection. J Clin Invest 1997; 100:1144–1149.

82. Pickles RJ, McCarty D, Matsui H, Hart PJ, Randell SH, Boucher RC. Limited entry of adenovirus vectors into well-differentiated airway epithelium is responsible for inefficient gene transfer. J Virol 1998; 72:6014–6023.

83. Pilewski JM, Engelhardt JF, Bavaria JE, Kaiser LR, Wilson JM, Albelda SM. Adenovirus-mediated gene transfer to human bronchial submucosal glands using xenografts. Am J Physiol 1995; 268:L657–665.

84. Zabner J, Zeiher BG, Friedman E, Welsh MJ. Adenovirus-mediated gene transfer to ciliated airway epithelia requires prolonged incubation time. J Virol 1996; 70:6994–7003.

85. Matsui H, Johnson LG, Randell SH, Boucher RC. Loss of binding and entry of

liposome-DNA complexes decreases transfection efficiency in differentiated airway epithelial cells. J Biol Chem 1997; 272:1117–1126.

86. Flotte TR, Solow R, Owens RA, Afione S, Zeitlin PL, Carter BJ. Gene expression from adeno-associated virus vectors in airway epithelial cells. Am J Respir Cell Mol Biol 1992; 7:349–356.

87. Flotte TR, Afione SA, Conrad C, McGrath SA, Solow R, Oka H, Zeitlin PL, Guggino WB, Carter BJ. Stable in vivo expression of the cystic fibrosis transmembrane conductance regulator with an adeno-associated virus vector. Proc Natl Acad Sci USA 1993; 90:10613–10617.

88. Flotte TR, Afione SA, Solow R, Drumm ML, Markakis D, Guggino WB, Zeitlin PL, Carter BJ. Expression of the cystic fibrosis transmembrane conductance regulator from a novel adeno-associated virus promoter. J Biol Chem 1993; 268:3781–90.

89. Flotte TR. Prospects for virus-based gene therapy for cystic fibrosis. J Bioenerg Biomembr 1993; 25:37–42.

90. Flotte TR, Carter BJ. Adeno-associated virus vectors for gene therapy. Gene Ther 1995; 2:357–362.

91. Summerford C, Samulski RJ. Membrane-associated heparan sulfate proteoglycan is a receptor for adeno-associated virus type 2 virions. J Virol 1998; 72:1438–1445.

92. Qing K, Mah C, Hansen J, Zhou S, Dwarki V, Srivastava A. Human fibroblast growth factor receptor 1 is a co-receptor for infection by adeno-associated virus 2. Nat Med 1999; 5:71–77.

93. Summerford C, Bartlett JS, Samulski RJ. AlphaVbeta5 integrin: a co-receptor for adeno-associated virus type 2 infection. Nat Med 1999; 5:78–82.

94. Duan D, Yue Y, Yan Z, Yang J, Engelhardt JF. Endosomal processing limits gene transfer to polarized airway epithelia by adeno-associated virus. J Clin Invest 2000; 105:1573–1587.

95. Halbert CL, Alexander IE, Wolgamot GM, Miller AD. Adeno-associated virus vectors transduce primary cells much less efficiently than immortalized cells. J Virol 1995; 69:1473–1479.

96. Ferrari FK, Samulski T, Shenk T, Samulski RJ. Second-strand synthesis is a rate-limiting step for efficient transduction by recombinant adeno-associated virus vectors. J Virol 1996; 70:3227–3234.

97. Alexander IE, Russell DW, Miller AD. DNA-damaging agents greatly increase the transduction of nondividing cells by adeno-associated virus vectors. J Virol 1994; 68:8282–8287.

98. Rabinowitz JE, Samulski RJ. Adeno-associated virus expression systems for gene transfer. Curr Opin Biotechnol 1998; 9:470–475.

99. Russell DW, Alexander IE, Miller AD. DNA synthesis and topoisomerase inhibitors increase transduction by adeno-associated virus vectors. Proc Natl Acad Sci USA 1995; 92:5719–5723.

100. Coffin JM. Retroviridae: the viruses and their replication. In: Fields BN, Knippe DM, Howley PM, eds. Fields Virology. Philadelphia: Lippincott-Raven, 1996; pp. 1767–1847.

101. Trono D. Lentiviral vectors: turning a deadly foe into a therapeutic agent. Gene Ther 2000; 7:20–23.

102. Miller AD, Rosman GJ. Improved retroviral vectors for gene transfer and expression. Biotechniques 1989; 7:980–982, 984–986, 989–990.
103. Naldini L. Lentiviruses as gene transfer agents for delivery to non-dividing cells. Curr Opin Biotechnol 1998; 9:457–463.
104. Naldini L, Blomer U, Gallay P, Ory D, Mulligan R, Gage FH, Verma IM, Trono D. In vivo gene delivery and stable transduction of nondividing cells by a lentiviral vector. Science 1996; 272:263–267.
105. Naldini L, Blomer U, Gage FH, Trono D, Verma IM. Efficient transfer, integration, and sustained long-term expression of the transgene in adult rat brains injected with a lentiviral vector. Proc Natl Acad Sci USA 1996; 93:11382–11388.
106. Zufferey R, Nagy D, Mandel RJ, Naldini L, Trono D. Multiply attenuated lentiviral vector achieves efficient gene delivery in vivo. Nat Biotechnol 1997; 15:871–875.
107. Delviks KA, Hu WS, Pathak VK. Psi-vectors: murine leukemia virus-based self-inactivating and self-activating retroviral vectors. J Virol 1997; 71:6218–6224.
108. Zufferey R, Dull T, Mandel RJ, Bukovsky A, Quiroz D, Naldini L, Trono D. Self-inactivating lentivirus vector for safe and efficient in vivo gene delivery. J Virol 1998; 72:9873–9880.
109. Leigh MW, Kylander JE, Yankaskas JR, Boucher RC. Cell proliferation in bronchial epithelium and submucosal glands of cystic fibrosis patients. Am J Respir Cell Mol Biol 1995; 12:605–612.
110. Olsen JC. Gene transfer vectors derived from equine infectious anemia virus. Gene Ther 1998; 5:1481–1487.
111. Wang G, Slepushkin V, Zabner J, Keshavjee S, Johnston JC, Sauter SL, Jolly DJ, Dubensky TW, Jr., Davidson BL, McCray PB, Jr. Feline immunodeficiency virus vectors persistently transduce nondividing airway epithelia and correct the cystic fibrosis defect. J Clin Invest 1999; 104:R55–62.
112. Miller DG, Adam MA, Miller AD. Gene transfer by retrovirus vectors occurs only in cells that are actively replicating at the time of infection. Mol Cell Biol 1990; 10:4239–4242.
113. Burns JC, Friedmann T, Driever W, Burrascano M, Yee JK. Vesicular stomatitis virus G glycoprotein pseudotyped retroviral vectors: concentration to very high titer and efficient gene transfer into mammalian and nonmammalian cells. Proc Natl Acad Sci USA 1993; 90:8033–8037.
114. Wang G, Davidson BL, Melchert P, Slepushkin VA, van Es HH, Bodner M, Jolly DJ, McCray PB, Jr. Influence of cell polarity on retrovirus-mediated gene transfer to differentiated human airway epithelia. J Virol 1998; 72:9818–9826.
115. Zsengeller ZK, Halbert C, Miller AD, Wert SE, Whitsett JA, Bachurski CJ. Keratinocyte growth factor stimulates transduction of the respiratory epithelium by retroviral vectors. Hum Gene Ther 1999; 10:341–353.
116. Wang G, Xia H, Shao J, Davidson BL, McCray JPB. Post-binding steps impede gene transfer to differentiated airway epithelia from the apical surface. Mol Ther 2001; 3:S39.
117. Fuller S, von Bonsdorff CH, Simons K. Vesicular stomatitis virus infects and matures only through the basolateral surface of the polarized epithelial cell line, MDCK. Cell 1984; 38:65–77.

118. Johnson LG, Mewshaw JP, Ni H, Friedmann T, Boucher RC, Olsen JC. Effect of host modification and age on airway epithelial gene transfer mediated by a murine leukemia virus-derived vector. J Virol 1998; 72:8861–8872.

119. Johnson LG, Olsen JC, Naldini L, Boucher RC. Pseudotyped human lentiviral vector-mediated gene transfer to airway epithelia in vivo. Gene Ther 2000; 7:568–574.

120. Scherman D, Bessodes M, Cameron B, Herscovici J, Hofland H, Pitard B, Soubrier F, Wils P, Crouzet J. Application of lipids and plasmid design for gene delivery to mammalian cells. Curr Opin Biotechnol 1998; 9:480–485.

121. Ledley FD. Nonviral gene therapy: the promise of genes as pharmaceutical products. Hum Gene Ther 1995; 6:1129–1144.

122. Legendre JY, Szoka FC, Jr. Delivery of plasmid DNA into mammalian cell lines using pH-sensitive liposomes: comparison with cationic liposomes. Pharm Res 1992; 9:1235–1242.

123. Zhou X, Huang L. DNA transfection mediated by cationic liposomes containing lipopolylysine: characterization and mechanism of action. Biochim Biophys Acta 1994; 1189:195–203.

124. Ferkol T, Kaetzel CS, Davis PB. Gene transfer into respiratory epithelial cells by targeting the polymeric immunoglobulin receptor. J Clin Invest 1993; 92:2394–2400.

125. Ferkol T, Perales JC, Eckman E, Kaetzel CS, Hanson RW, Davis PB. Gene transfer into the airway epithelium of animals by targeting the polymeric immunoglobulin receptor. J Clin Invest 1995; 95:493–502.

126. Zabner J, Fasbender AJ, Moninger T, Poellinger KA, Welsh MJ. Cellular and molecular barriers to gene transfer by a cationic lipid. J Biol Chem 1995; 270:18997–19007.

127. Fasbender A, Zabner J, Zeiher BG, Welsh MJ. A low rate of cell proliferation and reduced DNA uptake limit cationic lipid-mediated gene transfer to primary cultures of ciliated human airway epithelia. Gene Ther 1997; 4:1173–1180.

128. Dong JY, Wang D, Van Ginkel FW, Pascual DW, Frizzell RA. Systematic analysis of repeated gene delivery into animal lungs with a recombinant adenovirus vector. Hum Gene Ther 1996; 7:319–331.

129. Kaplan JM, St George JA, Pennington SE, Keyes LD, Johnson RP, Wadsworth SC, Smith AE. Humoral and cellular immune responses of nonhuman primates to long-term repeated lung exposure to Ad2/CFTR-2. Gene Ther 1996; 3:117–127.

130. Look DC, Brody SL. Engineering viral vectors to subvert the airway defense response. Am J Respir Cell Mol Biol 1999; 20:1103–1106.

131. Otake K, Ennist DL, Harrod K, Trapnell BC. Nonspecific inflammation inhibits adenovirus-mediated pulmonary gene transfer and expression independent of specific acquired immune responses. Hum Gene Ther 1998; 9:2207–2222.

132. St George JA, Pennington SE, Kaplan JM, Peterson PA, Kleine LJ, Smith AE, Wadsworth SC. Biological response of nonhuman primates to long-term repeated lung exposure to Ad2/CFTR-2. Gene Ther 1996; 3:103–116.

133. van Ginkel FW, McGhee JR, Liu C, Simecka JW, Yamamoto M, Frizzell RA, Sorscher EJ, Kiyono H, Pascual DW. Adenoviral gene delivery elicits distinct

pulmonary-associated T helper cell responses to the vector and to its transgene. J Immunol 1997; 159:685–693.

134. Yang Y, Li Q, Ertl HC, Wilson JM. Cellular and humoral immune responses to viral antigens create barriers to lung-directed gene therapy with recombinant adenoviruses. J Virol 1995; 69:2004–2015.

135. Yei S, Mittereder N, Wert S, Whitsett JA, Wilmott RW, Trapnell BC. In vivo evaluation of the safety of adenovirus-mediated transfer of the human cystic fibrosis transmembrane conductance regulator cDNA to the lung. Hum Gene Ther 1994; 5:731–744.

136. Yei S, Mittereder N, Tang K, O'Sullivan C, Trapnell BC. Adenovirus-mediated gene transfer for cystic fibrosis: quantitative evaluation of repeated in vivo vector administration to the lung. Gene Ther 1994; 1:192–200.

137. Beck SE, Jones LA, Chesnut K, Walsh SM, Reynolds TC, Carter BJ, Askin FB, Flotte TR, Guggino WB. Repeated delivery of adeno-associated virus vectors to the rabbit airway. J Virol 1999; 73:9446–9455.

138. Halbert CL, Standaert TA, Aitken ML, Alexander IE, Russell DW, Miller AD. Transduction by adeno-associated virus vectors in the rabbit airway: efficiency, persistence, and readministration. J Virol 1997; 71:5932–5941.

139. Halbert CL, Standaert TA, Wilson CB, Miller AD. Successful readministration of adeno-associated virus vectors to the mouse lung requires transient immunosuppression during the initial exposure. J Virol 1998; 72:9795–9805.

140. Hernandez YJ, Wang J, Kearns WG, Loiler S, Poirier A, Flotte TR. Latent adeno-associated virus infection elicits humoral but not cell-mediated immune responses in a nonhuman primate model. J Virol 1999; 73:8549–8558.

141. Scheule RK, St George JA, Bagley RG, Marshall J, Kaplan JM, Akita GY, Wang KX, Lee ER, Harris DJ, Jiang C, Yew NS, Smith AE, Cheng SH. Basis of pulmonary toxicity associated with cationic lipid-mediated gene transfer to the mammalian lung. Hum Gene Ther 1997; 8:689–707.

142. Verma IM. A tumultuous year for gene therapy. Mol Ther 2000; 2:415–416.

143. Balter M. Gene therapy on trial. Science 2000; 288:951–957.

144. Armentano D, Zabner J, Sacks C, Sookdeo CC, Smith MP, St George JA, Wadsworth SC, Smith AE, Gregory RJ. Effect of the E4 region on the persistence of transgene expression from adenovirus vectors. J Virol 1997; 71:2408–2416.

145. O'Neal WK, Zhou H, Morral N, Langston C, Parks RJ, Graham FL, Kochanek S, Beaud et al. Toxicity associated with repeated administration of first-generation adenovirus vectors does not occur with a helper-dependent vector. Mol Med 2000; 6:179–195.

146. Mack CA, Song WR, Carpenter H, Wickham TJ, Kovesdi I, Harvey BG, Magovern CJ, Isom OW, Rosengart T, Falck-Pedersen E, Hackett NR, Crystal RG, Mastrangeli A. Circumvention of anti-adenovirus neutralizing immunity by administration of an adenoviral vector of an alternate serotype. Hum Gene Ther 1997; 8:99–109.

147. Mastrangeli A, Harvey BG, Yao J, Wolff G, Kovesdi I, Crystal RG, Falck-Pedersen E. "Sero-switch" adenovirus-mediated in vivo gene transfer: circumvention of anti-adenovirus humoral immune defenses against repeat adenovirus vector administration by changing the adenovirus serotype. Hum Gene Ther 1996; 7:79–87.

148. Scaria A, St George JA, Gregory RJ, Noelle RJ, Wadsworth SC, Smith AE, Kaplan JM. Antibody to CD40 ligand inhibits both humoral and cellular immune responses to adenoviral vectors and facilitates repeated administration to mouse airway. Gene Ther 1997; 4:611–617.

149. Yang Y, Trinchieri G, Wilson JM. Recombinant IL-12 prevents formation of blocking IgA antibodies to recombinant adenovirus and allows repeated gene therapy to mouse lung. Nat Med 1995; 1:890–893.

150. Piedimonte G, Pickles RJ, Lehmann JR, McCarty D, Costa DL, Boucher RC. Replication-deficient adenoviral vector for gene transfer potentiates airway neurogenic inflammation. Am J Respir Cell Mol Biol 1997; 16:250–258.

151. Teramoto S, Johnson LG, Huang W, Leigh MW, Boucher RC. Effect of adenoviral vector infection on cell proliferation in cultured primary human airway epithelial cells. Hum Gene Ther 1995; 6:1045–1053.

152. Chirmule N, Propert K, Magosin S, Qian Y, Qian R, Wilson J. Immune responses to adenovirus and adeno-associated virus in humans. Gene Ther 1999; 6:1574–1583.

153. Lee ER, Marshall J, Siegel CS, Jiang C, Yew NS, Nichols MR, Nietupski JB, Ziegler RJ, Lane MB, Wang KX, Wan NC, Scheule RK, Harris DJ, Smith AE, Cheng SH. Detailed analysis of structures and formulations of cationic lipids for efficient gene transfer to the lung. Hum Gene Ther 1996; 7:1701–1717.

154. Anderson JM, Van Itallie CM. Tight junctions and the molecular basis for regulation of paracellular permeability. Am J Physiol 1995; 269:G467–475.

155. Lutz KL, Siahaan TJ. Molecular structure of the apical junction complex and its contribution to the paracellular barrier. J Pharm Sci 1997; 86:977–984.

156. Hulbert WC, Man SF, Rosychuk MK, Braybrook G, Mehta JG. The response phase—the first six hours after acute airway injury by SO2 inhalation: an in vivo and in vitro study. Scanning Microsc 1989; 3:369–378.

157. Wang G, Zabner J, Deering C, Launspach J, Shao J, Bodner M, Jolly DJ, Davidson BL, McCray PB, Jr. Increasing epithelial junction permeability enhances gene transfer to airway epithelia in vivo. Am J Respir Cell Mol Biol 2000; 22:129–138.

158. Chu Q, St George JA, Lukason M, Cheng SH, Scheule RK, Eastman SJ. EGTA enhancement of adenovirus-mediated gene transfer to mouse tracheal epithelium in vivo. Hum Gene Ther 2001; 12:455–467.

159. Coyne CB, Kelly MM, Boucher RC, Johnson LG. Enhanced epithelial gene transfer by modulation of tight junctions with sodium caprate. Am J Respir Cell Mol Biol 2000; 23:602–609.

160. Coyne CB, Vanhook MK, Boucher RC, Johnson LG. Safety and efficiency of medium chain fatty acid–induced enhancement of airway epithelial gene transfer. Mol Ther 2001; 3:S89.

161. Douar AM, Poulard K, Stockholm D, Danos O. Intracellular trafficking of adeno-associated virus vectors: routing to the late endosomal compartment and proteasome degradation. J Virol 2001; 75:1824–1833.

162. Hansen J, Qing K, Srivastava A. Adeno-associated virus type 2-mediated gene transfer: altered endocytic processing enhances transduction efficiency in murine fibroblasts. J Virol 2001; 75:4080–4090.

163. Cosset FL, Morling FJ, Takeuchi Y, Weiss RA, Collins MK, Russell SJ. Retroviral retargeting by envelopes expressing an N-terminal binding domain. J Virol 1995; 69:6314–6322.

164. Dmitriev I, Krasnykh V, Miller CR, Wang M, Kashentseva E, Mikheeva G, Belousova N, Curiel DT. An adenovirus vector with genetically modified fibers demonstrates expanded tropism via utilization of a coxsackievirus and adenovirus receptor-independent cell entry mechanism. J Virol 1998; 72:9706–9713.

165. Douglas JT, Rogers BE, Rosenfeld ME, Michael SI, Feng M, Curiel DT. Targeted gene delivery by tropism-modified adenoviral vectors. Nat Biotechnol 1996; 14: 1574–1578.

166. Jiang A, Chu TH, Nocken F, Cichutek K, Dornburg R. Cell-type-specific gene transfer into human cells with retroviral vectors that display single-chain antibodies. J Virol 1998; 72:10148–10156.

167. Kasahara N, Dozy AM, Kan YW. Tissue-specific targeting of retroviral vectors through ligand-receptor interactions. Science 1994; 266:1373–1376.

168. Kitten O, Cosset FL, Ferry N. Highly efficient retrovirus-mediated gene transfer into rat hepatocytes in vivo. Hum Gene Ther 1997; 8:1491–1494.

169. Schreier H, Moran P, Caras IW. Targeting of liposomes to cells expressing CD4 using glycosylphosphatidylinositol-anchored gp120. Influence of liposome composition on intracellular trafficking. J Biol Chem 1994; 269:9090–9098.

170. Schwarzenberger P, Spence SE, Gooya JM, Michiel D, Curiel DT, Ruscetti FW, Keller JR. Targeted gene transfer to human hematopoietic progenitor cell lines through the c-kit receptor. Blood 1996; 87:472–478.

171. Watkins SJ, Mesyanzhinov VV, Kurochkina LP, Hawkins RE. The 'adenobody' approach to viral targeting: specific and enhanced adenoviral gene delivery. Gene Ther 1997; 4:1004–1012.

172. Wickham TJ, Lee GM, Titus JA, Sconocchia G, Bakacs T, Kovesdi I, Segal DM. Targeted adenovirus-mediated gene delivery to T cells via CD3. J Virol 1997; 71: 7663–7669.

173. Wickham TJ, Tzeng E, Shears LL, 2nd, Roelvink PW, Li Y, Lee GM, Brough DE, Lizonova A, Kovesdi I. Increased in vitro and in vivo gene transfer by adenovirus vectors containing chimeric fiber proteins. J Virol 1997; 71:8221–8229.

174. Yajima T, Kanda T, Yoshiike K, Kitamura Y. Retroviral vector targeting human cells via c-Kit-stem cell factor interaction. Hum Gene Ther 1998; 9:779–787.

175. Paillard F. Cell-specific targeting with retroviral vectors. Hum Gene Ther 1998; 9: 767–768.

176. Mason SJ, Paradiso AM, Boucher RC. Regulation of transepithelial ion transport and intracellular calcium by extracellular ATP in human normal and cystic fibrosis airway epithelium. Br J Pharmacol 1991; 103:1649–1656.

177. Hwang TH, Schwiebert EM, Guggino WB. Apical and basolateral ATP stimulates tracheal epithelial chloride secretion via multiple purinergic receptors. Am J Physiol 1996; 270:C1611–1623.

178. Drapkin PT, O'Riordan CR, Yi SM, Chiorini JA, Cardella J, Zabner J, Welsh MJ. Targeting the urokinase plasminogen activator receptor enhances gene transfer to human airway epithelia. J Clin Invest 2000; 105:589–596.

179. Ziady A, Kelley T, Davis P. SEC-R directed CFTR gene transfer in CF mouse

nasal epithelia partially corrects primary and secondary CF defects. Mo Ther 20001; 3:S12.

180. Pickles RJ, Kreda S, Olsen J, Johnson L, Gerard R, Segal D, Boucher RC. High efficiency gene transfer to polarized epithelial cells by re-targeting adenoviral vectors to P2Y$_2$ purinoceptors with bi-specific antibodies. Ped Pulmonol 1998; 17(Suppl):261.

181. Kreda SM, Pickles RJ, Lazarowski ER, Boucher RC. G-protein-coupled receptors as targets for gene transfer vectors using natural small-molecule ligands. Nat Biotechnol 2000; 18:635–640.

182. O'Riordan CR, Lachapelle A, Delgado C, Parkes V, Wadsworth SC, Smith AE, Francis GE. PEGylation of adenovirus with retention of infectivity and protection from neutralizing antibody in vitro and in vivo. Hum Gene Ther 1999; 10:1349–1358.

183. Zabner J, Chillon M, Grunst T, Moninger TO, Davidson BL, Gregory R, Armentano D. A chimeric type 2 adenovirus vector with a type 17 fiber enhances gene transfer to human airway epithelia. J Virol 1999; 73:8689–8695.

184. Bartlett JS, Kleinschmidt J, Boucher RC, Samulski RJ. Targeted adeno-associated virus vector transduction of nonpermissive cells mediated by a bispecific F(ab'-gamma)2 antibody. Nat Biotechnol 1999; 17:181–186.

185. Xiao W, Chirmule N, Berta SC, McCullough B, Gao G, Wilson JM. Gene therapy vectors based on adeno-associated virus type 1. J Virol 1999; 73:3994–4003.

186. Kaludov N, Brown KE, Walters RW, Zabner J, Chiorini JA. Adeno-associated virus serotype 4 (AAV4) and AAV5 both require sialic acid binding for hemagglutination and efficient transduction but differ in sialic acid linkage specificity. J Virol 2001; 75:6884–6493.

187. Rutledge EA, Halbert CL, Russell DW. Infectious clones and vectors derived from adeno-associated virus (AAV) serotypes other than AAV type 2. J Virol 1998; 72: 309–319.

188. Halbert CL, Allen JM, Miller AD. Adeno-associated virus type 6 (AAV6) vectors mediate efficient transduction of airway epithelial cells in mouse lungs compared to that of AAV2 vectors. J Virol 2001; 75:6615–6624.

189. Zabner J, Seiler M, Walters R, Kotin RM, Fulgeras W, Davidson BL, Chiorini JA. Adeno-associated virus type 5 (AAV5) but not AAV2 binds to the apical surfaces of airway epithelia and facilitates gene transfer. J Virol 2000; 74:3852–3858.

190. Walters RW, Yi SM, Keshavjee S, Brown KE, Welsh MJ, Chiorini JA, Zabner J. Binding of adeno-associated virus type 5 to 2,3-linked sialic acid is required for gene transfer. J Biol Chem 2001; 276:20610–20616.

191. Wagner JA, Reynolds T, Moran ML, Moss RB, Wine JJ, Flotte TR, Gardner P. Efficient and persistent gene transfer of AAV-CFTR in maxillary sinus. Lancet 1998; 351:1702–1703.

192. Wagner JA, Nepomuceno IB, Shah N, Messner AH, Moran ML, Norbash AM, Moss RB, Wine JJ, Gardner P. Maxillary sinusitis as a surrogate model for CF gene therapy clinical trials in patients with antrostomies. J Gene Med 1999; 1:13–21.

193. Yan Z, Zhang Y, Duan D, Engelhardt JF. Trans-splicing vectors expand the utility of adeno-associated virus for gene therapy. Proc Natl Acad Sci USA 2000; 97: 6716–6721.

194. Duan D, Yue Y, Yan Z, Engelhardt JF. Enhancement of recombinant type-2 AAV mediated gene expression through novel intermolecular cisactivation. Pediatr Pulmonol 2000; 20(Suppl):232.

195. Wang G, Sinn PL, McCray PB, Jr. Development of retroviral vectors for gene transfer to airway epithelia. Curr Opin Mol Ther 2000; 2:497–506.

196. Yang Y, Vanin EF, Whitt MA, Fornerod M, Zwart R, Schneiderman RD, Grosveld G, Nienhuis AW. Inducible, high-level production of infectious murine leukemia retroviral vector particles pseudotyped with vesicular stomatitis virus G envelope protein. Hum Gene Ther 1995; 6:1203–1213.

197. Ory DS, Neugeboren BA, Mulligan RC. A stable human-derived packaging cell line for production of high titer retrovirus/vesicular stomatitis virus G pseudotypes. Proc Natl Acad Sci USA 1996; 93:11400–11406.

198. Kafri T, van Praag H, Ouyang L, Gage FH, Verma IM. A packaging cell line for lentivirus vectors. J Virol 1999; 73:576–584.

199. Pitt BR, Schwarz MA, Pilewski JM, Nakayama D, Mueller GM, Robbins PD, Watkins SA, Albertine KH, Bland RD. Retrovirus-mediated gene transfer in lungs of living fetal sheep. Gene Ther 1995; 2:344–350.

200. Wang G, Slepushkin VA, Bodner M, Zabner J, van Es HH, Thomas P, Jolly DJ, Davidson BL, McCray PB, Jr. Keratinocyte growth factor induced epithelial proliferation facilitates retroviral-mediated gene transfer to distal lung epithelia in vivo. J Gene Med 1999; 1:22–30.

201. Goldman MJ, Lee PS, Yang JS, Wilson JM. Lentiviral vectors for gene therapy of cystic fibrosis. Hum Gene Ther 1997; 8:2261–2268.

202. Slepushkin VA, Staber PD, Wang G, McCray PB, Jr, Davidson BL. Infection of human airway epithelia with H1N1, H2N2, and H3N2 influenza A virus strains. Mol Ther 2001; 3:395–402.

203. Zhang L, Peeples ME, Boucher RC, Collins PL, Pickles RJ. Respiratory syncytial virus infection of human airway epithelial cells is polarized, specific to ciliated cells, and without obvious cytopathology. J Virol 2002; 76:5654–5666.

204. Morse KM, Olsen JC. Respiratory synctial virus infection of cultured well differentiated airway epithelial cells from cystic fibrosis patients. Pediatr Pulmonol 2000; 20(Suppl):229–230.

205. Wang G, Deering C, Macke M, Shao J, Burns R, Blau DM, Holmes KV, Davidson BL, Perlman S, McCray PB, Jr. Human coronavirus 229E infects polarized airway epithelia from the apical surface. J Virol 2000; 74:9234–9239.

206. Rai SK, DeMartini JC, Miller AD. Retrovirus vectors bearing jaagsiekte sheep retrovirus Env transduce human cells by using a new receptor localized to chromosome 3p21.3. J Virol 2000; 74:4698–4704.

207. Sinn PL, Jolly D, Sauter S, Sanders DA, Dubensky J, T.W., Staber P, Nosakowski J, Wang G, Davidson BL, McCray J, P.B. Pseudotyping feline immunodeficiency (fiv)–based vectors to target the apical surface of differentiated human airway epithelia. Pediatr Pulmonol 2000; 30(Suppl):233.

208. Kobinger GP, Weiner DJ, Yu QC, Wilson JM. Filovirus-pseudotyped lentiviral vector can efficiently and stably transduce airway epithelia in vivo. Nat Biotechnol 2001; 19:225–230.

209. Kollen WJ, Midoux P, Erbacher P, Yip A, Roche AC, Monsigny M, Glick MC,

Scanlin TF. Gluconoylated and glycosylated polylysines as vectors for gene transfer into cystic fibrosis airway epithelial cells. Hum Gene Ther 1996; 7:1577–1586.

210. Klink DT, Chao S, Glick MC, Scanlin TF. Nuclear translocation of lactosylated poly-1-lysine/cdna complex in cystic fibrosis airway epithelial cells. Mol Ther 2001; 3:831–841.

211. Ferrari S, Pettenazzo A, Garbati N, Zacchello F, Behr JP, Scarpa M. Polyethylenimine shows properties of interest for cystic fibrosis gene therapy. Biochim Biophys Acta 1999; 1447:219–225.

212. Funke M, Ziaday A, Davis P. Trafficking of sec-R targeted gene transfer. Pediatr Pulmonol 2001; 3:S13.

213. Yonemitsu Y, Kitson C, Ferrari S, Farley R, Griesenbach U, Judd D, Steel R, Scheid P, Zhu J, Jeffery PK, Kato A, Hasan MK, Nagai Y, Masaki I, Fukumura M, Hasegawa M, Geddes DM, Alton EW. Efficient gene transfer to airway epithelium using recombinant Sendai virus. Nat Biotechnol 2000; 18:970–973.

214. Li HO, Zhu YF, Asakawa M, Kuma H, Hirata T, Ueda Y, Lee YS, Fukumura M, Iida A, Kato A, Nagai Y, Hasegawa M. A cytoplasmic RNA vector derived from nontransmissible Sendai virus with efficient gene transfer and expression. J Virol 2000; 74:6564–6569.

215. Hall CB. Respiratory syncytial virus and parainfluenza virus. N Engl J Med 2001; 344:1917–1928.

216. Kass-Eisler A, Leinwand L, Gall J, Bloom B, Falck-Pedersen E. Circumventing the immune response to adenovirus-mediated gene therapy. Gene Ther 1996; 3: 154–162.

217. Bruder JT, Jie T, McVey DL, Kovesdi I. Expression of gp19K increases the persistence of transgene expression from an adenovirus vector in the mouse lung and liver. J Virol 1997; 71:7623–7628.

218. Kaplan JM, Pennington SE, St George JA, Woodworth LA, Fasbender A, Marshall J, Cheng SH, Wadsworth SC, Gregory RJ, Smith AE. Potentiation of gene transfer to the mouse lung by complexes of adenovirus vector and polycations improves therapeutic potential. Hum Gene Ther 1998; 9:1469–1479.

219. Jooss K, Turka LA, Wilson JM. Blunting of immune responses to adenoviral vectors in mouse liver and lung with CTLA4Ig. Gene Ther 1998; 5:309–319.

220. Wilson CB, Embree LJ, Schowalter D, Albert R, Aruffo A, Hollenbaugh D, Linsley P, Kay MA. Transient inhibition of CD28 and CD40 ligand interactions prolongs adenovirus-mediated transgene expression in the lung and facilitates expression after secondary vector administration. J Virol 1998; 72:7542–7550.

221. Croyle MA, Chirmule N, Zhang Y, Wilson JM. "Stealth" adenoviruses blunt cell-mediated and humoral immune responses against the virus and allow for significant gene expression upon readministration in the lung. J Virol 2001; 75:4792–4801.

222. Arcasoy SM, Latoche JD, Gondor M, Pitt BR, Pilewski JM. Polycations increase the efficiency of adenovirus-mediated gene transfer to epithelial and endothelial cells in vitro. Gene Ther 1997; 4:32–38.

223. Walters R, Welsh M. Mechanism by which calcium phosphate coprecipitation enhances adenovirus-mediated gene transfer. Gene Ther 1999; 6:1845–1850.

224. Walters RW, Duan D, Engelhardt JF, Welsh MJ. Incorporation of adeno-associated virus in a calcium phosphate coprecipitate improves gene transfer to airway epithelia in vitro and in vivo. J Virol 2000; 74:535–540.

13

Use of Adeno-Associated Virus in the Treatment of Cystic Fibrosis

THOMAS C. REYNOLDS

Zymogenetics
Seattle, Washington, U.S.A.

I. Adeno-Associated Virus for CF Gene Transfer

Adeno-associated virus (AAV) possesses many attributes that make it a good candidate as a gene transfer vector for the treatment of cystic fibrosis. AAV is a nonpathogenic human virus (1), and children are commonly exposed to this virus during the first 5 years of life without sequelae (2). AAV is a dependovirus, and it cannot usually replicate in the absence of a helper virus (3). There are six known AAV serotypes that have been isolated from primates, designated AAV-1–6 (2,4–6). Most gene transfer studies have focused on AAV-2, although more recent work suggests that other serotypes may also be of utility for airway gene transfer.

Vectors derived from AAV are commonly constructed by removing the only two viruses' encoded genes, *rep* and *cap* genes (7), further attenuating the potential for vector replication following administration. In this case, transduced cells cannot produce any AAV-derived proteins, and so the potential for an immune response directed against cells producing viral antigens is eliminated. AAV vectors have been shown to confer persistent gene transfer and expression in a wide variety of model systems, including the lung epithelium (8). Finally, a number of methods have been developed to produce and purify large quantities of AAV vectors for preclinical and clinical studies (9–11). These properties suggest that AAV vectors may have utility in developing gene transfer approaches for the treatment of cystic fibrosis.

The CFTR gene was isolated by positional cloning in 1989 (12). Subsequent studies suggested that transfer of the cDNA into cystic fibrosis transmembrane conductance regulator (CFTR)–deficient cells could correct the physiological defect (13), and that correction of as few as 6–10% of cells in an epithelial monolayer might suffice to restore normal physiology (14). Furthermore, only one to two copies of CFTR mRNA per cell is found in the airways of normal individuals (15), indicating that low-level CFTR expression is sufficient for appropriate physiological function. In mice, breeding studies of mutant animals have shown that 5% of normal levels of CFTR are sufficient to rescue 100% of the animals from the profound intestinal defect found in this model (16). These findings implied that the underlying molecular defect causing CF lung disease might be treated by transfer of the CFTR gene to the pulmonary tree.

II. AAV-CFTR Vector Development

Following the cloning of the human CFTR cDNA, it was immediately apparent that the cDNA encoding the 1480–amino acid human CFTR protein could pose difficulties in AAV vector generation due to packaging size limitations. The AAV-2 capsid is a relatively rigid structure of defined volume, placing constraints on the length of vector DNA that can be effectively packaged within each virion. The upper limit for the AAV-2 vector genome length has been defined as approximately 4.9–5.1 kilobases (kb) (17). The CFTR cDNA is approximately 4.5 kb in length, and the requisite AAV inverted terminal repeats (ITRs) comprise about 0.3 kb. This leaves only several hundred base pairs of sequence space to encompass all appropriate transcriptional regulatory signals. Several strategies have been employed to construct AAV vectors within these constraints.

Early studies demonstrated that AAV-2 vectors carrying marker genes could transduce immortalized cells lines derived from patients with CF, including the airway line IB3-1 (18). During evaluation of vectors utilizing the AAV-2 p5 promotor to drive transcription of a reporter gene, it was noted that a control vector containing the ITR alone produced reporter gene activity (19). This surprising result was replicated in vivo in the rat brain (20). Additional studies confirmed that the ITR could also drive CFTR expression in transduced cultures of IB3-1 cells as assessed by chloride efflux and immunofluorescence analyses. Patch clamp analysis (21) demonstrated restoration of small linear chloride conductance channels as well as activation of the outwardly rectifying chloride channels. Transcriptional activity of the ITR may be related to the presence of Sp1 binding sites within the ITR as well as homology to a consensus Inr sequence found within the ITR D region (22,23), although other studies have mapped this activity to a different region within the ITR (20).

More efficient expression of the CFTR gene within the confines of the AAV packaging limit has been approached by evaluating small promoters that can enhance transcriptional activity above that provided by the ITR alone. A number of promoter elements including the AAV-2 p5 promoter, simian virus 40 (SV40) early region promoter, and two herpes simplex virus (HSV) thymidine kinase minipromoters showed up to a 10-fold increase in activity relative to the ITR using a reporter gene construct. In particular, the p5 promoter driving the CFTR cDNA showed forskolin-induced conductance changes in transduced HeLa cells. Other small synthetic promoters capable of fitting within an AAV-CFTR construct have also demonstrated enhanced expression relative to the ITR alone (24).

An alternate approach to correcting the CF phenotype would be to employ a smaller CFTR minigene that would allow for the inclusion of larger and more powerful transcriptional elements. CFTR truncation mutants lacking the first four transmembrane domains have been shown to express functional chloride channel activity, albeit with a modestly reduced open channel probability and conductance (25). This approach would add approximately 350 bp of space within the vector backbone for additional transcriptional elements. A similar approach employing a 264–amino acid N-terminal deletion of CFTR resulted in functional chloride channel activity when coupled to a cytomegalovirus (CMV) enhance/chicken beta actin hybrid promoter and transfected into IB3 cells (26). A systematic study of deletions within the CFTR gene yielded several small regions that could be removed without deleterious consequences to halide efflux, resulting in up to about 250 bp of sequence removed (27).

Although promising, the minigene approach raises several questions. The linkage from a single gene defect to CF clinical pathophysiology is still unclear. Although the ion channel defect appears to play a central role (28) in the pathogenesis of CF, CFTR also appears to provide other functions in the cell. Data suggest that CFTR may be a receptor for *Pseudomonas* internalization in the airway (29,30). CFTR is also involved in a network of regulation of other cellular channels and proteins (31–35). It is unclear whether truncated or internally deleted minigenes possessing chloride channel activity will be able to complement these other CFTR functions.

III. Delivery of AAV Vectors to the Lung

Pulmonary delivery of AAV-2 vectors has been evaluated in a number of animal models. Initial studies were performed in the rabbit, which is large enough to allow direct instillation of vector to airways using a pediatric fiberoptic bronchoscope. AAV gene transfer to the airway was observed following a single administration of 10^{10} particles of SA306, an epitope-tagged CFTR vector, to the right lower lobe (8). Gene expression was monitored by reverse transcriptase–polymerase chain reaction (RT-PCR) and by immunostaining for the epitope tag or the human CFTR protein. Expression in the airway was initially observed 3 days following vector administration, and continued for up to 6 months, although there was a suggestion of waning expression in the last 3 months of the study. This study provided an initial proof of concept that AAV vectors might have utility for delivery of CFTR or other genes to the lung.

In contrast, a similar study using AAV vectors encoding the β-galactosidase or human placental alkaline phosphatase genes showed generally low levels of airway transduction as assessed by staining for relevant enzyme activity following instillation to the rabbit lung via balloon catheter (36). Transduction was maximal in focal areas possibly damaged by balloon inflation. Neutralizing antibodies to AAV-2 were also observed following vector administration, and repeated delivery of vector to the airway did not result in new transduction events. The study was confounded to some degree by the presence of wild-type AAV contaminants in the vector preparations, which was shown to inhibit transduction in this model and may have enhanced the generation of neutralizing antibodies.

A separate study of administration of an AAV β-galactosidase vector to neonatal rabbits showed dose-dependent reporter gene expression in the airways and alveoli at early time points, with data indicating transduction of the type II alveolar cell, which is thought to be an alveolar epithelial progenitor cell (37). No toxicity was observed throughout the 10-day study, and no change in cell counts or differential in pulmonary lavage fluids was detected.

Single-dose studies in the rhesus macaque evaluated both the safety and efficiency of gene transfer following direct instillation of a single dose of up to 10^{11} particles of AAV-CFTR vector to the right lower lobe airway by bronchoscope (38). The vector was well tolerated with no adverse clinical, functional, or biochemical findings. Persistent gene transfer in the airway epithelium as assessed by in situ PCR was observed for 180 days. RT-PCR and RNase protection demonstrated human CFTR mRNA expression throughout the duration of the study. Low-level vector dissemination, generally less than one copy per 100 cells, was observed in organs of some animals including the heart, liver, jejunum, kidney, lymph nodes, spleen, pancreas, and brain. No vector was detected in the gonads of any animal. Vector DNA was observed in the blood of some animals shortly following administration, indicating that hematogenous dissemination, possibly as a result of bronchoscopic trauma, probably was responsible for distant organ vector biodistribution.

The potential for long-term persistence of AAV vectors in the lung epithelium following pulmonary administration raised the possibility of vector rescue and replication if coinfection with wild-type AAV and adenovirus occurred. This possibility was tested empirically in the rhesus macaque by instilling either AAV-2 or an AAV-CFTR vector into the lung, and then subsequently administering the reciprocal virus or vector as well as adenovirus (39). Low-level rescue of vector following intranasal application of adenovirus occurred only when both vector and wild-type AAV-2 were administered to the same lung lobe. Administration of AAV-2 to the nose did not result in spread to the lower respiratory tract in the presence of adenovirus, and vector rescue and replication did not occur in this setting. These data suggest that rescue and replication of AAV-2 from the lower respiratory tract is unlikely, although this will need to be evaluated longitudinally in clinical studies.

For treatment of cystic fibrosis, the preferred route of administration to the lung is likely to be inhalation of aerosolized vector. Normal CFTR expression is largely confined to the airway and submucosal glands; this region of the pulmonary tree can be targeted using an aerosol droplet size range of 1–5 μm. Aerosol administration of AAV-CFTR was tested in nonhuman primates (40). A single dose of up to 10^{12} DNase-resistant particles (DRPs) was administered to rhesus macaques by oral aerosol inhalation using concurrent flow spirometry for dosimetry. No toxicity related to the vector was observed in the lung or any other organ. Dose-dependent gene transfer to the lung was observed without significant biodistribution to tissues other than the pulmonary tree and bronchial lymph nodes. Gene expression was detected by RT-PCR in a small number of samples. This study provided proof of concept that AAV vectors could be aerosolized and successfully delivered to the pulmonary tree.

A subsequent study of delivery of repeated doses of an aerosolized AAV-CFTR vector at 3-week intervals to the rhesus macaque was safe, with no changes in clinical or laboratory parameters (41). Exposure to the vector was associated with hyperplasia of lymphoid tissue in the pulmonary area, which was likely a physiological response to antigenic stimulation. There was significant gene transfer to the airway epithelium with up to one vector genome per diploid cell. Expression was seen in five of eight animals receiving vector as evaluated by RNA-specific PCR. Vector dissemination was observed in the upper gastrointestinal tract and lymphoid tissues of some animals, but was not seen in other organs such as the liver, heart, kidneys, or gonads. Repeated vector delivery did result in the development of serum neutralizing antibodies in some animals. However, induction of serum neutralizing antibodies was not dose dependent and did not correlate with the level of pulmonary gene transfer. Low-level neutralizing antibodies were also variably observed in bronchial wash fluid of some animals after the third vector dose.

Additional studies have addressed readministration of AAV vectors to the pulmonary epithelium. In mice, dose-dependent and persistent transduction was achieved in the distal airways following intratracheal administration of an AAV–alkaline phosphatase vector (42). However, this was paralleled by development of serum neutralizing antibodies to the vector, precluding repeated vector delivery. Transient immunosuppression at the time of initial vector delivery was required to successfully readminister vector. This is in contrast to a similar study in rabbits, where although repeated delivery of an AAV-CFTR vector produced elevations in serum neutralizing antibody, subsequent transduction with a green fluorescent protein (GFP) marker gene vector was not blocked (43). Development of an antibody response capable of blocking pulmonary administration may depend on many variables including species and strain, dose, interval, route of administration, quality of the vector preparation, and possibly transgene expression cassette. It is not clear that the presence of serum neutralizing antibodies reliably predicts blockage of pulmonary delivery of AAV vectors.

Persistent gene transfer and expression following pulmonary delivery of AAV has clearly been accomplished in a number of animal species with a marked lack of toxicity. Questions still remain regarding the efficiency of delivery, differential distribution to proximal as compared to distal airway, and induction of immune responses that may limit repeated administration to the lung. The robust vector safety profile, coupled with persistent gene transfer to the airway and lack of predictive animal models for CF lung disease, set the stage for early trials of AAV vectors in patients with CF.

IV. Clinical Studies

The first study of AAV vectors in humans was conducted in patients with CF. Initial studies began in 1995 and progressed relatively slowly, starting with low vector doses and with significant observation periods between patients and dose-escalation cohorts. Data generated from these studies have confirmed that administration of AAV-CFTR vectors to the respiratory epithelium appears safe and well tolerated, and initial data on biological and clinical activity are now under study in larger patient populations. A summary of the clinical trials of tgAAVCF, the only AAV vector administered to CF patients thus far, is found in Table 1.

The maxillary sinus has been proposed as a surrogate model for testing of CF gene therapy approaches (44,45). Patients with CF have an extremely high incidence of chronic sinusitis, approaching 100% in some studies (46). The maxillary sinus is lined by airway epithelium, and manifests the altered electrophysiology and microbiology seen in the lung. Advantages of the model include facile access following antrostomy for electrophysiological assessment and collection of fluid and biopsies; the availability of two sinuses in each patient allowing for simultaneous administration and evaluation of placebo and active agent; and the possibility of evaluating efficacy of active agents in preventing sinusitis relapse.

A Phase I/II study to evaluate direct instillation of tgAAVCF to the maxillary sinuses of patients with CF was performed at Stanford University (47). The

Table 1 Clinical Studies of tgAAVCF

Trial	Number of patients	Maximum dose (DRP)	Sites and investigators
Maxillary sinus			
Part 1	15	10^8	Stanford: P. Gardener, J. Wagner, R.
Part 2	23		Moss
Nose/lung	25	10^{12}	Johns Hopkins: P. Zeitlin
(bronchoscopy)			U. Florida: T. Flotte
Lung aerosol	12	10^{13}	Boston Children's Hosp: D. Waltz
(Phase I)			Stanford: R. Moss
			U. Washington: M. Aitkin
Lung aerosol	36	10^{13}	Boston Children's Hosp: D. Waltz
(Phase II)	(planned)		Johns Hopkins: P. Zeitlin
			Stanford: R. Moss
			U. Colorado: D. Rodman
			U. Florida: T. Spencer
			U. Washington: M. Aitkin

Phase I portion of the study was a simple dose escalation of tgAAVCF to a single maxillary sinus, with a starting dose of 100 replication units (RU), which is equivalent to roughly 2×10^5 DRP (48,49). The highest dose tested was 10^5 RU, which is equivalent to 2×10^8 DRP.

Ten patients received tgAAVCF to a total of 15 sinuses (five patients received separate instillations of vector to each sinus). Vector administration was well tolerated without evidence of increased acute or chronic inflammation in the sinus receiving vector. Significant changes in anti-AAV antibody titers were not observed in any patient.

Dose-dependent gene transfer was observed, with 0.1–1.0 vector genomes per diploid cell equivalent of DNA extracted from sinus epithelium biopsies 2 weeks following vector administration. In cases where the sinus was rebiopsied, vector persistence was confirmed for up to 70 days postinstillation. No vector-derived CFTR mRNA was detected by RT-PCR; however, high levels of vector DNA in some samples precluded clear analysis of gene expression owing to PCR amplification in the absence of reverse transcriptase.

Evidence of CFTR function was assessed by performing transepithelial potential difference (TEPD) measurements in the maxillary sinus. No changes in baseline TEPD values were observed following administration of tgAAVCF. However, dose-dependent hyperpolarization of the sinus epithelium was observed following administration of amiloride, low chloride, and isoproterenol 14 days after vector administration. This change was statistically significant ($P<.05$) in patients receiving 5×10^4 and 1×10^5 RU of tgAAVCF. It is unknown whether the magnitude of the change ($\sim +10$ mV) is significant, given that no TEPD data are available for normal maxillary sinus epithelium. However, the results suggest that functional CFTR protein was expressed in the sinus epithelium following a single administration of vector.

Following these encouraging results, 23 patients were enrolled in a double-blind study where 10^5 RU of tgAAVCF was administered to one sinus and placebo to the other on the same day (50). The primary endpoint was clinically defined, endoscopically diagnosed recurrent sinusitis during the 3-month period following study agent administration. Secondary endpoints included measures of safety, sinus fluid cell counts and cytokine measurements, TEPD, and evaluation of serum neutralizing antibodies.

No significant vector-related pulmonary toxicities were encountered during the study. One patient manifested an acute peripheral vestibulopathy shortly following vector administration; the event spontaneously resolved without sequelae. There were no changes in anti-AAV neutralizing antibody titers in any point.

Sinusitis recurrence rate or time to sinusitis was not different between sinuses receiving vector or placebo. This may have been confounded by both the difficulty in defining unilateral sinusitis, as well as a high proportion of patients receiving antibiotic treatment for nonsinusitis conditions following study agent administration but prior to sinusitis recurrence. The insensitivity of this model to unilateral sinusitis suggests that the more usual interpatient design, where both sinuses receive either vector or placebo, may be required in efficacy studies using recurrent sinusitis as an endpoint.

Of note was a large decrease in sinus interleukin-8 (IL-8) levels 14 days following administration of vector but not placebo. IL-8 secretion can be triggered by the binding of *Pseudomonas* pilin to receptors on airway epithelial cells, which are upregulated in cells with mutant CFTR (51–53). Alternatively, accumulation of mutant CFTR in the endoplasmic reticulum may trigger IL-8 secretion through the nuclear factor-κB (NF-κB) pathways (54). The decrease in IL-8 levels was correlated with a reduction in sinus neutrophil counts, as well as trend toward increased levels in anti-inflammatory IL-10 levels. These findings suggest that functional CFTR was being produced in the sinus following vector administration. However, no statistically significant changes in TEPD measurements were observed in vector-treated sinuses, and vector-derived CFTR mRNA was not measured.

The Phase I and II sinus studies demonstrated evidence of dose-dependent gene transfer to the sinus following a single direct administration of tgAAVCF. The vector was well tolerated, and no issues related to vector safety were identified. Indirect evidence of CFTR expression and function was observed, but the lack of a complete molecular chain of events (DNA→RNA→protein→function) makes it difficult to unequivocally conclude that a therapeutic proof of concept was achieved.

Although the maxillary sinus may be a useful model for CFTR gene transfer studies, the primary focus of CF gene therapy has been to develop treatments for the lethal pulmonary manifestations. An initial Phase I study of direct application of tgAAVCF directly to the nasal epithelium and a single lung lobe was recently completed (55). This dose-escalation study was designed primarily to evaluate the safety of vector application to the nose and lung, as well as to evaluate gene transfer, expression, biological activity, and immunological consequences. A total of 25 CF patients with relatively mild lung disease were enrolled, and they received one administration of vector to both the nasal epithelium by catheter and to the right lower lung lobe by fiberoptic bronchoscope. Starting doses were extremely low (30 RU, equivalent to roughly 6×10^4 DRP), and escalated in half-log increments to a maximal dose of 10^8 RU in the nose and 10^9 RU in the lung.

Vector administration was generally safe and well tolerated, with a total of 39 serious adverse events in 12 of the 25 patients. The majority of these events were related to the underlying CF lung disease or repeated bronchoscopies, although one pulmonary exacerbation in a high-dose patient was thought to be possibly related to vector administration. Little gene transfer was observed in the nose, and gene transfer in the lung was confounded by PCR-positive pretreatment samples in some patients. Given the high local concentrations of vector deposited on the nasal epithelium, it is surprising that gene transfer was not observed. However, efficient nasal gene transfer has also been difficult to achieve with other vector systems, including adenovirus (56,57) and lipid-DNA (58). The nasal epithelium may not be a useful site for evaluating potential gene therapy approaches to CF.

Patients receiving high doses of tgAAVCF did show a variable induction of neutralizing antibodies, which were not seen at lower doses. The threshold for this response was 10^8 RU administered to the lung. Shedding of infectious vector in the sputum 1 day following administration was also observed in a single patient receiving 10^8 RU of vector, but was not seen in other patients nor observed in urine or stool of any patient.

Direct application of the tgAAVCF vector to the nasal epithelium and a single lung lobe revealed no troubling safety issues, but it also did not provide evidence of efficient gene transfer or expression at the sites of administration. However, evaluation of aerosolized vector delivery to CF patients provided data that indicated that AAV vectors could produce gene transfer in the lung.

A Phase I single-dose–escalation study of aerosolized tgAAVCF was conducted in adult CF patients with mild lung disease (59). Three patients were enrolled in each of four-dose cohorts, receiving 10^{10}–10^{13} DRP of tgAAVCF in log dose increments. The primary objective of the study was evaluation of the safety of aerosolized vector administration to the lungs of CF patients. Additional endpoints included evaluation of gene transfer and expression, changes in markers of lung inflammation and function, and evaluation of vector shedding and immune responses.

Vector administration was safe and well tolerated by all subjects. Although over 240 adverse events were noted in the 12 CF patients, only 6 were serious. These included observation of a previously diagnosed supraventricular tachycardia, four episodes of pulmonary exacerbation in three patients, and one episode of hemoptysis. Three of the serious adverse events were thought to be possibly related to vector, although no clear dose or temporal relationships were noted. Longitudinal observation of changes in pulmonary function revealed no consistent pattern; two patients receiving low doses of vector showed transient declines in FEV_1 of approximately 10%, whereas one patient in the high-dose group showed a sustained improvement in FEV_1 of 30%. There were no significant changes in clinical laboratory results.

Dose-dependent gene transfer was observed by real-time PCR analysis of brushed airway cells. Samples were collected prior to and at several time points following vector administration from each of three separate lung regions at each time point. Significant gene transfer was observed in the 10^{12} and 10^{13} DRP cohorts, with a maximum of 0.1–0.6 vector copies per brushed cell diploid genome, similar to that observed in preclinical nonhuman primate studies (41). Gene transfer was maximal at the first sampling point 14 days following vector administration and slowly declined to <1 vector copy per 1000 diploid genomes by day 90. Vector gene expression was not detected in any sample by RT-PCR, although brushing could only be obtained from the upper airways, and evaluation of an endogenous control RNA suggested that the presence of protease and nuclease activities in the airway fluid could result in loss of amplifiable mRNA.

Transient shedding of infections vector in the sputum was observed 1 day following vector administration in most patients receiving 10^{11} DRP or more of tgAAVCF; no shedding was observed in urine or stool. Patients receiving 10^{12} or 10^{13} DRP of vector showed a serum neutralizing antibodies to AAV-2; however, no AAV-2 neutralizing activity was detected in the bronchial wash fluid of any patient. Evaluation of bronchial wash fluid cytokine levels was uninformative owing to the inflammatory nature of the repeated bronchoscopies during the 90-day study period.

In summary, single-dose aerosolized tgAAVCF was safe and well tolerated when administered to adult CF patients. Dose-dependent gene transfer was observed, but laboratory or clinical evidence of functional CFTR expression was not demonstrated. A study of repeated doses of tgAAVCF is currently in progress, and it may provide the first meaningful evaluation of this therapeutic approach from an efficacy perspective.

V. Future Directions for AAV-CFTR Gene Therapy

Preclinical and early clinical studies have shown that AAV-2 vectors can deliver genes, including CFTR, to the lung. However, a clear and unequivocal proof of efficacy of the current generation of vectors has yet to be established in patients with CF. It is difficult to assess at present whether therapeutic efficacy will be achieved with current vectors, or whether different vector constructs and serotypes, adjunctive therapies, or delivery methods will be required. A number of new approaches may enhance airway epithelium transduction with a fully functional CFTR gene are under development.

AAV-2 appears to enter cells by a receptor-mediated process, followed by endosomal trafficking, nuclear transport, uncoating, and conversion to an active transcriptional template. The presence of the heparin sulfate proteoglycan receptor (60) and FGFR-1 (61.) and $\alpha V \beta 5^{62}$ coreceptors have been localized predominantly to the basolateral surface of the airway epithelium, leading to inefficient AAV vector transduction from the luminal side of the airway (63). Recent work suggests that this inefficiency in transduction is caused by vector capsid ubiquitination followed by degradation in the proteasome (64). Concurrent administration of inhibitors of proteasome activity can increase productive transduction of the airway by 10- to 100-fold (64,65). This strategy may be amenable to clinical evaluation with suitable peptide or small molecule inhibitors of proteasome function.

Episomal genome persistence is thought to be the primary mechanism for long-term AAV transduction (66). However, AAV vectors have recently been shown to be capable of mediating homologous gene conversion events in target cells (67). This raises the possibility that specific CFTR mutations, most especially ΔF508, could be corrected in the airway epithelium. Such corrections would be passed on to daughter cells following cell division. Although the efficiency of homologous gene conversion is at present relatively low (68,69), enhancements in the efficiency of vector gene transfer and homologous recombination could lead to a promising therapeutic approach through CFTR gene correction.

Persistent gene transfer is a hallmark of AAV vector transduction. This appears to depend on the formation of high molecular weight concatemers that compromise multiple vector molecules (66). Cells transduced simultaneously with two separate vectors yield concatemers containing both types of vector (70,71). This raises the possibility that a dual vector approach might be applied to CF gene therapy. An AAV vector containing a full-length CFTR gene could be coadministered with a vector containing a substantial promoter/enhancer element, followed by concatemerization and high-level CFTR expression directed by the promoter/enhancer vector. Alternatively, vectors separately containing the 5′ and 3′ portions of the CFTR gene could be designed to concatemerize in a transsplicing configuration to yield efficient expression of a complete CFTR gene in the target cell. These approaches will require careful study in the airway to evaluate whether the efficiency of vector coadministration will be sufficient to produce robust CFTR expression.

Serotypes other than AAV2 have shown early promise for efficient lung transduction. In particular, AAV-5 (72) has shown particular tropism for the airway epithelium when administered from the luminal side (73), probably as a result of alternate receptor molecules found on the apical surface for this serotype (74). AAV-6 has also been successfully administered to the airway epithelium (75). Further studies of airway transduction by these serotypes will determine whether they are suitable candidates for therapeutic gene delivery to the lung.

Finally, increased physical delivery of AAV to the airways of patients with CF may be possible using aerosol generation devices with higher efficiency than conventional nebulizers. Alternatively, transduction adjuvants such as perfluorochemicals have shown promise in increasing gene delivery and expression to the lung (76).

The constellation of new AAV-based approaches directed toward optimizing gene transfer and expression of the CFTR gene in the lung bodes well for development of an effective therapeutic designed to address the underlying molecular defect in cystic fibrosis. In the absence of predictive animal models for this disease, these approaches will require early evaluation in patients with CF. Despite elucidation of many insights into the pathophysiology of cystic fibrosis over the last decade, a number of fundamental questions regarding a gene therapy approach to this disease still remain unanswered:

- How much normal CFTR mRNA or protein is required in transduced cells to produce a therapeutic effect?
- How many transduced cells are required to normalize the airway epithelium for all important functions, not just electrophysiological function?
- What part of the airway requires correction of the CFTR defect?
- How long is CFTR function required before clinical benefit can be manifested?

Future studies will therefore need to focus on well-characterized clinical surrogate endpoints, such as changes in FEV_1, to evaluate the potential for efficacy of AAV-CFTR vectors. The use of other noninvasive endpoints, such as high-resolution computed tomographic (CT) scans (77) or evaluation of inflammatory mediators in induced sputum (78), may also prove to be useful. Studies evaluating efficacy will need to move into patients with relatively good lung function, including children, once appropriate safety data have been generated.

Considerable progress has been made in the last decade toward developing CF gene therapy. Maturation of vector production technology, development of new analytical tools, and refinement of clinical trial design should accelerate the evaluation of AAV vectors carrying the CFTR gene for the treatment of cystic fibrosis.

References

1. Carter BJ. Adeno-associated virus vectors. Curr Opin Biotechnol 1992; 3:533–539.
2. Blacklow NR, Hoggan MD, Kapikian AZ, Austin JB, Rowe WP. Epidemiology of adenovirus-associated virus infection in a nursery population. Am J Epidemiol 1968; 88:368–378.
3. Atchison R, Casto BC, Hammon WM. Adenovirus-associated defective virus particles. Science 1965; 149:754–755.
4. Blacklow NR, Hoggan MD, Rowe WP. Serologic evidence for human infection with adenovirus-associated viruses. J Natl Cancer Inst 1968; 40:319–327.
5. Bantel-Schaal U, zur Hausen H. Characterization of the DNA of a defective human parvovirus isolated from a genital site. Virology 1984; 134:52–63.
6. Rutledge EA, Halbert CL, Russell DW. Infectious clones and vectors derived from adeno-associated virus (AAV) serotypes other than AAV type 2. J Virol 1998; 72: 309–319.
7. Muzyczka N. Use of adeno-associated virus as a general transduction vector for mammalian cells. Curr Top Microbiol Immunol 1992; 158:97–129.
8. Flotte TR, Afione SA, Conrad C, McGrath SA, Solow R, Oka H, Zeitlin PL, Guggino WB, Carter BJ. Stable in vivo expression of the cystic fibrosis transmembrane conductance regulator with an adeno-associated virus vector. Proc Natl Acad Sci USA 1993; 90:10613–10617.
9. Conway JE, Rhys CM, Zolotukhin I, Zolotukhin S, Muzyczka N, Hayward GS, Byrne BJ. High-titer recombinant adeno-associated virus production utilizing a recombinant herpes simplex virus type I vector expressing AAV-2 Rep and Cap. Gene Ther 1999; 6:986–993.
10. Debelak D, Fisher J, Iuliano S, Sesholtz D, Sloane DL, Atkinson EM. Cation-exchange high-performance liquid chromatography of recombinant adeno-associated virus type 2. J Chromatogr B Biomed Sci Appl 2000; 740:195–202.
11. Gao G, Qu G, Burnham MS, Huang J, Chirmule N, Joshi B, Yu QC, Marsh JA, Conceicao CM, Wilson JM. Purification of recombinant adeno-associated virus vectors by column chromatography and its performance in vivo. Hum Gene Ther 2000; 11:2079–2091.
12. Riordan JR, Rommens JM, Kerem B, Alon N, Rozmahel R, Grzelczak Z, Zielenski J, Lok S, Plavsic N, Chou JL. Identification of the cystic fibrosis gene: cloning and characterization of complementary DNA. Science 1989; 245:1066–1073.
13. Drumm ML, Pope HA, Cliff WH, Rommens JM, Marvin SA, Tsui LC, Collins FS, Frizzell RA, Wilson JM. Correction of the cystic fibrosis defect in vitro by retrovirus-mediated gene transfer. Cell 1990; 62:1227–1233.
14. Johnson LG, Olsen JC, Sarkadi B, Moore KL, Swanstrom R, Boucher RC. Efficiency of gene transfer for restoration of normal airway epithelial function in cystic fibrosis. Nat Genet 1992; 2:21–25.
15. Trapnell BC, Chu CS, Paakko PK, Banks TC, Yoshimura K, Ferrans VJ, Chernick

MS, Crystal RG. Expression of the cystic fibrosis transmembrane conductance regulator gene in the respiratory tract of normal individuals and individuals with cystic fibrosis. Proc Natl Acad Sci USA 1991; 88:6565–6569.

16. Dorin JR, Farley R, Webb S, Smith SN, Farini E, Delaney SJ, Wainwright BJ, Alton EW, Porteous DJ. A demonstration using mouse models that successful gene therapy for cystic fibrosis requires only partial gene correction. Gene Ther 1996; 3:797–801.

17. Dong JY, Fan PD, Frizzell RA. Quantitative analysis of the packaging capacity of recombinant adeno-associated virus. Hum Gene Ther 1996; 7:2101–2112.

18. Flotte TR, Solow R, Owens RA, Afione S, Zeitlin PL, Carter BJ. Gene expression from adeno-associated virus vectors in airway epithelial cells. Am J Respir Cell Mol Biol 1992; 7:349–356.

19. Flotte TR, Afione SA, Solow R, Drumm ML, Markakis D, Guggino WB, Zeitlin PL, Carter BJ. Expression of the cystic fibrosis transmembrane conductance regulator from a novel adeno-associated virus promoter. J Biol Chem 1993; 268:3781–3790.

20. Haberman RP, McCown TJ, Samulski RJ. Novel transcriptional regulatory signals in the adeno-associated virus terminal repeat A/D junction element. J Virol 2000; 74:8732–8739.

21. Egan M, Flotte T, Afione S, Solow R, Zeitlin PL, Carter BJ, Guggino WB. Defective regulation of outwardly rectifying Cl⁻ channels by protein kinase A corrected by insertion of CFTR (see comments). Nature 1992; 358:581–584.

22. DePamphilis ML. Transcriptional elements as components of eukaryotic origins of DNA replication. Cell 1988; 52:635–638.

23. Smale ST, Schmidt MC, Berk AJ, Baltimore D. Transcriptional activation by Sp1 as directed through TATA or initiator: specific requirement for mammalian transcription factor IID. Proc Natl Acad Sci USA 1990; 87:4509–4513.

24. Lynch C, Munson K, Stepan T, Feldhaus A. Small synthetic promoter elements increase expression of the full-length CFTR cDNA in AAV vectors. Meeting American Society of Gene Therapy, Seattle, 1999.

25. Carroll TP, Morales MM, Fulmer SB, Allen SS, Flotte TR, Cutting GR, Guggino WB. Alternate translation initiation codons can create functional forms of cystic fibrosis transmembrane conductance regulator. J Biol Chem 1995; 270:11941–11946.

26. Sirninger J, Hue H, Guggino WB, Flotte T. Restoration of CFTR chloride channel activity in IB3 cells with AAV-minigene constructs. Mol Ther 2001; 3:S184.

27. Zhang L, Wang D, Fischer H, Fan PD, Widdicombe JH, Kan YW, Dong JY. Efficient expression of CFTR function with adeno-associated virus vectors that carry shortened CFTR genes. Proc Natl Acad Sci USA 1998; 95:10158–10163.

28. Quinton PM. Cystic fibrosis: a disease in electrolyte transport. FASEB J 1990; 4:2709–2717.

29. Pier GB, Grout M, Zaidi TS, Goldberg JB. How mutant CFTR may contribute to Pseudomonas aeruginosa infection in cystic fibrosis. Am J Respir Crit Care Med 1996; 154:S175–182.

30. Pier GB, Grout M, Zaidi TS. Cystic fibrosis transmembrane conductance regulator

is an epithelial cell receptor for clearance of *Pseudomonas aeruginosa* from the lung. Proc Natl Acad Sci USA 1997; 94:12088–12093.

31. Schwiebert EM, Egan ME, Hwang TH, Fulmer SB, Allen SS, Cutting GR, Guggino WB. CFTR regulates outwardly rectifying chloride channels through an autocrine mechanism involving ATP. Cell 1995; 81:1063–1073.

32. Greger R, Mall M, Bleich M, Ecke D, Warth R, Riedemann N, Kunzelmann K. Regulation of epithelial ion channels by the cystic fibrosis transmembrane conductance regulator. J Mol Med 1996; 74:527–534.

33. Wei L, Vankeerberghen A, Cuppens H, Eggermont J, Cassiman JJ, Droogmans G, Nilius B. Interaction between calcium-activated chloride channels and the cystic fibrosis transmembrane conductance regulator. Pflugers Arch 1999; 438:635–641.

34. Wang S, Yue H, Derin RB, Guggino WB, Li M. Accessory protein facilitated CFTR-CFTR interaction, a molecular mechanism to potentiate the chloride channel activity. Cell 2000; 103:169–179.

35. Choi JY, Muallem D, Kiselyov K, Lee MG, Thomas PJ, Muallem S. Aberrant CFTR-dependent HCO_3-transport in mutations associated with cystic fibrosis. Nature 2001; 410:94–97.

36. Halbert CL, Standaert TA, Aitken ML, Alexander IE, Russell DW, Miller AD. Transduction by adeno-associated virus vectors in the rabbit airway: efficiency, persistence, and readministration. J Virol 1997; 71:5932–5941.

37. Zeitlin PL, Chu S, Conrad C, McVeigh U, Ferguson K, Flotte TR, Guggino WB. Alveolar stem cell transduction by an adeno-associated viral vector. Gene Ther 1995; 2:623–631.

38. Conrad CK, Allen SS, Afione SA, Reynolds TC, Beck SE, Fee-Maki M, Barrazza-Ortiz X, Adams R, Askin FB, Carter BJ. Safety of single-dose administration of an adeno-associated virus (AAV)–CFTR vector in the primate lung. Gene Ther 1996; 3:658–668.

39. Afione SA, Conrad CK, Kearns WG, Chunduru S, Adams R, Reynolds TC, Guggino WB, Cutting GR, Carter BJ, Flotte TR. In vivo model of adeno-associated virus vector persistence and rescue. J Virol 1996; 70:3235–3241.

40. McDonald R, Canfield D, Raabe O, Carter B, Reynolds T, Lynch C. Safety of aerosol administration of tgAAVCF vector for CF gene therapy in the non-human primate. American Thoracic Society, Toronto, 2000.

41. Munson K, Thompson S, Allen T, Dell'Aringa J, Gerard C, Klump W, Wilson L, Lynch C. Gene transfer and gene expression of tgAAVCF in nonhuman primates following repeated aerosolized administration. Mol Ther 2001; 3:S180.

42. Halbert CL, Standaert TA, Wilson CB, Miller AD. Successful readministration of adeno-associated virus vectors to the mouse lung requires transient immunosuppression during the initial exposure. J Virol 1998; 72:9795–9805.

43. Beck SE, Jones LA, Chesnut K, Walsh SM, Reynolds TC, Carter BJ, Askin FB, Flotte TR, Guggino WB. Repeated delivery of adeno-associated virus vectors to the rabbit airway. J Virol 1999; 73:9446–9455.

44. Wine JJ, King VV, Lewiston NJ. Method for rapid evaluation of topically applied agents to cystic fibrosis airways. Am J Physiol 1991; 261:L218–221.

45. Wagner JA, Nepomuceno IB, Shah N, Messner AH, Moran ML, Norbash AM, Moss

RB, Wine JJ, Gardner P. Maxillary sinusitis as a surrogate model for CF gene therapy clinical trials in patients with antrostomies. J Gene Med 1999; 1:13–21.

46. Moss RB, King VV. Management of sinusitis in cystic fibrosis by endoscopic surgery and serial antimicrobial lavage. Reduction in recurrence requiring surgery. Arch Otolaryngol Head Neck Surg 1995; 121:566–572.

47. Wagner JA, Moran ML, Messner AH, Daifuku R, Conrad CK, Reynolds T, Guggino WB, Moss RB, Carter BJ, Wine JJ. A phase I/II study of tgAAV-CF for the treatment of chronic sinusitis in patients with cystic fibrosis. Hum Gene Ther 1998; 9:889–909.

48. Wagner JA, Reynolds T, Moran ML, Moss RB, Wine JJ, Flotte TR, Gardner P. Efficient and persistent gene transfer of AAV-CFTR in maxillary sinus (letter). Lancet 1998; 9117.

49. Wagner JA, Messner AH, Moran ML, Daifuku R, Kouyama K, Desch JK, Manley S, Norbash AM, Conrad CK, Friborg S. Safety and biological efficacy of an adeno-associated virus vector-cystic fibrosis transmembrane regulator (AAV-CFTR) in the cystic fibrosis maxillary sinus. Laryngoscope 1999; 109:266–274.

50. Wagner J, Messner A, Moran M, Guggino W, Flotte T, Wine J, Carter B, Batson E, Moss R, Gardner P. A Phase II, Double-Blind, Randomized, Placebo-Controlled Clinical Trial of tgAAVCF using Maxillary Sinus Delivery in CF Patients with Antrostomies. 13th Annual North American Cystic Fibrosis Conference, Seattle, 1999.

51. Imundo L, Barasch J, Prince A, Al-Awqati Q. Cystic fibrosis epithelial cells have a receptor for pathogenic bacteria on their apical surface (published erratum appears in Proc Natl Acad Sci USA 1995 Nov 21; 92(24):11322). Proc Natl Acad Sci USA 1995; 92:3019–3023.

52. DiMango E, Zar HJ, Bryan R, Prince A. Diverse Pseudomonas aeruginosa gene products stimulate respiratory epithelial cells to produce interleukin-8. J Clin Invest 1995; 96:2204–2210.

53. Bryan R, Kube D, Perez A, Davis P, Prince A. Overproduction of the CFTR R domain leads to increased levels of asialoGM1 and increased *Pseudomonas aeruginosa* binding by epithelial cells. Am J Respir Cell Mol Biol 1998; 19:269–277.

54. DiMango E, Ratner AJ, Bryan R, Tabibi S, Prince A. Activation of NF-kappaB by adherent *Pseudomonas aeruginosa* in normal and cystic fibrosis respiratory epithelial cells. J Clin Invest 1998; 101:2598–2605.

55. Zeitlin P. AAV gene therapy for cystic fibrosis lung disease. Meeting American Society of Gene Therapy, Seattle, 2001.

56. Knowles MR, Hohneker KW, Zhou Z, Olsen JC, Noah TL, Hu PC, Leigh MW, Engelhardt JF, Edwards LJ, Jones KR. A controlled study of adenoviral-vector-mediated gene transfer in the nasal epithelium of patients with cystic fibrosis (see comments). N Engl J Med 1995; 333:823–831.

57. Grubb BR, Pickles RJ, Ye H, Yankaskas JR, Vick RN, Engelhardt JF, Wilson JM, Johnson LG, Boucher RC. Inefficient gene transfer by adenovirus vector to cystic fibrosis airway epithelia of mice and humans. Nature 1994; 371:802–806.

58. Noone PG, Hohneker KW, Zhou Z, Johnson LG, Foy C, Gipson C, Jones K, Noah TL, Leigh MW, Schwartzbach C. Safety and biological efficacy of a lipid-CFTR complex for gene transfer in the nasal epithelium of adult patients with cystic fibrosis. Mol Ther 2000; 1:105–114.

59. Reynolds T, Aitkin M, Moss R, Waltz D, Ramsey B, Carter B. A phase I study of aerosolized administration of tgAAVCF to CF patients with mild lung disease. Mol Ther 2000; 1:S145.

60. Summerford C, Samulski RJ. Membrane-associated heparan sulfate proteoglycan is a receptor for adeno-associated virus type 2 virions. J Virol 1998; 72:1438–1445.

61. Qing K, Mah C, Hansen J, Zhou S, Dwarki V, Srivastava A. Human fibroblast growth factor receptor 1 is a co-receptor for infection by adeno-associated virus 2. Nat Med 1999; 5:71–77.

62. Summerford C, Bartlett JS, Samulski RJ. AlphaVbeta5 integrin: a co-receptor for adeno-associated virus type 2 infection. Nat Med 1999; 5:78–82.

63. Duan D, Yue Y, Yan Z, McCray PB, Jr, Engelhardt JF. Polarity influences the efficiency of recombinant adeno-associated virus infection in differentiated airway epithelia. Hum Gene Ther 1998; 9:2761–2776.

64. Duan D, Yue Y, Yan Z, Yang J, Engelhardt JF. Endosomal processing limits gene transfer to polarized airway epithelia by adeno-associated virus. J Clin Invest 2000; 105:1573–1587.

65. Douar AM, Poulard K, Stockholm D, Danos O. Intracellular trafficking of adeno-associated virus vectors: routing to the late endosomal compartment and proteasome degradation. J Virol 2001; 75:1824–1833.

66. Vincent-Lacaze N, Snyder RO, Gluzman R, Bohl D, Lagarde C, Danos O. Structure of adeno-associated virus vector DNA following transduction of the skeletal muscle. J Virol 1999; 73:1949–1955.

67. Russell DW, Hirata RK. Human gene targeting by viral vectors. Nat Genet 1998; 18:325–330.

68. Inoue N, Hirata RK, Russell DW. High-fidelity correction of mutations at multiple chromosomal positions by adeno-associated virus vectors. J Virol 1999; 73:7376–7380.

69. Inoue N, Dong R, Hirata RK, Russell DW. Introduction of single base substitutions at homologous chromosomal sequences by adeno-associated virus vectors. Mol Ther 2001; 3:526–530.

70. Yang J, Zhou W, Zhang Y, Zidon T, Ritchie T, Engelhardt JF. Concatamerization of adeno-associated virus circular genomes occurs through intermolecular recombination. J Virol 1999; 73:9468–9477.

71. Miao CH, Nakai H, Thompson AR, Storm TA, Chiu W, Snyder RO, Kay MA. Nonrandom transduction of recombinant adeno-associated virus vectors in mouse hepatocytes in vivo: cell cycling does not influence hepatocyte transduction. J Virol 2000; 74:3793–3803.

72. Chiorini JA, Kim F, Yang L, Kotin RM. Cloning and characterization of adeno-associated virus type 5. J Virol 1999; 73:1309–1319.

73. Zabner J, Seiler M, Walters R, Kotin RM, Fulgeras W, Davidson BL, Chiorini JA. Adeno-associated virus type 5 (AAV5) but not AAV2 binds to the apical surfaces of airway epithelia and facilitates gene transfer. J Virol 2000; 74:3852–3858.

74. Walters RW, Yi SM, Keshavjee S, Brown KE, Welsh MJ, Chiorini JA, Zabner J. Binding of adeno-associated virus type 5 to 2,3-linked sialic acid is required for gene transfer. J Biol Chem 2001; 276:20610–20616.

75. Halbert CL, Rutledge EA, Allen JM, Russell DW, Miller AD. Repeat transduction

in the mouse lung by using adeno-associated virus vectors with different serotypes. J Virol 2000; 74:1524–1532.

76. Weiss DJ, Bonneau L, Allen JM, Miller AD, Halbert CL. Perfluorochemical liquid enhances adeno-associated virus-mediated transgene expression in lungs. Mol Ther 2000; 2:624–630.

77. Brody AS, Molina PL, Klein JS, Rothman BS, Ramagopal M, Swartz DR. High-resolution computed tomography of the chest in children with cystic fibrosis: support for use as an outcome surrogate. Pediatr Radiol 1999; 29:731–735.

78. Henig NR, Tonelli MR, Pier MV, Burns JL, Aitken ML. Sputum induction as a research tool for sampling the airways of subjects with cystic fibrosis. Thorax 2001; 56:306–311.

14

Use of Liposomes in the Treatment of Cystic Fibrosis

MYRA STERN and ERIC W. F. W. ALTON

Imperial College
National Heart and Lung Institute
London, England

I. Introduction

Cationic liposome–based gene therapy has been extensively studied for the treatment of cystic fibrosis (CF) where research has reached the stage of clinical trials. Liposomes represent just one strategy among a number used in nonviral gene therapy, ranging from intramuscular injection of naked DNA to the systemic or local administration of formulations comprising DNA and lipids, proteins, peptides, and polymers. Although the main limitation of nonviral gene transfer methods is their relatively low efficiency in vivo, both preclinical and clinical studies indicate that these methods exhibit safety profiles similar to conventional pharmaceutical and biological products. In this chapter, following a brief overview of lipid-mediated gene transfer, the progress of clinical studies for CF gene therapy are described.

II. Nonviral Vectors

Nonviral gene delivery systems currently in use for the development of pulmonary gene therapy have focused on cationic liposomes, with or without DNA-condensing agents or attached molecules intended to bind to receptors or to assist escape from endosomes. More recently, cationic polymers such as polyethylenimine (PEI) (1) and polyamidoamine dendrimers (2) have been used for gene transfer. Lipids and polymers are somewhat less efficient at gene transfer than recombinant viruses but lack their immunological and proinflammatory disadvantages and pose no risk of insertional mutagenesis. They can, moreover, accommodate large DNA plasmids. Current nonviral research aims to modify liposomes to incorporate advantageous viral features without introducing the inherent penalties of these vectors.

Cationic lipids vary in structure but are invariably composed of a hypdrophobic lipid anchor (an aliphatic chain or cholestrol ring), a positively charged head group that interacts with and condenses the DNA, and a linker that bridges these two components. The positively charged lipid forms a particle by condensing negatively charged DNA through ionic interactions. Particulate complexes subsequently form through further hydrophobic interactions among the bound lipids, and these may contain several plasmids. Within the complexes, the DNA is not simply encapsulated by lamellar lipid structures, rather freeze fracture electronmicroscopy reveals that the structure of lipid/DNA complexes is heterogeneous (3). Aggregated and fused liposomes together with tubular structures (composed of condensed DNA) give rise to the term *spagetti and meatballs*, and it has been suggested that the spaghetti could give rise to transfection due to its diameter ($\sim$10 nm), which is close to the diameter of the nuclear pore complexes ($\sim$7 nm).

DOTMA was the first synthetic cationic lipid used for gene transfer (4). Since then, a large number of cationic lipids have been assessed as transfer agents for lung gene delivery, and considerable progress has been achieved in improving efficiency. Some of those tested include the so-called first-generation vectors with structures analogous to DOTMA such as DMRIE (5) and DOTAP (6), cholestrol-containing cationic lipids such as DC-Chol/DOPE (7), and second-generation vectors which bear a polycationic headgroup (e.g., spermidine) like GL-67/DOPE/DMPE-PEG$_{500}$ (8). The basic mechanism of lipid-mediated transfection (Fig. 1), although poorly understood, involves an initial association between cationic lipids, usually in the form of liposomes and plasmid DNA as described above. The resulting complexes are then thought to bind to the cell by an electrostatic interaction between the cationic lipid and negatively charged components of the plasma membrane such as sialylated glycoproteins or possibly by coupling with sulfated membrane-associated proteoglycans (9). Following membrane association, entry of cationic lipid/DNA complexes into the cell is thought to occur via an endocytic process which differs from either receptor-mediated uptake or pinocytosis (10). Escape from the endosome is a limited factor for nonviral gene delivery, and is thought to occur via destablisation of the endosomal membrane. It has been postulated that destabilization results in the flip-flop of anionic lipids

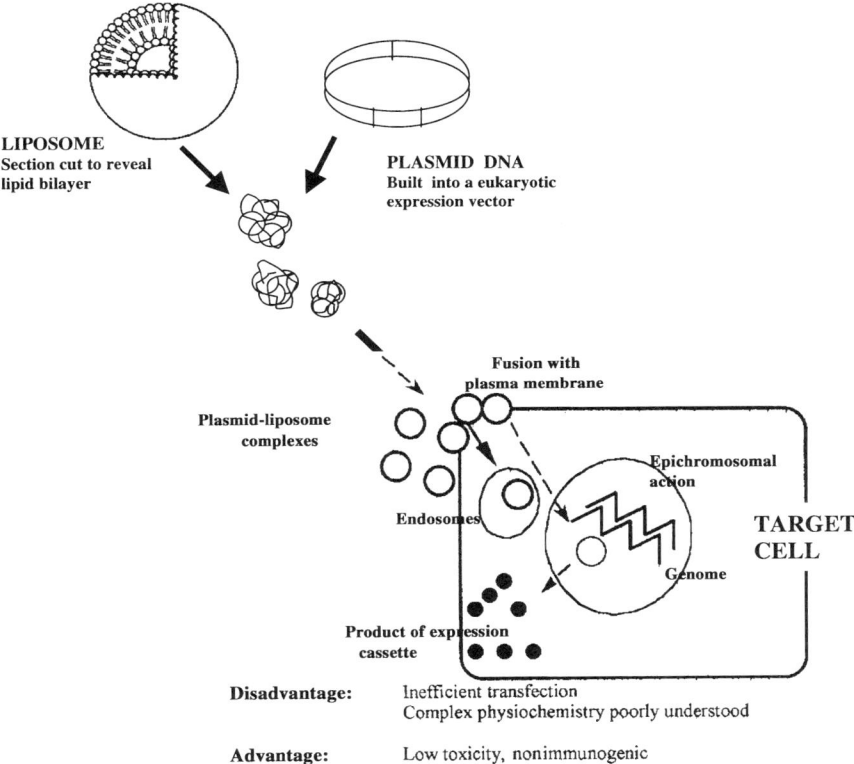

Figure 1 DNA-liposome complex design and gene transfer.

located principally in the cytoplasmic monolayer. These subsequently diffuse laterally into the complex where they form ion pairs with the cationic lipids, resulting in charge neutralization and release of DNA into the cytoplasm (11).

Intracellular trafficking and nuclear entry of the DNA is not, as yet, fully elucidated, although recent studies point to important roles for cytoskeletal elements, a number of nucleocytoplasmic transport factors, and the nuclear membrane. Thus, escape from the endosomal pathway is followed by important regulation by cytoskeletal elements of subsequent transfer of the DNA to the nucleus. The finding in vitro that inhibition of microfilament polymerisation significantly enhances gene expression irrespective of the magnitude of endosomal entrapment (10) supports a critical role for these elements. Nucleocytoplasmic transport factors (12), which include the nuclear-localizing signal (NLS) and their cognate receptors—importin-α, importin-β, and related proteins, are known to play an important role in the successful entry of exogenous DNA into the nucleus. Finally, synchronization of the cell into the G1 phase, likely to mimic conditions found in the terminally differentiated airway epithelium, has been shown significantly to attenuate gene expression (10), whereas mitotic nuclear disassembly has the opposite effect.

III. Gene Therapy for Cystic Fibrosis

CF is an autosomal recessive disease affecting more than 50,000 individuals worldwide, primarily, although not exclusively, white individuals. The disease affects epithelium-lined organs, such as the respiratory and intestinal tracts, of which the former are the site of major morbidity and mortality. Recurrent chest infections and colonization of the lower airways with organisms such as *Staphylococcus aureus* and *Pseudomonas aeruginosa* progress to subsequent bronchiectasis and finally respiratory failure, the most common cause of death.

Current treatment includes daily physiotherapy, vigorous antibiotic treatment of pulmonary infections, pancreatic enzyme supplementation for pancreatic insufficiency, and intensive dietary support. This combination has resulted in great improvements in life expectancy, but the treatment remains time consuming and intrusive for patients and is essentially symptomatic. In 1989, the gene mutated in CF was identified and the protein for which it codes—the cystic fibrosis transmembrane conductance regulator (CFTR)—was characterized (13). This opened the way for the development of gene therapy for the disease, offering the long-term possibility of a promising new and more effective approach to treatment.

The proposed strategies for gene therapy in CF are based on what is currently known about the molecular and biochemical pathology of the disease. CFTR functions as a cAMP-regulated chloride channel in the apical membrane of epithelial cells (14). Increases in intracellular cAMP result in increased chloride transport through CFTR followed by osmotic movement of water, and this probably contributes to maintenance of mucosal surface hydration. Mutations in the CF gene, located on the long arm of chromosome 7, result in CFTR that is either mislocalized or dysfunctional. This in turn results in disturbance of chloride transport across the epithelial cells of the airways, gut, pancreas, biliary tract, and sperm ducts. Secondary to the chloride transport defect there is also an increase in sodium absorption in the airways (15), although how this occurs is presently unclear.

The relationship between these defects and the clinical manifestations of cystic fibrosis still remains speculative. However, a reasonable hypothesis is that the ion transport defects may lead to suboptimal volumes of airways surface liquid resulting in impaired mucociliary clearance, bacterial colonization, and repeated infection. The idea of gene therapy was simply to administer the normal CF gene or protein as if it were a drug to the organ most affected yet apparently quite accessible—the lungs. In theory this should result in restoration of normal cellular function and so prevent or treat the disease. A vigorous research effort has therefore followed identification of the gene. The first reports of in vitro CFTR gene transfer appeared in 1990 (16), only 1 year after identification of the gene. Further in vitro studies (17) were followed by in vivo gene transfer to the airway epithelial cells of transgenic CF mice (18–19), confirming that it was possible to achieve some functional restoration of the ion transport defects in these cells following transgene expression. Within 4 years, at least four clinical studies of gene therapy in CF patients has been reported (20–23), and since then the number has risen to over 20; all Phase I safety studies.

Liposome/plasmid complexes have been tested in at least eight clinical trials (23–30). Of these, five were conducted in the United Kingdom and were all double-blind studies. Three trials with similar design showed partial correction of the chloride transport defect in the nose (23–25). In the first, Caplen et al. (23) tested a pSV-CFTR plasmid complexed with DC-Chol:DOPE in the nasal epithelium of ΔF508 homozygous CF patients. Three DNA doses were tested (10, 100, and 300 μg) in patient groups of three each, while a further six patients received only the equivalent lipid dose as control. No safety problems were encountered, and of eight biopsies taken from the treated patients evidence for the transgene was seen in all but one sample. In five of these seven positive samples, transgene expression was detected. The CF chloride secretory defect, as assessed by measurement of in vivo transepithelial potential difference (PD) (31), showed a significant 20% increase toward normal values, with two of the patients reaching the normal range for non-CF subjects. This change was maximal 3 days after gene administration and had reverted to pretreatment values after 7 days.

DC-Chol:DOPE was tested in a second trial of CFTR gene transfer to the nasal epithelium by Gill et al. (24). Again, DC-Chol:DOPE was used to deliver a CFTR-carrying plasmid driven by a RSV-LTR promoter to the nasal epithelium of 12 CF patients (mixed genotypes) by direct instillation. Two DNA doses were studied: 40 μg (four patients), 400 μg (four patients), and placebo (either buffer or lipid:plasmid encoding nonfunctional CFTR). No safety problems were encountered. Both in vivo nasal PD measurements and ex vivo SPQ analysis (32) of nasal epithelial cells obtained by brushings, were used as endpoints to assess the effect of gene transfer on ion transport. The combined results showed evidence of functional CFTR gene transfer in six out eight treated patients. Correction of the CF ion transport abnormalities were more sustained than those reported in the first trial above (23), lasting for 7 days in one patient and 15 days in another. No change was observed in sodium-related measurements.

In the third of these nasal trials (25), a single dose of 400 μg pCMV-CFTR complexed with 2.4 mg of DOTAP was administered to the nasal epithelium of

Table 1 Clinical Trials of Lipid-Mediated Gene Therapy for Cystic Fibrosis

Center	Gene delivery system	Target organ	Subjects	Reference
Royal Brompton Hospital, National Heart and Lung Institute, London, England	DC-Chol:DOPE	Nose	18	23
University of Oxford/University of Cambridge, England	DC-Chol:DOPE	Nose	19	24
MRC Human Genetics Unit, Western General Hospital, Royal Infirmary, University of Edinburgh, Edinburgh, Scotland	DOTAP	Nose	20	25
University of Iowa College of Medicine, Ames, IA	GL-67	Nose	21	26
Royal Brompton Hospital, National Heart and Lung Institute, London, England	GL-67	Nose and lungs	22	27
University of Alabama, Birmingham, AL	GL-67	Lungs	8	28
University of Oxford/University of Cambridge, England	DC-Chol:DOPE	Nose (repeat dose)	12	29
University of North Carolina at Chapel Hill, Chapel Hill, NC	GR213487B	Nose	23	30

CF patients (mixed genotype). Again, the trial was double-blind and placebo controlled, with eight patients receiving treatment and a further eight receiving buffer only. No safety problems were encountered. Vector-specific DNA was detected at 3 days and 7 days in seven of eight treated patients and at day 28 in two of these seven patients. Vector-derived mRNA was detected in two patients at days 3 and 7. Two treated patients demonstrated changes in their nasal PD following treatment consistent with partial correction of the chloride transport defect, with a mean change toward non-CF values of 20%.

The following three clinical trials (26–28) made use of a second-generation cationic lipid GL-67/DOPE/DMPE-PEG$_{500}$, shown to be nontoxic when administered by nebulization to the lungs of normal volunteers (33). Zabner et al. (26) administered naked DNA (1.25 mg of pCF1-CFTR driven by a cytomegalovirus [CMV]-promoter) to the epithelial surface of one nostril and the same dose of DNA but complexed with lipid Gl-67 to the other nostril in a randomized, double-blind fashion. Nine subjects were studied. Functional gene transfer was demonstrable by reverse transcriptase–polymerase chain reaction (RT-PCR) and in vivo nasal potential difference measurements, with little difference being observed between the two vector systems studied. In a further double-blind, placebo-controlled trial using GL-67, the complex was delivered to both nose and lungs of 16 CF patients by nebulization (27). Eight patients 4.2 mg of pCF1-CFTR complexed with 229 mg of the lipid administered to the lungs, and another eight patients received an equivalent dose of lipid alone. A lower dose (11.8 mg DNA) was nebulized into the nose. Using in vivo PD measurements and ex vivo SPQ fluorescence analysis, partial but significant correction of chloride transport was seen at both sites—approximately 25% correction toward normal values in the lungs and 20% in the nose. Furthermore, for the first time, a reduced binding of *Pseudomonas aeruginosa* to airway epithelial cells (34) was observed in both nose and lungs. Administration of the gene-lipid complexes to the lungs in this trial was associated with a transient febrile reaction which did not occur in the control group who received the lipid on its own. This side effect was thought to be attributable, at least in part, to the bacterial origin of the DNA (35). A similar syndrome was also reported by Ruiz et al. (28) following a dose-escalation trial of CFTR-cDNA complexed with GL-67 to the lungs of eight adult CF patients. Four of the eight patients developed a pronounced fever (maximum 103.3°F), associated with myalgia and arthralgia beginning within 6 hrs of gene administration. Serum interleukin-6 (IL-6) but not levels of IL-8, IL-1, tumor necrosis factor-α (TNF-α), or interferon-γ (IFN-γ) became elevated within 1–3 hr of gene administration. No antibodies to the cationic liposome or plasmid DNA were detected. It was found that plasmid DNA by itself elicited minimal proliferation of peripheral blood mononuclear cells taken from study patients, but led to brisk immune cell proliferation when complexed to a cationic lipid. This seemed to suggest that lipid and DNA were synergistic in causing this response. Further, cellular proliferation was seen with eukaryotic DNA, suggesting that at least part of the immunological response to lipid-DNA conjugates is independent of unmethylated (*Escherichia coli*–derived) CpG sequences that had previously been associated with this response. None of these studies showed any correction of the sodium transport defect, and vector-specific mRNA detected by RT-PCR was only inconsistently found.

A double-blind study to evaluate the safety and efficacy of multiple doses of CFTR-cDNA complexed with DC-Chol:DOPE to the nasal epithelium of CF patients has also been reported (29). Ten subjects received the complexed DNA, while a further two patients received placebo. Each subject received three doses, administered respectively at 4-week intervals. There was no evidence of inflammation, toxicity, or immunological response to either the complexes or to the expressed transgene. Endpoint assays included quantification of vector-specific DNA and mRNA, immunocytochemistry of CFTR protein, bacterial adherence to epithelial cells, in vivo nasal potential difference, and ex vivo SPQ analysis. On average, six of the treated subjects were positive for CFTR gene transfer after each dose. Of these, all subjects demonstrating some correction of the CF ion transport defect were also positive for plasmid-derived DNA, mRNA, and CFTR protein by immunocytochemistry. This study suggested that, unlike high-dose recombinant adenoviral gene therapy, cationic lipid/DNA complexex could be successfully readministered without apparent loss of efficacy.

Finally, a recently reported study using a novel second-generation cationic lipid, (p-ethyl-dimyristoylphosphatidylcholine [EDMPC] cholestrol) (30) reported that the lipid-DNA complex were safe but did not produce consistent evidence of gene transfer to the nasal epithelium.

IV. Future Considerations

Although a practical treatment using cationic lipid–mediated gene therapy has not yet been realized, a wealth of data have emerged from all of the above studies. These reflect both enormous progress, but they also bring to light numerous difficulties that were not anticipated. Gene transfer efficiency currently remains suboptimal, not only for cationic lipids, but also for the two viral systems tested clinically (recombinant adenovirus and AAV). Further progress will need resolution of a number of issues.

A. Target

CF affects the conducting airways rather than the alveoli. These include both the larger bronchial regions lined by a pseudostratified columnar epithelium and containing numerous submucosal glands and the small bronchiolar regions lined by a simple columnar epithelium devoid of glands. A central question for CF gene therapy is which cell type and which region (large or small) to target. Although ciliated superficial epithelium is abundant and displays the ion transport defects in patients with CF, the submucosal glands are the highest expressing CFTR cells in the lung and might well need to be targeted for clinical benefit. This raises considerations of delivery, since topical delivery will only reach these cells with difficulty and may therefore require systemic delivery of CFTR vectors. Further, most data suggest that small airways are both the initial and major site of disease in CF. Effective cDNA delivery to these areas is not inevitable using current nebulizer technology and remains an important strategic issue.

B. Barriers

An intrinsic function of the lining epithelium of the airways is to prevent penetration of the airways and interstitium by foreign material and invading organisms. Thus, a complex series of extracellular barriers, including a normal mucous layer which inhibits gene transfer (10), a glycocalyx, an apical cell membrane, and tight junctions between the cells, conspire to keep out intraluminally delivered materials including both viral and nonviral vectors. This problem is compounded in CF by the presence of thick, infected sputum, also known to inhibit gene transfer (36), and mucous plugging of the small airways. Removal of the mucous layer has been shown to increase transgene expression 25-fold in an ex vivo model of airway epithelium using native sheep trachea (10). Thus, the use of adjunctive mucolytic agents or abrogation of tight junction barrier function using either detergents or antibodies to intrinsic tight junction components are just two novel strategies being investigated to overcome these barriers.

The apical cell membrane presents another significant barrier, serving in vivo an important protective function by preventing entry of macromolecules into the cell. The extent of this barrier is however variable. Studies using airway epithelial cell cultures have shown that differentiated cells differ both in their surface charge and their ability to endocytose DNA-lipid complexes in comparison with dedifferentiated cells at the edge of the culture (37). These differences are paralleled by significantly more efficient gene transfer in the latter.

Once inside the cell, plasmid DNA is then subject to a further series of potential barriers, and unlike viruses, nonviral vectors lack any strategy to overcome intracellular barriers including the endosome and nuclear membrane. It is estimated that only 1 in 1000 liposome-delivered plasmids reach the nucleus and are expressed. It is difficult to quantify the relative importance of the different barriers facing lipid-mediated gene transfer. Further strategies to overcome the cell membrane and intracellular barriers might include (1) optimization of receptor-mediated endocytosis using polycations such as poly-L-lysine or protamine to condense the DNA together with receptor binding chemicals such as transferrin, antibodies to cell surface antigens like the polymeric IgA receptor, and viral entry proteins (38,39); (2) pH-sensitive ligands to encourage more efficient endosomal escape; (3) the use of nuclear proteins (e.g., HMG-1) to enhance trafficking of the DNA into the nucleus; and (4) the addition of relevant nuclear localization signals so that the DNA can enter the nucleus more efficiently.

C. Vectors

With respect to nonviral gene transfer, strategies aimed at improving gene transfer efficiency include the ongoing modification of lipid vectors currently in use. Third-generation synthetic vectors have been designed, and they include:

1. Dendrimers (2).

2. Ligand-polylysine-DNA complexes for receptor-mediated gene transfer; for example, lactosylated poly-L-lysine has been shown efficiently to transfer CFTR cDNA to CF airway epithelial cells in vitro (40).
3. DNA-gelatin nanospheres (41).
4. Polyethylenimine (PEI) (1), which has been shown to transfer genes both in vitro and in vivo. It has a number of chemical/structural properties which are quite different from cationic liposomes and may be advantageous for gene delivery. The size of PEI/DNA complexes is very small (<100 nm), potentially allowing for better distribution. It also appears to be efficient at endosomal escape, thus reducing DNA degradation.
5. Cationic detergents able to condense plasmid DNA into small uniform complexes (42).
6. ''Virosomes,'' which comprise liposomes with viral proteins such as Sendai virus hemagglutinin (HVJ liposomes). These complexes are thought to introduce DNA into the cytoplasm of the cell following hemaglutinin-mediated fusion of the liposome with the target cell membrane (43).

D. How Much Is Enough?

The vexing question of the level of gene expression needed to achieve clinical benefit remains unresolved, but it is likely that the level of transduced CFTR per cell required will be low. The percentage of CF cells which need to be corrected has been suggested by a study (44) demonstrating in vitro that 6–10% of cells within a monolayer must consist of "corrected CF cells" in order to restore normal chloride transport. The percentage required to correct the sodium transport defect is, however, much higher than this (45). The optimal strategy for functional correction would be to mimic normal expression; that is, to correct as close to 100% of cells as possible at low levels of expression per cell. This remains a challenging target with a realistic aim of achieving somewhere between 10 and 100% of cells.

Thus, although CFTR gene therapy using first- and second-generation nonviral vectors has essentially been shown to be quite safe and associated with some, albeit small, detectable functional correction of airway epithelial cells, it still remains elusive as a practical treatment for CF lung disease. However, the unresolved questions that remain to be answered for successful CF gene therapy have now been clearly defined—a prerequisite for overcoming the technical problems of efficient gene transfer in the right target cells. Gene therapy for CF remains the most promising possibility for curative rather than symptomatic therapy. It will likely prove to be most beneficial if given very early—prior to the onset of established infection/inflammation in the lungs. Although ongoing research worldwide aims to resolve the problems delineated above, questions about the execution and design of trials in the pediatric population, not studied thus far, will become the focus of new efforts. Rigorous measurement of gene transfer efficiency in vivo and the development of markers—both real and surrogate—of clinical benefit remain important challenges. One can still be optimistic that once gene transfer efficiency reaches the 10–100% target, clinical benefit when judged from an early stage of the disease will be easily apparent.

V. Conclusions

Non–virus mediated gene therapy for lung disease remains an attractive therapeutic strategy in view of its low toxicity and immunogenicity. A great deal of progress has been made within the field, and nonviral vectors have provided important proof-of-principle data, particularly for cystic fibrosis. However, gene transfer efficiency using nonviral vectors remains currently inadequate for clinical benefit, and ongoing research will focus on achieving optimum levels of transgene expression for therapeutic efficacy.

References

1. Ferrari S, Moro E, Pentenazzo A, et al. Exgen 500 is an efficient vector for gene delivery to lung epithelial cells in vitro and in vivo. Gene Ther 1997; 4:1100–1106.
2. Rudolph C, Lausier J, Naundorf S, et al. In vivo delivery to the lung using polyethylenimine and fractured polyamidoamine dendrimers. J Gene Med 2000; 2:269–278.
3. Sternberg B, Sorgi FL, Huang L. New structures in complex formation between DNA and cationic liposomes visualized by freeze-fracture electron microscopy. FEBS Lett 1994; 356:361–366.
4. Felgner PL, Gadek TR, Holm M, et al. Lipofection: A highly efficient lipid-mediated DNA-transfection procedure. Proc Natl Acad Sci USA 1987; 84:7413–7417.
5. Felgner JH, Kumar R, Sridhar CN, et al. Enhanced gene delivery and mechanism studies with a novel series of cationic lipid formulations. J Biol Chem 1994; 269: 2550–2561.
6. Leventis R, Silvius JR. Interactions of mammalian cells with lipid dispersions containing novel metabolizable cationic amphiphiles. Biochim Biophys Acta 1990; 1023:124–132.
7. Gao X, Huang L. A novel cationic liposome for efficient transfection of mammalian cells. Biochem Biophys Res Commun 1991; 179:280–285.
8. Lee ER, Marshall J, Siegel et al. Detailed analysis of structure and formulations of cationic lipids for efficient gene transfer to the lung. Hum Gene Ther 1996; 7:1701–1717.
9. Labat-Moleur F, Steffan AM, Brisson C, et al. An electron microscopy study into the mechanism of gene transfer with polyamines. Gene Ther 1996; 3:1010–1017.

10. Kitson C, Angel B, Judd D, et al. The extra- and intracellular barriers to lipid and adenovirus-mediated pulmonary gene transfer in native sheep airway epithelium. Gene Ther 1999; 6:534–546.

11. Xu Y, Szoka F. Mechanism of DNA release from cationic liposome/DNA complexes used in cell transfection. Biochemistry 1996; 35:5616–5623.

12. Wilson GL, Dean BS, Wang G, et al. Nuclear import of plasmid DNA in digitonin-permeabilised cells requires both cytoplasmic factors and specific DNA sequences. J Biol Chem 1999; 274:22025–22032.

13. Riordan JR, Rommens JM, Kerem BS, et al. Identification of the cystic fibrosis gene: cloning and characterization of complementary DNA. Science 1989; 245:1066–1073.

14. Welsh MJ. Abnormal regulation of ion channels in cystic fibrosis. FASEB J 1990; 4:2718–2725.

15. Knowles MR, Gatzy JT, Boucher RC. Increased bioelectric potential difference across respiratory epithelia in cystic fibrosis. N Engl J Med 1981; 305:1489–1495.

16. Drumm M, Pope HA, Cliff WH, et al. Correction of the CF defect in vitro by retrovirus-mediated gene transfer. Cell 1999; 62:1227–1233.

17. Rich DP, Anderson MP, Gregory RJ, et al. Expression of cystic fibrosis transmembrane conductance regulator corrects defective chloride channel regulation in cystic fibrosis airway epithelial cells. Nature 1990; 347:358–363.

18. Hyde SC, Gill DR, Higgins CF, et al. Correction of the ion transport defect in cystic fibrosis transgenic mice by gene therapy. Nature 1993; 362:250–255.

19. Alton EWFW, Middleton PG, Caplen NJ, et al. Non-invasive liposome-mediated gene delivery can correct the ion transport defect in cystic fibrosis mice. Nat Genet 1993; 5:135–142.

20. Zabner J, Couture RA, Gregory RJ, et al. Adenovirus-mediated gene transfer transiently corrects the chloride transport defect in nasal epithelia of patients with cystic fibrosis. Cell 1993; 75:207–216.

21. Crystal RG, McElvanehy LG, Rosenfeld MA, et al. Administration of an adenovirus containing the human CFTR cDNA to the respiratory tract of individuals with cystic fibrosis. Nat Genet 1994; 8:42–51.

22. Boucher RC, Knowles MR, Johnson LG, et al. Gene therapy for cystic fibrosis using E1-deleted adenovirus: a phase I trial in the nasal cavity. Hum Gene Ther 1994; 5:615–619.

23. Caplen NJ, Alton EW, Middleton PG, et al. Liposome-mediated CFTR gene transfer to the nasal epithelium of patients with cystic fibrosis. Nat Med 1995; 1:39–46.

24. Gill DR, Southern KW, Mofford KA, et al. A placebo controlled study of liposome-mediated gene transfer to the nasal epithelium of patients with cystic fibrosis. Gene Ther 1997; 4:199–209.

25. Porteus DJ, Dorin JR, McLachlan G, et al. Evidence for safety and efficacy of DOTAP cationic liposome-mediated CFTR gene transfer to the nasal epithelium of patients with cystic fibrosis. Gene Ther 1997; 4:210–218.

26. Zabner J, Cheng S, Meeker D, et al. Comparison of DNA-lipid complexes and DNA alone for gene transfer to cystic fibrosis airway epithelium in vivo. J Clin Invest 1997; 100:1529–1537.

27. Alton EWFW, Stern M, Farley R, et al. Cationic lipid-mediated CFTR gene transfer to the lungs and nose of patients with cystic fibrosis: a double-blind placebo-controlled trial. Lancet 1999; 353:947–954.

28. Ruiz FE, Clancy JP, Perricone MA, et al. A clinical inflammatory syndrome attributable to aerosolised lipid-DNA administration in cystic fibrosis. Hum Gene Ther 2001; 12:751–61.

29. Hyde SC, Southern KW, Gileadi U, et al. Repeat administration of DNA/liposomes to the nasal epithelium of patients with cystic fibrosis. Gene Ther 2000; 7:1156–1165.

30. Noone PG, Hohneker KW, Zhou Z, et al. Safety and efficacy of a lipid-CFTR complex for gene transfer in the nasal epithelium of adult patients with cystic fibrosis. Mol Med 2000; 1:105–114.

31. Middleton PG, Geddes DM, Alton EWFW. Protocols for in vivo measurement of the ion transport defects in cystic fibrosis epithelium. Eur Respir J 1994; 7:2050–2056.

32. Stern M, Munkonge F, Caplen NJ et al. Quantitative fluorescent measurements of chloride secretion in native airway epithelium from CF and non-CF subjects. Gene Ther 1995; 2:766–774.

33. Chadwick SL, Kingston HD, Stern M, et al. Safety of a single aerosol administration of escalating doses of the cationic lipid 67/DOPE/DMPE-PEG$_{500}$ formulation to the lungs of normal volunteers. Gene Ther 1997; 4:937–942.

34. Davies J, Stern M, Dewar A, et al. CFTR gene transfer reduces the binding of pseudomonas aeruginosa to cytic fibrosis epithelium. Am J Respir Cell Mol Biol 1997; 16:657–663.

35. Schwartz DA, Quinn TJ, Thorne PS, et al. CpG motifs in bacterial DNA cause inflammation in the lower respiratory tract. J Clin Invest 1997; 100:68–73.

36. Stern M, Caplen NJ, Browning JE, et al. The effect of mucolytic agents on gene transfer across a CF sputum barrier in vitro. Gene Ther 1998; 5:91–98.

37. Matsui H, Johnson LG, Randell SH, et al. Loss of binding and entry of liposome-DNA complexes decreases transfection efficiency in differentiated airway epithelial cells. J Biol Chem 1997; 272:1117–1126.

38. Wagner E, Zenke M, Cotten M, et al. Transferrin-polycation conjugates as carriers for DNA uptake into cells. Proc Natl Acad Sci USA 1990; 87:3410–3414.

39. Cotton M, Langle-Rouault R, Kirlappos H, et al. Transferrin-polycation-mediated introduction of DNA into human leukemic cells: stimulation by agents that affect the survival of transfected DNA or modulate transferrin receptor levels. Proc Natl Acad Sci USA 1990; 87:4033–4037.

40. Kollen WJ, Mulberg AE, Wei X, et al. High efficiency transfer of cystic fibrosis transmembrane conductance regulator into cystic fibrosis airway cells in culture using lactosylated polylysine as a vector. Hum Gene Ther 1999; 10:615–622.

41. Truong-Le VL, August JT, Leong KW. Controlled gene delivery by DNA-gelatin nanospheres. Hum Gene Ther 1998; 8:817–825.

42. Blessing T, Remy JS, Behr JP. Monomolecular collapse of plasmid DNA inot stable virus-like particles. Proc Natl Acad Sci USA 1998; 95:1427–1431.

43. Yonemitsu Y, Kaneda Y, Muraishi A, et al. HVJ (Sendai virus)–cationic liposomes:

a novel and potentially effective liposome-mediated technique for gene transfer to the airway epithelium. Gene Ther 1997; 4:631–638.

44. Johnson LG, Olsen JC, Sarkadi B. et al. Efficiency of gene transfer for restoration of normal airway epithelial function in cystic fibrosis. Nat Genet 1992; 2:21–25.

45. Johnson LG, Boyles SE, Wilson J, et al. Normalisation of raised sodium absorption and raised calcium-mediated chloride secretion by adenovirus-mediated expression of cystic fibrosis transmembrane conductance regulator in primary human cystic fibrosis airway epithelial cells. J Clin Invest 1995; 95:1377–82.

15

Delivery of Genes Through the Lung Circulation

DAVID M. RODMAN
and MARK BUCHHOLZ

University of Colorado Health Sciences
  Center
and The Children's Hospital
Denver, Colorado, U.S.A.

JAMES WEST

University of Colorado Health Sciences
  Center
Denver, Colorado, U.S.A.

I. Rationale and Therapeutic Targets

There are many reasons why delivering genes via the pulmonary circulation might prove to be useful. The most obvious of these reasons is to affect vascular function. Diseases of small and medium size pulmonary arteries, such as pulmonary hypertension, persistent pulmonary hypertension of the neonate, chronic thromboembolic disease, and vasculitis could be targets for pulmonary vascular gene therapy. Pulmonary capillary disorders, such as acute lung injury and reperfusion injury after lung transplantation could also be modulated by therapeutic gene delivery. Since the pulmonary circulation is exposed to 100% of cardiac output, the pulmonary circulation might also be used as a locus for production of secreted therapeutic proteins for a wide variety of systemic disorders.

Optimization of pulmonary vascular gene delivery requires that the following barriers be overcome: (1) selective targeting of transgene to the required cell type and location, (2) efficient, regulated transgene expression, (3) persistence of expression (if needed), and (4) control of host immune response to vector and transgene product. Several approaches to each of these barriers have been attempted or proposed with varying degrees of success. The approach to targeting and regulation is discussed elsewhere in this volume, and will only be reviewed briefly. Using the pulmonary circulation to deliver transgene to lung allografts is also discussed elsewhere in this volume. The major focus of this chapter will be on reviewing progress to date in optimizing vectors for pulmonary vascular gene delivery as well as detailing results of gene therapy for pulmonary hypertension in animal models.

II. Cell-Based Gene Delivery

Initial attempts at cell-based vascular gene delivery focused on the endothelial cell. Messina and coworkers cultured canine jugular vein endothelium, transducing these cells in culture with a murine amphotrophic retroviral vector containing genes coding for β-galactosidase (βgal) and neomycin resistance (1). The stably transfected endothelial cell population was then selected with the neomycin analog G418. These cells were injected into the hind limb of mice and expression detected for up to 28 days in lung and hind limb. However, no systematic analysis of lung expression and histology was reported.

More recently, Campbell et al. reported using vascular smooth muscle cells (SMCs) for cell-based gene delivery to the lung (2). Primary culture pulmonary artery SMCs from Fisher 344 rats were transfected with a plasmid encoding βgal under transcriptional control of the cytomagalovirus (CMV) enhancer/promotor. Then 5×10^5 cells/animal were injected by tail vein into syngeneic rats. Animals sacrificed after 24 hr demonstrated incorporation of injected SMC into the vascular wall of small pulmonary arterioles. Transgene expression was detected up to 14 days after injection. The investigators calculated that up to 15% of the injected cells persisted in the pulmonary circulation at 14 days.

To determine if a therapeutic gene of interest could be delivered to the pulmonary circulation using this approach, SMCs were transduced with a plasmid encoding the endothelial nitric oxide synthase (NOS3) gene under control of the CMV enhancer/promotor and injected into rats simultaneously with the endothelial cell toxin monocrotaline. Twenty-eight days after injection, the degree of pulmonary hypertension was assessed. Rats treated with NOS3-expressing SMCs, but not reporter gene–expressing controls, demonstrated a marked reduction in PA systolic pressure (33 ± 3 vs 50 ± 4 mmHg, $P < .01$). No evidence of host inflammatory response to the SMC injection or transgene was detected. However, the mechanism of clearance of the transduced cells was not established, and the feasibility of this technique for long-term gene expression is not known. Further, as the technique requires embolization of the pulmonary circulation by aggregated SMCs, the toxicity of this approach in an already hypertensive pulmonary circulation will need to be established. Still, this represents the first report of expression of therapeutically relevant levels of transgene via the pulmonary circulation, and thus provides a foundation for further optimization of pulmonary vascular gene delivery.

III. Nonviral Gene Delivery

Early investigations of systemic DNA-liposome gene delivery noted the preferential expression of transgene in the lung endothelium (3,4). Subsequently, many groups have investigated DNA-liposome (now termed "lipoplex") gene delivery to the pulmonary circulation. Several important observations have been common to these studies including: (1) lipid composition defines organ distribution after intravenous administration of lipoplex, (2) lipoplex is much more efficient than naked plasmid DNA, (3) lipoplex, but not naked plasmid DNA, induces a potent inflammatory response, and (4) transgene expression is transient and largely restricted to the pulmonary capillary endothelium.

Optimization of lipoplex for pulmonary vascular gene delivery has identified several factors that increase lung specificity (5–7). Higher cationic charge appears to produce more lung and less liver expression, possibly by increasing adhesion to and retention by the pulmonary microcirculation. However, toxicity may be seen when higher charge ratios are used. Addition of a neutral carrier lipid, particularly cholesterol, appears to be important as well. The mechanisms through which cholesterol improves lung expression are not clear, although prolonged retention in the circulation, improved integration into endothelial cell membranes, and altered binding to plasma proteins may all play a role (8). Li et al. have intensively investigated the use of lipid-protamine-DNA complexes for pulmonary gene delivery (9). They found that inclusion of the cationic protamine molecule improved efficiency, whereas addition of the neutral lipids DOPE and cholesterol decreased and increased, respectively, efficiency. Consistent with a hypothesis involving binding of plasma proteins, they found that DOPE increased binding to anionic proteins, whereas cholesterol did not. Others have suggested that binding of cholesterol stabilizes the complexes in serum, whereas DOPE binding leads to aggregation of complexes followed rapidly by disintegration and release of DNA (1).

Toxicity of lipoplex is a major problem limiting efficiency and utility. Dow et al. found that injection of small amounts of lipoplex induced CD69 expression on multiple cell types and activation of TH1 cytokines from both lung and spleen mononuclear cells. Neither naked plasmid DNA nor the lipids themselves induced this stereotypic inflammatory response (10). In mice, interferon-γ (INF-γ) levels peaked at 8 hr after injection and returned to control levels by 24 hr. In INF-γ knockout mice, peak levels of transgene expression were one to two orders of magnitude greater than in wild-type controls, although the rate of decline in expression did not differ (S. Dow, personal communication). Consistent with a role for inflammation in modulating expression efficiency, Tyler et al. found that mice treated with monocrotaline (producing localized pulmonary vascular inflammation) had markedly reduced transgene expression in response to lipoplex (11). The mechanism through which reduced expression occurs appeared to be promotor downregulation rather than inefficient delivery, and thus may be promotor specific.

Li et al found that injection of lipid-protamine-DNA complexes induced both interferon-γ and tumor necrosis factor-α (TNF-α) (12). Combined inhibition of these cytokines by neutralizing antibody prolonged transgene expression, adding further evidence that the systemic inflammatory response limits the expression of transgene. In that study, an increased rate of apoptosis of lung endothelial cells suggested enhanced clearance of transduced cells may also play a role in limiting the duration of expression. Following on this observation, Hofman et al. constructed synthetic expression plasmids eliminating unmethylated CpG motifs present in bacterial DNA (13). They found that induction of interleukin-12 (IL-12) and TNF-α was significantly reduced, and transgene expression increased. As an alternative, Tan et al. tested the effectiveness of sequential administration of lipid and DNA (14). Whereas sequential administration of DOTAP:chol liposomes followed by DNA produced a more than fivefold reduction in cytokine production, peak transgene expression tended to be slightly greater. Further, repeated administration was more effective, presumably due to the lack of initial inflammatory response.

Cationic polymers have also been used to complex and deliver DNA (polyplexes) to the pulmonary circulation. Best studied are polyethylenimine (PEI) complexes. Bragonzi et al. found that although PEI-DNA complexes injected systemically in mice produced relatively selective lung expression, they were not as effective as DOTAP lipoplexes (15). Li et al. found that PEI efficiency was related to structure, with linear PEI being much more efficient than branched PEI (9). They also tested the effect of adding a targeting antibody to the endothelial surface molecule platelet-endothelial cell adhesion molecule (PECAM) to the PEI polyplexes, funding that addition of the PECAM antibody to the complex resulted in a further 1-log increase in transgene expression (16). These complexes still induced a TH1 cytokine response, and pretreatment with the immunosuppressive dexamethasone produced a further increase in peak transgene expression.

There are few studies demonstrating the ability of nonviral vectors to deliver a therapeutically relevant transgene to the pulmonary circulation. Conary and coworkers tested the ability of lipoplex to deliver the prostaglandin G/H synthase gene in rabbits (17). They found increased production of prostacyclin and prostaglandin E2 (PGE2) in serum and lungs. Further, when these lungs were isolated, injury in response to endotoxin infusion was markedly reduced in transgene-expressing lungs. Thus, physiologically relevant expression of prostaglandin G/H synthase appears to have been achieved in rabbit lungs using lipoplex delivery. However, as other studies have demonstrated the reduced ability of lipoplex to transduce an inflamed pulmonary circulation, the utility of gene transfer for established lung inflammation or injury remains speculative.

It appears that nonviral vectors composed of either cationic lipid:cholesterol–DNA complexes or PEI-DNA complexes plus a targeting antibody both result in significant, lung-specific gene expression. The toxicity of lipoplex can be reduced by eliminating unmethylated DNA sequences, pretreatment with immunosuppressives, and possibly by sequential injection of lipid and DNA. However, despite these experimental advances, few reports of physiologically relevant levels of expression of therapeutic transgenes have been published to date. This may be due to two important limitations of non-viral delivery systems: (1) low level of efficiency despite incremental improvement in technology and (2) expression limited to the capillary bed rather than the small and medium sized pulmonary arteries involved in the pathogenesis of most forms of pulmonary vascular disease. Still, these delivery systems may find a role in the treatment of capillary disorders and metastatic cancer and for production of secreted therapeutic molecules.

IV. Viral Gene Delivery

Despite improvement in nonviral gene delivery systems, viral vectors continue to have higher efficiency in most experimental systems. Adenovirus, adeno-associated virus, retrovirus, lentivirus, herpes simplex virus, and others have been used both in the laboratory, and to a much lesser extent, in human trials. Of these potential vectors, studies of adenovirus in the pulmonary circulation are the only ones in the published literature.

LeMarchand and coworkers published the first report of adenovirus-mediated gene delivery to the pulmonary circulation in 1994 (18). In that initial report, the pulmonary circulation of sheep was surgically isolated and perfused with a virus-containing solution. Immunohistochemistry demonstrated gene expression both in the vasculature and airway. Vascular expression was restricted to endothelium. Subsequently, Rodman and coworkers tested the ability to deliver adenoviral vector to the pulmonary circulation via a PA catheter in rats (19). In that study, although lung expression was restricted to the lobe subtended by the catheter, even greater transgene expression was detected in liver. Further complicating that study was the finding of intense inflammatory response in the distal circulation and airspace. However, in contrast to systemic delivery of lipoplex, catheter-directed adenoviral gene delivery resulted in high level expression in the intima of pulmonary arteries up to 1 mm in diameter.

Reynolds and coworkers tested a different strategy for selective lung delivery of adenovirus. They modified a replication-defective adenoviral vector by complexing a bispecific antibody to an angiotensin-converting enzyme (ACE) antibody and the adenoviral fiber knob, thus redirecting expression to ACE-expressing cells (20). As the pulmonary capillary endothelium preferentially expresses ACE, this strategy was predicted to increase lung expression. Lung expression was increased up to 2000-fold by the directed virus compared to untreated adenovirus or blocked antibody. Although expression was reduced in other organs, the specificity was still only relative, and significant ectopic expression remained. Gene expression was detected primarily in pulmonary microvascular endothelium. No significant inflammatory response to the vector was noted in this study.

Continued improvement in adenoviral vectors may permit the use of this system to treat pulmonary vascular disease. To further reduce ectopic gene expression in liver and elsewhere, an endothelial cell specific promotor such as Flt-1 may be used. The inflammatory response can be mitigated by using more advanced vectors in which the full adenoviral DNA sequence has been deleted ("gutless" virus). It may also be useful to delete CpG motifs from the expression cassette by using mammalian promoters and transgene and synthetic elements for the remainder of the sequence. As with the nonviral vectors, no reports of successful expression of a physiologically relevant transgene have been published.

The utility of other viral vectors has not been reported in the literature. Adeno-associated virus appears to have very low infective potential in the circulation. Retrovirus may be useful in situations where there are replicating vascular cells in the lumen of pulmonary blood vessels. Thus, transduction of the developing lung circulation in utero could be possible. Lentivirus, another integrating vector, could be useful in nondividing cells, although its utility in the intact circulation has not been reported. Other viral vectors remain to be tested.

V. Using the Airway for Gene Therapy of Pulmonary Hypertension

Delivery of therapeutic genes via the airway in animal models of pulmonary hypertension has yielded some important, positive results. The rationale for using the airway as a delivery site is based on several empiric observations, including the fact that diffusible gases (such as O_2 and NO) and inhaled medications are able to affect the tone of small pulmonary arteries and that gene delivery via the airway restricts transgene expression to the lung without the need for complex, vector-targeting strategies.

Janssens and coworkers first demonstrated proof of principle for this approach using an adenovirus encoding the NOS3 gene (21). Rats inhaled 3×10^9 pfu of virus encoding NOS3. Four days after transfection, expression in distal airways was confirmed by immunostaining. Lung homogenates demonstrated an 86% increase in NOS activity. Acute hypoxic vasoconstriction was significantly reduced in NOS3-, but not LacZ-transduced rats (5 ± 1 vs 10 ± 1 mmHg, $P < .05$). Subsequently, the same group used a NOS2-encoding adenovirus (22). Aerosolization of 3×10^9 pfu of virus lead to a doubling of exhaled NO 3 days after transfection. Rats placed into 10% O_2 for 7 days immediately following transfection demonstrated significantly lower mean PA pressure (21 ± 1 vs 27 ± 1 mmHg, $P < .05$), as well as reduced RV hypertrophy and fewer muscular pulmonary arterioles.

Following a similar line of reasoning, Geraci and coworkers constructed an adenovirus encoding the prostacyclin synthase (PGIS) gene (23). They introduced this gene via the airway in rats, causing a significant reduction in hypoxic pulmonary vasoconstriction not seen in AdV-LacZ–treated controls. Attenuation of chronic hypoxic pulmonary hypertension was also seen, although the presence of inflammation in response to the vector makes interpretation of these results uncertain. Nagaya et al. introduced PGIS via the airway using HVJ liposomes 2 days before treatment with monocrotaline (24). They found a significant reduction in mean PA pressure (31 ± 1 vs 35 ± 1 mmHg, $P < .05$) and improved survival when vector was administered every 2 weeks.

The latter studies were directed at increasing endogenous vasodilator synthesis (either NO or PGI2) in the lung. Partovian and coworkers took a different approach, testing the ability of gene transfer of VEGF to inhibit the development of hypoxic pulmonary hypertension in rats (25). The rationale for this experiment was the observations that VEGF expression was increased in chronically hypoxic rat lungs and inhibition of VEGF, in the setting of chronic hypoxia, lead to marked intimal proliferation and pulmonary hypertension (26). They constructed a recombinant adenovirus encoding vascular endothelial growth factor-165 (VEGF-165) under control of the CMV promotor/enhancer. After aerosol delivery of 10^8 pfu, increased lung lavage VEGF could be detected both at 2 and 17 days after transfection. Mean PA pressure was reduced from 30 ± 2 mmHg in control to 25 ± 1 mmHg in AdV-VEGF treated rats ($P < .05$), along with a reduction in right ventricular hypertrophy. Preservation of lung NO production was found in Ad-VEGF–treated rats, suggesting that a mechanism of action of VEGF gene transfer may have been preservation of endothelial function. Subsequently the same group overexpressed the tissue inhibitor of metalloproteinase-1 (TIMP-1) gene and found a marked augmentation of hypoxic pulmonary hypertension (27). This suggests the possibility that expression of counterregulatory enzymes, such as matrix metalloproteinases (MMPs) might be useful in treating pulmonary hypertension.

Although the airway appears to be a suitable route of delivery for therapeutic genes in pulmonary hypertension, rodents appear to be far more amenable to viral vector transduction than is the human airway. Also, the toxicity of long-term overproduction of molecules such as NO and VEGF is unknown. Still, these provocative studies suggest that the airway should be considered a potential route of delivery for gene therapy of pulmonary vascular disorders.

VI. Conclusions

The technology of pulmonary vascular gene delivery has evolved significantly since the first edition of this book was published in 1997. The mechanisms through which nonviral vectors preferentially target the lung have been partially elucidated, and the inflammatory response to lipoplex has been carefully studied. Targeting strategies involving recognition of pulmonary endothelial cell surface proteins, such as PECAM and ACE, have been employed further to enhance lung selective expression. Despite these advances, several significant barriers to pulmonary vascular gene delivery remain, and few studies of therapeutic genes of interest have been published; none in humans. Once these barriers are overcome, we can expect studies of the utility of pulmonary vascular expression of a variety of genes of interest, including those which modulate vascular reactivity and structure (e.g., NOS, prostaglandin synthase, VEGF, MMPs, endothelin-1 [ET-1] antisense) and those which modulate the immune response (e.g., FAS-ligand, IL-10, bone morphogenic protein (BMP)) will be reported.

References

1. Messina M, Podrazik RM, Whitehill TA, et al. Adhesion and incorporation of lacZ-transduced endothelial cells into the intact capillary wall in the rat. Proc Natl Acad Sci USA 1992; 89:12018–12022.
2. Campbell AIM, Kuliszewski MA, Stewart DJ. Cell-based transfer to the pulmonary vasculature: endothelial nitric oxide synthase overexpression inhibits monocrotaline-induced pulmonary hypertension. Am J Respir Cell Mol Biol 1999; 21:567–575.
3. Zhu N, Liggitt D, Yong L, Debs R. Systemic gene expression after intravenous DNA delivery into adult mice. Science 1993; 261:209–212.
4. Brigham KL, Meyrick BO, Christman B, Magnuson M, King G, Berry LC Jr. Rapid communication: in vivo transfection of murine lungs with a functioning prokaryotic gene using a liposome vehicle. Am J Med Sci 1989; 296:278–281.
5. Floch V, Delepine P, Guillaume C, Loisel S, et al. Systemic administration of cationic phosphonolipids/DNA complexes and the relationship between formulation and lung transfection efficiency. Biochem Biophys Acta 2000; 1464:95–103.
6. Thierry AR, Lunardi-Iskandar Y, Dryant JL, et al. Systemic gene therapy: biodistribution and long-term expression of a transgene in mice. Proc Natl Acad Sci USA 1995; 92:9742–9746.
7. Solodin I, Brown CS, Bruno MS, et al. A novel series of amphiphilic imidazolinium

compounds for in vitro and in vivo gene delivery. Biochemistry 1995; 34:13537–13544.

8. Li S, Tseng WC, Stolz DB, et al. Dynamic changes in the characteristics of cationic lipidic vectors after exposure to mouse serum: implications for intravenous lipofection. Gene Ther 1999; 6:585–594.

9. Li S, Rizzo MA, Bhattacharya S, Huang L. Characterization of cationic lipid-protamine-DNA (LPD) complexes for intravenous gene delivery. Gene Ther 1998; 5:930–937.

10. Dow SW, Fradkin LG, Liggitt DH, et al. Lipid-DNA complexes induce potent activation of innate immune responses and antitumor activity when administered intravenously. J Immunol 1999; 163:1552–1561.

11. Tyler RC, Fagan KA, Unfer RC, et al. Vascular inflammation inhibits gene transfer to the pulmonary circulation in vivo. Am J Physiol (Lung Cell Mol Physiol 21) 1999; 277:L1199–L1204.

12. Li S, Wu S-P, Whitmore M, et al. Effect of immune response on gene transfer to the lung via systemic administration of cationic lipidic vectors. Am J Physiol (Lung Cell Mol Physiol 20) 1999; 276:L796–L804.

13. Hofman CR, Dileo JP, Li Z, et al. Efficient in vivo gene transfer by PCR amplified fragment with reduced inflammatory activity. Gene Ther 2001; 8:71–74.

14. Tan Y, Liu F, Li Z, et al. Sequential injection of cationic liposome and plasmid DNA effectively transfects the lung with minimal inflammatory toxicity. Mol Ther 2001; 3:673–682.

15. Bragonzi A, Boletta A, Biffi A, et al. Comparison between cationic polymers and lipids in mediating systemic gene delivery to the lungs. Gene Ther 1999; 6:1995–2004.

16. Li S, Tan Y, Viroonchatapan E, et al. Targeted gene delivery to the pulmonary endothelium by anti-PECAM antibody. Am J Physiol (Lung Cell Mol Physiol) 2000; 278:L504–L511.

17. Conary JT, Parker RE, Christman BW, et al. Protection of rabbit lungs from endotoxin injury by in vivo hyperexpression of the prostaglandin G/H synthase gene. J Clin Invest 1994; 93:1834–1840.

18. Lemarchand P, Jones M, Danel C, Yamada I, Mastrageli A, Crystal RG. In vivo adenovirus-mediated gene transfer to the lungs via pulmonary artery. J Appl Physiol 1994; 76:2840–2845.

19. Rodman DM, San H, Simari R, Stephan D, Tanner F, Yang Z, Nabel GJ, Nabel EG. In vivo gene delivery to the pulmonary circulation in rats: transgene distribution and vascular inflammatory response. Am J Respir Cell Mol Biol 1997; 16:640–649.

20. Reynolds PN, Zinn KR, Gavilyuk VD, Balyasnikova IV, et al. A targetable, injectable adenoviral vector for selective gene delivery to pulmonary endothelium in vivo. Mol Ther 2000; 2:562–578.

21. Janssens SP, Block KD, Nong Z, Gerard RD, et al. Adenoviral-mediated transfer of the human endothelial nitric oxide synthase gene reduces acute hypoxic vasoconstriction in rats. J Clin Invest 1996; 98:317–324.

22. Budts W, Pokreisz P, Nong Z, Van Pelt N, et al. Aerosol gene transfer with inducible nitric oxide synthase reduces hypoxic pulmonary hypertension and pulmonary vascular remodeling in rats. Circulation 2000; 102:2880–2885.

23. Geraci M, Gao B, Shepherd D, Allard J, et al. Pulmonary prostacyclin synthase overexpression by adenovirus transfection and in transgenic mice. Chest 1998; 114: 99S.

24. Nagaya N, Yokoyama C, Kyotani S, Shimonishi M, et al. Gene transfer of human prostacyclin synthase ameliorates monocrotaline-induced pulmonary hypertension in rats. Circulation 2000; 102:2005–2010.

25. Partovian C, Adnot S, Raffestin B, Louzier V, et al. Adenovirus-mediated lung vascular endothelial growth factor overexpression protects against hypoxic pulmonary hypertension in rats. Am J Respir Cell Mol Biol 2000; 23:762–771.

26. Taraseviciene-Stewart L, Kasahara Y, Alger L, Hirth P, et al. Inhibition of the VEGF receptor 2 combined with chronic hypoxia causes cell death-dependent pulmonary endothelial cell proliferation and severe pulmonary hypertension. FASEB J 2001; 15:427–438.

27. Vieillard-Baron A, Frisdal E, Edahibi S, Deprez I, et al. Inhibition of matrix metalloproteinases by lung TIMP-1 gene transfer or doxycycline aggravates pulmonary hypertension in rats. Circ Res 2000; 87:418–425.

16

Gene Therapy for α_1-Antitrypsin Deficiency

TERENCE R. FLOTTE

Powell Gene Therapy Center
and University of Florida Genetics Institute
University of Florida College of Medicine
Gainesville, Florida, U.S.A.

I. Introduction

α_1-Antitrypsin (AAT) is an abundant 52-kD serum protein that normally functions as a major serine proteinase inhibitor in the serum, counteracting the effects of neutrophil elastase (NE), cathespin G, proteinase-3, alpha defensins, and other neutrophil-derived proinflammatory molecules. AAT deficiency results in the accelerated loss of interstitial elastin from the pulmonary parenchyma, as well as increased air space inflammation, ultimately leading to the development of pulmonary emphysema. AAT deficiency could represent a very favorable target for gene therapy, since the primary function of this protein is in the extracellular environment, and since the threshold levels for protection of the lungs have been established at 11 μM, which is approximately 500–800 μg/mL. A number of groups have attempted to solve the problem of AAT gene therapy, utilizing vectors such as recombinant adenovirus (rAd), murine retrovirus, cationic liposomes, and naked DNA injection without a clear indication of success. The advantages and disadvantages of these systems are listed in Table 1. Recently, a new group of gene transfer modalities have been employed, including helper-dependent Ad (hd-Ad), chimeraplasty, simian virus 40 (SV40), and recombinant adeno-

Table 1 Advantages and Disadvantages of Some Commonly Used Gene Transfer
Vectors

Vector	Advantages	Disadvantages
Nonviral	High capacity	Low efficiency
	Safe (?)	Transient
Murine retrovirus	Stable	Require mitosis
		Insertional mutagenesis
Recombinant adenovirus	Efficient	Inflammation
(early generations)	Nondividing cells	Immune responses
Helper-dependent	Efficient	Some acute inflammation
adenovirus	Nondividing cells	Contamination with helper
	Stable	
	Less immunogenic	
	High capacity	
Adeno-associated virus	Efficient	Low capacity
	Stable	? Insertional mutagenesis
	Nondividing cells	
	Not proinflammatory	

associated virus (rAAV). In this chapter, the advantages and disadvantages of
each system and the status of proof-of-concept studies and preclinical development will be discussed.

II. Retrovirus Vectors

The first viruses to be adapted for eukaryotic gene transfer were the murine onco-
retroviruses, such as the Moloney murine leukemia virus (MMLV). MMLV is
an enveloped single-stranded RNA virus that requires reverse transcription from
RNA to DNA and subsequent integration of the cDNA provirus into the host
genome in order to complete its life cycle. The MMLV gene consists of two
genes, *gag-pol* and *env*. The *gag-pol* open reading frame encodes both the matrix
gag protein and the reverse transcriptase enzyme required for RNA-dependent
DNA polymerization. The *env* gene encodes the surface envelope glycoprotein.
These genes are flanked by two long terminal repeat (LTR) sequences, which
are required *in cis* for replication. The left-hand LTR also has promoter activity,
and just downstream from the left-hand LTR is the packaging signal, *psi*.

MMLV vectors were produced by deleting *gag-pol* and *env* and inserted
the transgene of interest into a *psi*$^+$, long terminal repeat-positive (LTR$^+$) cassette.
In order for such a construct to be packaged, it must be transfected into packaging
cell lines that constitutively express *gag-pol* and *env* from elsewhere in the nu-

cleus. The producer cell lines resulting from that transfection will bud recombinant virions off into the supernatant media. The vector virions, if packaged with the appropriate amphotrophic envelope, can transduce a range of mammalian cells. The major constraint on this system is that MMLV vectors require active cell mitosis in order to gain access to host cell DNA for integration.

These MMLV-based vectors have been extensively utilized to transfer eukaryotic genes, and were used for AAT gene transfer as well. Early studies focused on transplanting mouse fibroblasts that had been transduced to make them stable expressers of AAT (1,2). Subsequent studies utilized hepatocyte-directed AAT gene transfer in vivo (3) in mice after partial hepatectomy. The partial hepatectomy was used to induce hepatocyte proliferation. In a similar approach, hepatocytes removed after partial hepatectomy were reimplanted after retroviral-AAT transduction (4). Levels of AAT produced in these animals were significantly higher than had been previously seen, exceeding 1.4 µg/mL in the serum and were stable for 6 months after transduction. However, the levels were still well short of the therapeutic target of 500–800 µg/mL.

III. Recombinant Adenoviral Vectors

The rAV vectors that have been most extensively characterized in preclinical and clinical studies are based on the group C adenoviruses, serotypes 2 and 5. The viruses on which these vectors are based are nonenveloped, double-stranded DNA viruses that tend to cause transient mild inflammatory illnesses in the respiratory tract of normal individuals. Ad has evolved to be very efficient at cell attachment, entry, lysomal escape, and nuclear import. These viruses have been adapted for transferring genes to a wide range of target cell populations, including bronchial epithelial cells, hepatocytes, cardiac myocytes, and others, and have been used extensively in studies of the feasibility of AAT gene transfer.

The life cycle of Ad-15 has been well characterized. The fiber knob of the Ad-5 capsid binds to an initial attachment receptor, which has been identified as the coxsackie adenoviral receptor (CAR). A second interaction must then occur between the RGD (arginine-glycine-aspartate) motif on the penton base of Ad and its receptor, the α_v, β_5-integrin, in order for viral internalization to occur. Infection of permissive cells is followed within a few hours by the expression of the immediate early gene E1a, a multifunctional transcription regulator that controls the expression of an entire series of other early genes (E2a, E3, E4) which are required for viral DNA synthesis. After DNA replication, another series of genes, the late genes (L1, L2, L3) are expressed. These encode the structural components of the virion.

First-generation rAd vectors were produced by deleting portions of the immediate early gene, E1a. This produced a vector that can replicate conditionally within cells such as human embryonic kidney (HEK-293) cells, which express E1a, but not within the intended target cells. Some of these vectors are also deleted for E3, which is not required for replication of the virus. The resulting vectors still contained about 90% of the Ad genome, but could package up to 6 kb of exogenous DNA. First-generation rAd vectors were found to be highly efficient, albeit transient, gene transfer vehicles. rAd-AAT vectors were the first to be shown to be effective for gene transfer in vivo (5). Human AAT was detectable in the bronchoalveolar lavage fluid for 1 week after in vivo intratracheal injection of rAd-hAAT in cotton rats. The levels of AAT produced were low, but local expression within the lung was cited as a potential way to derive some benefit from these levels (6), since about two-thirds of the AAT produced from Ad vector–transduced cells was secreted from the apical surface. Subsequent studies showed that similar vectors were also efficient for gene transfer in nonhuman primates. In addition to lung delivery, it was shown that ectopic AAT secretion could be obtained after intraperitoneal or intradermal injection of rAd-AAT (7,8). However, the first-generation rAd vectors were limited by an immediate proinflammatory cytokine response, which represented an innate immune response, as well as by antigen-specific cytotoxic T-cell and antibody responses.

Later generation rAd vectors were then constructed by disabling or deleting other early genes, such as E2a and E4. These vectors were modestly less immunogenic, but still elicited proinflammatory cytokine responses and were generally not persistent over long periods of time. Most recently, new methods have been employed to delete all of the endogenous Ad genes. These helper-dependent Ad vectors may be particularly promising for AAT gene transfer, since they allow for the incorporation of large regions of genomic DNA including the endogenous AAT promoter sequence, which appears to promote persistence. The details of this system will be discussed in detail below.

IV. Helper-Dependent Adenoviral Vectors

In this context, hd-Ad vectors are considered separately, since their performance characteristics in vivo appear to be distinct from earlier generation rAd vectors. As mentioned above, the recombinant hd-Ad vector is deleted for all viral genes and retains only the small terminal repeats and packaging *psi* signal *in cis*. Packaging of these hdAd vectors, which are also known as high-capacity Ad, gutless Ad or gutted Ad, is accomplished by culturing them along with a second helper adenovirus which expresses all of the early and late genes required for replication and packaging of the vector. A number of techniques have been employed to enable the selective packaging of the vector genome instead of the helper genome. These strategies include the inclusion of *loxP* sites flanking the *psi* packaging signal in the helper virus, or the direct transfection of oversized Ad genomes to provide helper function.

The hd-Ad system has two major advantages over earlier rAd vectors. First, the amount of DNA that can be packaged is increased to over 30 kb, which allows for the incorporation of the entire AAT genomic locus. Second, the deletion of viral genes greatly reduces the host immune response to the vector. These two biological advantages combine to produce a system that has been shown to be capable of producing sustained serum levels of AAT within the therapeutic range in rodents and primates after delivery either to skeletal muscle or to liver (9,10). The major current limitation of this system is that there is some degree of contamination with the helper Ad, which ranges from 1 to 10% in most preparations.

V. Nonviral DNA Transfer

Cationic lipids are amphipathic molecules consisting of positively charged headgroups capable of interacting with the negatively charged backbone of DNA and hydrophobic tail groups that facilitate interaction with the cell membrane. Cationic lipid–DNA complexes (liposomes) often incorporate a neutral colipid to facilitate membrane fusion and endosomal escape. Cationic liposomes have been used successfully to transfer plasmid DNA containing the AAT cDNA to the lungs of rabbits (11–13). This method was not associated with any pathology in these early studies, but the levels of AAT produced were generally low, and expression was transient, necessitating repeated administration. Likewise, cationic liposome–mediated delivery of the AAT cDNA to the liver was generally well tolerated in experimental animals (14,15). Subsequent studies of aerosol delivery of cationic liposomes in cystic fibrosis patients has indicated that inflammatory responses are produced. These responses appear to be specific to the presence of undermethylated CpG motifs in the plasmid DNA.

Another mode of nonviral gene delivery that has been used to transfer AAT is gold-particle bombardment, also known as ballistic gene transfer, using a device known as a gene gun. In this method, naked plasmid DNA or RNA is coated onto gold spheres which are then propelled into cells or tissues using a pulse of compressed air. The gene gun technique was used to deliver the AAT mRNA to rodent liver. Levels of expression were detectable, but low, and expression was transient.

VI. Recombinant Adeno-Associated Vectors

The rAAV vectors have theoretical advantages as vehicles for human gene therapy, because they are based on a virus that is nonpathogenic and has a natural mechanism for long-term persistence in human cells (16–18). rAAV vectors were prepared by generating proviral rAAV vector plasmids deleted for the viral pro-

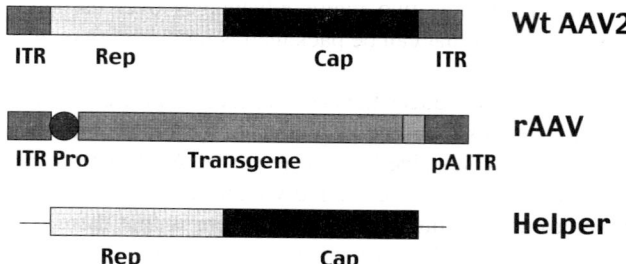

Figure 1 Simplified map of the recombinant AAV genome. The wild-type AAV-2 genome is shown in the top diagram, with "ITR" indicating the inverted terminal repeat sequences, "Rep" indicating the *rep* gene, and "Cap" gene. In the middle diagram, a recombinant AAV genome is depicted with an exogenous promoter (Pro) and polyadenylation signal (pA) inserted flanking the transgene of interest. In the bottom panel is shown the complementing helper plasmid which supplies Rep and Cap functions in trans to allow the rAAV vector to be packaged.

teins, *rep* and *cap*, and substituting the gene of interest (cystic fibrosis transmembrane conductance regulator [CFTR], AAT, or interleukin-10 [IL-10]) between the rAAV2 inverted terminal repeats (ITRs) (Fig. 1) with appropriate promoter and polyadenylation signal sequences. The packaging limit for such cassettes is approximately 5 kb. Recombinant AAV genomes are packaged into infectious virions using a cotransfection technique in which the vector plasmid is cotransfected into HEK-293 cells along with the helper plasmid, pDG, encoding the rAAV-2 *rep* and *cap* genes, as well as the necessary adenoviral helper functions (19). rAAV virions are released by lysing cells 48–72 hr after the transfection and purified using a combination of density gradient ultracentrifugation and/or affinity chromatography (20). All vector preparations are characterized with respect to their physical titer (total Dnase-resistant particles) and their biological titer (infectious units) and are screened for the presence of any contaminating replication-competent AAV prior to use in transduction experiments.

The rAAV system was first clinically exploited for gene therapy of cystic fibrosis (CF). A total of four clinical trials of the rAAV-CFTR vector have now been completed. These encompass 70 individuals with CF treated with doses from 6×10^4 to 1×10^{13} Dnase-resistant particles (drp) per administration to the surface of the nose, maxillary sinus, or bronchus (21–26). No vector-related adverse effects have been observed. Transgene expression has been detected at doses of 6×10^8 drp in the sinus or 1×10^{13} drp in the lung. Phase II trials are ongoing.

rAAV vectors have now been developed for the therapy of α_1-antitrypsin

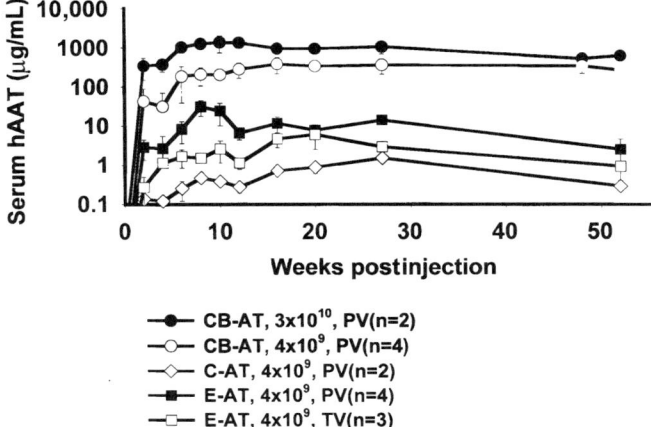

Figure 2 Stable expression of the human alpha 1-antitrypsin gene (AAT) after injection of rAAV vectors into the portal or systemic venous circulation in C57/B16 mice. Animals were treated with various rAAV-hAAT vectors at the doses indicated (C-AT = cytomegalovirus [CMV] immediate early promoter driving AAT, E-AT = human elongation factor 1 alpha promoter vector, CB-AT = CMV enhancer/chicken beta actin promoter hybrid construct; PV = portal vein injection; TV = tail vein injection). Doses of vector are indicated in infectious units. [Data from Ref. 31.]

(AAT) deficiency (27–29). Preparations of rAAV-hAAT have been extensively characterized in cell culture systems and animal models. In vivo studies in mice (29–31) have demonstrated long-term gene transfer and expression (>18 months for AAT) without any detectable pathology. These studies have also demonstrated that therapeutic levels of AAT can be achieved in mice by delivery to muscle (29,30), liver (31), or lung (32) (Fig. 2). The levels produced by intramuscular injection were approximately 0.8 mg/mL, which is above the threshold for lung protection, whereas the levels produced by direct portal vein injection reached 2 mg/mL. Interestingly, studies of rAAV-AAT in mice indicate that the vector DNA persists in long strings or concatemers that are episomal; that is, physically separate from the host cell chromosome (in contrast with the naturally occurring form of the virus) and that host cell factors, such as the DNA-dependent protein kinase play a role in this process (30,33–36). This could allow for the DNA to persist without incurring the potential risk of disrupting host cell genes. A phase I trial of rAAV-AAT in AAT-deficient patients is anticipated.

In preparation for Phase I trial, a series of additional formal preclinical toxicology and biodistribution studies have been performed in mice and nonhuman primates. In the first of these studies, a series of mice were injected with doses of rAAV2-hAAT vector ranging up as high as 3×10^{12} IU per animal (1.2×10^{14} IU p/kg; 2.5×10^{15} vector genomes/p kg). Animals were carefully studied with complete blood counts, serum chemistries, and timed necropsies out to 90 days after injection with complete histopathological examination of all organs. There was no evidence of any inflammation or other pathology in any of these animals. In a related study, vector dissemination was studied in cohorts of mice treated with doses again ranging up to 2.5×10^{15} vector genomes/kg either by the intramuscular or intravenous routes, and vector copy number was assessed in the blood, gonads, and various visceral organs at time points up to 60 days. Although vector DNA was present in the blood and in organs with high blood flow such as the liver, spleen, and kidney, these disseminated vector sequences did not persist past the first 10 days in any of the intramuscular injected animals, although persistence in the blood was seen in the highest dosage cohort of the intravenous injection group. Importantly, no vector sequences were noted in the gonads of any of the injected animals.

Another study was performed in baboons in order to determine whether vector dose ranging was appropriate and whether vector dissemination to the gonads might be different in a larger animal. These studies were initially performed with the same rAAV1-hAAT vector, but after the first four animals were injected, it was found that the animals developed antibodies to the human AAT. A baboon AAT vector was constructed with a C-terminal *myc* tag. Vector expression in animals injected with doses up to 3×10^{12} IU of this vector (equivalent to 5×10^{13} vector genomes or 5×10^{12} vector genomes/kg) was confirmed by immunostaining of the injected muscle. Once again there was no evidence of spread of vector DNA to the gonads. Based on all of these studies, a Phase I trial of intramuscular administration of rAAV-AAT is planned.

VII. Other Novel Systems

A number of other novel systems for gene augmentation or gene repair have been recently described in the AAT gene therapy literature. These include the use of SV40-derived vectors for direct delivery of the hAAT cDNA to the liver (37) and the use of RNA-DNA chimeras capable of single-nucleotide correction of genomic DNA (38,39). The potential advantages of the latter system are multiple, given the potential for complete physiological regulation of AAT gene expression. These vector systems are in the early stages of development, however, and the real potential of these for clinical gene therapy remains unclear.

VIII. Conclusions

Many studies have demonstrated the feasibility of using gene transfer technology to express the AAT gene. Some key studies with helper-dependent Ad and rAAV in animal models have shown that potentially therapeutic serum levels can be obtained and sustained for at least 6–18 months. Although the ability of these results to directly translate into clinical therapy remains far from proven, there is a definite indication that these agents will be available for investigational use in humans in the near future.

Acknowledgments

This work was supported by grants from the NHLBI (HL51811, HL59412), the NIDDK (DK51809, DK58327), the Cystic Fibrosis Foundation and the Alpha One Foundation.

References

1. Garver RI, Chytil A, Courtney M, Crystal RG. Clonal gene therapy: transplanted mouse fibroblast clones express human alpha 1-antitrypsin gene in vivo. Science 1987; 237:762–464.

2. Garver RI, Chytil A, Courtney M, Crystal RG. Clonal gene therapy: in vivo expression of a transplanted monoclonal population of murine fibroblasts containing a retrovirus inserted human alpha 1-antitrypsin gene. Trans Assoc Am Physicians 1987; 100:10–20.

3. Kay MA, Li Q, Liu TJ, Leland F, Toman C, Finegold M, Woo SL. Hepatic gene therapy: persistent expression of human alpha 1-antitrypsin in mice after direct gene delivery in vivo. Hum Gene Ther 1992; 3:641–647.

4. Kay MA, Baley P, Rothenberg S, Leland F, Fleming L, Ponder KP, Liu T, Finegold M, Darlington G, Pokorny W, Woo SL. Expression of human alpha 1-antitrypsin in dogs after autologous transplantation of retroviral transduced hepatocytes. Proc Natl Acad Sci USA 1992; 89:89–93.

5. Rosenfeld MA, Siegfried W, Yoshimura K, Yoneyama K, Fukayama M, Stier LE, Paakko PK, Gilardi P, Stratford-Perricaudet LD, Perricaudet M, Crystal RG. Adenovirus-mediated transfer of a recombinant alpha 1-antitrypsin gene to the lung epithelium in vivo. Science 1991; 252:431–434.

6. Siegfried W, Rosenfeld M, Stier L, Stratford-Perricaudet L, Perricaudet M, Pavirani A, Lecocq JP, Crystal RG. Polarity of secretion of alpha 1-antitrypsin by human respiratory epithelial cells after adenoviral transfer of a human alpha 1-antitrypsin cDNA. Am J Respir Cell Mol Biol 1995; 12:379–384.

7. Setoguchi Y, Jaffe HA, Danel C, Crystal RG. Ex vivo and in vivo gene transfer to the skin using replication-deficient recombinant adenovirus vectors. J Invest Dermatol 1994; 102:415–421.

8. Setoguchi Y, Jaffe HA, Chu CS, Crystal RG. Intraperitoneal in vivo gene therapy to deliver alpha 1-antitrypsin to the systemic circulation. Am J Respir Cell Mol Biol 1994; 10:369–377.

9. Morral N, Parks RJ, Zhou H, Langston C, Schiedner G, Quinones J, Graham FL, Kochanek S, Beaudet AL. High doses of a helper-dependent adenoviral vector yield

supraphysiological levels of alpha 1-antitrypsin with negligible toxicity. Hum Gene Ther 1998; 9:2709–2716.

10. Schiedner G, Morral N, Parks RJ, Wu Y, Koopmans SC, Langston C, Graham FL, Beaudet AL, Kochanek S. Genomic DNA transfer with a high-capacity adenovirus vector results in improved in vivo gene expression and decreased toxicity. Nat Genet 1998; 18:180–183.

11. Canonico AE, Plitman JD, Conary JT, Meyrick BO, Brigham KL. No lung toxicity after repeated aerosol or intravenous delivery of plasmid-cationic liposome complexes. J Appl Physiol 1994; 77:415–419.

12. Canonico AE, Conary JT, Meyrick BO, Brigham KL. Aerosol and intravenous transfection of human alpha 1-antitrypsin gene to lungs of rabbits. Am J Respir Cell Mol Biol 1994; 10:24–29.

13. Canonico AE, Brigham KL, Carmichael LC, Plitman JD, King GA, Blackwell TR, Christman JW. Plasmid-liposome transfer of the alpha 1-antitrypsin gene to cystic fibrosis bronchial epithelial cells prevents elastase-induced cell detachment and cytokine release. Am J Respir Cell Mol Biol 1996; 14:348–355.

14. Alino SF, Crespo J, Bobadilla M, Lejarreta M, Blaya C, Crespo A. Expression of human alpha 1-antitrypsin in mouse after in vivo gene transfer to hepatocytes by small liposomes. Biochem Biophys Res Commun 1994; 204:1023–1030.

15. Alino SF, Bobadilla M, Crespo J, Lejarreta M. Human alpha 1-antitrypsin gene transfer to in vivo mouse hepatocytes. Hum Gene Ther 1996; 7:531–536.

16. Berns KI, Linden RM. The cryptic life style of adeno-associated virus. Bioessays 1995; 17:237–245.

17. Blacklow NR, Hoggan MD, Kapikian AZ, Austin JB, Rowe WP. Epidemiology of adenovirus-associated virus infection in a nursery population. Am J Epidemiol 1968; 88:368–378.

18. Blacklow NR. Adeno-associated viruses of humans. In: Pattison JR, ed., Parvoviruses and Human Disease. Boca Raton, FL: CRC Press, 1988;165–174.

19. Grimm D, Kern A, Rittner K, Kleinschmidt JA. Novel tools for production and purification of recombinant adenoassociated virus vectors. Hum Gene Ther 1998; 9:2745–2760.

20. Zolotukhin S, Byrne BJ, Mason E, Zolotukhin I, Potter M, Chesnut K, Summerford C, Samulski RJ, Muzyczka N. Recombinant adeno-associated virus purification using novel methods improves infectious titer and yield. Gene Ther 1999; 6:973–985.

21. Flotte T, Carter B, Conrad C, Guggino W, Reynolds T, Rosenstein B, Taylor G, Walden S, Wetzel R. A phase I study of an adeno-associated virus–CFTR gene vector in adult CF patients with mild lung disease. Hum Gene Ther 1996; 7:1145–1159.

22. Virella-Lowell I, Poirier A, Chesnut KA, Brantly M, Flotte TR. Inhibition of recombinant adeno-associated virus (rAAV) transduction by bronchial secretions from cystic fibrosis patients. Gene Ther 2000; 7:1783–1789.

23. Wagner JA, Reynolds T, Moran ML, Moss RB, Wine JJ, Flotte TR, Gardner P. Efficient and persistent gene transfer of AAV-CFTR in maxillary sinus. Lancet 1998; 351:1702–1703.

24. Wagner JA, Moran ML, Messner AH, Daifuku R, Conrad CK, Reynolds T, Guggino

WB, Moss RB, Carter BJ, Wine JJ, Flotte TR, Gardner P. A phase I/II study of tgAAV-CF for the treatment of chronic sinusitis in patients with cystic fibrosis. Hum Gene Ther 1998; 9:889–909.

25. Wagner JA, Nepomuceno IB, Messner AH, Moran MI, Batson EP, Desch JK, Norbash AM, Conrad CK, Guggino WB, Flotte TR, Wine JJ, Carter BJ, Moss RB, Gardner P. A phase II, double-blind, randomized, placebo-controlled clinical trial of tgAAVCF using maxillary sinus delivery in CF patients with antrostomies. Human Gene Therapy 2002. In press.

26. Wagner JA, Messner AH, Moran ML, Daifuku R, Kouyama K, Desch JK, Manly S, Norbash AM, Conrad CK, Friborg S, Reynolds T, Guggino WB, Moss RB, Carter BJ, Wine JJ, Flotte TR, Gardner P. Safety and biological efficacy of an adeno-associated virus vector-cystic fibrosis transmembrane conductance regulator (AAV-CFTR) in the cystic fibrosis maxillary sinus. Laryngoscope 1999; 109:266–274.

27. Flotte TR, Afione SA, Conrad C, Mcgrath SA, Solow R, Oka H, Zeitlin PL, Guggino WB, Carter BJ. Stable in vivo expression of the cystic fibrosis transmembrane conductance regulator with an adeno-associated virus vector. Proc Natl Acad Sci USA 1993; 90:10613–10617.

28. Flotte TR, Carter BJ. Adeno-associated virus vectors for gene therapy of cystic fibrosis. Methods Enzymol 1998; 292:717–732.

29. Song S, Morgan M, Ellis T, Poirier A, Chesnut K, Wang J, Brantly M, Muzyczka N, Byrne BJ, Atkinson M, Flotte TR. Sustained secretion of human alpha 1-antitrypsin from murine muscle transduced with adeno-associated virus vectors. Proc Natl Acad Sci USA 1998; 95:14384–14385.

30. Song S, Laipis PJ, Berns KI, Flotte TR. Effect of DNA-dependent protein kinase on the molecular fate of the rAAV2 genome in skeletal muscle. Proc Natl Acad Sci USA 2001; 98:4084–4088.

31. Song S, Laipis P, Embury J, Berns K, Crawford J, Flotte TR. Stable therapeutic serum levels of human alpha-1 antitrypsin (AAT) after portal vein injection of recombinant adeno-associated virus (rAAV) vectors. Gene Ther 2001; 8:1299–1306.

32. Virella-Lowell I, Zusman B, Conlon T, Morgan M, Chesnut KA, Ferkol T, Flotte TR. A CMV/beta actin hybrid promoter enhances rAAV vector expression in the lung. Submitted.

33. Flotte TR, Afione SA, Zeitlin PL. Adeno-associated virus vector gene expression occurs in nondividing cells in the absence of vector DNA integration. Am J Respir Cell Mol Biol 1994; 11:517–521.

34. Afione SA, Conrad CK, Kearns WG, Chunduru S, Adams R, Reynolds TC, Guggino WB, Cutting GR, Carter BJ, Flotte TR. In vivo model of adeno-associated virus vector persistence and rescue. J Virol 1996; 70:3235–3241.

35. Kearns WG, Afione SA, Fulmer SB, Pang MC, Erikson D, Egan M, Landrum MJ, Flotte TR, Cutting GR. Recombinant adeno-associated virus (AAV-CFTR) vectors do not integrate in a site-specific fashion in an immortalized epithelial cell line. Gene Ther 1996; 3:748–755.

36. Hernandez YJ, Wang J, Kearns WG, Loiler S, Poirier A, Flotte TR. Latent adeno-associated virus infection elicits humoral but not cell-mediated immune responses in a nonhuman primate model. J Virol 1999; 73:8549–8558.

37. Zern MA, Ozaki I, Duan L, Pomerantz R, Liu SL, Strayer DS. A novel SV40-based vector successfully transduces and expresses an alpha 1-antitrypsin ribozyme in a human hepatoma-derived cell line. Gene Ther 1999; 6:114–120.
38. Kren BT, Parashar B, Bandyopadhyay P, Chowdhury NR, Chowdhury JR, Steer CJ. Correction of the UDP-glucuronosyltransferase gene defect in the gunn rat model of Crigler-Najjar syndrome type I with a chimeric oligonucleotide. Proc Natl Acad Sci USA 1999; 96:10349–10354.
39. Kren BT, Cole-Strauss A, Kmiec EB, Steer CJ. Targeted nucleotide exchange in the alkaline phosphatase gene of HuH-7 cells mediated by a chimeric RNA/DNA oligonucleotide. Hepatology 1997; 25:1462–1468.

17

Gene Therapy and Gene Transfer Approaches for Acute Lung Injury

DANIEL J. WEISS

Vermont Lung Center
University of Vermont College of Medicine
Burlington, Vermont, U.S.A.

I. Introduction

Efforts toward gene therapy of lung diseases have primarily focused on genetic lung diseases, such as cystic fibrosis (CF) and α_1-antitrypsin deficiency. For these diseases, the therapeutic goal is amelioration of a genetic defect and its physiological consequences by addition of the normal gene to affected cells. However, using gene transfer both to study and treat acute and acquired lung diseases and acute lung injury remains a potentially powerful and less well-explored approach.

There are many potential advantages for gene therapy of acute lung injury. For example, gene transfer can result in cell-specific expression of therapeutic molecules with the use of appropriate vectors and cell-specific promoters. Transgene expression that restores production of crucial biological mediators affected by the acute illness may be beneficial. Transfer of genes encoding for therapeutic intracellular or secreted substances that modulate inflammation accompanying acute lung disease may result in higher levels than administration of the substances themselves. Moreover, transgene expression need not be limited to naturally occurring biological products. For example, cDNA can be potentially constructed that will encode for novel synthetic antimicrobial peptides for use in sepsis or other infections.

419

In this context, gene therapy becomes a pharmacological tool in which the goal of gene transfer is transient high-level gene expression rather than prolonged lifelong expression. Although several of the problems associated with lifelong gene expression such as sustained transgene expression and how effectively to readminister vectors become less relevant, consideration of gene transfer for acute lung injury will be significantly influenced by approaches for effective gene delivery and expression in injured or diseased lung.

The following sections will discuss the approaches, potential problems, and available experimental evidence for using gene transfer techniques in acute lung injury.

II. Barriers to Airway Gene Delivery

Direct administration of gene transfer vectors to the lung airways provides a means of directly and specifically targeting gene expression in airway and alveolar epithelial cells. However, effective airway delivery of vectors in normal lung can be impeded by naturally occurring physical barriers that impede access to airway and alveolar epithelium. These include mucins and surfactants lining the airways and alveolar spaces, glycocalyceal proteins on the apical surface of airway epithelial cells, and tight junctions between epithelial surface cells that limit access of vectors to receptors on basolateral cell surface membranes (Fig. 1) (1–3). These barriers may be increased in acute lung injury in which edema, increased mucin production, and inflammatory cellular debris may further impede effective access of vectors to epithelial cells (Fig. 2) (2,4–6). The lung also has a highly developed innate immune response to introduction of foreign vector particles into the airways. Stimulation of inflammatory and immune pathways by both the vector itself and by expression of foreign genes can limit both the initial extent as well as the duration of epithelial cell gene expression (7–9). Alveolar macrophages have been demonstrated to phagocytose and inactive a large proportion of adenoviral and retroviral vectors following intratracheal administration to normal lung (10,11).

Physical and other barriers that can impede effective airway gene delivery have been mostly studied for adenoviral vectors. Less information is available for other viral vectors and for nonviral vectors. However, it is likely that many of the same barriers affecting adenoviral vector–mediated transduction of epithelial cells will also be applicable to other vectors. Additionally, nonviral vectors might be more affected by barriers than viral vectors. For example, normal mucins can significantly impede cationic liposome–mediated transfection but have less effect on transduction mediated by adenoviral vectors (2). Similarly, surfactants can decrease cationic liposome–mediated transfection by disruption of the liposomes with subsequent decrease in gene transfer (12), whereas administration of adenoviral vectors in surfactant can enhance gene expression (13,14).

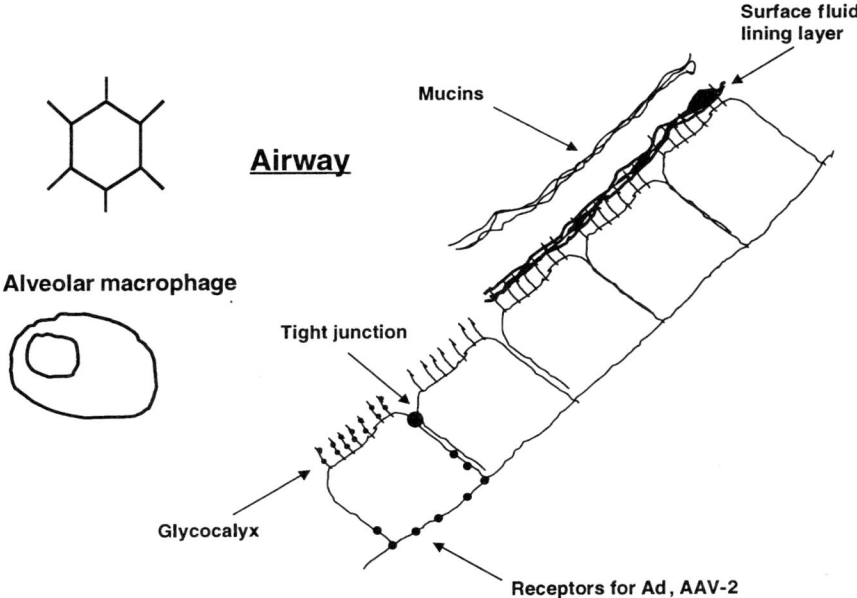

Figure 1 Barriers to delivery of gene transfer vectors in lung.

The inflammatory environment in an acutely injured lung may further impede vector access and expression. Inflammatory cytokines such as tumor necrosis factor-α (TNF-α) and interferon-γ (IFN-γ) as well as nitric oxide generated during acute lung injury can decrease adenoviral vector–mediated expression (6,9,15,16). Bronchial secretions and mucus from cystic fibrosis patients can interfere with adenoviral and cationic liposome–mediated transduction and contain proteolytic activity that can degrade adeno-associated virus 2 (AAV-2) vectors (2,5,17). Moreover, sputum from CF patients contains antiadenoviral antibodies that might also interfere with adenoviral vector–mediated transduction (18). Similar studies have not been done with secretions from acutely injured lung, but it is likely that these might similarly contain substances that can interfere with vector transduction or increase degradation of vectors.

There have been several attempts to develop methods to overcome some of these physical barriers. Intratracheal administration of EGTA has been used to open tight junctions transiently and enhance adenoviral vector–mediated gene expression in mouse lung epithelium by improving vector access to basolateral cell surface membrane receptors (19,20). Removal of the transmembrane mucin glycoprotein MUC-1 by treatment with neuraminidase was shown to improve subsequent adenovirus-mediated gene transfer to cultured human airway epithe-

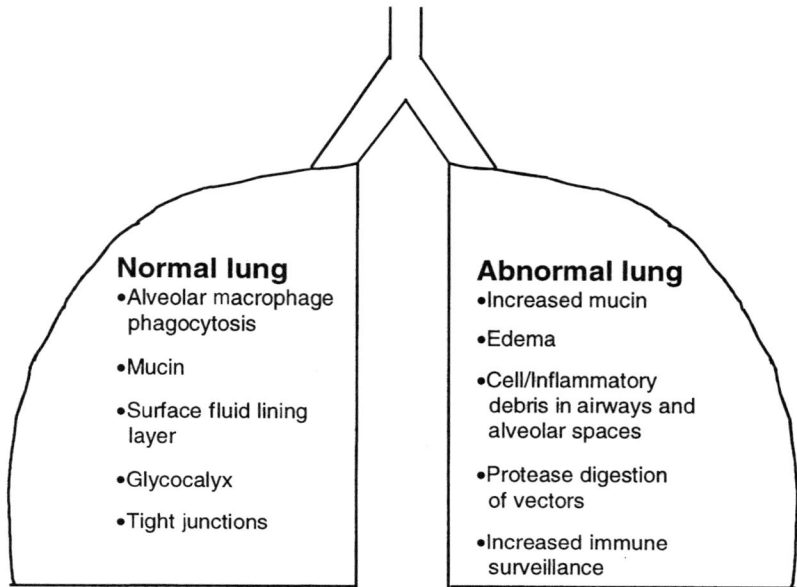

Normal lung
- Alveolar macrophage phagocytosis
- Mucin
- Surface fluid lining layer
- Glycocalyx
- Tight junctions

Abnormal lung
- Increased mucin
- Edema
- Cell/Inflammatory debris in airways and alveolar spaces
- Protease digestion of vectors
- Increased immune surveillance

Figure 2   Barriers to gene delivery and expression in normal and abnormal lung.

lial cells (21). Similarly, in cultured cells coated with sputum from cystic fibrosis patients, treatment with recombinant human DNAse but not mucolytic agents including N-acetylcysteine, alginase, or lysine improved adenoviral and cationic liposome–mediated gene transfer to these cells (5). In a related study using sheep trachea in organ culture, removal of mucin resulted in a 25-fold increase in cationic liposome–mediated gene expression (2). These studies illustrated the role tight junctions and mucin lining layers may play in impeding adenovirus- and liposome-mediated gene delivery to normal and injured lung, but have not yet suggested a clinically useful strategy for enhancing vector delivery.

Immune modulation has also been used to enhance lung gene expression, predominantly inhibition of T-cell responses to administration of adenoviral vectors (9,22–26). Whether this proves to be a clinically safe and useful strategy, particularly in the setting of acute lung injury, has not been determined.

III.   Vectors for Use in Acute Lung Injury: Airway-Based Delivery

A hypothetical ideal vector for airway-based gene delivery in acute lung injury would require the characteristics listed in Table 1. Other considerations for an

Table 1 Hypothetical Ideal Vector for Use in Acute Lung Injury

Tropism for respiratory epithelium resulting in transduction of enough epithelial cells
 or sufficient expression of soluble mediators to result in therapeutic effect
Ability to target the desired population of respiratory epithelial cells
Rapid onset of gene expression
Relatively short duration of gene expression
Ability to survive in a hostile inflammatory environment in the airways of an injured
 lung
No provocation or augmentation of inflammatory events occurring in the setting of
 lung injury

ideal vector are similar to those for use in the correction of genetic defects; that is, the ability to package the appropriately sized DNA sequences and a manufacturing process that can produce large amounts of clinical grade vectors. A number of both viral and nonviral vectors have been used for gene transfer to the lung. A review of these vectors and consideration of their potential use in acute lung injury follows.

A. Viral Vectors

Retrovirus and Lentivirus

Several aspects of retrovirus-mediated transduction make them less attractive vectors for use in acute lung injury. As vectors that integrate into the host genome, gene expression is more likely to be sustained rather than transient. Moreover, initial studies with Moloney murine leukemia retroviral vectors demonstrated low levels of transduction in normal nonproliferating airway epithelium (27–29). Higher levels of transduction were observed in cultures of proliferating airway epithelial cells and in wounded regenerating regions of trachea (29). The use of adjunct agents such as keratinocyte growth factor to increase airway epithelium proliferation in vivo can increase retrovirus-mediated transduction (30,31). Administration of retroviral vector in utero to fetal sheep lungs also demonstrates that retroviral vector–mediated transduction is more effective in actively proliferating lung epithelial cells (32). Additionally, the majority of receptors for Moloney murine leukemia virus–based vectors may reside on the basolateral cell surface membrane of epithelial cells, making them more resistant to transduction with airway delivery of vectors (30).

Less is known about administration of retroviral vectors to injured lung. Retroviral vectors are phagocytosed and inactivated by alveolar macrophages in normal lung (11). It is unclear if this clearance is increased or whether retroviruses are stable following administration to injured lungs. Administration of retroviral vector to lungs of mice with SO_2-induced acute lung injury resulted in gene expression in only a small percentage of tracheal epithelial cells (33). In contrast, one potential use of retroviral vectors in acquired lung disease is for lung cancer through either direct tumor injection or by ex vivo modification of immune cells (34,35).

Similarly lentiviral vectors also integrate and are more likely to result in sustained gene expression (36,37). Moreover, levels of expression following airway administration of lentiviral vectors are low, and there is little information about the efficacy of lentiviruses in injured lung (36,37).

Adeno-Associated Virus

Adeno-associated virus (AAV) vectors are trophic for respiratory epithelium and do not induce acute inflammatory responses in normal lung. As such, AAV vectors have undergone much recent investigation for use in cystic fibrosis as well as for use in other diseases such as hemophilia and several retinopathies (38,39). However, a major characteristic of AAV vector–mediated expression that is attractive for these diseases, that is, sustained duration of transgene expression for periods of months, makes them less potentially applicable for use in acute lung injury (40–42). Moreover, there is a long latency following airway vector administration with transgene expression usually not detected before approximately 3–4 weeks (40–42). Several adjunct techniques for AAV-mediated gene expression have resulted in earlier transgene expression but still require at least 1–2 weeks for detection of potentially therapeutic levels of gene expression (43). Different AAV serotypes preferentially interact with receptors predominantly localized on either apical or on basolateral cell surface membranes, so choice of serotype becomes important (44–46). AAV vectors are also limited by the size of cDNA that can be carried (42).

AAV vectors may not survive in acutely injured lungs. Bronchial secretions obtained from cystic fibrosis patients contain proteolytic activity that degrades AAV-2 (17). Comparable studies of AAV vector administration to more acutely injured lungs have not yet been done, but may likely also demonstrate increased clearance or destruction of AAV vectors. Reactive oxygen intermediates can increase AAV vector–mediated transduction in vitro by altering cellular redox states resulting in increased integration of AAV vectors (47). Although not yet evaluated, similar generation of reactive oxygen intermediates during acute lung injury could possibly increase AAV vector transduction in vivo.

Adenovirus

Adenoviruses are trophic for respiratory epithelium and are able to transduce virtually all types of epithelial cells from trachea to alveoli. The receptors for adenoviral vectors, the coxsackie-adenoviral receptor (CAR) and the $\alpha_v\beta_{3/5}$ integrins, are predominantly located on basolateral cell surface membranes of airway epithelial cells (1,48). Tight junction complexes between airway epithelial cells can limit access of adenoviral vectors to these receptors (19,20). Apical surface glycocalyx proteins may also impede vector access (3). Moreover, alveolar macrophages can phagocytose and inactivate a substantial proportion of adenoviral vector delivered to airways of normal animals (10,49). Whether this clearance is increased during acute lung injury has not yet been determined. Increasing the contact time of adenoviral vector with nasal and airway epithelium has also been shown to increase the level of gene expression (2,50,51).

Despite these obstacles, gene transfer using adenoviral vectors results in the highest level of airway and alveolar epithelial gene expression of any viral vector. Adenoviral vector–mediated expression in lung has a short latency with transgene expression often detected within 1 day of vector administration (52,53). Transgene expression generally peaks at 3–4 days and then tapers off over a period of several weeks. Readministration of adenoviral vectors is hampered by development of neutralizing antiadenoviral antibodies, which can significantly reduce repeat transduction of epithelial cells (23,54). This would likely be less relevant for use of adenoviral vectors in acute lung injury in which ideally only one administration of vector would be performed.

Adenoviral vectors have been well described to provoke acute inflammatory and subsequent immunological responses following airway delivery to normal lung and to lungs of patients with cystic fibrosis (7–9,54). Moreover, expression of foreign proteins also can contribute to inflammatory and immune responses (9,55–57). However, two recent investigations have demonstrated that administration of adenoviral vectors does not provoke any additional inflammation in lungs of mice with experimentally induced acute lung injury resulting from administration of endotoxin or of bleomycin (58,59). These studies suggest that adenoviral vectors may be less inflammatory when used in acutely injured lung. Moreover, most studies with adenoviral vectors have utilized first- or second-generation vectors that contain endogenous adenoviral sequences that contribute to acute inflammatory responses when expressed. Use of helper-dependent high-capacity adenoviral vectors containing no endogenous adenoviral coding sequences may prove less inflammatory in lung (60,61). Similarly, modification of the adenoviral capsid either by replacement of capsid proteins with other ligands that can interact with epithelial cell surface receptors or by coating of the capsid with polyethylene glycol ("pegylation") may also decrease host inflammatory and immune responses (62,63).

Most studies of adenoviral vector delivery to lung have been done in either normal lung or in lungs of cystic fibrosis patients with mild lung disease without current exacerbation. A smaller number of studies have utilized airway delivery of adenoviral vectors to animals or patients with lung cancer (64–66). There are fewer studies on vector delivery to acutely injured lung. Theoretically in the setting of acute lung injury where airway and alveolar epithelial cells may be damaged or sloughed and tight junctions disrupted, adenoviral vectors may have increased access to basolateral cell surface membrane receptors. Moreover, increased expression of α_v integrins occurs in regenerating lung epithelium, and injured epithelium is more susceptible to adenoviral vector–mediated transduction (67). However, increased mucins, edema, or inflammatory debris in airway and alveolar spaces may impede access of vectors to the epithelial cells. For example, sputum from CF patients impedes adenoviral vector–mediated transduction in cultured sheep trachea (2). Preexisting antiadenoviral antibodies in sputum from some CF patients may contribute to this inhibitory effect (18). Increased nitric oxide, a reactive metabolite generated during acute lung inflammation, has been demonstrated to reduce adenoviral vector–mediated transduction in mouse lungs (6). Adenoviral vector–mediated gene expression in murine nasal and airway epithelium was decreased in animals with bronchopulmonary inflammation induced by prior inoculation with a mucoid *Pseudomonas aeruginosa* (4). Nonspecific inflammatory changes and elevation of proinflammatory cytokines in bronchoalveolar lavage fluid have also been associated with decreased adenoviral vector–mediated gene transfer and expression in rodent lung (7). Treatment of animals with dexamethasone to reduce inflammation was accompanied by increased adenovirus-mediated gene expression in lung (7). The use of adjunct methods for airway delivery of adenoviral vectors, for example, delivering vector with surfactant or with perfluorochemical liquid, has also been demonstrated to enhance gene expression in both normal lungs and in acutely injured lungs (13,14,59,69–71).

Other Viruses

Several other viral vectors including Sendai and influenza viruses have recently been investigated for use in the lung (72,73). It is unclear at present whether these will prove advantageous to currently available viral vectors, particularly in lung injury.

B.   Nonviral Vectors

In general, nonviral vectors have resulted in less effective airway and alveolar epithelial gene expression following airway administration to normal lung than have the viral vectors, particularly adenoviral vectors. Although not well studied, naked DNA and complexes of DNA with cationic liposomes (lipoplexes) or with cationic polymers (polyplexes) are more likely to be degraded or inactivated in an inflammatory environment or impeded by increased mucins or surfactants found in injured lung. Moreover, cationic liposomes can provoke significant inflammatory and systemic responses when administered to lung by either airway or intravenous routes (74–79). This results in part from immune stimulation by unmethylated CpG bacterial sequences in the plasmid DNA (9,80,81). Nonviral vectors are likely to be less useful for intratracheal administration to acutely injured or diseased lung.

Naked DNA

Several studies have demonstrated a low level of airway epithelial gene expression following instillation of naked DNA to normal murine airways (82–84). However, transgene expression mediated by naked DNA in normal mouse lungs was decreased when the DNA was administered with a synthetic surfactant solution (Exosurf) (85). Other effects of physical barriers on transduction mediated by naked DNA are generally unknown, and it is likely that the inflammatory environment, including DNAses released by injured or necrotic cells in an acutely injured lung, may significantly reduce naked DNA–mediated expression.

Cationic Liposomes

There are a wide variety of liposomes that have been investigated for airway gene delivery to normal lung. Physicochemical properties of the component lipids as well as size and charge of the liposome-DNA complex (lipoplex) can significantly influence the ability of the liposomal vector to transfect airway and alveolar epithelial cells (86,87). However, at best, gene expression mediated by liposomal vectors generally occurs in only a small percentage of epithelial cells. Transfection mediated by liposomal vectors generally has a rapid onset with gene expression being frequently detected within 24 hr (86,88). Moreover gene expression usually tapers off after several weeks (86,88,89). Airway epithelium has been shown to be relatively resistant to liposomal vector–mediated transfection, although this depends on the formulation of liposome utilized (2,90,91). This may result from inefficient intracellular trafficking of internalized liposome-DNA complexes or from a low proliferative rate in differentiated epithelial cells (2,92,93). Mucins lining the airway epithelium in normal lung have been demonstrated to reduce liposome-mediated transduction in cultured sheep trachea (2). Similarly surfactant has been shown to inhibit expression mediated by cationic liposomes in cultured lung epithelial cells (12,94). It has been postulated that mixing of surfactant components with those in the cationic liposomes resulted in disruption of the liposomes with subsequent decrease in gene transfer (12).

Cationic liposomes complexed with plasmid DNA encoding for cystic fibrosis transmembrane conductance regulator (CFTR) have been administered to nasal epithelium and to airways of patients with mild cystic fibrosis (76,95–97). However, only low levels of gene expression or activity were detected. Moreover, administration of the vectors provoked local and systemic inflammatory responses in several patients (76,96). It is not known whether the inflammatory environment in the CF airways degraded or inactivated the liposomal vectors.

Sputum from CF patients has been demonstrated to inhibit cationic liposomal vector–mediated transfection of cultured cells and cultured sheep trachea (2,5). There has been little study of airway administration of polyplexes to more acutely injured lungs.

Cationic Polymer and Molecular Conjugates

Plasmid DNA complexed or conjugated with a variety of cationic ligands (polyplexes), organic solvents (solvoplexes), or ligands that recognize receptors on the apical surface of epithelial cells such as the polymeric immunoglobulin receptor have also been investigated for airway gene delivery (84,98–103). In general, although potentially effective in vitro, most of these vectors result in only a low level of airway and alveolar epithelial gene expression following airway administration to normal lungs and have not been evaluated in injured lungs.

One potentially promising polyplex, polyethyleneimine (PEI) has recently been demonstrated to result in a higher level of gene expression following aerosol delivery to rodent lung than a number of comparably delivered lipoplexes (104,105). Aerosol delivery of a PEI-p53 complex in a murine melanoma metastasis model was demonstrated to inhibit growth of metastases (106). Aerosol delivery of PEI does elicit transient inflammatory response in normal lung and has not yet been evaluated in acutely injured lungs (107).

IV. Vectors for Use in Acute Lung Injury: Intravenous Delivery

Intravenous (IV) administration has also been used to deliver vectors to the lung. With this approach, the primary target is the pulmonary vascular endothelium rather than the airway and alveolar epithelium. Transgene activity has been described in airway and alveolar epithelial cells following IV administration of cationic liposomal and adenoviral vectors (88,108). However, expression is usually sparse and sporadic.

IV vector administration is more likely to be useful for diseases affecting the pulmonary vascular endothelium such as pulmonary hypertension (66). The endothelium may also be a good locus for transgene-mediated expression of soluble mediators for use in acute lung injury. However, this has been less well explored (66). The only two vectors that have received significant study for targeting lung after IV delivery are the adenoviral and cationic liposomal vectors.

A. Cationic Liposomes

Cationic liposomes (lipoplexes) exhibit a tropism for pulmonary vascular endothelium that goes beyond a first-pass effect following systemic IV administration

(109). As with airway administration of lipoplexes, targeting of vascular endothelium is influenced by physicochemical properties of the component lipids as well as size and charge of the lipoplex (110,111). Lipoplexes can also be constructed containing ligands that target endothelial cell surface membrane receptors (112,113). However, less is known about the effectiveness of IV administration of cationic liposomes for transfecting pulmonary vascular endothelium or airway and alveolar epithelium in the setting of acute lung injury. Serum proteins may interfere with cationic liposomal vector–mediated transduction and a significant proportion of liposomes are taken up and cleared by Kupffer's cells in the liver following IV administration (114,115). Moreover, systemic administration of cationic liposomes can provoke a significant inflammatory response mediated by bacterial CpG sequences (75,78,116).

B. Adenovirus

Adenoviral vectors can also transduce pulmonary vascular endothelium (66). Modification of the adenoviral capsid to express ligand that interacts with endothelial cell surface receptors improves endothelial transduction (117–119). However, systemic administration of adenoviral vectors can provoke acute inflammatory responses (120). As with the cationic vectors, little is known about the effectiveness of adenoviral vectors for transducing vascular endothelium or airway or alveolar epithelium in the setting of acute lung injury (66,121).

V. Methods of Airway Gene Delivery

Current techniques of delivering gene transfer vectors to airway and alveolar epithelia include nasal deposition of vector, direct instillation of vector into the trachea or lower airways using a catheter or bronchoscope (122,123), and aerosolization and inhalation of vectors (124,125). Nasal deposition in obligate nasal breathers such as rodents can be effective in distributing vector throughout the lower airways (126). However, in humans, gene expression resulting from nasal deposition of vector is generally limited to nasal epithelia (96,127). There is little experience with nasal deposition and delivery of vectors to acutely injured lungs.

There are several approaches to direct vector instillation into the trachea or lower airways. In small animal models, transtracheal puncture with a small-gauge needle is commonly used (71,128), whereas bronchoscopic administration of vector is usually performed in larger animal models (primates) and in human patients (122,129). Whatever the method, direct vector instillation generally results in heterogeneous distribution to limited portions of lung (122,123,129). Multiple instillations are required to achieve more widespread vector distribution. Moreover, the resulting transgene expression is usually more evident in epithelium of larger proximal airways. Catheter-directed instillation, particularly when using a bronchoscope, generally also requires topical analgesia and sedation to be performed comfortably and safely. A recent technique has been developed using a spray device directed through a bronchoscope (130). This approach allows for positioning of the bronchoscope at the carina or in either of the mainstem bronchi and spraying vector solution more effectively into more distal airways. Although this method has met with some success, it has not been widely utilized.

Most studies of direct instillation of vectors have been done either in normal animal models or patients or in CF patients with mild disease and no acute inflammatory exacerbation. There is less experience with direct instillation into more acutely injured lungs, although it has been shown that adenoviral vector–mediated gene expression was decreased following instillation into lungs of mice with mucoid *Pseudomonas* infection compared to that in normal controls (4). Even less is known about effective methods to enhance gene delivery and expression in acutely injured lungs, although both surfactant and perfluorochemical liquid delivery vehicles have been demonstrated to enhance adenoviral vector–mediated gene expression in rodent models of lung injury (59,70).

Inhalation of aerosolized vector solutions can result in more diffuse transgene distribution throughout the lung and in increased distribution to distal airway and alveolar epithelium (91,124,125,131,132). This approach is also easier to apply clinically. However, large amounts of vector are required, as material is lost by deposition in the aerosolization equipment and on oropharyngeal or nasopharyngeal, laryngeal, or upper airway mucosa (124,125,131,133). This can be rate limiting for viral vectors. Moreover, cationic liposomes may be disrupted during the aerosolization process (134). As with direct instillation, most studies of aerosol vector administration have been done either in normal animal models or human patients or in CF patients with mild disease and no acute inflammatory exacerbation (91,124,125,131,132). There is little information available about the effectiveness of aerosol delivery of vectors to acutely injured lungs.

VI. Adjunct Methods for Airway Gene Delivery

Several techniques have been demonstrated to augment expression following direct airway instillation of vectors, particularly viral vectors. Although the clinical applicability of some of these approaches is unclear, methods utilizing surfactant and the perfluorochemical liquids are based on established clinical use of each of these for treatment of acute lung injury.

A. Calcium Phosphate

Precipitating adenovirus or AAV-2 vectors with calcium phosphate ($CaPo_4$) results in a complex that exhibits increased nonspecific uptake on the apical surface of airway epithelial cells (135–137). This approach abrogates the need to pass vectors through the tight junctions to access the more predominant basolateral receptors for each of these vectors and enhances transgene expression in both cultured lung epithelial cells and in mouse lung in vivo with no apparent toxicity (135–137). CaPo$_4$ precipitation of vectors may also increase viral release from endosomes following vector internalization by cells. This approach has not yet been demonstrated to have efficacy in injured lung.

B. EGTA

The rationale for airway administration of EGTA is that localized calcium chelation will disrupt calcium-dependent proteins in the tight junction complex and increase permeability of tight junctions to small molecules including vectors. Application of EGTA to cultured lung epithelial cells does increase tight junction permeability to retroviral and adenoviral vectors and increases the amount bound to basolateral surface receptors (19,30). The use of EGTA has been demonstrated to enhance adenoviral vector–mediated transgene expression in mouse lung (20) and adenovirus- and retrovirus-mediated transduction in rabbit trachea and human nasal epithelium (19). This approach also has not yet been demonstrated to have efficacy in injured lung.

C. Detergent

Airway administration of a phospholipid detergent can also disrupt tight junctions between mature ciliated airway epithelial cells, and it has been demonstrated to increase adenovirus-mediated transgene expression in murine nasal epithelium (68). Whether this approach is applicable in either normal or injured lung is undetermined.

D. Surfactant

Surfactant can be safely administered to the airways, and it has become a mainstay of treatment for respiratory failure in premature infants (138). Airway delivery of drugs in surfactant vehicles has been successfully utilized to enhance drug deposition in the lung (139). Administering adenoviral vectors in either 10 or 25 mg/mL solutions of the synthetic surfactant Survanta increased gene expression in rabbit lung parenchyma (13,14). Expression in trachea and main bronchi was decreased, suggesting that the surfactant vehicle resulted in more effective distribution of vector to the lower airways (13). Similar findings have been observed delivering adenoviral vector in a 50% Survanta solution to rat lungs (69). In contrast, transgene expression mediated by naked DNA in mouse lungs was decreased when the DNA was administered with a different synthetic surfactant solution (Exosurf) (85). The mechanism by which gene expression was inhibited remains unclear. Survanta had no effect on naked DNA–mediated gene expression in cultured lung epithelial cells or cultured lung fibroblasts, but it did inhibit expression mediated by cationic liposomes (94). Naturally occurring bovine and rabbit surfactants also inhibited cationic liposome-mediated gene expression in cultured lung epithelial cells (12). In these studies, mixing of surfactant components with those in the cationic liposomes probably resulted in disruption of the liposomes with subsequent decrease in gene transfer (12).

Most recently, administering adenoviral vector in a (50%) Survanta solution enhanced gene expression in rat lungs with experimentally induced pulmonary edema (70). This finding suggests that the use of surfactants during airway vector delivery may be effective in other forms of acute lung injury as well.

E. Perfluorochemical Liquid

Perfluorochemical (PFC) liquids are chemically inert fluorinated carbon chain liquids that are excellent solvents for O_2, CO_2, and other gases yet are immiscible with aqueous and lipid solutions (140,141). Other properties include high density and low surface tension which allow PFC liquids to distribute throughout communicating airways and spread over alveolar walls following instillation into lungs (141). PFC liquids have been subsequently used for supporting gas exchange in acutely injured lungs; that is, liquid ventilation (141,142). Clinical experience with the PFC liquid perflubron (LiquiVent; Alliance Pharmaceuticals, San Diego) in both children and adults demonstrated that this compound can be safely instilled in intubated, mechanically ventilated patients with minimal toxicity (142). This liquid ventilation allows effective gas exchange, and the volatile PFC liquids clear by evaporation within 24 hrs.

PFC liquids also have anti-inflammatory effects in injured lung. Clinical studies of liquid ventilation as well as observations in animals with experimentally induced lung injury undergoing liquid ventilation demonstrate that, in addition to improving oxygenation and lung mechanics, the use of perflubron decreased the amount of lung injury observed on histopathological specimens (143). Moreover, the use of perflubron decreased the amount of edema, bleeding, and neutrophilic influx into injured lungs (144,145). The level of the proinflammatory cytokines interleukin-1β (IL-1β) and IL-6 as well as total white cell and neutrophilic count were reduced in bronchoalveolar lavage (BAL) fluid collected from patients with acute respiratory distress syndrome (ARDS) undergoing liquid ventilation compared to levels in BAL fluid from ARDS patients undergoing gas ventilation (146). These collected observations suggest that the use of PFC liquid may be beneficial in the setting of acute lung injury.

The use of perflubron and other PFC liquids during vector administration has been demonstrated to enhance adenovirus-mediated gene expression in intubated, ventilated rabbits and adenovirus, AAV-2, and cationic liposomal vector–

mediated expression into lungs of spontaneously breathing normal rodents (71,128,147,148). Total transgene expression was increased and transgene distribution was enhanced within and between lung lobes (71,128,148). Transgene expression was particularly improved in distal airways and alveoli (71,128). Most recently, it has been demonstrated that a single dose of PFC liquid administered through a bronchoscope to nonhuman primates (rhesus macaques) was both well tolerated by the animals and resulted in improved adenoviral vector–mediated gene distribution in the lung (149,150).

The PFC liquids likely act by propelling droplets of vector solutions further into and more uniformly throughout the lung than can be accomplished with either catheter-directed or aerosol administration of vectors. The PFC liquids may also transiently displace mucins, allowing better access of vectors to epithelial cells (151). Additional effects of PFC liquids may also contribute to enhanced gene expression. PFC liquids are taken up by alveolar macrophages following instillation into lung (152). The macrophages are subsequently less able to phagocytose and inactivate adenoviral vectors, presumably allowing for more vector available for epithelial cell transduction (152). Instillation of PFC liquid also can transiently increase tight junction permeability and presumably allow increased access of adenoviral and AAV vectors to basolateral cell surface membrane receptors sites (153).

PFC liquids have also been demonstrated to enhance adenoviral vector–mediated transgene expression in models of both acute (bleomycin) and chronic (granulocyte-macrophage colony-stimulating factor [GM-CSF] knockout mice with alveolar proteinosis) lung injury (59,151). A significant part of PFC liquid action in these models is likely to be transient displacement of inflammatory debris from the airway and alveolar spaces, allowing better access of vector to epithelial cells. Other actions of PFC liquids may also be important but have not yet been studied in injured lungs.

VII. Experience with Gene Transfer in Acute Lung Injury

There is a growing literature describing both airway and intravenous delivery of gene transfer vectors in models of acute and acquired lung diseases. Consideration of gene transfer approaches for several conditions including pneumonia, pulmonary hypertension, lung cancer, and lung transplantation appears in other chapters in this volume. Gene transfer approaches for other acquired lung diseases such as bronchiolitis obliterans, pulmonary alveolar proteinosis, and radiation pneumonitis suggest that these also might be amenable to gene therapy (154–158). Discussed below is the rationale and experience with gene transfer approaches for acute lung injury and acute respiratory distress syndrome.

A.   Acute Lung Injury and Acute Respiratory Distress Syndrome

Acute lung injury (ALI) and ARDS are syndromes characterized clinically by severe hypoxemia requiring intubation and assisted mechanical ventilation, diffuse radiographic infiltrates, and reduced pulmonary compliance in the absence of congestive heart failure or hydrostatic pulmonary edema (159,160). ARDS was first described in 1967 and affects anywhere from 15,000 to 150,000 patients per year in the United States. Mortality remains high at approximately 40–50%, and aggressive supportive care and appropriate ventilator management to reduce ventilator-induced lung injury remain the mainstays of treatment (161,162).

Histologically, ALI and ARDS are characterized by diffuse alveolar damage, hyaline membrane formation, noncardiogeneic pulmonary edema, loss of normal surfactant function, diffuse interstitial inflammation, and diffuse pulmonary vascular damage (159,160). Survivors of the early phase of ARDS frequently go on to develop excess collagen deposition and pulmonary fibrosis (159,160). Determining a single pathogenesis for ARDS has been proven to be difficult, as multiple clinical conditions including sepsis, pneumonia, trauma, inhalation injury, and pancreatitis can lead to development of ARDS (159,160). The different inciting events appear to converge into a common pathway wherein an initial appropriate inflammatory response is followed by an overexuberant sustained inflammatory response leading to inappropriate recruitment of inflammatory cells to the lung and generation of the histopathological and physiological abnormalities characteristic of ARDS. A number of deranged metabolic pathways have been described in ALI/ARDS including complement activation, generation of reactive oxygen and nitrogen species, and generation of a number of inflammatory cytokines and other mediators that lead to platelet aggregation, coagulopathy, and neutrophilic recruitment to airway and alveolar spaces (159,160). Capillary endothelial integrity is disrupted resulting in leakage of fluid and proteins into alveolar spaces.

A number of attempts to alter the course of ALI/ARDS pharmacologically have not been proven to be successful. These include the use of exogenous surfactant, glucocorticoids, antioxidant (n-acetylcysteine), prostaglandin and leukotriene synthesis inhibitors (ketoconazole, ibuprofen), prostaglandin E1, inhaled nitric oxide, and pentoxifylline (159,160). Trials with antibodies aimed at blocking inflammation provoked by endotoxin, TNF-α, and IL-1 have also not been proven to be successful (159,160). Part of the failure of these antibody trials may result from the temporal complexity of cytokine and inflammatory responses in which an initial elevation of proinflammatory cytokines is an appropriate part of the normal host response to the inciting injury (159,160). Overall, the failure of individual pharmacological interventions highlights the difficulty in singling out any one pathway for therapeutic intervention in ALI/ARDS.

Why then gene therapy for ALI/ARDS? The rationale for gene transfer approaches is that localized expression of therapeutic molecules may be more effective than systemic expression, particularly if expression can be localized to specific target airway or alveolar epithelial cells. Epithelial cell expression of therapeutic cytokines or other substances will likely also be more effective than airway administration of cytokine or other proteins, as these may be degraded in the inflammatory environment of the airways and alveolar spaces in acutely injured lungs. Moreover, as the temporal sequences of deranged metabolic pathways in ARDS are further elucidated, gene expression can be coordinated to maximize potential therapeutic benefit. Moreover, gene transfer need not be limited to expression of single gene products. Several potentially therapeutic substances can be delivered in a coordinated fashion with gene transfer approaches.

The vectors that will likely be most useful in ARDS are those that result in rapid gene expression such as adenoviral or cationic liposomal vectors. These vectors also result in nonsustained gene expression in lung that is potentially also useful for timing gene expression with underlying pathology. Moreover, incorporation of molecular switches such as the tetracycline regulator can further coordinate gene expression with the underlying pathology (163). The use of appropriate promoters, for example, surfactant promoters or the cytokeratin promoter which will result in expression in specific airway or alveolar epithelial cells only, can help target gene expression to specific cells (164,165).

Acutely injured or regenerating lung may provide a better target for gene transfer than normal lung. Regenerating lung epithelial cells have been shown to be targeted preferentially by adenoviral vectors in vitro (67,166). Part of this observation may result from disruption of tight junctions between the injured cells that allows better access of vectors to basolateral cell surface membrane receptors. Regenerating epithelial cells also have increased expression of cell surface integrins including those utilized for adenoviral internalization (67,166). Similarly, fibroblast growth factor (FGF) receptors are upregulated in type 2 epithelial cells following hyperoxic lung injury (167). Retargeting adenoviral vectors to interact with FGF receptors has been demonstrated to increase transduction of cells otherwise refractory to adenoviral vector–mediated transduction and may be useful for targeting gene expression in injured lungs (168–170). However, one of the hurdles to gene transfer approaches for acute lung injury and ARDS is effective delivery of vector to injured lungs. An adjunct delivery method such as use of surfactant or PFC liquids is likely to be necessary.

Summarized below is a description of gene transfer efforts for acute lung injury and ARDS.

B. Cytokine Gene Transfer

As multiple overlapping cytokine pathways are involved in the pathogenesis of acute lung injury and ARDS, targeted airway or alveolar epithelial expression of any one cytokine or cytokine antagonist is likely to be an overly simplistic approach. Nonetheless, targeted expression of various cytokines in lung by adenoviral vector–mediated gene expression has helped elucidate specific pathogenic or anti-inflammatory roles of each cytokine (66,171,172). For example, overexpression of IL-6 in rat lungs resulted in lymphocytic infiltrates and peribronchial lymphocytic hyperplasia (173,174). Similarly, overexpression of TNF-α in rat lungs resulted in a severe acute lung injury that developed into pulmonary fibrosis (175). Overexpression of GM-CSF or of transforming growth factor-β (TGF-β) in airway epithelium similarly induces pulmonary fibrosis in rat lungs (176,177). In contrast, overexpression of TNF-α in airway epithelium has proven to be effective in increasing bacterial clearance and survival in gram-negative pneumonia and improving survival and host defense to gram-negative lung infection in a murine model of sepsis (178,179). Similarly, overexpression of IL-12 in mouse airway epithelium decreased mortality from gram-negative lung infection (180).

A potentially useful strategy for acute lung injury may be to use targeted cytokine expression to boost immune responses in the lung by augmenting airway mucosal production of immunoglobulins. Adenoviral vector–mediated expression of IL-5 and IL-6 resulted in enhanced local and systemic levels of IgG and IgA in normal rodent lungs (181,182). This approach has not yet been evaluated in injured lungs.

One promising approach is gene transfer–mediated expression of IL-10. IL-10 is pleiotrophic cytokine with a broad range of anti-inflammatory effects (183). Both animal and human studies demonstrate that systemic administration of IL-10 can reduce inflammatory responses in response to pneumonia or sepsis (184,185). However, IL-10 has a short half-life in vivo and gene transfer may provide a better mechanism of sustained IL-10 expression. To date, although there is good evidence for the efficacy of IL-10 expressed in other organs, there is only limited experience with in vivo IL-10 gene expression in lung. For example, intramuscular injection of an IL-10–expressing adenoviral vector resulted in suppression of proinflammatory cytokines in endotoxemic mice (186). Intraperitoneal injection of IL-10–expressing adenoviral vector resulted in increased survival and suppressed TNF-α expression in models of gram-negative bacterial infection or endotoxin challenge (187,188). Intraperitoneal administration of an IL-10 expressing liposome decreased both inflammatory changes as well as development of lung fibrosis in response to intratracheal administration of bleomycin (189). Intracardiac administration of an IL-10–expressing adenoviral vector prolonged cardiac allograft survival (190). Intratracheal administration of an IL-10–expressing cationic liposomal vector to mouse lungs resulted in improved mortality and decreased lung inflammation in response to endotoxin challenge (191). Intratracheal administration of naked DNA encoding IL-10 suppressed nitric oxide synthetase levels and decreased exhaled nitric oxide in a rat lung transplant model (192). Adenoviral vector–mediated expression of IL-10 in mouse lung decreased the inflammation provoked by instillation of the vector itself (193). This may prove to be a useful strategy for use in combination with adenoviral vector–mediated delivery of other transgenes (194).

C. Regulation of Free Radical Production and Oxidant Stress

A potentially more promising approach for gene therapy of ALI/ARDS involves targeted overexpression of antioxidants such as superoxide dismutase or catalase. This approach may be particularly useful in the setting of critically ill intubated and mechanically ventilated patients in whom increased reactive oxygen species resulting from hyperoxia and localized shunting of pulmonary vasculature (i.e., ischemia-reperfusion) may overwhelm normal antioxidant function. Adenoviral vector–mediated overexpression of glutathione reductase protected cultured Chinese hamster ovary cells against oxidant injury (195,196). Similarly, cationic liposomal vector–mediated expression of superoxide dismustase (SOD) in rat lung epithelial cells protected against paraquat- and xanthine oxidase–mediated superoxide anion injury (197). Adenoviral vector–mediated expression of SOD in cultured human lung epithelial cells decreased apoptosis in response to irradiation injury (198). Subsequent in vivo studies demonstrated that overexpression of superoxide dismustase in mouse lung airway epithelial cells protected against radiation-induced acute pneumonitis (156).

Overexpression of heme oxygenase in cultured human lung epithelial cells improved survival following hyperoxic exposure (199). Subsequent adenoviral vector–mediated expression of heme oxygenase in rat airway epithelium protected against hyperoxic lung injury with significant reductions in inflammation, neutrophilic apoptosis, edema, and hemorrhage (200). Similarly, overexpression of catalase and of SOD in rat lung epithelium protected against hyperoxia but not ischemia-reperfusion–mediated induced lung injury (201). Concommitant overexpression of antioxidants in pulmonary vascular endothelium may also be necessary for protection against ischemia-reperfusion–induced lung injury. Adenoviral vector–mediated catalase expression in cultured human umbilical vein endothelial cells improved survival and decreased injury following oxidant injury (202). However, a similar effect in pulmonary vascular endothelium has not yet been demonstrated.

D. Pulmonary Edema

Early ALI/ARDS is characterized by injury to both the alveolar epithelial and pulmonary capillary endothelial membranes that results in leak of fluid and proteins into the alveolar spaces (159,160,203). Reabsorption of pulmonary edema fluid is also impaired in ALI/ARDS (204). One of the key mediators of active water reabsorption across the alveolar epithelium is Na$^+$, K$^+$-ATPase in the epithelial cell membrane (203,204). Activity of this enzyme can be deranged in acute lung inflammation and injury by direct injury to epithelial cells, trauma from mechanical ventilation, and reactive oxygen and nitrogen species generated during acute inflammation (203,204). Adenoviral vector–mediated expression of the β_1 subunit of Na^+, K^+-ATPase in rat lungs increased clearance of intratracheally administered isotonic saline (69). Adenoviral vector–mediated expression of the β_1 subunit of Na^+, K^+-ATPase in cultured fetal rat lung distal epithelial cells similarly mitigated the decrease in sodium transport caused by oxidant injury (205). Another approach has been to enhance expression of the β_2-adrenergic receptor. β-Adrenergic receptor activation has been demonstrated to increase Na^+, K^+-ATPase expression and activity and to increase Na^+ transport in lung. Adenoviral vector–mediated expression of the β_2-adrenergic receptor has been demonstrated to increase fluid transport and edema clearance in cultured lung epithelial cells and in rat lung (206). Cationic liposome–mediated expression of the α and β subunits of Na^+, K^+-ATPase in mouse lungs has also been shown to increase edema clearance in a model of pulmonary edema induced by intraperitoneal administration of thiourea (207).

Another potential approach to gene therapy of pulmonary edema may be targeted overexpression of aquaporin water channels. Adenoviral vector– and AAV vector–mediated expression of aquaporin 1 in cultured human and rat salivary gland epithelial cells and in rat salivary glands in vivo resulted in increased transepithelial fluid movement (208–210). Conversely, adenoviral vector–mediated expression of vascular endothelial growth factor (VEGF) in mouse lungs increased pulmonary edema, suggesting a role of VEGF in the pathogenesis of pulmonary edema in acute lung injury (211).

One potential hurdle to gene transfer approaches for pulmonary edema is effective airway delivery of vector to an edematous lung. However, it has recently been demonstrated that administration of adenoviral vector in a 50:50 surfactant: saline mixture enhanced gene delivery in a rat model of acute pulmonary edema (70). The use of perfluorochemical liquids during vector administration may also be useful for gene delivery in the setting of pulmonary edema and acute and chronic lung injury (59,151).

E. Other Airway-Based Gene Transfer Approaches for ALI/ARDS

There are a number of other potential targets for gene transfer in ALI/ARDS. Adenoviral vector–mediated expression of atrial natriuretic peptide in rat lung airway and alveolar epithelium reduced development of pulmonary hypertension after hypoxic challenge (212). Adenovirus-mediated expression of a neutrophilic elastase inhibitor has been demonstrated in rat lung but not yet evaluated for efficacy in acute lung injury (213). Cationic liposome–mediated expression of α_1-antitrypsin in cultured CF bronchial epithelial cells decreased injury resulting from exposure to neutrophil elastase (214). Gene transfer that interferes with NF-κB function, a key intracellular intermediary for proinflammatory cytokine action, has been found to decrease TNF-α–mediated IL-8 secretion in cultured CF airway epithelial cells and in cultured lung cancer cells (215,216). Similar approaches might be useful for acute lung injury.

Surfactant metabolism is altered in ALI/ARDS and levels of several surfactant proteins are decreased (159,160). Attempts at replacement with the use of replacement therapy using artificial surfactant, although successful in inflammatory lung diseases in premature infants (217), have not been proven to be useful for ALI/ARDS (159,160). Gene transfer–mediated surfactant expression may be a more effective means of replenishing necessary surfactant proteins. Adenovirus vector–mediated expression of surfactant proteins A and B has been demonstrated in cultured lung epithelial cells and in normal rat lungs (218,219). This strategy has not yet been evaluated in models of lung injury.

Ex vivo transduction of alveolar macrophages may also be a useful strategy for increasing macrophage proliferation for potential use in acute lung injury, particularly for immunocompromised patients (220,221).

F. Gene Transfer Approaches for ALI/ARDS Targeting the Pulmonary Vascular Endothelium

Intravenous administration of vectors targeting the pulmonary vascular endothelium may have a role in acute lung injury, although this has been less well explored. Cationic liposome–mediated expression of prostaglandin G/H synthase reduced hypotension, pulmonary edema, and thromboxane B_2 release in response to endotoxin challenge in rabbit lungs (222). Expression of neutrophil inhibitory factor in mouse pulmonary vascular endothelium prevented endotoxin-stimulated infiltration of neutrophils into the lung as well as decreased vascular leak across the alveolar-capillary barrier (223). Overexpression of antioxidant molecules in vascular endothelium may also be useful in acute lung injury. Adenoviral vector–mediated catalase expression in cultured human umbilical vein endothelial cells improved survival and decreased injury following oxidant injury (202). Similarly, adenoviral vector–mediated catalase expression in rabbit heart decreased cardiac ischemia-reperfusion injury (224). Comparable studies evaluating antioxidant expression in pulmonary vascular endothelium in the setting of acute lung injury could potentially show comparable beneficial effect. However, one potential difficulty with IV administration of adenoviral vectors is the lack of specificity for targeting the pulmonary vasculature and the inflammation provoked by systemic administration of adenovirus vectors. Similarly, cationic liposomal vectors provoke inflammatory responses when administered systemically. The use of less inflammatory (high-capacity or pegylated) vectors or vectors retargeted to interact specifically with receptors on the pulmonary vascular endothelial cell membranes

(117,118) may help overcome some of these hurdles. Direct delivery of vectors to the pulmonary capillary circulation, for example, through indwelling pulmonary artery catheters, may also help direct expression to the pulmonary vascular endothelium. However, the choice of catheter is important, as not all catheter materials are compatible with adenoviral vector delivery (225,226).

VIII. Conclusions

The use of gene transfer techniques for acute lung injury is an exciting method for both probing mechanisms involved in acute inflammatory injury as well as providing potential therapeutic approaches. However, there are a number of hurdles to be overcome including developing methods for effectively delivering vectors to the acutely injured lung as well as developing a strategy for specific therapeutic gene expression.

References

1. Walters RW, Grunst T, Bergelson JM, Finberg RW, Wlesh MJ, Zabner J. Basolateral localization of fiber receptors limits adenovirus infection from the apical surface of airway epithelia. J Biol Chem 1999; 274:10219–10226.
2. Kitson C, Angel B, Judd D, Rothery S, Severs NJ, Dewar A, et al. The extra- and intracellular barriers to lipid and adenovirus-mediated pulmonary gene transfer in native sheep airway epithelium. Gene Ther 1998; 6:534–546.
3. Pickles RJ, Fahrner JA, Petrella JM, Boucher RC, Bergelson JM. Retargeting the coxsackievirus and adenovirus receptor to the apical surface of polarized epithelial cells reveals the glycocalyx as a barrier to adenovirus-mediated gene transfer. J Virol 2000; 74:6050–6057.
4. van Heeckeren A, Ferkol T, Tosi M. Effects of bronchopulmonary inflammation induced by pseudomonas aeruginosa on adenovirus-mediated gene transfer to airway epithelial cells in mice. Gene Ther 1998; 5:345–351.
5. Stern M, Caplen NJ, Browning JE, Griesenbach U, Sorgi F, Huang L, et al. The effect of mucolytic agents on gene transfer across a CF sputum barrier in vitro. Gene Ther 1998; 5:91–98.
6. Haddad IY, Sorscher EJ, Garver RI, Hong J, Tzeng E, Matalon S. Modulation of adenovirus-mediated gene transfer by nitric oxide. Am J Respir Cell Mol Biol 1997; 16:501–509.
7. Otake K, Ennist DL, Harrod K, Trapnell BC. Nonspecific inflammation inhibits adenovirus-mediated pulmonary gene transfer and expression independent of specific acquired immune responses. Hum Gene Ther 1998; 9:2207–2222.
8. Look DC, Brody SL. Engineering viral vectors to subvert the airway defense response. Am J Respir Cell Mol Biol 1999; 20:1103–1106.
9. Bromberg JS, Debruyne LA, Qin L. Interactions between the immune system and

gene therapy vectors: bidirectional regulation of response and expression. Adv Immunol 1998; 69:353–409.

10. Worgall S, Leopold PL, Wolff G, Ferris B, Van Roijen N, Crystal RG. Role of alveolar macrophages in rapid elimination of adenovirus vectors administered to the epithelial surface of the respiratory tract. Hum Gene Ther 1997; 8:1675–1684.

11. McCray PB, Wang G, Kline JN, Zabner J, Chada S, Jolly DJ, et al. Alveolar macrophages inhibit retrovirus-mediated gene transfer to airway epithelia. Hum Gene Ther 1997; 8:1087–1093.

12. Duncan JD, Whitsett JA, Horowitz AD. Pulmonary surfactant inhibits cationic liposome-mediated gene delivery to respiratory epithelial cells in vitro. Hum Gene Ther 1997; 8:431–438.

13. Jobe AH, Ueda T, Whitsett JA, Trapnell BC, Ikegami M. Surfactant enhances adenovirus-mediated gene expression in rabbit lungs. Gene Ther 1996; 3:775–779.

14. Katkin JP, Husser RC, Langston C, Welty SE. Exogenous surfactant enhances the delivery of recombinant adenoviral vectors to the lung. Hum Gene Ther 1997; 8:171–176.

15. Zhang H-G, Zhou T, Yang P, Edwards CKI, Curiel DT, Mountz JD. Inhibition of tumor necrosis factor α decreases inflammation and prolongs adenovirus gene expression in lung and liver. Hum Gene Ther 1998; 9:1875–1884.

16. Sung RS, Qin L, Bromberg JS. TNFα and IFNγ induced by innate anti-adenoviral immune responses inhibit adenovirus-mediated transgene expression. Mol Ther 2001; 3:757–767.

17. Virella-Lowell I, Poirier A, Chesnut KA, Brantly M, Flotte TR. Inhibition of recombinant adeno-associated virus (rAAV) transduction by bronchial secretions from cystic fibrosis patients. Gene Ther 2000; 7:1783–1789.

18. Perricone MA, Rees DD, Sacks CR, Smith KA, Kaplan JM, St. George JA. Inhibitory effect of cystic fibrosis sputum on adenovirus-mediated gene transfer in cultured epithelial cells. Hum Gene Ther 2000; 11:1997–2008.

19. Wang G, Zabner J, Deering C, Launspach J, Shao J, Bodner M, et al. Increasing epithelial junction permeability enhances gene transfer to airway epithelia in vivo. Am J Respir Cell Mol Biol 2000; 22:129–138.

20. Chu Q, St. George JA, Lukason M, Cheng SH, Scheule RK, Eastman SJ. EGTA enhancement of adenovirus-mediated gene transfer to mouse tracheal epithelium in vivo. Hum Gene Ther 2001; 12:455–467.

21. Arcasoy SM, Latoche J, Gondor M, Watkins SC, Henderson RA, Hughey R, et al. MUC1 and other sialoglycoconjugates inhibit adenovirus-mediated gene transfer. Am J Respir Cell Mol Biol 1997; 17:422–435.

22. Lei D, Lehmann M, Shellito JE, Nelson S, Siegling A, Volk HD, et al. Nondepleting anti-CD4 antibody treatment prolongs lung-directed E1-deleted adenovirus-mediated gene expression in rats. Hum Gene Ther 1996; 7:2273–2279.

23. Kaplan JM, Smith AE. Transient immunosuppression with deoxyspergualin improves longevity of transgene expression and ability to readminister adenoviral vector to the mouse lung. Hum Gene Ther 1997; 8:1095–1104.

24. Scaria A, St. George JA, Gregory RJ, Noelle RJ, Wadsworth SC, Smith AE, et al.

Antibody to CD40 ligand inhibits both humoral and cellular immune responses to adenoviral vectors and facilitates repeated administration to mouse airway. Gene Ther 1997; 4:611–617.

25. Shean MK, Baskin G, Sullivan D, Schurr J, Cavender DE, Shellito JE, et al. Immunomodulation and adenoviral-mediated gene transfer to the lungs of non-human primates. Hum Gene Ther 2000; 11:1047–1055.

26. Rahman A, Tsai V, Goudreau A, Shinoda JY, Wen SF, Ramachandra M, et al. Specific depletion of human anti-adenovirus antibodies facilitates transduction in an in vivo model for systemic gene therapy. Mol Ther 2001; 3:768–778.

27. Engelhardt JF, Yankaskas JR, Wilson JM. In vivo retroviral gene transfer into human bronchial epithelia of xenografts. J Clin Invest 1992; 90:2598–2607.

28. Olsen JC, Johnson LG, Stutts MJ, Sarkadi B, Yankaskas JR, Swanstrom R, et al. Correction of the apical membrane chloride permeability defect in polarized cystic fibrosis airway epithelia following retroviral mediated gene transfer. Hum Gene Ther 1992; 3:253–266.

29. Halbert CL, Aitken ML, Miller AD. Retroviral vectors efficiently transduce basal and secretory airway epithelial cells in vitro resulting in persistent gene expression in organotypic culture. Hum Gene Ther 1996; 7:1871–1881.

30. Wang G, Davidson BL, Melchert P, Slepushkin VA, van Es HHG, Bodner M, Jolly DL, McCray PB. Influence of cell polarity on retrovirus-mediated gene transfer to differentiated human airway epithelial epithelia. J Virol 1998; 72:9818–9826.

31. Zsengeller ZK, Halbert C, Miller AD, Wert SE, Whitsett JA, Bachurski CJ. Keratinocyte growth factor stimulates transduction of the respiratory epithelium by retroviral vectors. Hum Gene Ther 1999; 10:341–353.

32. Pitt BR, Schwarz MA, Pilewski JM, Nakayama D, Mueller GM, Robbins PD, et al. Retrovirus-mediated gene transfer in lungs of living fetal sheep. Gene Ther 1995; 2:344–350.

33. Johnson LG, Mewshaw JP, Ni H, Friedman T, Boucher RC, Olsen JC. Effect of host modification and age on airway epithelial gene transfer mediated by a murine leukemia virus–derived vector. J Virol 1998; 72:8861–8872.

34. Fujiwara T, Cai DW, Georges RN, Mukhopadhyay T, Grimm EA, Roth JA. Therapeutic effect of a retroviral wild-type p53 expression vector in an orthotopic lung cancer model. J Natl Cancer Inst 1994; 86:1458–1462.

35. Roth JA, Nguyen D, Lawrence DD, Kemp BL, Carrasco CH, Ferson DZ, et al. Retrovirus-mediated wild-type p53 gene transfer to tumors of patients with lung cancer. Nat Med 1996; 2:985–991.

36. Goldman MJ, Lee PS, Yang JS, Wilson JM. Lentiviral vectors for gene therapy of cystic fibrosis. Hum Gene Ther 1997; 8:2261–2268.

37. Lever AM. Lentiviral vectors: progress and potential. Curr Opin Mol Therapeut 2000; 2:488–496.

38. White GC, Roberts HR. Gene therapy for hemophilia: a step closer to reality. Mol Ther 2000; 1:207–208.

39. Green ES, Rendahl KG, Zhou S, Ladner M, Coyne M, Srivastava R, et al. Two animal models of retinal degeneration are rescued by recombinant adeno-associated virus-mediated production of FGF-5 and FGF-18. Mol Ther 2001; 3:507–515.

40. Conrad CK, Allen SS, Afione SA, Reynolds TC, Beck SE, Fee-Maki M, et al.

Safety of single-dose administration of an adeno-associated virus (AAV)–CFTR vector in the primate lung. Gene Ther 1996; 3:658–668.

41. Flotte TR, Solow R, Owens RA, Afione SA, Zeitlin PL, Carter BJ. Gene expression from adeno-associated virus vectors in airway epithelial cells. Am J Respir Cell Mol Biol 1992; 7:349–356.

42. Flotte TR, Carter BJ. Adeno-associated virus vectors for gene therapy. Gene Ther 1995; 2:357–362.

43. Munson KL, Weiss DJ, Strandjord TP, Lynch CM. Improved detection of AAV transduction in lung. Pediatr Pulmonol 1999; 19(suppl):231.

44. Duan D, Yue Y, Yan Z, McCray PBJ, Engelhardt JF. Polarity influences the efficiency of recombinant adeno-associated virus infection in differentiated airway epithelia. Hum Gene Ther 1998; 9:2761–2776.

45. Chao H, Liu Y, Rabinowitz J, Li C, Samulski RJ, Walsh CE. Several log increase in therapeutic transgene delivery by distinct adeno-associated viral serotype vectors. Mol Ther 2000; 2:619–623.

46. Walters R, Yi SM, Keshavjee S, Brown K, Welsh MJ, Chiorini J, et al. Binding of adeno-associated virus type 5 to 2,3-linked sialic acid is required for gene transfer. Mol Ther 2001; 3:S231.

47. Sanlioglu S, Engelhardt JF. Cellular redox state alters recombinate adeno-associated virus transduction through tyrosine phosphatase pathways. Gene Ther 1991; 6:1427–1437.

48. Pickles RJ, McCarty D, Matsui H, Hart PJ, Randell SH, Boucher RC. Limited entry of adenovirus vectors into well-differentiated airway epithelium is responsible for inefficient gene transfer. J Virol 1998; 72:6014–6023.

49. Worgall S, Wolff G, Falck-Pedersen E, Crystal RG. Innate immune mechanisms dominate elimination of adenoviral vectors following in vivo administration. Hum Gene Ther 1997; 8:37–44.

50. Zabner J, Zeiher BG, Friedman E, Welsh MJ. Adenovirus-mediated gene transfer to ciliated airway epithelia requires prolonged incubation time. J Virol 1996; 70: 6994–7003.

51. Jiang C, Akita GY, Colledge WH, Ratcliff RA, Evans MJ, Hehir KM, et al. Increased contact time improves adenovirus-mediated CFTR gene transfer to nasal epithelium of CF mice. Hum Gene Ther 1997; 8:671–680.

52. Engelhardt JF, Yang Y, Stratford-Perricaudet LD, Allen ED, Kozarsky K, Perricaudet M, et al. Direct gene transfer of human CFTR into human bronchial epithelia of xenografts with E1-deleted adenoviruses. Nat Genet 1993; 4:27–34.

53. Rosenfeld MA, Yoshimura K, Trapnell BC, Yoneyama K, Rosenthal ER, Dalemans W, et al. In vivo transfer of the human cystic fibrosis transmembrane conductance regulator gene to the airway epithelium. Cell 1992; 68:143–155.

54. Kaplan J, St. George JA, Pennington SE, Keyes LD, Johnson RP, Wadsworth SC, et al. Humoral and cellular immune responses of nonhuman primates to long-term repeated lung exposure to Ad2/CFTR-2. Gene Ther 1996; 3:117–127.

55. Morral N, O'Neial W, Zhou H, Langston C, Beaudet A. Immune responses to reporter proteins and high viral dose limit duration of expression with adenoviral vectors: comparison of E2a wild type and E2a deleted vectors. Hum Gene Ther 1997; 8:1275–1286.

56. Song W, Kong H-L, Traktman P, Crystal RG. Cytotoxic T lymphocyte responses to proteins encoded by heterologous transgenes transferred in vivo by adenoviral vectors. Hum Gene Ther 1997; 8:1207–1217.

57. Yang Y, Jooss KU, Su Q, Ertl HC, Wilson JM. Immune responses to viral antigens versus transgene product in the elimination of recombinant adenovirus-infected hepatocytes in vivo. Gene Ther 1996; 3:137–144.

58. Thorne PS, McCray PB, Howe TS, O'Neill MA. Early-onset inflammatory responses in vivo to adenoviral vectors in the presence or absence of lipopolysaccharide-induced inflammation. Am J Respir Cell Mol Biol 1999; 20:1155–1164.

59. Weiss DJ, Bonneau L, Liggitt D. Use of perfluorochemical liquid allows earlier detection and use of less adenovirus vector for gene expression in normal lung and enhances gene expression in acutely injured lung. Mol Ther 2001; 3:734–745.

60. Morsy MA, Gu MC, Motzel S, Zhao J, Lin J, Su Q, et al. An adenoviral vector deleted for all viral coding sequences results in enhanced safety and extended expression of a leptin transgene. Appl Biol Sci 1998; 95:7866–7871.

61. Morral N, Parks RJ, Zhou H, Langston C, Schiedner G, Quinones J, et al. High doses of a helper-dependent adenoviral vector yield supraphysiological levels of α_1-antitrypsin with negligible toxicity. Hum Gene Ther 1998; 9:2709–2716.

62. Chillón M, Lee JH, Fasbender A, Welsh MJ. Adenovirus complexed with polyethylene glycol and cationic lipid is shielded from neutralizing antibodies in vitro. Gene Ther 1998; 5:995–1002.

63. O'Riordan CR, Lachapell A, Delgado C, Parkes V, Wadsworth SC, Smith AE, et al. PEGylation of adenovirus with retention of infectivity and protection from neutralizing antibody in vitro and in vivo. Hum Gene Ther 1999; 10:1349–1358.

64. Tursz T, Cesne AL, Opolon P, Schatz C, Pavirani A, Courtney M, et al. Phase I study of a recombinant adenovirus-mediated gene transfer in lung cancer patients. J Natl Cancer Inst 1996; 88:1857–1863.

65. Carbone DP, Adak S, Schiller J, Kubba S, Slovis B, Coffee K, et al. Objective responses from adenovirus p53 administered by bronchoalveolar lavage in patients with bronchioalveolar cell lung carcinoma (BAC). Lung Cancer 2000; 29:103.

66. Albelda SM, Wiewrodt R, Zuckerman JB. Gene therapy for lung disease: hype or hope? Ann Intern Med 2000; 132:649–660.

67. Pilewski JM, Latoche JD, Arcasoy SM, Albelda SM. Expression in integrin cell adhesion receptors during human airway epithelial repair in vivo. Am J Physiol 1997; 273:L256–L263.

68. Parsons DW, Grubb BR, Johnson LG, Boucher RC. Enhanced in vivo airway gene transfer via transient modification of host barrier properties with a surface-active agent. Hum Gene Ther 1998; 9:2661–2672.

69. Factor P, Saldias F, Ridge K, Dumasius V, Zabner J, Jaffe HA, et al. Augmentation of lung liquid clearance via adenovirus-mediated transfer of a Na, K-ATPase betal subunity gene. J Clin Invest 1998; 102:1421–1430.

70. Factor P, Mendez M, Mutlu G, Dumasius V. Gene transfer to severely injured rat lungs. Mol Ther 2001; 3:S337–S338.

71. Weiss DJ, Strandjord TP, Jackson JC, Clark JG, Liggitt D. Perfluorochemical liquid-enhanced adenoviral vector distribution and expression in lungs of spontaneously breathing rodents. Exp Lung Res 1999; 25:317–333.

72. Yonemitsu Y, Kitson C, Ferrari S, Farley R, Griesenbach U, Judd D, et al. Efficient gene transfer to airway epithelium using recombinant Sendai virus. Nat Biotechnol 2000; 18:970–973.

73. Slepushkin VA, Staber PD, Wang G, McCray PB, Jr, Davidson BL. Infection of human airway epithelia with H1N1, H2N2, and H3N2 Influenza A virus strains. Mol Ther 2001; 3:395–402.

74. Scheule RK, St. George JA, Bagley RG, Marshall J, Kaplan JM, Akita GY, et al. Basis of pulmonary toxicity associated with cationic lipid-mediated gene transfer to the mammalian lung. Hum Gene Ther 1997; 8:689–707.

75. Tan Y, Liu F, Li Z, Li S, Huang L. Sequential injection of cationic liposome and plasmid DNA effectively transfects the lung with minimal inflammatory toxicity. Mol Ther 2001; 3:673–682.

76. Ruiz FE, Clancy JP, Perricone MA, Bebok Z, Hong JS, Cheng SH, et al. A clinical inflammatory syndrome attributable to aerosolized lipid-DNA administration in cystic fibrosis. Hum Gene Ther 2001; 12:751–761.

77. Freimark BD, Blezinger HP, Florack VJ, Nordstrom JL, Long SD, Deshpande DS, et al. Cationic lipids enhance cytokine and cell influx levels in the lung following administration of plasmid:cationic lipid complexes. J Immunol 1998; 160:4580–4586.

78. Li S, Wu SP, Whitmore M, Loeffert EJ, Wang L, Watkins SC, et al. Effect of immune response on gene transfer to the lung via systemic administration of cationic lipidic vectors. Am J Physiol 1999; 276:L796–L804.

79. Yew NS, Zhao H, Wu IH, Song A, Tousignant JD, Przybylska M, et al. Reduced inflammatory response to plasmid DNA vectors by elimination and inhibition of immunostimulatory CpG motifs. Mol Ther 2000; 1:255–262.

80. Yew NS, Wang KX, Przybylska M, Bagley RG, Stedman M, Marshall J, et al. Contribution of plasmid DNA to inflammation in the lung after administration of cationic lipid:pDNA complexes. Hum Gene Ther 1999; 10:223–234.

81. Krieg AM. Minding the Cs and Gs. Mol Ther 2000; 1:209–210.

82. Tsan MF, White JE, Shepard B. Lung-specific direct in vivo gene transfer with recombinant plasmid DNA. Am J Physiol 1995; 268:L1052–L1056.

83. Tsan MF, White JE, Pastore JN, Hayes VD, Shepard BA, Lee CY. Pulmonary response to plasmid DNA and immunohistochemical localization of transgene expression. Exp Lung Res 1996; 22:651–666.

84. Kukowska-Latallo JF, Raczka E, Quintana A, Chen C, Rymaszewski M, Baker JR. Intravascular and endobronchial DNA delivery to muring lung tissue using a novel, nonviral vector. Hum Gene Ther 2000; 11:1385–1395.

85. Raczka E, Kukowska-Latallo JF, Rymaszewski M, Chen C, Baker JR. The effect of synthetic surfactant Exosurf on gene transfer in mouse lung in vivo. Gene Ther 1998; 5:1333–1339.

86. Yew NS, Wysokenski DM, Wang KX, Ziegler RJ, Marshall J, McNeilly D, et al. Optimization of plasmid vectors for high-level expression in lung epithelial cells. Hum Gene Ther 1997; 8:575–584.

87. Fasbender AJ, Zabner J, Welsh MJ. Optimization of cationic lipid-mediated gene transfer to airway epithelia. Am J Physiol 1995; 269:L45–L51.

88. Griesenbach U, Chonn A, Cassady R, Hannam V, Ackerley C, Post M, et al. Com-

parison between intratracheal and intravenous administration of liposome-DNA complexes for cystic fibrosis lung gene therapy. Gene Ther 1998; 5:181–188.

89.   Debs R, Pian M, Gaensler K, Clements J, Friend DS, Dobbs L. Prolonged transgene expression in rodent lung cells. Am J Respir Cell Mol Biol 1992; 7:406–413.

90.   Matsui H, Johnson LG, Randell SH, Boucher RC. Loss of binding and entry of liposome-DNA complexes decreases transfection efficiency in differentiated airway epithelial cells. J Biol Chem 1997; 272:1117–1126.

91.   Stribling R, Brunette E, Liggitt D, Gaensler K, Debs R. Aerosol gene delivery in vivo. Proc Natl Acad Sci USA 1995; 89:11277–11281.

92.   Zabner J, Fasbender AJ, Moninger T, Poellinger KA, Welsh MJ. Cellular and molecular barriers to gene transfer by a cationic lipid. J Biol Chem 1995; 270:18997–19007.

93.   Fasbender A, Zabner J, Zeiher BG, Welsh MJ. A low rate of cell proliferation and reduced DNA uptake limit cationic lipid-mediated gene transfer to primary cultures of ciliated human airway epithelia. Gene Ther 1997; 4:1173–1180.

94.   Tsan MF, Tsan GL, White JE. Surfactant inhibits cationic liposome-mediated gene transfer. Hum Gene Ther 1997; 8:817–825.

95.   Zabner J, Cheng SH, Meeker D, Launspach J, Balfour R, Perricone MA, et al. Comparison of DNA-lipid complexes and DNA alone for gene transfer to cystic fibrosis airway epithelia in vivo. J Clin Invest 1997; 100:1529–1537.

96.   Alton EWFW, Stern M, Farley R, Jaffe A, Chadwick SL, Phillips J, et al. Cationic lipid-mediated CFTR gene transfer to the lungs and nose of patients with cystic fibrosis: a double-blind placebo-controlled trial. Lancet 1999; 353:947–954.

97.   Noone PG, Hohneker KW, Zhou Z, Johnson LG, Foy C, Gipson C, et al. Safety and biological efficacy of a lipid-CFTR complex for gene transfer in the nasal epithelium of adult patients with cystic fibrosis. Mol Ther 2000; 1:105–114.

98.   Harris CE, Agarwal S, Hu P, Wagner E, Curiel DT. Receptor-mediated gene transfer to airway epithelial cells in primary culture. Am J Respir Cell Mol Biol 1993; 9:441–447.

99.   Gao L, Wagner E, Cotten M, Agarwal S, Harris C, Romer M, et al. Direct in vivo gene transfer to airway epithelium employing adenovirus-polylysine-DNA complexes. Hum Gene Ther 1993; 4:17–24.

100. Fajac I, Briand P, Monsigny M, Midoux P. Sugar-mediated uptake of glycosylated polylysines and gene transfer into normal and cystic fibrosis airway epithelial cells. Hum Gene Ther 1999; 10:395–406.

101. Schughart K, Bischoff R, Rasmussen UB, Ali Hadji D, Perraud F, Accart N, et al. Solvoplex: A new type of synthetic vector for intrapulmonary gene delivery. Hum Gene Ther 1999; 10:2891–2905.

102. Gene transfer into the airway epithelium of animals by targeting the polymeric immunoglobulin receptor. J Clin Invest 2001; 95:493–502.

103. Gupta S, Eastman J, Silski C, Kerkol T, Davis PB. Single chain Fv: a ligand in receptor-mediated gene delivery. Gene Ther 2001; 8:586–592.

104. Gautam A, Densmore CL, Golunski E, Xu B, Waldrep JC. Transgene expression in mouse airway epithelium by aerosol gene therapy with PEI-DNA complexes. Mol Ther 2001; 3:551–556.

105. Gautam A, Densmore CL, Xu B, Waldrep JC. Enhanced gene expression in mouse lung after PEI-DNA aerosol delivery. Mol Ther 2000; 2:63–70.
106. Gautam A, Densmore CL, Waldrep JC. Inhibition of experimental lung metastasis by aerosol delivery of PEI-p53 complexes. Gene Ther 2000; 2:318–323.
107. Gautam A, Densmore CL, Waldrep JC. Pulmonary cytokine responses associated with PEI-DNA aerosol gene therapy. Gene Ther 2001; 8:254–257.
108. Huard J, Lochmuller H, Acsadi G, Jani A, Bassie B, Karpati G. The route of administration is a major determinant of the transduction efficiency of rat tissues by adenoviral recombinants. Gene Ther 1995; 2:107–115.
109. McLean JW, Fox EA, Baluk P, Bolton PB, Haskell A, Pearlman R, et al. Organ-specific endothelial cell uptake of cationic liposome-DNA complexes in mice. Am J Physiol (Heart Circ Physiol) 1997; 273:H387–H404.
110. Templeton NS, Lasic DD, Frederik PM, Strey HH, Roberts DD, Pavlakis GN. Improved DNA: liposome complexes for increased systemic delivery and gene expression. Nat Biotechnol 1997; 15:647–652.
111. Mahato RI, Anwer K, Tagliaferri F, Meaney C, Leonard P, Wadhwa MS, et al. Biodistribution and gene expression of lipid/plasmid complexes after systemic administration. Hum Gene Ther 1998; 9:2083–2099.
112. Hughes BJ, Kennel S, Lee R, Huang L. Monoclonal antibody targeting of liposomes to mouse lung in vivo. Cancer Res 1989; 49:6214–6220.
113. Maruyama K, Holmberg E, Kennel SJ, Klibanov A, Torchilin VP, Huang L. Characterization of in vivo immunoliposome targeting to pulmonary endothelium. J Pharm Sci 1990; 79:978–984.
114. Litzinger DC, Brown JM, Wala I, Kaufman SA, Van GY, Farrell CL, et al. Fate of cationic liposomes and their complex with oligonucleotide in vivo. Biochim Biophys Acta 1996; 1281:139–149.
115. Schughart K, Bischoff R, Ali Hadji D, Boussif O, Perraud F, Accart N, et al. Effect of liposome-encapsulated clodronate pretreatment on synthetic vector-mediated gene expression in mice. Gene Ther 1999; 6:448–453.
116. Rodman DM, San H, Simari R, Stephan D, Tanner F, Yang Z, et al. In vivo gene delivery to the pulmonary circulation in rats: transgene distribution and vascular inflammatory response. Am J Respir Cell Mol Biol 1997; 16:640–649.
117. Reynolds PN, Zinn KR, Gavrilyuk VD, Balyasnikova IV, Rogers BE, Buchsbaum DJ, et al. A targetable, injectable adenoviral vector for selective gene delivery to pulmonary endothelium in vivo. Mol Ther 2000; 2:562–578.
118. Nettelbeck DM, Miller DW, Jérôme J, Zuzart M, Watkins SJ, Hawkins RE, et al. Targeting of adenovirus to endothelial cells by a bispecific single-chain diabody directed against the adenovirus fiber knob domain and human endoglin (CD105). Mol Ther 2001; 3:882–891.
119. Varga CM, Wickham TJ, Lauffenburger DA. Receptor-mediated targeting of gene delivery vectors: insights from molecular mechanisms for improved vehicle design. Biotechnol Bioeng 2000; 70:593–605.
120. Zhang Y, Chirmule N, Gao GP, Qian R, Croyl M, Joshi B, et al. Acute cytokine response to systemic adenoviral vectors in mice is mediated by dendritic cells and macrophages. Mol Ther 2001; 3:697–707.

121. Tyler RC, Fagan KA, Unfer RC, Gorman C, McClarrion M, Bullock C, et al. Vascular inflammation inhibits gene transfer to the pulmonary circulation in vivo. Am J Physiol 1999; 277:L1199–L1204.

122. Simon RH, Engelhardt JF, Yang Y, Zepeda M, Weber-Pendleton S, Grossman M, et al. Adenovirus-mediated transfer of the CFTR gene to lung of nonhuman primates: toxicity study. Hum Gene Ther 1993; 4:771–780.

123. Engelhardt JF, Simon RH, Yang Y, Zepeda M, Weber-Pendleton S, Doranz B, et al. Adenovirus-mediated transfer of the CFTR gene to lung of nonhuman primates: biological efficacy study. Hum Gene Ther 1993; 4:759–769.

124. Sene C, Bout A, Imler JL, Schultz H, Willemot JM, Hennebel V, et al. Aerosol-mediated delivery of recombinant adenovirus to the airways of nonhuman primates. Hum Gene Ther 1995; 6:1587–1593.

125. McDonald RJ, Lukason MJ, Raabe OG, Canfield DR, Burr EA, Kaplan JM, et al. Safety of airway gene transfer with Ad2/CFTR2: aerosol administration in the nonhuman primate. Hum Gene Ther 1997; 8:411–422.

126. Halbert CL, Standaert TA, Wilson CB, Miller AD. Successful readministration of adeno-associated virus vectors to the mouse lung requires transient immunosuppression during the initial exposure. J Virol 1998; 72:9795–9805.

127. Zabner J, Ramsey BW, Meeker DP, Aitken ML, Balfour RP, Gibson RL, et al. Repeat administration of an adenovirus vector encoding cystic fibrosis transmembrane conductance regulator to the nasal epithelium of patients with cystic fibrosis. J Clin Invest 1996; 97:1504–1511.

128. Weiss DJ, Bonneau L, Allen JM, Miller AD, Halbert CL. Perfluorochemical liquid enhances adeno-associated virus-mediated transgene expression in lung. Mol Ther 2000; 2:624–630.

129. Zuckerman JB, Robinson CB, McCoy KS, Shell R, Sferra TJ, Chirmule N, et al. A Phase I study of adenovirus-mediated transfer of the human cystic fibrosis transmembrane conductance regulator gene to a lung segment of individuals with cystic fibrosis. Hum Gene Ther 1999; 10:2973–2985.

130. Harvey BG, Leopold PL, Hackett NR, Grasso TM, Williams PM, Tucker AL, et al. Airway epithelial CFTR mRNA expression in cystic fibrosis patients after repetitive administration of a recombinant adenovirus. J Clin Invest 1999; 104:1165–1166.

131. Katkin JP, Gilbert BE, Langston C, French K, Beaudet AL. Aerosol delivery of a β-galactosidase adenoviral vector to the lungs of rodents. Hum Gene Ther 1995; 6:985–995.

132. Bellon G, Michel-Calemard L, Thouvenot D, Jagneaux V, Poitevin F, Malcus C, et al. Aerosol administration of a recombinant adenovirus expressing CFTR to cystic fibrosis patients: a phase I clinical trial. Hum Gene Ther 1997; 8:15–25.

133. Eastman SJ, Tousignant JD, Lukason MJ, Chu Q, Cheng SH, Scheule RK. Aerosolization of cationic lipid:pDNA complexes in vitro optimization of nebulizer parameters for human clinical studies. Hum Gene Ther 1998; 9:43–52.

134. Brown AR, Chowdhury SI. Propellant-driven aerosols of DNA plasmids for gene expression. J Aerosol Med 1997; 10:129–146.

135. Lee JH, Zabner J, Welsh MJ. Delivery of an adenovirus vector in a calcium phos-

phate coprecipitate enhances the therapeutic index of gene transfer to airway epithelia. Hum Gene Ther 1999; 10:603–613.

136. Fasbender A, Lee JH, Walters RW, Moninger TO, Zabner J, Welsh MJ. Incorporation of adenovirus in calcium phosphate precipitates enhances gene transfer to airway epithelia in vitro and in vivo. J Clin Invest 1998; 102:184–193.

137. Walters RW, Duan D, Engelhardt JF, Welsh MJ. Incorporation of adeno-associated virus in a calcium phosphate coprecipitate improves gene transfer to airway epithelia in vitro and in vivo. J Virol 2000; 74:535–540.

138. Greenough A. Expanded use of surfactant replacement therapy. Eur J Pediatr 2001; 159:635–640.

139. Kharasch VS, Sweeny TD, Fredberg J, Lehr J, Damokosh AI, Avery ME, et al. Pulmonary surfactant as a vehicle for intratracheal delivery of technetium sulfur colloid and pentamidine in hamster lungs. Am Rev Respir Dis 1991; 144:909–913.

140. Clark LC, Jr, Gollan F. Survival of mammals breathing organic liquids equilibrated with oxygen at atmospheric pressure. Science 1966; 152:1755–1756.

141. Shaffer TH, Wolfson MR, Clark LC. Liquid ventilation. Pediatr Pulmonol 1992; 14:102–109.

142. Leach CL, Greenspan JS, Rubenstein SD, Shaffer TH, Wolfson MR, Jackson JC, et al. Partial liquid ventilation with perflubron in premature infants with severe respiratory distress syndrome. N Engl J Med 1996; 335:761–767.

143. Blackwell TS, Blackwell TR, Holden EP, Christman BW, Christman JW. In vivo antioxidant treatment suppresses nuclear factor-κB activation and neutrophilic lung inflammation. J Immunol 1996; 157:1630–1637.

144. Papo MC, Paczan PR, Fuhrman BP, Steinhorn DM, Hernan LJ, Leach CL, et al. Perfluorocarbon-associated gas exchange improves oxygenation, lung mechanics, and survival in a model of adult respiratory distress syndrome. Crit Care Med 1996; 24:466–474.

145. Colton DM, Till GO, Johnson KJ, Dean SB, Bartlett RH, Hirschl RB. Neutrophil accumulation is reduced during partial liquid ventilation. Crit Care Med 1998; 26:1716–1724.

146. Croce MA, Fabian TC, Patton JH, Melton SM, Moore M, Trenthem LL. Partial liquid ventilation decreases the inflammatory response in the alveolar environment of trauma patients. J Trauma Injury Infect Crit Care 1998; 45:273–282.

147. Lisby DA, Ballard PL, Fox WW, Wolfson MR, Shaffer TH, Gonzales LW. Enhanced distribution of adenovirus-mediated gene transfer to lung parenchyma by perfluorochemical liquid. Hum Gene Ther 1997; 8:919–928.

148. Weiss DJ, Niven RW, Strandjord TP, Liggitt D, Clark JG. Perfluorochemical liquid-enhanced liposomal-mediated gene transfer to lungs of spontaneously breathing rats. Pediatr Pulmonol 1998; 17:269.

149. Weiss DJ, Baskin GB, Shean MK, Blanchard JL, Kolls JK. Use of perfluorochemical liquid to enhance adenoviral-mediated gene expression in lungs of spontaneously breathing non-human primates: feasibility and initial studies. Pediatr Pulmonol 2000; 20 (Suppl):235–236.

150. Weiss DJ, Baskin GB, Shean MK, Blanchardt JL, Kolls JK. Perflubron enhances

adenovirus-mediated gene expression in lungs of spontaneously breathing non-human primates. Mol Ther 2001; 3:S338.

151. Weiss DJ, Strandjord TP, Liggitt D, Clark JG. Perflubron enhances adenoviral-mediated gene expression in lungs of transgenic mice with chronic alveolar filling. Hum Gene Ther 1999; 10:2287–2293.

152. Bonneau L, Shaffer TH, Lukason M, St. George J, Wolfson MR, Weiss DJ. Ingestion in vivo by alveolar macrophages of perfluorochemical (PFC) liquid correlates with altered pro-inflammatory cytokine release. Am J Respir Crit Care Med 2000; 161:A902.

153. Weiss DJ, Bonneau L, Liggitt D. Instillation of perfluorochemical (PFC) liquid to lungs of spontaneously breathing mice transiently opens tight junctions between airway epithelial cells: a possible mechanism for enhancement of gene expression using PFC liquids. Mol Ther 2001; 3:S337.

154. Boehler A, Chamberlain D, Xing Z, Slutsky AS, Jordana M, Gauldie J, et al. Adenovirus-mediated interleukin-10 gene transfer inhibits post-transplant fibrous airway obliteration in an animal model of bronchiolitis obliterans. Hum Gene Ther 1998; 9:541–551.

155. Zsengeller ZK, Reed JA, Bachurski CJ, LeVine AM, Forry-Schaudies S, Hirsch R, et al. Adenovirus-mediated granulocyte-macrophage colony-stimulating factor improves lung pathology of pulmonary alveolar proteinosis in granulocyte-macrophage colony-stimulating factor-deficient mice. Hum Gene Ther 1998; 9: 2101–2109.

156. Epperly M, Bray J, Kraeger S, Zwacka R, Engelhardt J, Travis E, et al. Prevention of late effects of irradiation lung damage by manganese superoxide dismutase gene therapy. Gene Ther 1998; 5:196–208.

157. Epperly MW, Travis EL, Sikora C, Greenberger JS. Manganese (correction of magnesium) superoxide dismutase (MnSOD) plasmid/liposome pulmonary radioprotective gene therapy: modulation of irradiation-induced mRNA for IL-I, TNF-alpha, and TGF-beta correlates with delay of organizing alveolitis/fibrosis. Biol Blood Marrow Transplant 1999; 5:204–214.

158. Epperly MW, Bray JA, Krager S, Berry LM, Gooding W, Engelhardt JF, et al. Intratracheal injection of adenovirus containing the human MnSOD transgene protects athymic nude mice from irradiation-induced organizing alveolitis. Int J Radiat Oncol Biol Phys 1999; 43:169–181.

159. Kollef MH, Schuster DP. Acute respiratory distress syndrome. N Engl J Med 1995; 332:27–38.

160. Fulkerson WJ, MacIntyre N, Stamler J, Crapo JD. Pathogenesis and treatment of the adult respiratory distress syndrome. Arch Intern Med 1996; 156:29–38.

161. International consensus conferences in intensive care medicine: Ventilator-associated lung injury in ARDS. Am J Respir Crit Care Med 2001; 160:2118–2124.

162. The Acute Respiratory Distress Syndrome Network. Ventilation with lower tidal volumes as compared with traditional tidal volumes for acute lung injury and the acute respiratory distress syndrome. N Engl J Med 2000; 342:1301–1308.

163. Ye L, Chan S, Chow YH, Tsui LC, Hu J. Regulated expression of the human CFTR gene in epithelial cells. Mol Ther 2001; 3:723–733.

164. Smith MJ, Rousculp MD, Goldsmith KT, Curiel DT, Garver RI. Surfactant protein

A-directed toxin gene kills lung cancer cells in vitro. Hum Gene Ther 1994; 5:29–35.

165. Chow YH, Plumb J, Wen Y, Steer BM, Lu Z, Buchwald M, et al. Targeting transgene expression to airway epithelia and submucosal glands, prominent sites of human CFTR expression. Mol Ther 2000; 2:359–367.

166. Dupuit F, Zahm JM, Pierrot D, Brezillon S, Bonnet N, Imler JL, et al. Regenerating cells in human airway surface epithelium represent preferential targets for recombinant adenovirus. Hum Gene Ther 1995; 6:1185–1193.

167. Buch S, Han RNN, Liu J, Moore A, Edelson JD, Freeman BA, et al. Basic fibroblast growth factor and growth factor receptor gene expression in 85% O_2-exposed rat lung. Am J Physiol (Lung Cell Mol Physiol) 1995; 268:L455–L464.

168. Goldman CK, Rogers BE, Douglas JT, Sosnowski BA, Ying W, Siegal GP, et al. Targeted gene delivery to Kaposi's sarcoma cells via the fibroblast growth factor receptor. Cancer Res 1997; 57:1447–1451.

169. Sosnowski BA, Gonzalez AM, Chandler LA, Buechler YJ, Pierce GF, Baird A. Targeting DNA to cells with basic fibroblast growth factor (FGF2). J Biol Chem 1996; 271:33647–33653.

170. Hoganson DK, Sosnowski BA, Pierce GF, Doukas J. Uptake of adenoviral vectors via fibroblast growth factor receptors involves intracellular pathways that differ from targeting ligand. Mol Ther 2001; 3:105–112.

171. Gauldie J, Graham F, Xing Z, Braciak T, Foley R, Sime PJ. Adenovirus-vector–mediated cytokine gene transfer to lung tissue. Ann NY Acad Sci 1996; 796:235–244.

172. West J, Rodman DM. Gene therapy for pulmonary diseases. Chest 2001; 119:613–617.

173. Xing Z, Braciak T, Jordana M, Croitoru K, Graham FL, Gauldie J. Adenovirus-mediated cytokine gene transfer at tissue sites. J Immunol 1994; 153:4059–4069.

174. Yoshida M, Sakuma J, Hayashi S, Abe K, Saito I, Harada S, et al. A histologically distinctive interstitial pneumonia induced by overexpression of the interleukin 6, transforming growth factor β1, or platelet-derived growth factor B gene. Proc Natl Acad Sci USA 1995; 92:9570–9574.

175. Sime PJ, Marr RA, Gauldie D, Xing Z, Hewlett BR, Graham FL, et al. Transfer of tumor necrosis factor-alpha to rat lung induces severe pulmonary inflammation and patchy interstitial fibrogenesis with induction of transforming growth factor-beta 1 and myofibroblasts. Am J Pathol 1998; 153:825–832.

176. Xing Z, Tremblay GM, Sime PJ, Gauldie J. Overexpression of granulocyte-macrophage colony-stimulating factor induces pulmonary granulation tissue formation and fibrosis by induction of transforming growth factor-beta 1 and myofibroblast accumulation. Am J Pathol 1997; 150:59–66.

177. Sime PJ, Xing Z, Graham FL, Csaky KG, Gauldie J. Adenovector-mediated gene transfer of active transforming growth factor-β1 induces prolonged severe dibrosis in rat lung. J Clin Invest 1997; 100:768–776.

178. Standiford TJ, Wilkowski JM, Sisson TH, Hattori N, Mehrad B, Bucknell KA, et al. Intrapulmonary tumor necrosis factor gene therapy increases bacterial clearance and survival in murine gram-negative pneumonia. Hum Gene Ther 1999; 10:899–909.

179. Chen GH, Reddy RC, Newstead MW, Tateda K, Kyasapura BL, Standiford TJ. Intrapulmonary TNF gene therapy reverses sepsis-induced suppression of lung antibacterial host defense. J Immunol 2000; 165:6496–6503.

180. Greenberger MJ, Kunkel SL, Strieter RM, Lukacs NW, Bramson J, Gauldie J, et al. IL-12 gene therapy protects mice in lethal Klebsiella pneumonia. J Immunol 1996; 157:3006–3012.

181. Xing Z, Braciak T, Chong D, Feng X, Schroeder JA, Gauldie J. Adenoviral-mediated gene transfer of interleukin-6 in rat lung enhances antiviral immunoglobulin A and G responses in distinct tissue compartments. Biochem Biophys Res Commun 1999; 258:332–335.

182. Braciak TA, Gallichan WS, Graham FL, Richards CD, Ramsay AJ. Recombinant adenovirus vectors expressing interleukin-5 and -6 specifically enhance mucosal immunoglobulin a responses in the lung. Immunology 2000; 101:388–396.

183. Ding Y, Qin L, Kotenko SV, Pestka S, Bromberg JS. A single amino acid determines the immunostimulatory activity of interleukin 10. J Exp Med 2000; 191: 213–223.

184. Sawa T, Corry DB, Gropper MA, Ohara M, Kurahashi K, Wiener-Kronish JP. IL-10 improves lung injury and survival in Pseudomonas aeruginosa pneumonia. J Immunol 1997; 159:2858–2866.

185. Chernoff AE, Granowitz EV, Shapiro L, Vannier E, Lonnemann G, Angel JB, et al. A randomized, controlled trial of IL-10 in humans: inhibition of inflammatory cytokine production and immune responses. J Immunol 1995; 154:5492–5499.

186. Xing Z, Ohkawara Y, Jordana M, Graham FL, Gauldie J. Adenoviral vector–mediated interleukin-10 expression in vivo: intramuscular gene transfer inhibits cytokine responses in endotoxemia. Gene Ther 1997; 4:140–149.

187. Takakuwa T, Endo S, Shirakura Y, Yokoyama M, Tamatani M, Tohyama M, et al. Interleukin-10 gene transfer improves the survival rate of mice inoculated with *Escherichia coli*. Crit Care Med 2000; 28:2685–2689.

188. Drazan KE, Wu L, Bullington D, Shaked A. Viral IL-10 gene therapy inhibits TNF-alpha and IL-beta, not IL-6, in the newborn endotoxemic mouse. J Pediatr Surg 1996; 31:411–414.

189. Arai T, Abe K. Introduction of the interleukin-10 gene into mice inhibited bleomycin-induced lung injury in vivo. Am J Physiol (Lung Cell Mol Physiol) 2000; 278: L914–L922.

190. Qin L, Ding Y, Pahud DR, Robson ND, Shaked A, Bromberg JS. Adenovirus-mediated gene transfer of viral interleukin-10 inhibits the immune response to both alloantigen and adenoviral antigen. Hum Gene Ther 1997; 8:1365–1374.

191. Rogy MA, Auffenberg T, Espat NJ, Philip R, Remick D, Wollenberg GK, et al. Human tumor necrosis factor receptor (p55) and interleukin 10 gene transfer in the mouse reduces mortality to lethal endotoxemia and also attenuates local inflammatory responses. J Exp Med 1995; 181:2289–2293.

192. Itano H, Zhang W, Ritter JH, McCarthy TJ, Yew NS, Mohanakumar T, et al. Endobronchial transfection of naked viral interleukin-10 gene in rat lung allotransplantation. Ann Thorac Surg 2001; 71:1126–1133.

193. Minter RM, Rectenwald JE, Fukuzuka K, Tannahill CL, La Face D, Tsai V, et al.

TNF-α receptor signaling and IL-10 gene therapy regulate the innate and humoral immune responses to recombinant adenovirus in the lung. J Immunol 2000; 164: 443–451.

194. Virella-Lowell I, Mason E, Ferkol T, Flotte TR. Anti-inflammatory gene therapy for cystic fibrosis with a RAAV-IL-10 vector. Pediatr Pulmonol 2000; 20(Suppl):231.

195. O'Donovan DJ, Katkin JP, Tamura T, Husser R, Xu X, Smith CV, et al. Gene transfer of mitochondrially targeted glutathione reductase protects H441 cells from t-butyl hydroperoxide-induced oxidant stresses. Am J Respir Cell Mol Biol 1999; 20:256–263.

196. O'Donovan DJ, Katkin JP, Tamura T, Smith CV, Welty SE. Attenuation of hyperoxia-induced growth inhibition in H441 cells by gene transfer of mitochondrially targeted glutathione reductase. Am J Respir Cell Mol Biol 2000; 22:732–738.

197. Komada F, Nishiguchi K, Tanigawara Y, Wu XY, Iwakawa S, Okumura K. Effect of transfection with a superoxide dismutase expression plasmid on xanthine/xanthine oxidase-induced cytotoxicity in cultured rat lung cells. Biol Pharm Bull 1996; 19:1100–1102.

198. Engelhardt JF, Zwacka RM, Dudus L, Epperly MW, Greenberger JS. Redox gene therapy protects human IB-3 lung epithelial cells against ionizing radiation-induced apoptosis. Hum Gen Ther 1998; 9:1381–1386.

199. Lee PJ, Alam J, Wiegand GW, Choi AMK. Overexpression of heme oxygenase-1 in human pulmonary epithelial cells results in cell growth arrest and increased resistance to hyperoxia. Proc Natl Acad Sci USA 1996; 93:10393–10398.

200. Otterbein LE, Kolls JK, Mantell LL, Cook JL, Alam J, Choi AM. Exogenous administration of heme oxygenase-1 by gene transfer provides protection against hyperoxia-induced lung injury. J Clin Invest 1999; 103:1047–1054.

201. Danel C, Erzurum SC, Prayssac P, Eissa NT, Crystal RG, Hervé P, et al. Gene therapy for oxidant injury-related diseases: adenovirus-mediated transfer of superoxide dismutase and catalase cDNAs protects against hyperoxia but not against ischemia-reperfusion lung injury. Hum Gene Ther 1998; 9:1487–1496.

202. Erzurum SC, Lemarchand P, Rosenfeld MA, Yoo JH, Crystal RG. Protection of human endothelial cells from oxidant injury by adenovirus-mediated transfer of the human catalase cDNA. Nucleic Acids Res 1993; 21:1607–1612.

203. Sznajder JI. Alveolar edema must be cleared for the acute respiratory distress syndrome patient to survive. Am J Respir Crit Care Med 2001; 163:1293–1294.

204. Ware LB, Matthay MA. Alveolar fluid clearance is impaired in the majority of patients with acute lung injury and the acute respiratory distress syndrome. Am J Respir Crit Care Med 2001; 163:1376–1383.

205. Thome U, Chen L, Factor P, Dumasius V, Freeman B, Sznajder JI, et al. Na,K-ATPase gene transfer mitigates an oxidant-induced decrease of active sodium transport in rat fetal ATII cells. Am J Respir Cell Mol Biol 2001; 24:245–252.

206. Dumasius V, Wantroba Z, Azzam Z, Sznajder JI, Factor P. Helper-dependent adenovirus-mediated overexpression of a β2-adrenergic receptor increases receptor expression and function in rat lungs without causing lung injury. Am J Respir Crit Care Med 2001; 163:A526.

207. Stern M, Ulrich K, Robinson C, Copeland J, Griesenbach U, Masse C, et al. Pre-

treatment with cationic lipid-mediated transfer of the Na⁺,K⁺-ATPase pump in a
mouse model in vivo augments resolution of high permeability pulmonary oedema.
Gene Ther 2000; 7:960–966.

208. Delporte C, O'Connell BC, He X, Ambudkar IS, Agre P, Baum BJ. Adenovirus
mediated expression of Aquaporin-5 in epithelial cells. J Biol Chem 1996; 271:
22070–22075.
209. Delporte C, O'Connell BC, He X, Lancaster HE, O'Connell AC, Agre P, et al.
Increased fluid secretion after adenoviral-mediated transfer of the aquaporin-1
cDNA to irradiated rat salivary glands. Proc Natl Acad Sci USA 1997; 94:3268–
3273.
210. Braddon VR, Chiorini JA, Wang S, Kotin RM, Baum BJ. Adeno-associated virus-
mediated transfer of a functional water channel into salivary epithelial cells in vitro
and in vivo. Hum Gene Ther 1998; 9:2777–2785.
211. Kaner RJ, Ladetto JV, Singh R, Fukuda N, Matthay MA, Crystal RG. Lung overexpression of the vascular endothelial growth factor gene induces pulmonary edema.
Am J Respir Cell Mol Biol 2000; 22:657–664.
212. Louzier V, Eddahibi S, Raffestin B, Déprez I, Adam M, Levame M, et al. Adenovirus-mediated atrial natriuretic protein expression in the lung protects rats from
hypoxia-induced pulmonary hypertension. Hum Gene Ther 2001; 12:503–513.
213. Sallenave JM, Xing Z, Simpson AJ, Graham FL, Gauldie J. Adenovirus-mediated
expression of an elastase-specific inhibitor (elafin): a comparison of different promoters. Gene Ther 1998; 5:352–360.
214. Canonico AE, Brigham KL, Carmichael LC, Plitman JD, King GA, Blackwell TR,
et al. Plasmid-liposome transfer of the alpha 1 antitrypsin gene to cystic fibrosis
bronchial epithelial cells prevents elastase-induced cell detachment and cytokine
release. Am J Respir Cell Mol Biol 1996; 14:348–355.
215. Griesenbach U, Scheid P, Hillery E, de Martin R, Huang L, Geddes DM, et al.
Anti-inflammatory gene therapy directed at the airway epithelium. Gene Ther 2000;
7:306–313.
216. Batra RK, Guttridge DC, Brenner DA, Dubinett SM, Baldwin AS, Boucher RC.
I kappa β alpha gene transfer is cytotoxic to squamous-cell lung cancer cells and
sensitizes them to tumor necrosis factor-alpha-mediated cell death. Am J Respir
Cell Mol Biol 1999; 12:238–245.
217. Spragg RG. Surfactant replacement therapy. Clin Chest Med 2001; 21:531–541.
218. Yei S, Bachurski CJ, Weaver TE, Wert SE, Trapnell BC, Whitsett JA. Adenoviral-
mediated gene transfer of human surfactant protein B to respiratory epithelial cells.
Am J Respir Cell Mol Biol 1994; 11:329–336.
219. Korst RJ, Bewig B, Crystal RG. In vitro and in vivo transfer and expression of
human surfactant SP-A- and SP-B-associated protein cDNAs mediated by replication-deficient, recombinant adenoviral vectors. Hum Gene Ther 1995; 6:277–
287.
220. Ferkol T, Mularo F, Hilliard J, Lodish S, Perales JC, Ziady A, et al. Transfer of
the human alpha 1-antitrypsin gene into pulmonary macrophages in vivo. Am J
Respir Cell Mol Biol 1998; 18:591–601.
221. Worgall S, Singh R, Leopold PL, Kaner RJ, Hackett NR, Topf N, et al. Selective
expansion of alveolar macrophages in vivo by adenovirus-mediated transfer of the

murine granulocyte-macrophage colony-stimulating factor cDNA. Blood 1999; 93: 655–666.

222. Conary JT, Parker RE, Christman BW, Faulks RD, King GA, Meyrick BO, et al. Protection of rabbit lungs from endotoxin injury by in vivo hyperexpression of the prostaglandin G/H synthase gene. J Clin Invest 1994; 93:1834–1840.

223. Zhou MY, Lo SK, Bergenfeldt M, Tiruppathi C, Jaffe A, Xu N, et al. In vivo expression of neutrophil inhibitory factor via gene transfer prevents lipopolysaccharide-induced lung neutrophil infiltration and injury by a β_2 integrin–dependent mechanism. J Clin Invest 1998; 101:2427–2437.

224. Zhu HL, Stewart AS, Taylor MD, Vijayasarathy C, Ardner TJ, Sweeney HL. Blocking free radical production via adenoviral gene transfer decreases cardiac ischemia-reperfusion injury. Mol Ther 2000; 2:470–475.

225. Tsui LV, Zayek N, Frey D, Mello C, Banik G, Falotico R, et al. Stability of adenoviral vectors following catheter delivery. Mol Ther 2001; 3:122–125.

226. Marshall DJ, Palasis M, Lepore JJ, Leiden JM. Biocompatibility of cardiovascular gene delivery catheters with adenovirus vectors: an important determinant of the efficiency of cardiovascular gene transfer. Mol Ther 2000; 1:423–429.

18

Gene Therapy for Lung Transplantation

SAMER A. KANAAN, BENJAMIN D. KOZOWER, and G. ALEXANDER PATTERSON

Washington University School of Medicine
St. Louis, Missouri, U.S.A.

STEPHEN D. CASSIVI

Mayo Medical School
and Mayo Clinic
Rochester, Minnesota, U.S.A.

I. Introduction

The results of lung transplantation have improved for the treatment of many end-stage pulmonary diseases. However, they continue to lag behind other solid organ transplants. The 1-, 2-, and 5-year survival for lung transplantation are 70, 60, and 46%, respectively (1). The major obstacle to better long-term survival is bronchiolitis obliterans or chronic rejection. Ischemia reperfusion injury and acute rejection are also associated with significant morbidity and mortality and are risk factors for bronchiolitis obliterans. The treatment of these acute lung injuries remains imprecise and has done little to improve long-term outcome. Gene therapy strategies aimed at prevention and management of ischemia reperfusion injury and acute rejection may reduce chronic rejection and ultimately improve long-term survival.

II. Clinical Overview

A. Lung Transplantation

Hardy reported the first human lung transplant at the University of Mississippi in 1963 (2,3). Following this initial report, approximately 40 human lung transplants were attempted at various centers. Only two recipients lived longer than 1 month without any true long-term survivor (4). The first successful long-term lung transplant was performed by the Toronto Lung Transplant Group in 1983 (5). Since that time, over 8500 human lung transplants have been performed worldwide (6). The indications for lung transplantation have expanded to include a variety of end-stage lung diseases such as chronic obstructive pulmonary disease, cystic fibrosis, idiopathic pulmonary fibrosis, α_1-antitrypsin deficiency emphysema, primary pulmonary hypertension, eisenmenger's syndrome, bronchiectasis, sarcoidosis, lymphangiomyomatosis, and eosinophilic granuloma of the lung (7).

The majority of donor organs for lung transplantation are harvested from brain-dead donors. Unfortunately, this limited donor supply has not been able to meet the increased demand for lung transplantation. Although demand continues to increase, the number of brain-dead organ donors in the United States has remained fixed at 4500–5000 annually (8). Compounding this problem, only 20% of multiorgan donors have lungs that are suitable for transplantation (9,10). The donor lung shortage has increased the median waiting time for lung transplantation to over 700 days in the United States (11). This extended waiting time has led to 10–15% of patients dying on the waiting list (8).

Several alternative strategies have been developed to alleviate the donor lung shortage. First, living-related donors are being used to a limited degree in a few lung transplant centers (12,13). Although no donor mortality has been reported, this approach subjects a healthy organ donor to potential operative risk without any appreciable improvement in overall results (14). Second, experimental xenotransplantation has been investigated as a source for donor lungs. Unfortunately, problems related to hyperacute rejection currently limit this option (15,16). Finally, non–heart beating donors have been evaluated. Although there has been success reported in a few cases, this strategy has not been widely accepted or applied (17,18).

B. Ischemia Reperfusion Injury in Lung Transplantation

Ischemia reperfusion injury continues to have a significant impact on lung transplantation. Various mediators have been implicated on its pathogenesis, including activated neutrophils and platelets, the complement cascade, arachidonic acid metabolites, and free oxygen radicals (19–22). The damage caused by this process is mediated by the interaction between neutrophils and the pulmonary endothelium through a complex system of adhesion molecules (23). These interactions result in neutrophilic sequestration in the pulmonary capillaries and emigration into alveoli. Neutrophils release oxygen free radicals, cytokines, and proteases which damage the pulmonary graft endothelium (24,25). This damage exposes the basement membrane, alters vascular tone, and increases pulmonary capillary permeability. Together these factors can result in acute graft dysfunction.

Despite improvements in organ preservation and perioperative management, ischemia reperfusion injury remains the most common cause for morbidity and mortality within the first month of lung transplantation (26,27). Severe early graft dysfunction results from increased pulmonary vascular permeability and alveolar type II cell dysfunction (28–30). Histologically, there is diffuse alveolar damage as well as organizing pneumonia (31,32).

Ischemia reperfusion injury leads to severe graft dysfunction, known as the reimplantation response, in 10–20% of lung transplant recipients (28). This noncardiogenic pulmonary edema manifests as severe hypoxia and pulmonary infiltrates and may require prolonged mechanical ventilatory support. Treatment consists of ventilatory support, positive end-expiratory pressure, diuresis, and inhaled nitric oxide and may require extracorporeal membrane oxygenation (33,34).

C. Acute Rejection in Lung Transplantation

Although acute rejection is rarely a cause of early mortality, it is the most important predictor of long-term survival (35). Most patients experience at least one episode of acute rejection during the first few weeks after transplant (7). Frequency and severity of rejection have been repeatedly identified as principal risk factors for chronic rejection or the development of bronchiolitis obliterans (36,37).

Acute rejection is primarily a phenomenon of cell-mediated inflammation as the recipient immune system recognizes the foreign transplanted organ (38). T lymphocytes are the major effectors of acute rejection. T lymphocytes infiltrate lung allografts soon after implantation and are increased during acute rejection episodes. In addition, proinflammatory cytokines are increased during allograft rejection (39,40). Cytokines play a critical role in mediating and amplifying the immune response via paracrine and autocrine mechanisms (41). T helper lymphocytes secrete cytokines causing the proliferation of cytotoxic T lymphocytes which infiltrate and injure the graft (42).

In the early years of lung transplantation, the diagnosis and treatment of acute allograft rejection were imprecise. Current techniques of transbronchial biopsy and bronchioalveolar lavage are invasive but improve diagnostic accuracy. Unfortunately, the treatment of acute allograft rejection remains unfocused and relies upon generalized immunosuppression with triple therapy: steroids, cyclosporin, or tacrolimus and azathioprine or mycophenolate mofetil.

Most initial episodes of acute rejection are readily reversible. Induction and maintenance immunosuppression are the primary means for preventing acute rejection complemented by augmentation of immunosuppression during acute rejection episodes. However, morbidity occurs secondary to the loss of pulmonary function and the side effects of immunosuppression. These side effects include renal failure, thrombocytopenia, osteoporosis, glucose intolerance, and poor wound healing (43). Immunosuppressant agents are nonspecific and predispose the recipient to infection, toxicity to other organ systems, and neoplasia.

D. Chronic Rejection

The primary cause for reduced survival in lung transplantation is bronchiolitis obliterans, which is thought to be a manifestation of chronic rejection (44,45). Bronchiolitis obliterans develops in 75% of recipients surviving 5 years (46). Although first described in the posttransplantation setting over 17 years ago, this injury remains the single most important obstacle to long-term survival following lung transplantation (47–49). In a recent series of lung transplant recipients, the presence of bronchiolitis obliterans increased mortality by 200% (50).

Bronchiolitis obliterans manifests as deteriorating graft function that develops 3 months or more after transplantation. Patients typically present with increasing dyspnea and progressive airflow obstruction (51). It is characterized histologically by inflammation of the small airways with partial or complete occlusion by fibrous tissue (52,53). The pathophysiology is likely related to repeated immune-mediated injury to the bronchiolar epithelium. This injury results in epithelial cell loss, uncontrolled repair, and eventually to luminal occlusion by fibroproliferative tissue (50,54). There is no known effective treatment for bronchiolitis obliterans. It causes progressive graft failure and ultimately leads to the death of the transplant recipient.

III. Therapeutic Approach Using Gene Therapy

A. Rationale

Gene transfer or transfection is under intense investigation, because it offers hope for the future treatment of a wide variety of diseases including ischemia reperfusion injury and acute allograft rejection in transplantation (55–57). Unfortunately, achieving prolonged gene expression remains one of the most difficult problems faced in gene therapy. Ischemia reperfusion injury and acute rejection are early inflammatory lung injuries that may avoid this limitation and be altered by short-term gene expression. However, treatment of bronchiolitis obliterans will likely require prolonged gene expression.

Lung transplantation offers a unique opportunity for the study of transfection. Both in vivo and ex vivo transfection strategies exist. In vivo transfection targets the donor prior to harvest or the recipient before or after transplantation. Ex vivo transfection targets the harvested organ. The lung conducts aerobic metabolism during moderate hypothermic storage conditions, which may permit transfection after harvest and during transport from the donor site (58,59). This provides an excellent application for ex vivo gene transfer in clinical lung transplantation. In addition, lung transplantation is unique, because access to the airway allows transfection to be performed during transplantation or any time thereafter.

B. Vectors

A key component of gene therapy is the vector used to deliver the therapeutic agent. The ideal vector would be easily produced in pure form at high titers. It would efficiently and stably transduce nonproliferating cells in vivo and would enable long-term transgene expression without producing cytotoxic effects, inflammation, or immune responses (60). Although such a vector does not exist, many potential vectors have been investigated. Lung transplantation has focused primarily on three vector strategies: adenovirus, liposomes, and naked plasmid (61–63). Although gene transfer using viral vectors is technically termed transduction, this chapter uses the term transfection for both viral and non-viral vectors.

Adenovirus

Adenovirus is the most widely studied and employed viral vector (64). Its main advantages are high transduction efficiency, high titer production capability, and amenability to purification and concentration. Its principal disadvantage is the strong host immune response limiting the duration of expression and effective retransfection (64–66). Transgene expression is limited, because adenoviruses do not incorporate into the host DNA. Unfortunately, adenoviruses cause mild to moderate host inflammation and a strong secondary immune response which limits the effectiveness of readministration of a vector of the same serotype (67).

The use of second-generation adenoviruses (deletion of E1 and E4 regions) and standard immunosuppression decrease the inflammatory reaction caused by the adenovirus. Cassivi et al. demonstrated that immunosuppression attenuates the host immune response after adenovirus-mediated transfection of rodent lungs (68). In addition, they showed that transgene expression after adenovirus-mediated retransfection is increased and prolonged by transplant immunosuppression (69). This is especially promising in lung transplantation, because patients receive immunosuppression to prevent graft rejection. Newer generation and targeted adenovirus hold the promise to create a vector which delivers genes selectively and safely and with little immune response (70). The future will also be influenced by drug-regulated gene therapies with great potential to expand the efficacy and safety of gene therapy (71).

Liposomes

Nonviral vectors such as liposomes and naked plasmid may be safer than viral vectors yet demonstrate significantly lower transfection efficiency (72,73). Liposomes are nonpathogenic and consist of a cationic amphophile and a neutral phospholipid. They bind and condense DNA, transfecting cells by endocytosis (74). Liposomal transfection is less efficient than adenovirus and results in varying levels of gene expression. Nonetheless, work by Boasquevisque et al. documented transgene expression 28 days after transfection (75). However, the transgene expression is dose dependent. At higher concentrations needed for therapeutic benefit, Nagahiro et al. illustrated that cell lysis and pulmonary inflammation occur (76).

The feasibility of liposomal transfection for use in lung transplantation has been studied. Boasquevisque et al. demonstrated that liposome-mediated gene transfer in vivo and ex vivo allows for significant transgene expression in lung isografts with minimal effects on graft function (77). Lee et al. compared liposome-mediated gene transfer via the ex vivo pulmonary artery and intravenous routes (78). The ex vivo route provided prolonged, lung-specific gene expression. Finally, Yano et al. showed significant transgene expression in proximal pulmonary artery segments after exposure with ex vivo liposome-mediated chloramphenicol acetyl transferase (79).

Naked Plasmid

Naked plasmid DNA gene transfer is one of the simplest transfection techniques available. Naked plasmid produces a minimal host immune response, but expression is transient. Uptake of the plasmid is through endocytosis and significant degradation occurs by lysosomes (73). The purified DNA, in the form of plasmids, has been used primarily for DNA vaccine protocols, since naked plasmid can be effectively readministered. Similar to liposomes, it is nonpathogenic and is reported to have a lower transfection efficiency (80). Transgene expression has been detected 7 days after transfection (81).

Other Vectors

Other vectors such as adeno-associated virus (AAV) and lentivirus may be useful in lung transplantation. AAV induces a mild immune response allowing long-term expression. However, AAV possesses a small packaging capacity that limits the genes that may be employed. In addition, a high seroprevalence exists in humans with up to 80% of the population being positive for antibodies to AAV. This may limit its use in gene therapy and lung transplantation (82).

Lentiviruses produce no immune response and stably transduce close to 100% of target cells. They possess a large cloning capacity and a broad target spectrum. The main drawbacks are that lentiviruses are derived from human immunodeficiency virus (HIV) and have potential mutagenesis precluding clinical use at this time (83).

C. Delivery Routes

The goal of successful transfection is to produce the desired gene product while minimizing systemic expression and complications (55). Many different routes have been described with variable success in lung transplantation models (Table 1). The feasibility of gene transfer using both in vivo and ex vivo routes has been described.

In vivo routes of delivery have been limited by organ specificity and duration of expression. For example, intravenous administration results in transfection of multiple organs and limited duration of expression (77,78). When treating ischemia reperfusion injury in lung grafts, transgene expression is required at the time of reperfusion. This has only been accomplished with in vivo transfection, because ex vivo transfection requires up to 24 hr for protein expression (84–86). Recently, Cassivi and Kanaan reported that airway transfection has improved organ specificity and transgene expression (87,88). Airway or endobronchial transfection is highly efficient and holds great promise for future clinical application (89,90). It is relatively easy and could be performed in the intensive care unit prior to lung harvest or after transplantation.

In contrast, ex vivo gene transfer occurs during or after harvest and before implantation. Chapelier et al. and others argue that ex vivo gene transfer is easier during lung harvest, increases gene transfer efficiency secondary to longer incubation time between the graft and vector, is more organ-specific, and provides

Table 1 Lung Transplantation Gene Transfer Delivery Routes

Delivery route	Description	Vector used
Endobronchial	Highly efficient gene transfer route	Adenovirus and naked plasmid in vivo
Intramuscular	Administered to the gluteal or gastrocnemius muscles	Adenovirus in vivo
Intrapulmonary artery	Used in proximal pulmonary artery segment	Adenovirus and liposome in vivo and ex vivo
Intrapulmonary vein	Improved gene transfer efficiency compared to intrapulmonary artery route	Adenovirus in vivo
Intravenous	Injection via the internal jugular vein; transfects multiple organs	Adenovirus in vivo

for prolonged gene expression (78,91,92). Several studies by Yano et al. demonstrated the feasibility of ex vivo pulmonary artery transfection, and Jeppsson et al. showed that ex vivo gene transfer through the pulmonary vein is more efficient than through the pulmonary artery (62,79,93–95).

Intramuscular gene transfection is a novel recipient-based approach that releases gene product into the bloodstream to produce its systemic effect. Intramuscular gene transfer to the recipient prior to transplantation is feasible (96). Clinically, it could be used for a lung transplant recipient as soon as a donor is identified. It is the easiest delivery strategy and focuses the vector-related inflammatory reaction to the transfected muscle rather than the lung graft.

D. Functional Results/Animal Studies

Gene Therapy for Ischemia Reperfusion Injury

Therapy targeted at reducing ischemia reperfusion injury requires in vivo transfection strategies. Because reperfusion injury begins immediately, transgene expression must be present at the time of transplantation to improve ischemia reperfusion injury. This can only be accomplished with in vivo transfection, because ex vivo transfection requires up to 24 hr for gene expression (94). Donor endobronchial transfection and recipient intramuscular transfection are the in vivo strategies with the most promise for reducing ischemia reperfusion injury.

As the components of ischemia reperfusion injury have been identified, strategies to reduce this injury have evolved. Gene therapy using heat shock protein 70, nitric oxide synthase, and interleukin-10 have successfully reduced experimental lung transplant ischemia reperfusion injury. In all of these experiments, gene transfer was performed in vivo prior to reperfusion. Although gene expression has been transient, lasting 1–3 weeks, it enables the therapeutic protein to reduce this acute lung injury. In addition, gene transfer provides a single administration treatment for proteins with a short half-life.

Heat shock protein 70 is a heat stress protein with many cytoprotective effects. Hiratsuka et al. intravenously injected donor animals with adenovirus-mediated heat shock protein 70 24 hr prior to lung harvest (84). Twenty-four hours after lung transplantation, heat shock protein 70 improved lung oxygenation, decreased parenchymal edema, and reduced neutrophil sequestration.

Endothelial nitric oxide synthase regulates vascular tone and inhibits platelet aggregation and leukocyte adhesion. Suda et al. demonstrated that intravenous adenovirus-mediated endothelial nitric oxide synthase gene transfer improved lung graft oxygenation and reduced neutrophilic sequestration (85).

Interleukin-10 is a potent anti-inflammatory cytokine secreted by macrophages and T lymphocytes. Its two principal anti-inflammatory functions are the inhibition of macrophage cytokine production and the reduction of T-lymphocyte activation. Itano et al. used an intravenous donor protocol to demonstrate that interleukin-10 gene transfer ameliorates ischemia reperfusion injury (86). Preliminary work by Tagawa et al. shows that low-dose donor endobronchial gene transfer of interleukin-10 ameliorates ischemia reperfusion injury in rat lung isografts by improving lung graft oxygenation and reducing neutrophilic sequestration (97).

Kozower et al. demonstrated that recipient intramuscular gene transfer of adenovirus-mediated interleukin-10 produced sufficient interleukin-10 overexpression in plasma (98). This improved lung graft oxygenation and reduced neutrophilic sequestration and edema of lung isografts. Finally, Daddi et al. used intramuscular gene transfer of naked plasmid transforming growth factor-β1 (TGF-β1) and interleukin-10 to ameliorate lung isograft ischemia reperfusion injury after prolonged ischemia. They also showed superior mean arterial oxygenation and significantly reduced neutrophilic sequestration in the cotransfected group versus transfection with either gene alone. Furthermore, there was a synergistic reduction in proinflammatory cytokine levels in the cotransfected group versus transfection with either gene alone (99).

Gene Therapy in Acute Rejection

More focused strategies aimed at the prevention and management of acute rejection have lead to the investigation of gene therapy. Cytokines such as TGF-β1 have inherent immunosuppressive functions and are not increased during episodes of acute rejection. Thus, anti-inflammatory cytokines can suppress the initial immune response and may play a significant role in improving allograft survival.

TGF-β1 suppresses the proliferation of B and T cells, inhibits inflammatory cytokines, and inhibits natural killer cells. Mora et al. used ex vivo transfer of liposome-mediated TGF-β1 to improve graft oxygenation and reduce both vascular and airway rejection scores (100). In addition, they demonstrated that exhaled nitric oxide correlates with experimental lung transplant rejection (101). Yano et al. delivered TGF-β1 ex vivo to a segment of the pulmonary artery hypothesizing that the secreted protein would have a beneficial effect downstream (94). Boasquevisque et al. showed that ex vivo pulmonary vein gene transfer of liposome-mediated TGF-β1 produced superior arterial oxygenation compared to either in vivo intravenous gene transfer of liposome-mediated TGF-β1 or ex vivo pulmonary vein gene transfer of naked plasmid TGF-β1 (92).

D'Ovidio et al. delivered naked plasmid TGF-β1 via endobronchial transfection. They demonstrated selective airway transfection, improved lung graft oxygenation, and reduced rejection scores (102). Suda et al. demonstrated that in vivo intramuscular gene transfer of adenovirus-mediated TGF-β1 attenuated acute allograft rejection (96).

Fas ligand and nitric oxide synthase gene transfer have also been investigated for the reduction of acute rejection. Schmid et al. reported that Fas ligand ex vivo gene transfer in combination with cyclosporin improved oxygenation and reduced rejection scores versus cyclosporin alone (103). Jeppsson et al. successfully transfected rodent airways with endothelial nitric oxide synthase but was unable to detect any improvement in acute rejection (89).

These acute rejection studies have utilized a major antigen mismatch model resulting in profound rejection within 1 week. Therefore, the long-term effects of gene therapy using this model have not been investigated. Furthermore, it is important to recognize that chronic overexpression of TGF-β1 may result in fibrosis, and the results of this cytokine on acute rejection require further investigation (104).

Gene Therapy for Chronic Rejection/Bronchiolitis Obliterans

Bronchiolitis obliterans was first described in the posttransplant setting over 17 years ago. This manifestation of chronic rejection remains the most important obstacle to long-term survival following lung transplantation (105). Gene therapy has the potential to reduce this critical obstacle. As vector technology improves and gene expression is prolonged, the therapeutic potential of gene therapy may be realized.

A heterotopic tracheal transplant model has been used to investigate bronchiolitis obliterans (106,107). Although the model is not vascularized, it produces fibrous obliteration with a similar morphology to clinical bronchiolitis obliterans. Using this model, Boehler et al. demonstrated that intramuscular interleukin-10 gene therapy inhibits posttransplant fibrous airway obliteration (108). The interleukin-10 gene was delivered 5 days after transplantation, corresponding with lymphocytic infiltration. However, when interleukin-10 was delivered at the time of transplantation, it did not reduce the fibrous airway obliteration. The mechanism behind this remains unclear, and given the impact of clinical bronchiolitis obliterans, the use of gene therapy to reduce this injury warrants further investigation.

IV. Potential Human Use

Since the early experimental success with gene therapy in the 1990s, the clinical use of gene therapy has been proven to be difficult. Phase I clinical trials for pulmonary diseases have focused primarily on cystic fibrosis and more recently on lung cancer (109,110). Although gene therapy for lung transplantation has seen increased experimental success, no clinical trials have been conducted.

V. Conclusions

Anderson's landmark paper on human gene therapy outlined criteria that must be achieved in order to rationalize and realize a specific gene therapy approach

(111). A thorough understanding of the pathogenesis of the targeted disease must be attained in order to develop a strategy for gene therapy. As our understanding of ischemia reperfusion injury, acute rejection, and bronchiolitis obliterans improves, investigators will determine the appropriate genes to administer. Currently, gene therapy has investigated the physiological effects of several different genes and vector strategies in lung transplantation. In addition, vectors with prolonged gene expression and reduced inflammation are being developed. The combination of improved vectors and optimal gene selection may help overcome the obstacles confronting lung transplantation.

References

1. Hosenpud JD, Bennett LE, Keck BM, Boucek MM, Novick RJ. The Registry of the International Society for Heart and Lung Transplantation: seventeenth official report—2000. J Heart Lung Transplant 2000; 19:909–931.
2. Hardy JD, Webb WR, Dalton ML, Walker GR. Lung homotransplantation in man: report of the initial case. JAMA 1963; 186:1965–1974.
3. Blumenstock DA, Lewis C. The first transplantation of the lung in a human revisited. Ann Thorac Surg 1993; 56:1423–1425.
4. Veith FJ, Montefusco C, Kamholz SL, Mollenkopf FP. Lung transplantation. Heart Transplant 1983; 2:155–164.
5. The Toronto Lung Transplant Group. Unilateral lung transplantation for pulmonary fibrosis. N Engl J Med 1986; 314:1140–1145.
6. Pohl MS, Cooper JD. The international status of lung transplantation. Clin Transpl 1995; 11:85–89.
7. Trulock EP. Lung Transplantation. Am J Respir Crit Care Med 1997; 155:789–818.
8. Division of Transplantation, Bureau of Health Resources Development. Annual Report of the U.S. Scientific Registry for Transplant Recipients and the Organ Procurement and Transplantation Network—Transplant Data: 1988–1994. Health Resources and Services Administration, U.S. Department of Health and Human Services, Rockville, MD, 1995.
9. Egan TM, Boychuk J, Rosato K, Cooper JD. Whence the lungs? A study to assess suitability of donor lungs for transplantation. Transplantation 1992; 53:420–422.
10. Sundaresan S, Semenkovich J, Ochoa L, Richardson G, Trulock EP, Cooper JD, Patterson GA. Successful outcome of lung transplantation is not compromised by the use of marginal donor lungs. J Thorac Cardiovasc Surg 1995; 109:1075–1080.
11. United Network for Organ Sharing—Organ Procurement and Transfer Network. Waiting List and Removal Files. UNOS, Richmond, VA, 2000.
12. Starnes VA, Barr ML, Cohen RG. Lobar transplantation: indications, technique, and outcome. J Thorac Cardiovasc Surg 1994; 108:403–411.
13. Couetil JP, Tolan MJ, Loulmet DF, Guinvarch A, Chevalier PG, Achkar A, Birmbaum P, Carpentier AF. Pulmonary bipartitioning and lobar transplantation: a new approach to donor organ shortage. J Thorac Cardiovasc Surg 1997; 113:529–537.
14. Starnes VA, Barr ML, Cohen RG, Hagen JA, Wells WJ, Horn MV, Schenkel FA.

Living-donor lobar lung transplantation experience: intermediate results. J Thorac Cardiovasc Surg 1996; 112(5):1284–1291.

15. Kaplon RJ, Platt JL, Kwiatkowski PA, Edwards NM, Xu H, Shah AS, Masroor S, Michler RE. Absence of hyperacute rejection in pig-to-primate orthotopic pulmonary xenografts. Transplantation 1995; 59:410–416.

16. Pierson III RN, Kaspar-Konig W, Tew DN, Young VK, Braidley PC, White DJ, Wallwork J. Profound pulmonary hypertension characteristic of pig lung rejection by human blood is mediated by xenoreactive antibody independent of complement. Transplant Proc 1995; 27:274.

17. D'Alessandro AM, Hoffmann RM, Knechtle SJ, Eckhoff DE, Love RB, Kalayoglu M, Sollinger HW, Belzer FO. Controlled non-heart-beating donors: a potential source of extrarenal organs. Transplant Proc 1995; 27(1):707–9.

18. Steen S, Sjoberg T, Pierre L, Liao Q, Eriksson L, Algotsson L. Transplantation of lungs from a non-heart-beating donor. Lancet 2001; 357:825–829.

19. Kennedy TP, Rao NV, Hopkins C, Pennington L, Tolley E, Hoidal JR. Role of reactive oxygen species in reperfusion injury of the rabbit lung. J Clin Invest 1989; 83:1326–1335.

20. Detterbeck FC, Keagy BA, Paull DE, Wilcox BR. Oxygen free radical scavengers decrease reperfusion injury in lung transplantation. Ann Thorac Surg 1990; 50: 204–210.

21. Novick RJ, Menkis AH, McKenzie FN. New trends in lung preservation: a collective review. J Heart Lung Transplant 1992; 11:377–392.

22. Christie NA, Smith DE, DeCampos KN, Slutsky AS, Patterson GA, Tanswell AK. Lung oxidant injury in a model of lung storage and extended reperfusion. Am J Respir Crit Care Med 1994; 150:1032–1037.

23. Horgan MJ, Ge M, Gu J, Rothlein R, Malik AB. Role of ICAM-1 in neutrophil-mediated lung vascular injury after occlusion and reperfusion. Am J Physiol 1991; 261:H1578–H1584.

24. Horgan MJ, Wright SD, Malik AB. Antibody against leukocyte integrin (CD18) prevents reperfusion-induced lung vascular injury. Am J Physiol 1990; 259:L315–L319.

25. Lefer AM, Lefer DJ. Pharmacology of the endothelium in ischemia-reperfusion and circulatory shock. Annu Rev Pharm Toxicol 1993; 33:71–90.

26. Lee KH, Martich GD, Boujoukos AJ, Keenan RJ, Griffith BP. Predicting ICU length of stay following single lung transplantation. Chest 1996; 110:1014–1017.

27. Eriksson LT, Steen S. Induced hypothermia in critical respiratory failure after lung transplantation. Ann Thorac Surg 1998; 65:827–829.

28. Novick RJ, Gehman KE, Ali IS, Lee J. Lung preservation: the importance of endothelial and alveolar type II cell integrity. Ann Thorac Surg 1996; 62:302–314.

29. Kaplan JD, Trulock EP, Cooper JD, Schuster DP. Pulmonary vascular permeability after lung transplantation. A positron emission tomographic study. Am Rev Respir Dis 1992; 145:954–957.

30. Hunter DN, Morgan CJ, Yacoub M, Evans TW. Pulmonary endothelial permeability following lung transplantation. Chest 1992; 102:417–421.

31. Cooper JD, Vreim CE. Biology of lung preservation for transplantation. Am Rev Respir Dis 1992; 146:803–807.

32. Yousem SA, Duncan SR, Griffith BP. Interstitial and airspace granulation tissue reactions in lung transplant recipients. Am J Surg Pathol 1992; 16:877–884.

33. Meyers BF, Sundt TM III, Henry S, Trulock EP, Guthrie T, Cooper JD, Patterson GA. Selective use of extracorporeal membrane oxygenation is warranted after lung transplantation. J Thorac Cardiovasc Surg 2000; 120:20–28.

34. Date H, Triantafillou AN, Trulock EP, Pohl MS, Cooper JD, Patterson GA. Inhaled nitric oxide reduces human allograft dysfunction. J Thorac Cardiovasc Surg 1996; 111:913–919.

35. King-Biggs MB. Acute pulmonary allograft rejection. Clin Chest Med 1997; 18: 301–310.

36. Bando K, Paradis IL, Similo S, Konishi H, Komatsu K, Zullo TG, Yousem SA, Close JM, Zeevi A, Duquesnoy RJ. Obliterative bronchiolitis after lung and heart-lung transplantation. An analysis of risk factors and management. J Thorac Cardiovasc Surg 1995; 110:4–13.

37. Clelland C, Higenbottam T, Otulana B, Stewart S, Igboaka G, Scott J, Smyth R, Wallwork J. Histologic prognostic indicators for the lung allografts of heart-lung transplants. J Heart Transplant 1990; 9:177–185.

38. Halloran PF, Broski AP, Batiuk TD, Madrenas J. The molecular immunology of acute rejection: an overview. Transplant Immunol 1993; 1:3–27.

39. Hall BM. Cells mediating allograft rejection. Transplantation 1991; 51:1141–1151.

40. Zhai Y, Ghobrial RM, Busuttil RW, Kupiec-Weglinski JW. Th1 and Th2 cytokines in organ transplantation: paradigm lost? Crit Rev Immunol 1999; 19:155–172.

41. Kita Y, Li XK, Ohba M, Funeshima N, Enosawa S, Tamura A, Suzuki K, Amemiya H, Hayashi S, Kazui T, Suzuki S. Prolonged cardiac allograft survival in rats systemically injected with adenoviral vectors containing CTLA4Ig-gene. Transplantation 1999; 68:758–766.

42. VanBuskirk AM, Pidwell DJ, Adams PW, Orosz CG. Transplant immunology. JAMA 1997; 278:1993–1999.

43. Harmon KR, Hertz MI. Immune suppression: Background and considerations in lung transplantation. In: Patterson GA, Couraud L, eds. Current Topics in General Thoracic Surgery—Lung Transplantation, vol. 3. Amsterdam: Elsevier, 1994, pp. 333–360.

44. Berry GJ, Brunt EM, Chamberlain D, Hruban RH, Sibley RK, Stewart S, Tazelaar HD. A working formulation for the standardization of nomenclature in the diagnosis of heart and lung rejection: lung rejection study group. J Heart Transplant 1990; 9:593–601.

45. Yousem SA, Berry GJ, Cagle PT, Chamberlain D, Husain AN, Hruban RH, Marchevsky A, Ohori NP, Ritter J, Stewart S, Tazelaar HD. Revision of the 1990 working formulation for the classification of pulmonary allograft rejection: lung rejection study group. J Heart Lung Transplant 1996; 15:1–15.

46. Smith MA, Sundaresan S, Mohanakumar T, Trulock EP, Lynch JP, Phelan DL, Cooper JD, Patterson GA. Effect of development of antibodies to HLA and cytomegalovirus mismatch on lung transplantation survival and development of bronchiolitis obliterans syndrome. J Thorac Cardiovasc Surg 1998; 116(5):812–820.

47. Levine SM, Bryan CL. Bronchiolitis obliterans in lung transplant recipients. The "thorn in the side" of lung transplantation. Chest 1995; 107:894–897.

48. Scott JP, Peters SG, McDougall JC, Beck KC, Midthun DE. Posttransplantation

physiologic features of the lung and obliterative bronchiolitis. Mayo Clinic Proc 1997; 72:170–174.

49. Boehler A, Kesten S, Weder W, Speich R. Bronchiolitis obliterans after lung transplantation. Chest 1998; 114:1411–1426.

50. Sundaresan S, Trulock EP, Mohanakumar T, Cooper JD, Patterson GA, and the Washington University Lung Transplantation Group. Prevalence and outcome of bronchiolitis obliterans syndrome after lung transplantation. Ann Thorac Surg 1995; 60:1341–1347.

51. Paradis I, Yousem S, Griffith B. Airway obstruction and bronchiolitis obliterans after lung transplantation. Clin Chest Med 1993; 14:751–763.

52. Stewart S. Lung transplant pathology. In: Hammond EH, ed. Solid organ transplantation pathology. Philadelphia: Saunders, 1994:133–158.

53. Chamberlain DW. Lung transplantation pathology: allograft evaluation. In: Patterson GA, Couraud L, eds. Current Topics in General Thoracic Surgery—Lung Transplantation. Amsterdam: Elsevier, 1995:307–324.

54. Kelly K, Hertz MI. Obliterative bronchiolitis. In: Maurer JR, ed. Surgical approaches to end-stage disease: Lung transplantation and volume reduction. Philadelphia: WB Saunders, 1997:319–338.

55. Romano G, Pacilio C, Giordano A. Gene transfer technology in therapy: current applications and future goals. Stem Cells 1999; 17:191–202.

56. Blaese RM, Culver KW, Anderson WF. The ADA human gene therapy clinical protocol. Hum Gen Ther 1990; 1:331–337.

57. Anderson WF. End-of-year potpourri-1995. Hum Gene Ther 1995; 1505–1506.

58. Date H, Matsumura A, Manchester JK, Obo H, Lima O, Cooper JM, Sundaresan S, Lowry OH, Cooper JD. Evaluation of lung metabolism during successful twenty-four hour canine lung preservation. J Thorac Cardiovasc Surg 1993; 105:480–491.

59. Date H, Matsumura A, Manchester JK, Cooper JM, Lowry OH, Cooper JD. Changes in alveolar oxygen and carbon dioxide concentration and oxygen consumption during lung preservation. J Thorac Cardiovasc Surg 1993; 105:492–501.

60. Kaji EH, Leiden JM. Gene and stem cell therapies. JAMA 2001; 285:545–550.

61. Schmid RA, Narita M, Boasquevisque CH, Ando K, Botney M, Cooper JD, Schwartz AL, Patterson GA. Adenovirus mediated gene transfer into rat lung grafts at the time of harvest. Eur J Cardiothorac Surg 1997; 11:1023–1028.

62. Yano M, Hiratsuka M, Mora BN, Scheule R, Patterson GA. Transfection of pulmonary artery segments in lung isografts during storage. Ann Thorac Surg 1999; 68: 1810–1814.

63. D'Ovidio F, Daddi N, Suda T, Grapperhaus K, Patterson GA. Efficient naked plasmid cotransfection of lung grafts by extended lung plasmid exposure time. Ann Thorac Surg 2001; 71:1817–1824.

64. Mulligan RC. The basic science of gene therapy. Science 1993; 260:926–932.

65. Gojo S, Cooper DK, Iacomini J, LeGuern C. Gene therapy and transplantation. Transplantation 2000; 69(10):1995–1999.

66. Kitson C, Alton E..Gene therapy for cystic fibrosis. Exp Opin Invest Drugs 2000; 9(7):1523–1535.

67. Gilgenkrantz H, Duboc D, Juillard V, Couton D, Pavirani A, Guillet JG, Briand

P, Kahn A. Transient expression of genes transferred in vivo into heart using first-generation adenoviral vectors: role of the immune response. Hum Gene Ther 1995; 6:1265–1274.

68. Cassivi SD, Liu M, Boehler A, Pierre A, Tanswell AK, O'Brodovich H, Mullen JB, Slutsky AS, Keshavjee SH. Transplant immunosuppression increases and prolongs transgene expression following adenoviral-mediated transfection of rat lungs. J Heart Lung Transplant 2000; 19(10):984–994.

69. Cassivi SD, Liu M, Boehler A, Tanswell AK, Slutsky AS, Keshavjee S, Todd STRJ. Transgene expression after adenovirus-mediated retransfection of rat lungs is increased and prolonged by transplant immunosuppression. J Thorac Cardiovasc Surg 1999; 117(1):1–7.

70. Wickham TJ. Targeting adenovirus. Gene Ther 2000; 7:110–114.

71. Clackson T. Regulated gene expression systems. Gene Ther 2000; 7:120–125.

72. West J, Rodman DM. Gene therapy for pulmonary diseases. Chest 2001; 119:613–617.

73. Li S, Huang L. Nonviral gene therapy: promises and challenges. Gene Ther 2000; 7:31–34.

74. Gao X, Huang L. Cationic liposome-mediated gene transfer. Gene Ther 1995; 2:710–722.

75. Boasquevisque CH, Mora BN, Bernstein BS, Osburn WO, Nietupski J, Scheule RK, Cooper JD, Botney M, Patterson GA. Ex vivo liposome mediated gene transfer to lung isografts. J Thorac Cardiovasc Surg 1998; 115:38–44.

76. Nagahiro I, Mora BN, Boasquevisque CHR, Scheule RK, Patterson GA. Toxicity of cationic liposome-DNA complex in lung isografts. Transplantation 2000; 69:1802–1805.

77. Boasquevisque CH, Lee TC, Mora BN, Peterson D, Osburn WO, Bernstein M, Zhang W, Nietupski JB, Scheule RK, Cooper JD, Botney MD, Patterson GA. Liposome-mediated gene transfer to lung isografts. J Thorac Cardiovasc Surg 1997; 114:783–792.

78. Lee R, Boasquevisque CH, Boglione MM, Hiratsuka M, Scheule RK, Cooper JD, Patterson GA. Isolated lung liposome-mediated gene transfer produces organ-specific transgenic expression. Ann Thorac Surg 1998; 66:903–907.

79. Yano M, Boasquevisque CHR, Scheule RK, Botney MD, Cooper JD, Patterson GA. Successful in vivo and ex vivo transfection of pulmonary artery segments in lung isografts. J Thorac Cardiovasc Surg 1997; 114(5):793–802.

80. Fry JW, Wood KJ. Gene therapy: potential applications in clinical transplantation. Expert Rev Mol Med 1999; June: 1–24.

81. Knechtle SJ, Wang J, Jiao S, Geissler EK, Sumimoto R, Wolff J. Induction of specific tolerance by intrathymic injection of recipient muscle cells transfected with donor class I major histocompatibility complex. Transplantation 1994; 57(7):990–996.

82. Monahan PE, Samulski RJ. AAV vectors: is clinical success on the horizon? Gene Ther 2000; 7:24–30.

83. Trono D. Lentiviral vectors: turning a deadly foe into a therapeutic agent. Gene Ther 2000; 7:20–23.

84. Hiratsuka M, Mora BN, Yano M, Mohanakumar T, Patterson GA. Gene transfer

of heat shock protein 70 protects lung grafts from ischemia-reperfusion injury. Ann Thorac Surg 1999; 67:1421–1427.

85. Suda T, Mora BN, D'Ovidio F, Cooper JA, Hiratsuka M, Zhang W, Mohanakumar T, Patterson GA. In vivo adenovirus-mediated endothelial nitric oxide synthase gene transfer ameliorates lung allograft ischemia-reperfusion injury. J Thorac Cardiovasc Surg 2000; 119:297–304.

86. Itano H, Zhang W, Mohanakumar T, Patterson GA. Adenovirus-mediated gene transfer of human interleukin-10 ameliorates reperfusion injury of rat lung isografts. J Thorac Cardiovasc Surg 2000; 120:947–956.

87. Cassivi SD, Cardella JA, Fischer S, Liu M, Slutsky AS, Keshavjee S. Transtracheal gene transfection of donor lungs prior to organ procurement increases transgene levels at reperfusion and following transplantation. J Heart Lung Transplant 1999; 18:1181–1188.

88. Kanaan SA, Suda T, Kozower BD, Daddi N, Tagawa T, Mohanakumar T, Patterson GA. Intratracheal adenovirus mediated gene transfer is the optimal delivery route for use in experimental lung transplantation. 87th Clinical Congress of the American College of Surgeons, Surgical Forum, New Orleans, Oct 10, 2001.

89. Jeppsson A, Pellegrini C, O'Brien T, Miller VM, Tazelaar HD, Taner CB, McGregor CG. Transbronchial gene transfer of endothelial nitric oxide synthase to transplanted lungs. Ann Thorac Surg 1998; 66:318–324.

90. Jeppsson A, Lee R, Pellegrini C, O'Brien T, Tazelaar HD, McGregor CG. Gene therapy in lung transplantation: effective gene transfer via the airway. J Thorac Cardiovasc Surg 1998; 115:638–643.

91. Chapelier A, Danel C, Mazmanian M, Bacha EA, Sellak H, Gilbert MA, Herve P, Lemarchand P. Gene therapy in lung transplantation: feasibility of ex vivo adenovirus-mediated gene transfer to the graft. Hum Gene Therapy 1996; 7:1837–1845.

92. Boasquevisque CH, Mora BN, Boglione M, Ritter JK, Scheule RK, Yew N, Debruyne L, Qin L, Bromberg JS, Patterson GA. Liposome-mediated gene transfer in rat lung transplantation: a comparison between the in vivo and ex vivo approaches. J Thorac Cardiovasc Surg 1999; 117:8–15.

93. Yano M, Hiratsuka M, Nagahiro I, Mora BN, Scheule RK, Patterson GA. Ex vivo transfection of pulmonary artery segments in lung isografts. Ann Thorac Surg 1999; 68:1805–1809.

94. Yano M, Mora BN, Ritter JM, Scheule RK, Yew NS, Mohanakumar T, Patterson GA. Ex vivo transfection of transforming growth factor-beta1 gene to pulmonary artery segments in lung grafts. J Thorac Cardiovasc Surg 1999; 117:705–713.

95. Jeppsson A, Pellegrini C, Lee R, O'Brien T, Miller VM, Tazelaar HD, McGregor CG. Improved efficiency of gene transfer to the transplanted lung by retrograde vascular gene delivery. Transpl Int 2000; 13:241–246.

96. Suda T, D'Ovidio F, Daddi N, Ritter JH, Mohanakumar T, Patterson GA. Recipient intramuscular gene transfer of active transforming growth factor-beta1 attenuates acute lung rejection. Ann Thorac Surg 2001; 71:1651–1656.

97. Tagawa T, Suda T, Daddi N, Kozower BD, Kanaan SA, Mohanakumar T, Patterson GA. Low dose endobronchial gene transfer to ameliorate lung graft ischemia-reperfusion injury. J Thorac Cardiovasc Surg 2002; 123:795–802.

98. Kozower BD, Daddi N, Kanaan SA, Tagawa T, Suda T, Patterson GA. Recip-

ient intramuscular transfection of adenovirus interleukin-10 reduces lung graft ischemia-reperfusion injury. 87th Clinical Congress of the American College of Surgeons, Surgical Forum, New Orleans, Oct 10, 2001.

99. Daddi N, Suda T, Kozower BD, Kanaan S, Mohanakumar TS, Patterson GA. Recipient intramuscular cotransfection of naked plasmid TGF beta1 and IL-10 ameliorates lung graft ischemia-reperfusion injury. American Association for Thoracic Surgery, San Diego, May 9, 2001.

100. Mora BN, Boasquevisque CHR, Boglione M, Ritter JM, Scheule RK, Yew NS, Debruyne L, Qin L, Bromberg JS, Patterson GA. Transforming growth factor-beta1 gene transfer ameliorates acute lung allograft rejection. J Thorac Cardiovasc Surg 2000; 119:913–920.

101. Mora BN, Boasquevisque CH, Uy G, McCarthy TJ, Welch MJ, Boglione M, Patterson GA. Exhaled nitric oxide correlates with experimental lung transplant rejection. Ann Thorac Surg 2000; 69:210–215.

102. D'Ovidio F, Yano M, Ritter JH, Mohanakumar T, Patterson GA. Endobronchial transfection of naked TGF-beta1 cDNA attenuates acute lung rejection. Ann Thorac Surg 1999; 68:1008–1013.

103. Schmid RA, Stammberfer U, Hillinger S, Gaspert A, Boasquevisque CH, Malipiero U, Fontana A, Weder W. Fas ligand gene transfer combined with low dose cyclosporine A reduces acute lung allograft rejection. Transpl Int 2000; 13(Suppl 1):S324–S328.

104. Sime PJ, Xing Z, Graham FL, Csaky KG, Gauldie J. Adenovector-mediated gene transfer of active transforming growth factor-beta1 induces prolonged severe fibrosis in rat lung. J Clin Invest 1997; 100(4):768–776.

105. Burke CM, Theodore J, Dawkins KD, Yousem SA, Blank N, Billingham ME, Van Kessel A, Jamieson SW, Oyer PE, Baldwin JC. Post-transplant obliterative bronchiolitis and other late lung sequelae in human heart-lung transplantation. Chest 1984; 86:824–829.

106. Huang XH, Reichenspurner H, Shorthouse R, Cao W, Berry G, Morris R. Heterotopic tracheal allograft transplantation: a new model to study the molecular events causing obliterative airway disease in rats. J Heart Lung Transplant 1995; 14:S49.

107. Boehler A, Chamberlain D, Kesten S, Slutsky AS, Liu M, Keshavjee S. Lymphocytic airway infiltration as a precursor to fibrous obliteration in a rat model of bronchiolitis obliterans. Transplantation 1997; 64:311–317.

108. Boehler A, Chamberlain D, Xing Z, Slutsky AS, Jordana M, Gauldie J, Liu M, Keshavjee S. Adenoviral-mediated interleukin-10 gene transfer inhibits post-transplant fibrous airway obliteration in an animal model of bronchiolitis obliterans. Hum Gene Ther 1998; 9:541–551.

109. Boucher BC. Status of gene therapy for cystic fibrosis lung disease. J Clin Invest 1999; 103:441–445.

110. Swisher SG, Roth JA. Adenoviral-mediated p53 gene transfer in advanced non-small cell lung cancer. J Natl Cancer Inst 1999; 91:763–771.

111. Anderson WF. Prospects for human gene therapy. Science 1984; 226(4673):401–409.

AUTHOR INDEX

Italic numbers give the page on which the complete reference is listed.

A

Abbas AE, 150, *163*
Abboud CN, 242, *269*, 296, *313*
Abdullah L, 324, *353*
Abe A, 296, *313*
Abe K, 222, 225, 226, *229*, *230*, 436, *451, 452*
Abraham GN, 296, *313*
Abramowicz D, 196, *212*
Abrams J, 196, *212*
Accart N, 320, *350*, 428, 429, *446, 447*
Accurso FJ, 322, *352*
Achkar A, 458, *467*
Achong MK, 174, *185*
Ackerley C, 101, 102, 103, *114*, 427, *445*
Ackerman V, 320, *350*
Acland GM, 69, *89*
Acsadi G, 8, *25*
Adachi Y, 134, 135, *143*
Adak S, 425, *444*
Adam MA, 330, *357*, 438, *454*
Adams LB, 196, *212*
Adams PW, 459, *469*
Adams R, 368, *379*
Adamson IY, 220, 221, *229*

Addison CL, 175, *186*, 250, 260, 261, *279, 287, 288*
Adida C, 244, *271*
Adid C, 304, *316*
Adler S, 54, 63, *79*
Adnot S, 175, *186*, 403, *406*
Afek A, 134, *143*
Afione S, 62, 63, 65, 70, 74, *85, 86, 92*, 319, 327, *349, 356*, 366, 367, *378*, 424, *443*
Afione SA, 61, 64, 70, *84, 90*, 365, 368, *377, 379*, 413, *417*, 424, *442*
Agbandje-McKenna M, 54, *80*
Aggarwal AK, 65, *87*
Aggarwal S, 122, *139*, 428, *446*
Agre P, 438, *454*
Aguilar-Cordova E, 156, *165*, 302, *315*
Aguirre GD, 69, *89*
Agus D, 243, *270*
Ahmad A, 94, *112*
Ahmadzadeh M, 253, *281*
Aikawa M, 103, *113*
Aitken M, 373, *381*
Aitken ML, 65, 70, *87*, 320, 333, 334, *351, 359*, 368, 376, *379, 382*, 423, 429, *442, 448*
Ait-Yahia S, 197, *213*

Akita GY, 103, 105, 106, *115, 116,*
   333, *359,* 425, 426, *443, 445*
Akiyama T, 243, *270*
Akkaraju G, 7, *25*
Alam J, 437, *453*
Alam S, 52, *79*
Alavi A, 301, *315*
Alavi JB, 249, *277,* 302, *315*
Al-Awqati Q, 371, *380*
Albelda SM, 108, 111, *117,* 150, 156,
   163, 165, 246, 257, *273, 285,* 294,
   296, 297, 300, 302, 303, 307, 308,
   312, 313, 314, 315, 316, 318, 327,
   355, 425, 426, *444*
Albert R, 346, *364*
Alcami A, 198, *214*
Alderson MR, 249, *278*
Alemany R, 122, 130, 131, 132, 134,
   135, *138, 143,* 147, 150, *162, 164,*
   303, *315*
Alexander IE, 54, 65, 70, 72, *79, 87,*
   91, 328, 333, 334, *356, 359,* 368, *379*
Alger L, 403, *406*
Algotsson L, 458, *468*
Al-Hendry A, 302, *315*
Ali Hadji D, 428, 429, *446, 447*
Ali IS, 459, *468*
Alijagic S, 253, *281*
Alino SF, 411, *416*
Alitalo K, 256, *284*
Allard J, 403, *406*
Allavena P, 255, *283*
Allen ED, 325, *354,* 425, *443*
Allen H, 326, *355*
Allen JM, 65, 69, 73, 74, *87, 90,* 110,
   118, 224, *230,* 338, *362,* 376, *381,*
   382, 429, *448*
Allen SS, 70, *90,* 367, 368, *378, 379,*
   424, *442*
Allen T, 369, 373, *379*
Allet B, 196, *211*
Alleva DG, 247, *275*
Allione A, 249, *275*
Allred DC, 121, *138*
Alon N, 366, *377*
Alonso C, 156, *165*

Alston J, 64, *86*
Altieri DC, 244, *271,* 304, *316*
Altmann KH, 244, *271*
Alton EW, 111, *118,* 308, *318,* 320,
   321, 322, 345, *350, 351, 352, 364,*
   366, *378,* 461, *470*
Alton EWFW, 100, 103, 104, 106, 111,
   114, 116, 387, *394, 395,* 427, *446*
Al-Tweigeri T, 302, *315*
Alvarez D, 177, *187*
Alvarez R, 243, *270*
Alvarez RD, 120, 123, 125, 131, *138,*
   140, 142
Alvira M, 39, 43, *48*
Amalfitano A, 42, *49,* 326, *354*
Ambrosini G, 244, *271,* 304, *316*
Ambudkar IS, 438, *454*
Amemiya H, 459, *469*
Amin KM, 108, 111, *117,* 150, 156,
   163, 165, 245, *272,* 296, 297, 300,
   302, 303, 307, 308, *314, 315, 316,*
   317, 318
Amin P, 158, *166*
Amin S, 238, *267*
Ampel NM, 205, *215, 216*
Anand V, 65, 73, *87*
Andersen P, 207, *217*
Anderson B, 131, *143*
Anderson FA, 148, *163*
Anderson JM, 335, *360*
Anderson KD, 181, *190*
Anderson LJ, 207, *218*
Anderson MP, 319, *349,* 387, *394*
Anderson PJ, 3, *24*
Anderson R, 68, *89*
Anderson WF, 12, *26,* 136, *144,* 460,
   466, *470, 473*
Ando K, 461, *470*
Andrews JJ, 195, *210*
Anello R, 245, *272*
Angel B, 70, *90,* 385, *394,* 422, 425,
   427, *440*
Angel JB, 436, *452*
Angiolillo AL, 260, *287*
Anthony DC, 179, *189,* 222, *229*
Anton M, 326, *354*

Anttila M, 205, *216*
Anttila S, 303, *315*
Anwer K, 101, 102, *114*, 429, *447*
Apparailly F, 197, *212*
Apte RN, 249, *276*
Arai T, 222, 226, *229, 230*, 436, *452*
Araki K, 178, *189*
Araki N, 157, *165*
Arand M, 254, *282*
Arcasoy SM, 324, 347, *353, 364*, 422,
    426, *441, 444*
Ardner TJ, 439, *455*
Arduzzoni A, 308, *318*
Arenberg DA, 255, 256, 259, 260, 261,
    283, 284, 287, 288
Armentano D, 36, *45*, 127, *141*, 325,
    326, 333, 338, *354, 359, 362*
Armitage RJ, 198, *214*
Arnold F, 257, *285*
Arruda V, 6, 14, *24, 26*
Arruda VR, 110, *117*
Arseneau J, 151, *164*
Aruffo A, 346, *364*
Asakawa M, 346, *364*
Ascadi G, 428, *447*
Asher AL, 249, *276*
Asikainen T, 303, *315*
Askin FB, 333, 334, *359*, 368, 370, *379*
Astoul P, 305, *317*
Atchison RW, 53, 60, *79*, 365, *377*
Athappilly FK, 33, *45*
Atkins CJ, 307, *317*
Atkinson EM, 58, 68, *82, 89*, 366, *377*
Atkinson G, 245, *272*, 304, *316*
Atkinson M, 413, *417*
Atkinson N, 120, 122, *138*
Atochina EN, 126, *141*
Audouy S, 100, *113*
Auerbach R, 256, *284*
Auerbach W, 256, *284*
Auffenberg T, 436, *452*
August JT, 392, *395*
Aukerman SL, 124, *140*
Auriault C, 197, *212*
Auricchio A, 6, *24*, 66, 68, *87, 89*
Ausprunk DH, 257, *285*

Austin EA, 294, *312*
Austin JB, 65, *87*, 365, *377*, 411, *416*
Austin LL, 39, *47*
Avery ME, 431, *449*
Avis FP, 194, *209*
Awata N, 157, *165*
Aymard M, 320, *350*
Azzam Z, 438, *453*

B

Baas IO, 235, *266*
Baba T, 101, *114*
Bacha EA, 464, 465, *472*
Bachofen M, 174, *185*
Bachurski CJ, 330, *357*, 423, 433, 439,
    442, 450, 454
Bacon K, 174, *185*
Bagby GJ, 183, *190*, 196, 197, 202,
    212, 213, 215
Baggiolini M, 259, *287*
Bagley RG, 105, 106, *115*, 333, *359*,
    426, 427, *445*
Bailey-Wilson JE, 234, 249, *265*
Bains MS, 293, *312*
Bainton B, 196, *212*
Baird A, 123, 124, 136, *139, 140, 144*,
    435, *451*
Bai Y, 259, *287*
Bajpai A, 57, 62, *81*
Bakacs T, 125, *140*, 337, *361*
Baker AH, 128, 134, *142, 144*
Baker JR, 427, *445*
Baker PJ, 240, *268*
Balague C, 55, *80*, 147, *162*, 303, *315*
Balbay M, 260, *287*
Baldacci P, 238, *267*
Baldeyrou P, 264, *290*
Baldwin AJ, 245, *273*
Baldwin ASJ, 245, *273*, 439, *454*
Baldwin JC, 466, *473*
Baldwin SL, 207, *217*
Baley P, 409, *415*
Balfour R, 103, 104, 106, 111, *116*,
    320, 321, *351*, 427, *446*
Balfour RP, 320, 321, *351*, 429, *448*

Ballard PL, 74, *91*, 433, *449*
Bals R, 71, *91*
Balter M, 333, *359*
Baltimore D, 19, *27*, 367, *378*
Baluk P, 101, 102, 107, *114*, 429, *447*
Balyasnikova IV, 126, 127, 134, *140, 141, 143*, 402, *405*, 429, *447*
Bancheeau J, 253, *281*
Bandholtz L, 205, *216*
Bando K, 459, *469*
Bandyopadhyay P, 414, *418*
Banik G, 440, *455*
Bankert RB, 240, *269*
Banks TC, 366, *377*
Bantel-Schall U, 54, 65, 79, 365, *377*
Bantra R, 244, *271*
Bao S, 175, *186*
Baradet T, 135, *144*
Barasch J, 371, *380*
Barbot A, 37, *46*
Bar-Eli M, 260, *287*
Barenholz Y, 99, *113*
Bargon J, 319, *350*
Barker JWCN, 256, *284*
Barker PM, 326, *355*
Barnes MJ, 41, *48*
Barnes MN, 120, 123, *138*
Barraza EM, 32, *45*
Barrazza-Ortiz X, 368, *379*
Barr D, 39, 43, *47*
Barrett J, 199, *214*
Barrett JB, 100, *113*
Barr ML, 458, *467*
Barron LG, 102, 104, *115*
Barry MA, 128, *142*
Barsomian G, 126, 128, *140*
Barsoum J, 135, *144*, 308, *318*
Barst RJ, 126, *141*
Bartlett JS, 57, 58, 72, 74, *82*, *91*, 136, *144*, 328, 338, *356*, *362*, 375, *381*
Bartlett RH, 432, *449*
Basbaum C, 176, *187*, 324, *353*
Baskin G, 422, *442*
Baskin GB, 433, *449*
Bassie B, 428, *447*
Batiuk TD, 459, *469*

Batra RK, 120, 122, *138*, 233, 234, 240, 245, 249, 261, *265*, *266*, *269*, *273*, 289, 294, *313*, 439, *454*
Batson E, 371, *380*
Batson EP, 412, *417*
Battini JL, 262, *290*
Baumann B, 244, *271*
Baumann H, 174, 175, *185*, *186*
Baum BJ, 438, *454*
Baumeister W, 72, *91*
Baumgartner I, 16, *27*
Bavaria JE, 327, *355*
Beaman L, 205, *216*
Beard P, 62, 77, *85*, *92*
Beart RW, 136, *144*
Beaton A, 55, *80*
Beaucage SL, 427, *445*
Beaudet A, 39, 43, *47*, 425, *443*
Beaudet AL, 411, *415*, *416*, 430, *448*
Bebok Z, 100, 103, 104, 105, 106, 111, *114*, *116*, 426, *445*
Beck JM, 194, 195, *210*
Beck KC, 460, *469*
Beck LA, 15, *26*
Beck SE, 65, 73, *87*, 333, 334, *359*, 368, 370, *379*, 424, *442*
Beegen H, 10, *25*
Behera AK, 183, *190*
Behrens C, 234, 249, *266*
Behr JP, 345, *364*, 392, *395*
Beitz JG, 256, *284*
Bejarano GC, 205, *215*
Belcastro R, 102, 104, *115*
Belin D, 194, *209*
Belinksy S, 237, *267*
Belisle JT, 207, *217*
Belladonna ML, 250, *279*
Bell JA, 32, *45*
Bell JR, 15, *26*
Bellon G, 320, *350*, 430, *448*
Belousova N, 120, 129, 131, 132, *137*, *142*, *143*, 337, *361*
Belperio J, 256, *284*
Belzer FO, 458, *468*
Benjamini E, 205, *216*
Benner DA, 245, *273*

Bennett B, 196, *212*
Bennett J, 65, 73, *87*, 195, *211*
Bennett LE, 457, *467*
Bennett M, 193, *209*
Bennink JR, 247, *274*
Benson PK, 58, *82*
Bepler G, 240, *268*
Berencsi K, 5, *24*, 39, 41, *47*, *48*, 196, *211*, 326, *354*
Bergelson JM, 33, *45*, 70, *91*, 120, 121, 122, 131, *137*, *138*, 262, *289*, 324, 326, *353*, *355*, 420, 425, *440*
Bergenfeldt M, 439, *455*
Berger M, 12, *26*
Berg P, 19, *27*
Berg RK, 9, *25*
Berk AJ, 243, *270*, 367, *378*
Berke G, 247, *274*
Berkner K, 325, *354*
Berkowitz R, 127, *141*
Bermudes D, 148, *163*
Bernacki SH, 324, *353*
Bernon H, 320, *350*
Berns A, 239, *268*
Berns AJ, 252, *281*
Berns KI, 51, 54, 55, 56, 59, 60, 61, 63, 64, *78*, *79*, *80*, *81*, *83*, *84*, *86*, 411, 413, *416*, *417*
Bernstein BS, 461, *471*
Beroiza T, 249, *278*
Berry GJ, 177, *188*, 460, 466, *469*, *473*
Berry LC, 399, *404*
Berry LM, 433, *450*
Bertacca G, 235, *266*
Berta SC, 338, *362*
Bertran J, 65, *86*
Berzofsky JA, 247, *274*
Bessodes M, 331, *358*
Bett AJ, 326, *355*
Beusechem VW, 124, *140*
Beutler B, 183, *191*, 194, 196, *209*, *211*, *212*
Beven MJ, 205, *216*, 254, *282*
Bewig B, 439, *454*
Bewley MC, 122, *138*
Bhardwaj R, 256, *284*

Bhattacharya S, 399, *405*
Bianchi R, 250, *279*
Biederer CH, 151, *164*
Bienvenu J, 320, *350*
Biffi A, 400, *405*
Bignon J, 305, *317*
Billingham ME, 466, *473*
Bilton D, 320, 321, *351*
Bilyk N, 251, *280*
Biraud C, 60, *83*
Birkebak T, 110, *118*
Birmbaum P, 458, *467*
Birnstiel ML, 11, *25*
Bischoff JR, 151, *164*, 243, *270*
Bischoff R, 428, 429, *446*, *447*
Bishop DK, 16, *27*, 252, *280*
Bishop GA, 427, *445*
Bistoni F, 194, *210*
Bjorklund A, 68, *89*
Black CM, 194, *209*
Black HB, 39, 43, *47*
Black HR, 322, *352*
Black ME, 303, *315*
Black RA, 197, *213*
Blacklow NR, 53, 54, 65, *79*, *87*, 365, *377*
Blackwell JL, 120, 131, *137*, *138*, *142*
Blackwell TR, 411, *416*, 432, 439, *449*, *454*
Blackwell TS, 432, *449*
Blaese RM, 12, *26*, 38, *46*, 156, *165*, 245, *272*, 296, 302, *313*, *315*, 460, *470*
Blair R, 16, *27*
Blanchard DK, 196, *212*
Blanchard JL, 433, *449*
Blanchard K, 200, *215*
Blanche F, 37, *46*
Blank N, 466, *473*
Blau DM, 343, *363*
Blaya C, 411, *416*
Bleich M, 367, *379*
Blessing T, 392, *395*
Blezinger HP, 105, *115*, 426, *445*
Blezinger P, 103, *115*
Blobe GC, 225, *230*

Block KD, 402, *405*
Blomer U, 3, *24*, 262, *289*, 329, 330, 341, *357*
Bloom BR, 195, 206, *210*, *217*, 346, *364*
Blumenstock DA, 457, *467*
Boasquevisque CH, 175, *186*, 461, 464, 465, 466, *470*, *472*, *473*
Boatman BG, 134, *143*
Bobadilla M, 411, *416*
Boczkowski D, 253, *282*
Bodey GP, 201, *215*
Bodmer H, 247, *274*
Bodner M, 123, *139*, 330, 336, 341, *357*, *360*, *363*, 421, 423, 425, 431, *441*, *442*
Boehler A, 197, *212*, 433, *450*, 460, 461, 466, *470*, *471*, *473*
Boehme R, 294, *313*
Boehm T, 257, *285*
Boger DL, 259, *287*
Boglione M, 175, *186*, 461, 464, 465, *471*, *472*, *473*
Bohl D, 64, 75, *85*, 375, *381*
Bohlen P, 258, *286*
Bolden S, 233, 234, 249, *265*
Boletta A, 400, *405*
Bolhuis RL, 306, *317*
Bolivar R, 201, *215*
Bolton ES, 249, *278*
Bolton PB, 101, 102, 107, *114*, 429, *447*
Bonato VL, 207, *217*
Bonavida B, 196, *211*
Boncyk L, 205, *216*
Bonfil TL, 322, *352*
Bongartz G, 306, *317*
Bonham L, 110, *118*
Bonneau L, 69, 74, *90*, 123, *139*, 224, *230*, 376, *382*, 425, 429, 430, 433, *444*, *448*, *450*
Bonnet N, 326, *355*, 435, *451*
Boon T, 246, *273*, *274*
Border WA, 180, *189*
Borgland SL, 263, *290*
Boris-Lawrie K, 262, *289*
Borthwick DW, 70, *90*, 320, *350*
Bosma GC, 240, *268*

Bosma MJ, 240, *268*, *269*
Bost T, 322, *352*
Botney M, 461, *470*, *471*
Bottazzi B, 249, *276*
Boucek MM, 457, *467*
Boucher C, 424, *442*
Boucher DW, 54, 65, *79*
Boucher R, 240, 244, 245, 261, *269*, *271*, *289*
Boucher RC, 13, *26*, 70, 72, 74, *91*, 120, 122, 123, 125, 126, 136, *137*, *138*, *139*, *140*, *144*, 294, *313*, 319, 320, 322, 323, 324, 326, 327, 330, 331, 333, 336, 338, 341, 343, *349*, *350*, *351*, *352*, *353*, *355*, *357*, *358*, *360*, *361*, *362*, *363*, 366, 373, *377*, *380*, 386, *394*, 425, 426, 427, 439, *440*, *443*, *444*, *446*, *454*
Boucher Y, 258, *286*
Bouck N, 258, *286*
Boujoukos AJ, 459, *468*
Boulanger P, 132, *143*
Boussif O, 429, *447*
Bousso P, 12, *26*
Bout A, 37, *46*, 100, *114*, 297, *314*, 429, *448*
Boutin C, 305, *317*
Bowden DH, 220, 221, *229*
Bowen GP, 263, *290*
Bowman R, 306, *317*
Bowne WB, 247, *275*
Bowton DL, 202, *215*
Boychuk J, 458, *467*
Boyer HW, 19, *27*
Boyle JO, 235, *266*
Boyles SE, 392, *396*
Braciak T, 173, 174, 175, 179, *185*, *186*, 201, *215*, 436, *451*, *452*
Braddon VR, 438, *454*
Bragonzi A, 400, *405*
Braidley PC, 458, *468*
Braileanu G, 302, *315*
Braithwaite AW, 151, *164*
Brambilla E, 243, *271*
Bramson JL, 173, 184, *185*, *191*, 195, *211*, 250, *279*, 436, *452*

Brandley M, 305, *317*
Brandt CD, 207, *218*
Brandts CH, 151, *164*
Brantly M, 70, *91*, 323, *353*, 412, 413, *416*, *417*, 421, 424, *441*
Braquet P, 196, *211*
Brasfield D, 320, *350*
Bray JA, 245, *273*, 433, 437, *450*
Braybrook G, 336, *360*
Brecher SM, 148, *163*
Brees DK, 180, *189*
Brekken J, 259, *287*
Brekken RA, 258, *286*
Brennan D, 149, *163*
Brennan PJ, 207, *217*
Brenneise IE, 176, *187*
Brenner DA, 439, *454*
Breslow JL, 61, *83*
Brewer HB, 13, *26*
Brezillon S, 326, *355*, 435, *451*
Briand P, 38, *46*, *47*, 428, *446*, 461, *470*
Briathwaite AW, 243, *270*
Brie A, 131, *143*
Brigham KL, 399, *404*, 411, *416*, 439, *454*
Briles DE, 198, *214*
Bringas P, 181, 182, *189*, *190*
Briscoe H, 207, *217*
Brisson C, 384, *393*
Britton WJ, 207, *217*
Broad R, 245, *273*
Brockelmann TJ, 224, *230*
Brody AS, 376, *382*
Brody SL, 13, *26*, 333, *358*, 425, *440*
Broekelmann TJ, 178, *189*
Bromberg JS, 175, *186*, 197, *212*, 262, *289*, 421, 425, 436, *440*, *441*, *452*, 464, 465, *472*, *473*
Brookes R, 207, *217*
Brooks G, 150, *164*
Brooks P, 257, *285*
Brooks PC, 257, *285*
Broski AP, 459, *469*
Brosman MJ, 134, *144*

Brough DE, 120, 122, 129, *137*, *142*, 158, *166*, 269, *291*, 325, 337, *354*, *361*
Brown AR, 430, *448*
Brown CS, 399, *404*
Brown JA, 183, *190*, 204, *215*
Brown JF, 195, *210*
Brown JM, 429, *447*
Brown KE, 57, *82*, 338, 339, *362*, 376, *381*, 424, *443*
Brown M, 149, *163*
Brown MP, 207, *218*
Brown R, 245, *273*
Brown SL, 122, *138*, 245, *272*
Brown SM, 150, *163*
Browne J, 2, *23*
Browning JE, 103, 104, 106, 111, *116*, 308, *318*, 320, 321, 322, *351*, *352*, 389, *395*, 422, 425, *440*
Brownstein DG, 193, *209*
Bruder JT, 325, 346, *354*, *364*
Brunda MJ, 195, *210*, 250, *279*
Brundage JF, 32, *45*
Brunette EN, 194, 195, *210*, 427, 430, *446*
Brunham RC, 206, *216*
Brunner N, 121, *138*
Bruno MS, 399, *404*
Brunori M, 158, *167*
Brunt EM, 460, *469*
Bruso P, 151, *165*
Bruyns C, 196, *212*
Bryan CL, 460, *469*
Bryan R, 371, *380*
Bryant JL, 101, 102, *114*
Bubb VJ, 235, *266*
Bucana CD, 260, *288*
Buchanan A, 243, *270*
Buchanan JA, 38, *46*
Buch S, 435, *451*
Buchsbaum DJ, 120, 123, 126, *137*, *138*, *141*, 429, *447*
Buchwald M, 135, *144*, 435, *451*
Buckely S, 181, *189*
Bucknell KA, 183, *190*, 200, *215*, 436, *451*

Bu D, 181, *189*
Bucy RP, 120, *138*
Budker V, 8, *25*
Budts W, 402, *405*
Buechler YJ, 435, *451*
Bui J, 64, *86*
Bukovsky A, 330, *357*
Bukowski R, 245, *273*
Bukowski RM, 251, *280*
Bukreyev A, 207, *218*
Bukreyev N, 207, *218*
Bullington D, 436, *452*
Bullock C, 102, 110, *115*, 429, *448*
Bunch D, 42, *49*
Bunn HF, 200, *215*
Bunn PJ, 243, *270*
Burda J, 5, *24*, 326, *354*
Burda JF, 62, *85*
Burdick MD, 255, 260, *283*, *287*, *288*
Burg MA, 136, *144*
Burger CJ, 247, *275*
Burke CM, 466, *473*
Burkle A, 65, *86*
Burnett RM, 33, *45*
Burnham MS, 68, *89*, 366, *377*
Burns JC, 330, *357*
Burns JL, 376, *382*
Burns R, 343, *363*
Burr EA, 429, *448*
Burrascano M, 330, *357*
Burrows SR, 15, *26*
Burt ME, 293, *312*
Burton M, 110, *117*
Bussey LB, 102, 110, *115*
Busuttil RW, 197, *212*, 459, *469*
Butterfield L, 253, *281*
Buttrick PM, 39, 43, *48*
Byrne BJ, 67, *88*, 366, *377*, 412, 413,
    416, *417*
Byrne PS, 305, *317*

C

Cagle PT, 460, *469*
Cai D, 15, *26*, 241, *269*
Cai DW, 424, *442*

Cai Z, 33, *45*
Cajal SR, 156, *165*
Callahan JE, 195, *211*
Cameron B, 37, *46*, 331, *358*
Caminischi I, 294, 307, *312*, *317*
Campain JA, 123, *139*
Campbell AIM, 398, *404*
Campbell JB, 147, *162*
Camplejohn R, 304, *316*
Canchola JG, 207, *218*
Canfield D, 369, *379*
Canfield DR, 429, *448*
Cano A, 156, *165*
Canonico AE, 411, *416*, 439, *454*
Cao G, 249, *277*
Cao L, 67, *88*
Cao W, 466, *473*
Cao X, 52, 68, *78*
Capaccio A, 308, *318*
Caparelli DJ, 150, *163*
Caplen NJ, 100, *114*, 320, 322, *350*,
    352, 387, *394*, *395*, 422, 425, *440*
Capogrossi M, 310, *318*
Cappelletti M, 60, 61, *83*
Caras IW, 337, *361*
Carasco CH, 15, *26*
Carbone D, 234, 242, *265*, *269*
Carbone DP, 247, *274*, 425, *444*
Carbone M, 311, *318*
Carby FA, 235, *266*
Cardella J, 126, 128, *140*, 338, *361*
Cardella JA, 463, *472*
Cardoso WV, 181, *190*
Cardoza LM, 325, *354*
Carducci MA, 15, *26*
Carey FA, 235, *266*
Carey K, 101, 102, *114*
Carlier Y, 198, *214*
Carmeliet P, 256, *284*
Carmen IH, 302, *315*
Carmichael LC, 411, *416*, 439, *454*
Carothers AD, 320, 321, *351*
Carpenter H, 333, *359*
Carpentier AF, 458, *467*
Carrasco CH, 424, *442*
Carrigan PE, 176, *187*

Carrion ME, 127, *141*
Carroll AM, 240, *269*
Carroll TP, 367, *378*
Carroll WR, 120, *137, 138*
Carter B, 7, *25*, 76, *92*, 369, 371, 373,
    379, 380, 381, 412, *416*, 424, *443*
Carter BJ, 54, 55, 59, 60, 62, 65, *79,
    80, 82, 84*, 319, 320, 327, 333, 334,
    349, 351, 356, 359, 365, 366, 367,
    368, 370, *377, 378, 379, 380*, 412,
    413, *417*
Carter CA, 62, *85*
Carter CS, 12, *26*
Caruso M, 296, 303, *313, 315*
Carvajal J, 124, *140*
Casanova JL, 12, *26*
Cascino CJ, 148, *162*
Caskey C, 263, *290*
Caskey CT, 326, *355*
Cassady R, 101, 102, 103, *114*, 427,
    445
Cassell WA, 146, 147, *161, 162*
Cassiman JJ, 367, *379*
Cassivi SD, 461, 463, *471, 472*
Castanos-Velez E, 205, *216*
Castel D, 134, *143*
Castleden S, 296, *313*
Castleden SA, 304, *316*
Casto BC, 53, 60, *79*, 365, *377*
Castranova V, 175, *186*
Catalano A, 310, *318*
Catanzaro A, 198, *214*
Caterini J, 206, *216*
Caterson B, 261, *289*
Cathomen T, 65, *87*
Catterall JR, 194, *209*
Caux C, 198, *214*
Cavazzana-Calvo M, 12, *26*
Cavender A, 243, *270*
Cavender DE, 422, *442*
Cayanis E, 126, *141*
Celio MR, 303, *316*
Celluzzi CM, 253, 254, *282*
Centofanti R, 308, *318*
Cerami A, 194, 196, *209, 211, 212*
Cerasoli F, 109, *117*

Certain S, 12, *26*
Cesne A, 264, *290*
Cesne AL, 425, *444*
Chada S, 323, *353*, 420, 423, *441*
Chadeuf G, 55, *81*
Chadwick SL, 103, 104, 106, 111, *116*,
    320, 321, *351*, 389, *395*, 427, *446*
Chaires JB, 56, *81*, 99, *113*
Chamberlain D, 197, *212*, 433, *450*,
    460, 466, *469, 473*
Chamberlain DW, 460, *470*
Chamberlain JS, 42, *49*, 326, *354*
Chan J, 206, *217*
Chan SH, 250, *279*, 326, *355*, 435, *450*
Chan VW, 255, *282*
Chandler LA, 435, *451*
Chang AE, 194, *209*, 252, *280*
Chang CD, 95, 96, *113*
Chang F, 309, *318*
Chang HC, 3, *24*
Chang JF, 252, *281*, 309, *318*
Chang K, 303, *316*
Chang L, 12, *26*
Chang LS, 54, 63, 67, *79, 88*
Chang MY, 108, 111, *117*, 150, *163*,
    261, *289*, 300, 307, *315, 317*
Chang SM, 323, *353*
Chang YN, 158, *166*
Chanock RM, 207, *218*, 325, *354*
Chao H, 424, *443*
Chao S, 345, *364*
Chaplier A, 464, *472*
Chapman HA, 183, *190*
Charlton D, 158, *166*
Chartier C, 43, *49*
Chasse JF, 38, *46*
Chatterjee S, 61, 64, *84*
Chaussabel D, 198, *214*
Chazen GD, 249, *278*
Chedrese PJ, 302, *315*
Chehimi J, 250, *279*
Chejanovsky N, 55, 65, *80*
Chen C, 255, 256, *283*, 427, *445*
Chen D, 254, *282*
Chen F, 175, *186*
Chen GA, 247, *274*

Chen GH, 202, *215*, 436, *452*
Chen H, 242, *269*
Chen HH, 326, *355*
Chen HL, 253, *281*
Chen JJ, 257, *285*
Chen L, 54, 65, 66, *80*, 175, *186*, 326, *354*, 438, *453*
Chen SH, 106, *115*, 121, *138*, 296, 304, *314*, *316*
Chen SJ, 5, *24*, 326, *354*
Chen W, 196, *212*
Chen Y, 158, *166*, 246, 247, *274*
Chen ZH, 136, *144*
Chen ZY, 110, *118*
Cheng H, 245, *273*
Cheng SH, 93, 94, 96, 98, 99, 100, 101, 103, 104, 105, 106, 107, 109, 110, 111, *112*, *113*, *114*, *115*, *116*, *117*, 123, *139*, 319, 320, 321, 333, 334, 336, 346, *349*, *351*, *359*, *360*, *364*, 387, *394*, 421, 425, 426, 427, 430, *441*, *445*, *446*, *448*
Chensue SW, 175, *186*
Cheresh D, 257, *285*, 326, *355*
Cheresh DA, 122, *138*, *139*, 259, 262, *287*, *289*
Chernick MS, 366, *377*
Chernoff AE, 436, *452*
Cherry M, 98, 103, 106, 110, *113*, *116*
Chesnoy S, 93, 99, *112*
Chesnut KA, 65, 70, 73, *87*, *91*, 323, 333, 334, *353*, *359*, 370, *379*, 412, 413, *416*, *417*, 421, 424, *441*
Chevalier PG, 458, *467*
Chew AJ, 6, 14, *24*, *26*
Chiang Y, 12, *26*
Chiang YL, 158, *166*
Chiang YW, 195, *210*
Chiarelli C, 303, *316*
Chillon M, 123, *139*, 338, *362*, 425, *444*
Chiocca EA, 157, *165*
Chiorini JA, 62, *85*, 126, 128, *140*, 338, 339, *361*, *362*, 376, *381*, 424, 438, *443*, *454*

Chirmule N, 41, *48*, 54, 65, 66, 73, *79*, *87*, *88*, 135, *144*, 263, *290*, 333, 338, 347, *360*, *362*, *364*, 366, *377*, 429, *447*, *448*
Chiu W, 110, *118*, 375, *381*
Chizzonite R, 250, *279*
Choi AMK, 437, *453*
Choi EA, 249, *277*
Choi H, 5, *24*, 326, *354*
Choi JY, 367, *379*
Chomarat P, 197, *213*
Chong D, 175, *186*, 436, *452*
Chong H, 296, 304, *313*, *316*
Chong W, 8, *25*
Chonn A, 101, 102, 103, *114*, 427, *445*
Chou JL, 366, *377*
Chou SH, 56, *81*
Chow YH, 135, *144*, 435, *450*, *451*
Chowdhury JR, 414, *418*
Chowdhury NR, 414, *418*
Chowdhury SI, 430, *448*
Christ M, 39, 42, 43, *48*, *49*
Christian L, 205, *216*
Christie NA, 458, *468*
Christman B, 399, *404*
Christman BW, 400, *405*, 432, 439, *449*, *455*
Christman JW, 411, *416*, 432, *449*
Christmas T, 305, *317*
Christofidou-Solomidou M, 257, *285*
Chu BY, 56, *81*
Chu CS, 13, *26*, 320, *350*, 366, *377*, 410, *415*
Chu Q, 123, *139*, 336, *360*, 421, 425, 430, *441*, *448*
Chu S, 102, 104, *115*, 368, *379*
Chu TH, 337, *361*
Chunduru S, 368, *379*, 413, *417*
Chung AS, 151, *164*
Chung I, 158, *166*
Chung LW, 158, *166*
Chung RY, 157, *165*
Chytil A, 409, *415*
Cicala C, 311, *318*
Cichutek K, 337, *361*

Ciernik IF, 247, 252, *274*, *280*
Cieslewicz G, 177, *187*
Ciliberto G, 61, 65, 67, *84*, *86*
Cinquegrana A, 308, *318*
Clackson T, 109, *117*, 461, 462, *471*
Clairmont C, 148, *163*
Clancy JP, 103, 104, 106, 111, *116*, 387, 389, *395*, 426, *445*
Clark BJ, 13, *26*
Clark J, 238, *268*
Clark JG, 74, *92*, 426, 429, 433, *444*, *449*, *450*
Clark KR, 65, 67, 68, *86*, *88*
Clark LC, 432, *449*
Clark R, 257, *285*
Clark SC, 195, *210*
Clarke MF, 157, *165*
Claude F, 103, *115*
Clelland C, 459, *469*
Clemens PR, 326, *355*
Clements J, 427, *446*
Clements V, 249, *278*
Clerici M, 12, *26*
Cliff WH, 319, *349*, 366, *377*, 386, 387, *394*
Clifford KN, 198, *214*
Clift SM, 15, *26*, 252, *281*
Cline MG, 2, *23*
Close JM, 459, *469*
Clow K, 100, *113*
Cochran A, 247, *275*
Coffee K, 425, *444*
Coffey MC, 147, *162*
Coffin JM, 328, *356*
Cohen GI, 148, *162*
Cohen J, 194, *209*
Cohen JL, 198, *214*
Cohen LK, 15, *26*, 252, *281*
Cohen RG, 458, *467*
Cohen S, 245, *272*
Cohen SN, 19, *27*
Cohn JA, 320, *350*
Cohn ZA, 193, *208*
Coker RK, 178, *189*
Colby TV, 178, *189*, 224, *230*

Cole KE, 260, *288*
Cole NM, 76, *92*
Cole-Strauss A, 414, *418*
Collaco RF, 52, 68, *78*
Collart MA, 178, *188*, 194, *209*
Collector MI, 320, *350*
Colledge WH, 111, *118*, 320, 321, *351*, 425, *443*
Collete D, 65, *87*
Colley DG, 207, *218*
Collins FM, 207, *217*
Collins FS, 319, *349*, 366, *377*
Collins MK, 123, *139*, 262, *290*, 337, 338, *361*
Collins PL, 207, *218*, 343, *363*
Collis P, 67, *88*
Coll J, 304, *316*
Colombo MP, 249, *276*
Colotta F, 249, *276*
Colston MJ, 206, *217*, 307, *317*
Colton DM, 432, *449*
Colubjatnikov R, 205, *216*
Columbo JP, 2, *23*
Compere SJ, 238, *267*
Compton D, 255, *283*
Conary JT, 400, *405*, 411, *416*, 439, *455*
Conceicao CM, 366, *377*
Condos R, 182, *190*
Conlon T, 54, *80*, 413, *417*
Connelly C, 36, 37, *45*
Connick E, 249, *278*
Connors M, 207, *218*
Conover J, 427, *445*
Conrad C, 7, *25*, 76, *92*, 327, *356*, 365, 368, 371, *377*, *379*, *380*, 412, 413, *416*, *417*
Conrad CK, 63, 70, *85*, *90*, 320, *351*, 370, *380*, 412, *416*, *417*, 424, *442*
Consalvo M, 244, 249, *271*, *275*
Constantino P, 103, *115*
Content J, 207, *217*
Conway JE, 67, *88*, 366, *377*
Cook JL, 437, *453*

Cooper AM, 182, *190*, 195, 206, *211*, *216*
Cooper CA, 235, *266*
Cooper DK, 461, *470*
Cooper JA, 463, *472*
Cooper JD, 458, 459, 460, 461, *467*, *468*, *469*, *470*
Cooper JM, 461, *470*
Copeland J, 438, *453*
Copenhaver SC, 322, *352*
Corbett T, 68, *89*
Cordier L, 66, 69, *88*, *89*
Cork J, 198, *213*
Corraliza I, 193, *209*
Corry DB, 197, 205, *213*, *216*, 436, *452*
Cortese R, 61, 65, 67, *84*
Cosset FL, 123, *139*, 262, *290*, 337, 338, *361*
Costa DL, 333, *360*
Costello E, 62, *85*
Cosyn JP, 148, *163*
Cotran RS, 256, *284*
Cotten M, 11, *25*, 122, *139*, 391, *395*, 428, *446*
Couetil JP, 458, *467*
Coughlin CM, 251, *280*
Coughlin SR, 251, *280*
Coukos G, 150, *163*
Coulie PG, 246, *274*
Courage NL, 109, *117*
Courtney M, 306, *317*, 320, *350*, 409, *415*, 425, *444*
Coutelle C, 100, *114*, 124, *140*, 320, *350*
Couto LB, 6, 14, *24*, *26*, 61, 64, *84*, 110, *117*
Couton D, 461, *470*
Couture KK, 326, *354*
Couture LA, 38, *46*, 320, 325, *350*, *354*
Couture RA, 387, *394*
Cox AL, 246, 247, *274*
Cox G, 174, 179, *185*
Cox RA, 205, *216*
Coyle A, 177, *187*
Coyne CB, 336, *360*

Coyne M, 424, *442*
Craig C, 243, *270*
Crapo JD, 434, 437, *450*
Crawford J, 413, *417*
Crawford SE, 258, *286*
Crawford-Miksza L, 32, 40, *45*
Crellin N, 302, *315*
Crespo J, 411, *416*
Crispens MA, 260, *288*
Croce MA, 432, *449*
Croitoru K, 174, 175, 177, *185*, *186*, *188*, 436, *451*
Cronin K, 249, *276*
Cronin L, 249, *276*
Cross S, 15, *26*
Crossley J, 174, *185*
Crouzet J, 331, *358*
Crowe JE, 207, *218*
Crowell RL, 120, 122, *137*, 326, *355*
Croyle MA, 135, *144*, 263, *290*, 347, *364*
Croyl M, 429, *447*
Cruciani AR, 308, *318*
Cruickshank G, 149, *163*
Crystal RG, 13, *26*, 38, 40, *46*, *48*, 120, 126, 127, 135, *137*, *141*, *144*, 158, *166*, 202, *215*, 262, 263, *289*, *290*, 320, 322, 323, 324, *350*, *351*, *352*, *353*, 366, *378*, 387, *394*, 401, *405*, 409, *415*, 420, 425, 437, 438, 439, *441*, *443*, *444*, *453*, *454*
Csaky KG, 180, 181, *189*, 225, *230*, 436, *451*, 466, *473*
Cuervo N, 126, *141*
Cui L, 245, *273*
Cui ZH, 197, *213*
Cullis PR, 100, *113*
Culver KW, 12, *26*, 38, *46*, 296, *313*, 460, *470*
Cunningham C, 243, *270*
Cunningham JA, 33, *45*, 120, 122, *137*, 262, *289*, 326, *355*
Cuppens H, 367, *379*
Curiel C, 303, *315*
Curiel D, 302, *315*

Curiel DT, 11, *25*, 43, *49*, 120, 122, 123, 124, 126, 127, 128, 129, 130, 131, 132, 134, *137*, *138*, *139*, *140*, *141*, *142*, *143*, *144*, 150, *164*, 269, *291*, 309, *318*, 337, *361*, 421, 428, 435, *441*, *446*, *450*
Curiel TC, 147, *162*
Curiel TJ, 123, *140*
Cusack JJ, 245, *273*
Cusack S, 122, 132, *138*
Custer MC, 249, *278*
Custer RP, 240, *268*
Cuthbert AW, 320, 321, *351*
Cuthbertson A, 101, 102, *114*
Cutting GR, 367, *378*, *379*, 413, *417*
Cyster JG, 255, *282*
Czuprynski CJ, 195, *210*

D

Dabouis G, 305, *317*
Daddi N, 461, 463, 465, *470*, *472*, *473*
Dai Y, 326, *354*
Daifuku R, 320, *351*, 370, 371, *380*, 412, *416*, *417*
Dalemans W, 207, *217*, 319, *349*, 425, *443*
Dalesio O, 235, *266*
D'Alessandro AM, 458, *468*
Dalton DK, 206, *216*, *217*
Dalton ML, 457, *467*
D'Amico G, 255, *283*
D'Andrea A, 250, *279*
D'Andrea M, 124, *140*
Damokosh AI, 431, *449*
Danel C, 13, *26*, 38, *47*, 401, *405*, 437, *453*, 464, *472*
Danforth JM, 184, *191*, 196, 197, *211*, *213*
Daniels B, 249, *276*
Daniel T, 260, *287*
Danilov SM, 126, *141*
Danos O, 64, 75, *85*, 102, *115*, 336, *360*, 375, *381*
Danthinne X, 34, 35, *45*

Darlington G, 409, *415*
Das HK, 61, *83*
Dash PR, 100, *113*
Date H, 459, 461, *469*, *470*
Davatelis G, 196, *211*
Davidson A, 294, *312*
Davidson B, 296, *314*
Davidson BL, 39, 43, *47*, 70, *91*, 123, 131, *139*, *143*, 175, *186*, 263, *290*, 296, *313*, 323, 330, 336, 338, 339, 341, 342, 343, *353*, *357*, *360*, *362*, *363*, 376, *381*, 423, 426, *442*, *445*
Davidson DJ, 100, 102, 103, 105, *114*
Davidson H, 320, 321, *351*
Davidson JA, 306, *317*
Davidson-Smith H, 100, 102, 103, 105, *114*, 320, 321, *351*
Davies DE, 181, *190*
Davies J, 103, 104, 106, 111, *116*, 320, 321, *351*, 389, *395*
Davies MG, 103, 104, 106, 111, *116*, 320, 321, *351*
Davies PB, 321, *352*
Davis A, 297, *314*
Davis AR, 207, *218*, 294, *312*
Davis CW, 322, *352*
Davis M, 256, *284*
Davis MD, 65, *86*
Davis PB, 322, 332, 335, 338, 345, *352*, *358*, *361*, *364*, 371, *380*, 428, *446*
Davis RW, 19, *27*
Davis S, 255, *283*
Davis ST, 294, *312*
Dawkins KD, 466, *473*
Dazin P, 102, *115*
Dean BS, 385, *394*
Dean SB, 432, *449*
De Bartolomeis A, 311, *318*
Debelak D, 68, *89*, 366, *377*
Debruyne L, 175, *186*, 464, 465, *472*, *473*
Debruyne LA, 425, *440*
Debs R, 102, *115*, 399, *404*, 427, *446*
Debs RJ, 194, 195, *210*
De Buitrago GG, 156, *165*

DeCampos KN, 458, *468*
Deck RR, 207, *217*
Dedieu JF, 42, *49*, 131, *143*
Deering C, 123, *139*, 336, 343, *360*, *363*, 421, 425, 431, *441*
Defrance T, 197, *212*
De Glovanni C, 244, *271*
De Greve J, 242, *270*
De Gruijl TD, 124, 125, *140*
Degtyareva N, 60, 61, *83*
Deisenhofer J, 129, *142*
Dei Tos AP, 303, *316*
Dejana E, 256, *284*
De Jonge J, 198, *214*
De Kossodo S, 194, *209*
DeKruyff RH, 177, *188*
De La Maza LM, 54, *79*, 195, *210*
De La Monte SM, 184, *191*
Delaney SJ, 366, *378*
Deleage G, 136, *144*, 262, *289*
DeLeij L, 100, *113*
Delepine P, 103, *115*, 399, *404*
Delgado C, 135, *144*, 338, *362*, 425, *444*
DeLisser HM, 257, *285*
Dell'Aringa J, 369, 373, *379*
Dell J, 245, *272*
Delman K, 157, *165*
Delmastro P, 61, 65, *84*
Delogu G, 207, *217*
Delporte C, 438, *454*
DeLuca NA, 7, *25*
Delvaux A, 196, *212*
De Martin R, 439, *454*
DeMarzo AM, 158, *166*
DeMatteo R, 62, *85*
Demayo F, 239, *268*
Demayo FJ, 109, *117*
Demeneix BA, 94, *112*
Demers B, 151, *164*
Demers GW, 150, *164*
Deng JC, 196, *211*
Deng W, 320, *350*
Deng Z, 126, *141*
Denis O, 207, *217*
Denkers EY, 193, *209*

Densmore CL, 428, *446*, *447*
Denzler KL, 176, *187*
DePalma M, 308, *318*
DePamphilis ML, 367, *378*
De Plaen E, 246, *274*
Deprez I, 403, *406*, 438, *454*
Derin RB, 367, *379*
Der Meulen-Muileman I, 124, *140*
De Saint Basile G, 12, *26*
Desch JK, 320, *351*, 371, *380*, 412, *417*
Deshane J, 243, *270*
Deshpande DS, 103, 105, *115*, 426, *445*
Desmouliere A, 179, *189*
Desseroth AB, 158, *166*
Detels R, 203, *215*
Detorie N, 158, *166*
Detterbeck FC, 458, *468*
Devalarja M, 260, *288*
Devalarja R, 260, *288*
De Veerman M, 198, *214*
De Vries JE, 196, *212*
De Waal Malefyt R, 196, *212*
De Waal MR, 196, *212*
Dewald B, 259, *287*
Dewar A, 389, *395*, 422, 425, 427, *440*
DeWeese TL, 158, *166*
Dhanani S, 249, *278*
Di Battista JA, 197, *213*
Dickinson P, 100, 102, 103, 105, *114*
DiCosmo B, 172, *184*
DiCosmo BF, 176, *187*
Dietrich PY, 306, *317*
Dieu MC, 255, *283*
DiGiovine B, 261, *288*
Dignam SS, 56, *81*
Dileo JP, 107, *117*, 400, *405*
Dilley J, 158, *166*
DiMango E, 371, *380*
Ding L, 60, *83*
Ding W, 66, *88*
Ding Y, 197, *212*, 436, *452*
DiPersio L, 240, *268*
Divangahi M, 176, *187*
Dix BR, 151, *164*, 243, *270*
Djeu JY, 196, *212*
Djossou O, 197, *213*

Dmitriev I, 120, 128, 129, 131, 132, *137*, *138*, *142*, *143*, 337, *361*
Dobbs L, 427, *446*
Dodge RW, 205, *216*
Doglioni C, 303, *316*
Doh SG, 101, *114*
Dohadwala M, 253, *281*
Dokka S, 175, *186*
Dolin PJ, 206, *216*
Dolormente MM, 15, *26*
Dominiczak AF, 134, *144*
Dong J, 100, 103, 105, *114*, 158, *166*
Dong JY, 74, *92*, 333, *358*, 366, 367, *378*
Dong R, 375, *381*
Dong Z, 249, 259, *277*, *286*
Donsante A, 77, *92*
Doranz B, 41, *48*, 220, *229*, 326, *354*, 429, *448*
Doring G, 320, *350*
Dorin JR, 70, *90*, 100, 102, 103, 105, *114*, 320, 321, *350*, *351*, 366, *378*, 387, *394*
Dornburg R, 337, *361*
Doronin K, 150, *164*
Dorval T, 306, *317*
Dottorini M, 194, *210*
Douar AM, 336, *360*, 375, *381*
Doucet L, 107, *117*
Dougherty G, 245, *272*
Douglas JT, 119, 120, 123, 124, 125, 126, 128, 132, *137*, *138*, *139*, *140*, *141*, *143*, 269, *291*, 337, *361*, 435, *451*
Douillard JT, 305, *317*
Doukas J, 124, *139*, *140*, 435, *451*
Douvdevani A, 249, *276*
D'Ovidio F, 461, 463, 465, *470*, *472*, *473*
Dower WJ, 128, *142*
Downey G, 102, 104, *115*
Dow SW, 108, *117*, 263, *290*, 399, *405*
Dozy A, 262, *289*
Dozy AM, 119, 128, *137*, 337, *361*
Dranoff G, 15, *26*, 176, *187*, 249, *276*
Drapkin PT, 126, 128, *140*, 338, *361*

Drazan KE, 197, *212*, 436, *452*
Dressman D, 69, *89*
Driever W, 330, *357*
Driscoll K, 174, 179, *185*, 201, *215*
Droal C, 103, *115*
Droguett G, 33, *45*, 120, 122, *137*, 262, *289*, 326, *355*
Droogmans G, 367, *379*
Drumm ML, 319, 327, *349*, *356*, 366, *377*, *378*, 386, 387, *394*
Dryant JL, 399, *404*
Drynda A, 262, *289*
D'Souza C, 207, *217*
Du J, 260, *288*
Duan D, 52, 57, 58, 59, 62, 63, 64, 66, 69, 70, 71, 73, 74, 75, 76, *78*, 82, *85*, 88, *90*, *92*, 324, 328, 339, 347, *353*, *356*, *362*, *363*, *364*, 375, *381*, 424, 430, 431, *443*, *449*
Duan L, 414, *418*
Dubensky J, 343, *363*
Dubensky TW, 330, *357*
Dubielzig R, 55, 60, *80*
Dubinett SM, 233, 234, 245, 246, 247, 249, 253, *265*, *266*, *273*, *275*, *278*, *281*, 439, *454*
Duboc D, 461, *470*
Dubois B, 198, *214*
Dubois PJ, 15, *26*
Dubois R, 253, *281*
Du Bois RM, 178, *189*
Ducharme S, 102, 104, *115*
Duda DG, 251, *280*
Dudley ME, 247, *275*
Dudus L, 63, 64, 70, 75, *85*, *90*, 93, 99, *112*, 437, *453*
Dull T, 330, *357*
Dumasius V, 426, 430, 432, 438, *444*, *453*
Dummer R, 120, *138*
Dumont JE, 257, *285*
Duncan JD, 420, 432, *441*
Duncan SR, 459, *469*
Dunn P, 206, *216*
Dupressoir T, 61, *84*
Dupuit F, 43, *49*, 326, *355*, 435, *451*

Duque PM, 156, *165*
Duquesnoy RJ, 459, *469*
Durand I, 198, *214*
Durham SR, 103, 104, 106, 111, *116*, 320, 321, *350*, *351*
During MJ, 67, 69, *88*, *90*
Dutheil N, 61, *84*
Dutia BM, 193, *209*
Dwarki V, 57, *82*, 328, *356*, 375, *381*
Dyall J, 60, 61, *83*
Dzarniecki CW, 195, *210*

E

Eastman J, 428, *446*
Eastman SJ, 95, 96, 103, 104, 106, 107, 109, 111, *113*, *115*, *116*, *117*, 123, *139*, 320, 321, 336, *351*, *360*, 421, 425, 430, *441*, *448*
Ebrahimi B, 193, *209*
Eck SL, 249, *277*, 296, 297, 302, *314*, *315*
Ecke D, 367, *379*
Eckhoff DE, 458, *468*
Eckman E, 332, *358*
Edahibi S, 403, *406*, 438, *454*
Edelson JD, 435, *451*
Edington HD, 250, *279*
Edwards CD, 235, *266*
Edwards CKI, 421, *441*
Edwards EA, 54, 65, *79*
Edwards LJ, 13, *26*, 320, *350*, 373, *380*
Edwards NM, 458, *468*
Eeles R, 235, *266*
Efstathiou S, 198, *214*
Efthimiou J, 320, *351*
Egan JJ, 320, *351*
Egan M, 319, *349*, 367, *378*, 413, *417*
Egan ME, 367, *379*
Egan TM, 458, *467*
Egawa M, 158, *166*
Eggermont AM, 306, *317*
Eggermont J, 367, *379*
Ehlert J, 260, *287*
Eigen H, 320, *350*
Einfeld DA, 122, 132, *138*

Eisenbach L, 247, *274*
Eisenlohr LC, 146, *162*
Eisenstein M, 247, *274*
Eissa NT, 437, *453*
Eissa T, 13, *26*
Eitzman DT, 224, *230*
Ekman MR, 205, *216*
Elbash M, 297, *314*
Elfenbein DH, 39, 43, *48*
Elgert KD, 247, *275*
Elias JA, 172, 176, 183, *185*, *187*, *190*, 220, *229*
Ellem KA, 15, *26*
Ellinger C, 52, 68, *78*
Ellinger S, 52, 68, *78*
Ellis T, 413, *417*
Elshami AA, 150, *163*, 245, *272*, 296, 297, *313*, *314*
Elston RC, 234, 249, *265*
Embree LJ, 346, *364*
Embry M, 158, *166*
Embury J, 413, *417*
Emi N, 296, *313*
Emmendorffer A, 195, *210*
Emoto M, 182, *190*
Emtage PCR, 174, *185*
Endo S, 436, *452*
Endo Y, 257, *285*
Engdahl RK, 37, *46*
Engelhardt JF, 5, 13, *24*, *26*, 41, *48*, 52, 57, 58, 59, 62, 63, 64, 66, 69, 70, 71, 73, 74, 75, 76, *78*, *82*, *85*, *88*, *90*, *91*, *92*, 93, 99, *112*, 120, *137*, 220, 228, *229*, *230*, 320, 324, 325, 326, 327, 328, 339, 347, *350*, *352*, *353*, *354*, *355*, *356*, *362*, *363*, *364*, 373, 375, *380*, *381*, 423, 424, 425, 429, 430, 431, 433, 437, *442*, *443*, *448*, *449*, *450*, *453*
Engerman R, 256, *284*
Engler H, 151, *164*
Ennist DL, 333, *358*, 425, *440*
Enosawa S, 459, *469*
Epperly MW, 245, *273*, 433, 437, *450*, *453*
Erbacher P, 344, *363*

Erickson AM, 184, *191*
Erikson D, 61, 65, *84*, 413, *417*
Eriksson L, 458, *468*
Eriksson LT, 459, *468*
Ernst SA, 320, *350*
Ertl HC, 39, *47*, 262, *289*, 333, *359*, 425, *444*
Erzurum SC, 437, *453*
Esakof DD, 17, *27*
Esandi MC, 297, *314*
Espat NJ, 436, *452*
Espevik T, 250, *279*
Espino PC, 325, *354*
Esposito V, 311, *318*
Esquivel F, 253, *281*
Esty AC, 3, *24*
Eto H, 259, *287*
Eura M, 247, *274*
Evans MJ, 111, *118*, 320, 321, *351*, 425, *443*
Evans TW, 459, *468*
Eve B, 260, *287*
Eyre JH, 234, 249, *265*

F

Fabbro D, 244, *271*
Fabian TC, 432, *449*
Fabrega A, 70, *91*, 120, 122, *137, 139*, 327, *355*
Faccioli LH, 207, *217*
Factor P, 426, 430, 432, 438, *444, 453*
Fadok V, 174, *186*
Fagan KA, 400, *405*, 429, *448*
Faha B, 150, *164*
Fahrner JA, 70, *91*, 120, 125, *137*, 324, *353*, 425, *440*
Fainstein V, 201, *215*
Fair DS, 223, *229*
Fairweather NF, 124, *140*
Fajac I, 428, *446*
Fakharai H, 305, *317*
Falck-Pedersen E, 39, 40, 43, *48*, 120, 127, 135, *138, 141*, 333, 346, *359*, *364*, 425, *443*
Fallaux FJ, 37, *46*

Falloon J, 249, *278*
Falo LD, 253, 254, *282*
Falotico R, 440, *455*
Fan PD, 74, *92*, 366, 367, *378*
Fang B, 120, 122, *138*, 310, *318*
Fang SL, 93, 99, *112*
Fanslow WC, 198, *214*
Farassati F, 150, *163*
Farber JM, 260, *287, 288*
Farini E, 366, *378*
Farjo A, 39, 43, *47*
Farley R, 103, 104, 106, 111, *116, 118*, 320, 321, 345, *351, 364*, 366, *378*, 387, *395*, 426, 427, *445, 446*
Farmer SC, 176, *187*
Farrell CL, 429, *447*
Farson D, 42, *49*
Fasbender A, 96, 101, *113, 114*, 123, *139*, 320, 321, 346, *351, 364*, 425, 427, 430, 431, *444, 446, 449*
Fasbender AJ, 332, *358*, 427, *445, 446*
Fattaey A, 151, *164*
Fattori E, 61, *83*
Fauci AS, 203, *215*
Faulks RD, 439, *455*
Faust LZ, 67, *88*
Favrot M, 304, *316*
Fawell SE, 135, *144*
Fay WP, 224, *230*
Fearon E, 247, 249, *275, 277*
Febbraio M, 258, *286*
Fee-Maki M, 368, *379*, 424, *442*
Feiden KL, 22, *27*
Feldhaus A, 367, *378*
Feldman M, 247, *274*
Felgner PL, 8, 9, 11, *25*, 94, 100, 101, 103, 105, *112, 113, 114*, 384, *393*
Felip E, 244, *271*
Fell A, 15, *26*
Fels AOS, 193, *208*
Feng CG, 207, *217*
Feng GJ, 193, *209*
Feng M, 123, *139*, 269, *291*, 337, *361*
Feng X, 175, *186*, 436, *452*
Ferara N, 256, *284*
Ferber S, 134, *143*

Ferec C, 107, *117*
Ferguson D, 39, 43, *47*
Ferguson K, 368, *379*
Ferkol T, 10, *25*, 321, 323, 332, 335, *352*, *353*, *358*, 413, *417*, 425, 437, 439, *440*, *453*, *454*
Fernando MB, 148, *162*
Ferrans VJ, 366, *377*
Ferrari FK, 62, 68, *85*, *88*, 328, *356*
Ferrari G, 249, *276*
Ferrari ME, 100, *113*
Ferrari S, 111, *118*, 345, *364*, 384, *393*
Ferris B, 135, *144*, 323, *353*, 420, 425, *441*
Ferry N, 337, *361*
Fersh M, 65, 73, *87*
Ferson DZ, 15, *26*, 424, *442*
Fidler IJ, 240, 249, 259, 260, *268*, *277*, *286*, *288*
Fields PA, 110, *117*
Fields RC, 254, *282*
Fiers W, 257, *285*
Fife KH, 55, *81*
Figdor CG, 196, *212*
Figlin R, 293, *312*
Filaci G, 247, *275*
Finberg RW, 70, *91*, 120, 122, 131, *137*, *138*, 262, *289*, 326, *355*, 420, 425, *440*
Finegold M, 239, *268*, 409, *415*
Finegold MJ, 304, *316*
Finer MH, 42, *49*, 326, *354*
Fink DJ, 7, *25*
Finkbeiner WE, 93, 99, *112*
Finke R, 69, *89*
Finn CC, 15, *26*
Finn OJ, 324, *353*
Fiorentino DF, 196, *212*
Fipaldini C, 61, 65, 67, *84*
Firestone CY, 207, *218*
Fischer A, 12, *26*
Fischer H, 76, *92*, 367, *378*
Fischer I, 320, *350*
Fischer S, 463, *472*
Fischer SG, 126, *141*

Fisher AB, 126, *141*
Fisher DE, 241, *269*
Fisher J, 68, *89*, 366, *377*
Fisher KJ, 5, *24*, 40, *48*, 59, 62, 64, 66, 75, *82*, *85*, *86*, *88*, 326, *354*
Fisher RE, 53, *79*
Fisher-Adams G, 61, 64, *84*
Fishman GI, 296, *313*
Fitz L, 195, *210*, 250, *279*
Fitzgerald D, 11, *25*
Fitzgerald DJ, 326, *355*
Fitzjohn EM, 320, *351*
Flake AW, 6, 14, *24*, *26*
Flanagan JM, 122, *138*
Flanders KC, 178, *189*
Flavell RA, 39, 43, *48*, 172, 176, *184*, *185*, 187, 198, *214*, 220, *229*
Fleisher T, 12, *26*
Fleming L, 409, *415*
Floch V, 107, *117*, 399, *404*
Flockhart JH, 70, *90*
Florack VJ, 103, 105, *115*, 426, *445*
Flores-Degaldo G, 181, *190*
Flores-Romo L, 197, *213*
Flory CM, 207, *217*
Flotte T, 7, *25*, 66, 70, 74, *87*, *91*, *92*, 319, 339, *349*, *362*, 367, 371, *378*, *380*, 412, *416*, 437, *453*
Flotte TR, 63, 64, 70, 74, *85*, *86*, *90*, 320, 323, 327, 333, 334, *351*, *353*, *356*, *359*, 365, 366, 367, 368, 370, *377*, *378*, *379*, 412, *417*, 421, 424, *441*, *443*
Flynn JL, 182, *190*, 195, 206, *210*, *217*
Foley R, 173, 174, 179, *185*, 201, *215*, 436, *451*
Folkman J, 255, 256, 257, 258, *283*, *284*, *285*, *286*
Fong Y, 157, *165*
Fontana A, 466, *473*
Force SD, 108, 111, *117*, 156, *165*, 243, *270*, 302, 307, *315*, *317*
Ford H, 156, *165*
Forman SJ, 61, 64, *84*
Fornerod M, 341, *363*

Forney Prescott M, 136, *144*
Forry-Schaudies S, 433, *450*
Forsyth PA, 147, *162*
Fortunati E, 100, *114*
Foskett JK, 322, *352*
Fossiez F, 197, *213*
Foster PS, 177, *188*
Fox B, 102, 103, 110, *113*, *115*
Fox EA, 101, 102, 103, 107, *113*, *114*, 429, *447*
Fox WW, 74, *91*, 433, *449*
Foy C, 320, *351*, 373, *380*, 427, *446*
Fradkin LG, 102, 108, 110, *115*, *117*, 263, *290*, 399, *405*
Fraley DM, 65, *86*
Francis GE, 135, *144*
Frank AA, 207, *217*
Frank I, 250, *279*
Franke FE, 126, *141*
Franke-Ullmann G, 195, *210*
Franklin L, 326, *355*
Franklin WA, 234, 243, 249, *266*, *270*
Fraser NW, 7, *25*, 150, *163*
Fredberg J, 431, *449*
Frederik PM, 99, *113*, 429, *447*
Freeman BA, 435, 438, *451*, *453*
Freeman SM, 242, 245, *269*, *272*, 294, 296, 304, *312*, *313*, *316*
Freimark BD, 103, 105, *115*, 426, *445*
Freimuth P, 70, *91*, 120, 122, *137*, *138*, *139*, 327, *355*
Fremont DH, 199, *214*
French K, 430, *448*
French M, 101, 102, *114*
Frey D, 440, *455*
Freytag SO, 156, *165*, 245, *272*
Friborg S, 320, *351*, 371, *380*, 412, *417*
Fridkin M, 247, *274*
Fridman WH, 306, *317*
Friedland JS, 174, *185*
Friedman E, 70, *90*, 327, *355*, 425, *443*
Friedman M, 196, *212*
Friedmann T, 3, *24*, 330, 331, 341, *357*, *358*, 424, *442*
Friend DS, 427, *446*

Frisdal E, 403, *406*
Frizzell RA, 74, *92*, 100, 103, 105, *114*, 319, 333, *349*, *358*, 366, *377*, *378*
Frizelle SP, 309, *318*
Frost P, 249, *277*
Fry JW, 461, *471*
Fry TJ, 249, *278*
Fu SM, 198, *214*
Fuchs HJ, 194, 195, *210*
Fueto J, 130, 131, *143*, 150, *164*
Fuhrman BP, 432, *449*
Fuji M, 180, *189*, 225, *230*
Fujiwara T, 241, 242, *269*, 424, *442*
Fukayama M, 410, *415*
Fuks Z, 256, *284*
Fukuda N, 438, *454*
Fukumura M, 345, 346, *364*
Fukuzuka K, 437, *452*
Fulgeras W, 339, *362*, 376, *381*
Fulkerson WJ, 434, *450*
Fuller S, 331, *357*
Fulmer SB, 61, 64, *84*, 367, *378*, *379*, 413, *417*
Funeshima N, 459, *469*
Fung-Leung WP, 240, *269*
Funke M, 345, *364*
Furney SK, 207, *217*
Furth EE, 39, *47*
Furukawa K, 249, *277*
Furuya S, 135, *144*
Fusco U, 308, *318*

G

Gabbiani F, 179, *189*
Gabbiani G, 179, *189*
Gabizon A, 10, *25*
Gabrilovich DI, 253, *281*
Gadek TR, 101, 102, *114*, 384, *393*
Gaensler K, 427, *446*
Gagandeep S, 296, *313*
Gage FH, 3, *24*, 262, *289*, 329, 330, 341, *357*, *363*
Gagne L, 102, 103, 104, *115*
Gahery-Segard H, 39, 43, *47*, 264, *290*

Gajewska B, 177, *187*
Gajewska BU, 177, *188*
Gajewski TF, 246, *274*
Galand P, 257, *285*
Gale NW, 255, *283*
Galer CE, 126, 128, *140*
Galgiani JN, 205, *215, 216*
Gallay P, 3, *24*, 262, *289*, 329, 330, 341, *357*
Gallichan WS, 436, *452*
Gallimore PH, 151, *164*
Gall JGD, 40, *48*, 346, *364*
Gallo RC, 101, 102, *114*
Gallup MW, 176, *187*
Galt T, 180, *189*
Gamble JR, 196, *211*
Ganapathi R, 245, *273*
Ganly I, 151, *164*
Ganly P, 235, *266*
Gansbacher B, 249, *276*
Gao B, 403, *406*
Gao GP, 5, 6, *24*, 37, 42, *46, 49*, 62, 66, *85, 87, 88*, 135, *144*, 263, *290*, 300, 308, *315, 318*, 338, *362*, 366, *377*, 429, *447*
Gao L, 428, *446*
Gao X, 100, *114*, 320, *350*, 384, *393*, 461, *471*
Garbati N, 345, *364*
Garcia E, 197, *212*
Garcia I, 178, *189*
Garcia M, 243, *270*
Garcia-Ribas I, 304, *316*
Garcia SB, 239, *268*
Gardner P, 320, 339, *351, 362*, 370, 371, *380*, 412, *416, 417*
Gardner R, 320, *350*
Gardner TA, 158, *166*
Garlepp M, 294, 305, *312, 317*
Garlepp MJ, 305, 307, *317*
Garrett RE, 146, *161*
Garver RI, 409, *415*, 425, 435, *440, 450*
Gaspert A, 466, *473*
Gaston J, 39, 43, *47*
Gately MK, 195, *210*, 250, *279*
Gates AL, 107, 109, *117*

Gatzy JT, 322, *352*, 386, *394*
Gauldie D, 179, *189*, 222, *229*
Gauldie J, 173, 174, 175, 179, 180, 181, 182, 184, *185, 186, 187, 189, 190, 191*, 195, 197, *211, 212*, 222, 225, *229, 230*, 250, *279*, 433, 436, 438, *450, 451, 452, 454*, 466, *473*
Gaumer R, 294, *312*
Gautam A, 428, *446, 447*
Gavrilyuk VD, 126, 127, *140, 141*, 402, 405, 429, *447*
Gaydos JC, 32, *45*
Gazdar AF, 150, *163*, 234, 249, *266*
Gazzeri S, 243, *271*
Gazzinelli RT, 195, *211*
Ge M, 458, *468*
Ge Y, 66, *87*
Geba GP, 172, 176, *184, 185, 187*
Geddes D, 100, *114*
Geddes DM, 103, 104, 106, 111, *116, 118*, 308, *318*, 320, 321, 322, 345, *351, 352, 364*, 387, *395*, 439, *454*
Gee MS, 251, *280*
Geertsen R, 120, *138*
Gehman KE, 459, *468*
Geionoz A, 179, *189*
Geissler EK, 461, *471*
Geletneky K, 51, *78*
Gelfand EW, 176, 177, *187*
Gellene RA, 194, *210*
Gemmill RM, 235, *266*
Geng Y, 196, *211*
George CX, 94, *112*
Georges R, 241, *269*
Georges RN, 424, *442*
Georgiou A, 207, *218*
Geraci M, 403, *406*
Geradts J, 309, *318*
Gerard C, 196, *212*, 369, 373, *379*
Gerard R, 338, *362*
Gerard RD, 125, 129, *140, 142*, 402, 405
Gerritsen WR, 123, 127, 132, *140, 142, 143*
Gerwig GJ, 322, *352*
Getzy DM, 195, *211*

Ghobrial RM, 459, *469*
Giangreco A, 320, *350*
Gibbs JB, 243, *270*
Gibson M, 3, *23*
Gibson RL, 320, *351*, 429, *448*
Giese NA, 207, *218*
Gilardi P, 410, *415*
Gilbert BE, 430, *448*
Gilbert JD, 156, *165*
Gilbert MA, 464, 465, *472*
Gilbert SC, 207, *217*
Gilboa E, 247, 249, 253, *274*, *276*, *282*
Gileadi U, 320, *351*, 387, 389, *395*
Gilgenkrantz H, 461, *470*
Gilkey L, 102, 110, *115*
Gill DR, 320, 321, *351*, 387, *394*
Gillenwater AM, 151, *165*
Gillenwater JY, 158, *166*
Gillespie GY, 120, 123, *137*, 149, *163*
Gilliand G, 200, *215*
Gillies C, 223, *229*
Gilliet M, 253, *281*
Gillis S, 249, *278*
Gillmore LK, 32, *44*
Gilly B, 320, *350*
Gilly R, 320, *350*
Gilman M, 109, *117*
Gimbrone MA, 256, *284*
Ginsberg H, 11, *25*
Ginsberg HS, 325, *354*
Ginsburg D, 224, *230*
Giordano A, 311, *318*, 460, *470*
Gipson C, 320, *351*, 373, *380*, 427, *446*
Giraud C, 51, *78*
Girgis KR, 253, *281*
Girod A, 54, *80*, 136, *144*
Giuliano M, 310, *318*
Giuliano MT, 311, *318*
Gjerset R, 305, *317*
Glader B, 6, 14, *24*, *26*
Gladson CL, 223, *229*
Glass M, 260, *288*
Glasser SW, 172, *184*
Glick MC, 322, 344, 345, *352*, *363*, *364*
Glorioso JC, 7, *25*, 51, 66, *78*, 147, *162*
Gluzman R, 64, 75, *85*, 375, *381*

Godbey WT, 94, *112*
Goddard CA, 320, *351*
Godfrin D, 39, 43, *47*
Godowski P, 101, 102, *114*
Godwin D, 293, *312*
Godwin SG, 55, 65, *80*
Goebeler M, 256, *284*
Goemann MM, 158, *166*
Goey SH, 306, *317*
Goff SP, 3, *24*
Goins WF, 7, *25*
Gojo S, 461, *470*
Gold LI, 178, *188*
Goldberg I, 134, *143*
Goldberg J, 259, *287*
Goldberg JB, 367, *378*
Goldman CK, 123, 124, *139*, 435, *451*
Goldman M, 197, *213*
Goldman MJ, 70, *91*, 326, 327, 341, 342, *354*, *355*, *363*, 424, *442*
Goldsmith KT, 435, *450*
Goldstein MM, 195, *210*
Goldwasser E, 39, 43, *47*
Golightly D, 158, *166*
Gollan F, 432, *449*
Golumbek P, 253, *281*
Golunski E, 428, *446*
Gomella L, 146, *162*
Gomez-Manzano C, 150, *164*
Gomez-Navarro J, 120, 123, 129, 131, *138*, *142*
Gonczol E, 5, *24*, 39, 41, *47*, *48*, 196, *211*, 326, *354*
Gondor M, 324, 347, *353*, *364*, 422, *441*
Gonen A, 134, *143*
Gong J, 254, *282*
Gonzales LW, 74, *91*, 433, *449*
Gonzalez AM, 124, *140*, 435, *451*
Good MF, 15, *26*
Good SS, 294, *312*
Gooding LR, 326, *354*
Gooding W, 433, *450*
Goodleski JJ, 174, *185*
Goodman JC, 296, *314*
Goodman RE, 197, *213*

Goodrum FD, 156, *165*
Gooi HC, 320, *351*
Gooya JM, 337, *361*
Gordon D, 16, *27*
Gordon EM, 136, *144*
Gore M, 151, *164*
Gorgoni B, 60, 61, *83*
Gorman C, 102, 110, *115*, 429, *448*
Gorman CM, 102, 103, 110, *113*, *115*
Gorziglia MI, 40, *48*
Goto Y, 193, *209*
Gotzos V, 303, *316*
Goudreau A, 422, *442*
Govers R, 72, *91*
Govoni D, 249, *276*
Goya S, 222, 226, *229*, *230*
Grabowski D, 245, *273*
Grabstein KH, 249, *278*
Graham BS, 207, *218*
Graham FL, 5, *24*, 35, 37, *45*, *46*, 147,
  162, 173, 174, 175, 179, 180, 181,
  184, *185*, *186*, *189*, *191*, 197, *212*,
  222, 225, *229*, *230*, 250, 263, *279*,
  290, 326, 333, *354*, *355*, *359*, 411,
  415, *416*, 436, 438, *451*, *452*, *454*,
  466, *473*
Graham RW, 100, *113*
Graham SM, 38, *46*, 320, *350*
Grand RJ, 151, *164*
Granger DN, 126, *141*
Granowitz EV, 436, *452*
Grant AJ, 249, *278*
Grant DS, 257, *285*
Grapperhaus K, 461, *470*
Grasso TM, 430, *448*
Gratama JW, 306, *317*
Grau GE, 178, *188*, 193, 196, *208*,
  211
Gray T, 324, *353*
Greber UF, 59, *82*, 262, *289*
Greelish JP, 69, *89*
Green ES, 424, *442*
Greenbaum D, 239, *268*
Greenberg S, 183, *191*, 194, *209*
Greenberg SM, 260, *287*

Greenberger JS, 245, *273*, 433, 437,
  450, *453*
Greenberger MJ, 184, *191*, 195, 197,
  211, *213*, 436, *452*
Greenberger S, 134, *143*
Greenblatt JJ, 12, *26*
Greenburg G, 42, *49*
Greene G, 249, *277*
Greening AP, 320, 321, *351*
Greenlee RT, 233, 234, 249, *265*
Greenough A, 431, *449*
Greenspan JS, 74, *91*, 432, *449*
Greenstein RJ, 94, *112*
Greger R, 367, *379*
Gregory RJ, 38, *46*, 319, 320, 325, 326,
  333, 338, 346, *349*, *350*, *354*, *359*,
  360, *362*, *364*, 387, *394*, 422, *441*
Grenet C, 259, *287*
Grewal IS, 39, 43, *48*, 198, *214*
Griesenbach U, 101, 102, 103, *114*,
  322, 345, *352*, *364*, 422, 425, 426,
  427, 438, 439, *440*, *445*, *453*, *454*
Griffin GE, 174, *185*
Griffin JP, 206, *216*
Griffith BP, 459, 460, *468*, *469*, *470*
Grifman M, 128, *142*
Grill J, 127, *142*
Grim J, 309, *318*
Grimley PM, 311, *318*
Grimm D, 55, 60, 65, 67, 68, *80*, *86*,
  88, 412, *416*
Grimm E, 241, *269*
Grimm EA, 424, *442*
Grizzle WE, 134, 135, *143*
Grohamm U, 250, *279*
Gromeier M, 148, *163*
Gropper MA, 197, *213*, 436, *452*
Groshen S, 136, *144*
Gross F, 12, *26*
Grossman M, 13, *26*, 220, 228, 229,
  230, 429, *448*
Grossman R, 296, *314*
Grossman RG, 296, *314*
Grosveld G, 341, *363*
Grout M, 367, *378*

Groves M, 124, *140*
Grubb BR, 120, 123, *137, 139*, 320,
  322, 323, *352, 353*, 373, *380*, 426,
  444
Gruenert DC, 100, *114*, 197, *213*, 322,
  352
Grunst T, 70, *91*, 96, *113*, 120, 122,
  131, *137, 139*, 262, *289*, 338, *362*,
  420, 425, *440*
Grzelczak Z, 366, *377*
Gu DL, 124, *140*
Gu J, 244, *271*, 458, *468*
Gu M, 263, *290*, 326, *355*
Gu MC, 425, *444*
Guedez L, 249, *278*
Guerin JC, 305, *317*
Guggino W, 7, *25*, 371, *380*, 412, *416*
Guggino WB, 70, *90*, 319, 320, 327,
  333, 334, 338, *349, 351, 356, 359,
  361*, 365, 366, 367, 368, 370, *377,
  378, 379, 380*, 412, 413, *416, 417*
Guiggio VM, 325, *354*
Guillaume C, 103, *115*, 399, *404*
Guillet JG, 39, 43, *47*, 461, *470*
Guinvarch A, 458, *467*
Guiterrez-Ramos J, 177, *187*
Guo X, 36, 37, *45*
Guo ZS, 247, *274*
Gupta JW, 250, *279*
Gupta P, 309, *318*
Gupta S, 428, *446*
Gurnani M, 245, *272*
Gurunathan S, 198, *214*
Guthrie T, 459, *469*
Gutin PH, 148, *163*
Guttridge DC, 245, *273*, 439, *454*
Gyorffy S, 175, *187*
Gyulai Z, 196, *211*

H

Haberman RP, 367, *378*
Habetz S, 183, *190*, 204, *215*
Hacien-Bey S, 12, *26*
Hack AA, 66, 69, *88, 89*

Hackett NR, 120, *138*, 333, *359*, 430,
  439, *448, 454*
Haczku A, 176, 177, *187*
Haddad IY, 425, *440*
Hadji DA, 122, 132, *138*
Hadley D, 149, *163*
Haecker SE, 39, 43, *47*
Haendle I, 246, *273*
Haenel T, 294, 306, *312, 317*
Hagen JA, 458, *467*
Hagiwara K, 158, *166*
Hagstrom JN, 110, *117*
Hahn DL, 205, *216*
Haisma HJ, 124, 127, 132, *140, 142,
  143*
Hajian G, 245, *272*
Haku T, 251, *280*
Halbert CL, 65, 69, 70, 73, 74, *87, 90*,
  110, *118*, 224, *230*, 328, 330, 333,
  334, 338, *356, 357, 359, 362*, 365,
  368, 369, 376, *377, 379, 381, 382*,
  423, 429, *442, 448*
Hall AR, 151, *164*, 243, *270*
Hall BM, 459, *469*
Hall CB, 346, *364*
Hall FL, 136, *144*
Hall S, 245, *272*
Hall SJ, 304, *316*
Hallek M, 54, *80*, 136, *144*
Hallenback PL, 147, *162*
Hallenbeck PL, 158, *166*
Halloran PF, 459, *469*
Hamelmann E, 177, *187*
Hamid Q, 177, *187*
Hamilton JM, 16, *27*
Hammon WM, 53, 60, *79*, 365, *377*
Hamper UM, 158, *166*
Han CI, 15, *26*
Han RNN, 435, *451*
Handa H, 62, *84*
Haney J, 234, 249, *266*
Hannam V, 101, 102, 103, 104, *114,
  115*, 427, *445*
Hannavy K, 320, *351*
Hann BC, 151, *164*

Hann N, 240, *268*
Hansen J, 57, 58, *82*, 328, 337, *356*, *360*, 375, *381*
Hanson RW, 10, *25*, 332, *358*
Hara N, 122, *139*
Hara S, 249, *277*
Harada JN, 243, *270*
Harada S, 225, 226, *230*, 436, *451*
Haralabopoulos GC, 257, *285*
Harari OA, 127, *141*
Harats D, 134, *143*
Hardwick N, 304, *316*
Hardy JD, 457, *467*
Hardy S, 326, *354*
Hargrove P, 65, *86*
Harlan JM, 196, *211*
Harland J, 149, *163*
Harmon KR, 460, *469*
Harmsen A, 196, *212*
Harmsen AG, 198, *214*
Harnett G, 306, *317*
Harris A, 324, *353*
Harris CE, 428, *446*
Harris DJ, 93, 95, 96, 100, 103, 105, *112*, *113*, *115*, 134, *143*, 333, 334, *359*, 360
Harrison L, 245, *272*, 294, *312*
Harrison LH, 305, *317*
Harris-Stansil T, 326, *354*
Harrod K, 333, *358*, 425, *440*
Harshaw DW, 126, *141*
Hart IR, 296, 304, *313*, *316*
Hart PJ, 70, *91*, 120, *137*, 327, *355*, 425, *443*
Hart SL, 104, *115*
Hartigan-O'Connor D, 254, *282*, 326, *354*
Hartikka J, 101, *114*
Harvey BG, 135, *144*, 262, *289*, 333, *359*, 430, *448*
Hasan MK, 345, *364*
Hase H, 252, *281*
Hasegawa M, 346, *364*
Hasegawa T, 296, *313*, 345, *364*
Hasegawa Y, 244, *271*, 296, *313*
Hashida M, 101, *114*

Hashio M, 157, *165*
Haskard DO, 127, *141*
Haskell A, 101, 102, 107, *114*, 429, *447*
Hasleton P, 235, *266*
Haslett C, 174, *186*
Hastings G, 258, *286*
Hattori N, 183, *190*, 200, *215*, 224, *230*, 436, *451*
Hauda KM, 15, *26*
Haura EB, 233, 249, *265*
Hauser MA, 76, *92*
Hauser P, 238, *267*
Hautala T, 122, *139*
Havell EA, 196, *212*
Hawkins L, 150, *164*
Hawkins RE, 127, 128, *142*, 337, *361*, 429, *447*
Hay C, 158, *166*
Hay JG, 13, *26*, 156, *165*, 320, *350*, *351*
Hayakawa T, 64, *86*, 256, *285*
Hayashi H, 256, *284*
Hayashi S, 222, 225, 226, *229*, *230*, 436, *451*, 459, *469*
Hayashi T, 198, *214*
Hayes TL, 125, *140*
Hayes VD, 427, *445*
Hayward GS, 67, *88*, 366, *377*
Hazama S, 249, *276*
He C, 244, *271*
He CY, 110, *118*, 326, *355*
He X, 438, *454*
He Y, 197, *213*
Hearing P, 40, *48*
Heath TD, 108, *117*, 263, *290*
Hecht SS, 238, *267*
Hedrick JA, 255, *282*
Heelan R, 246, *273*
Hehir K, 325, *354*
Hehir KM, 93, 99, *112*, 326, *354*, 425, *443*
Heike C, 151, *164*
Heike Y, 247, *275*
Heilbronn R, 59, 65, *82*, *86*
Heinter S, 156, *165*
Heinzel FP, 195, *210*

Heise C, 147, 150, 151, *162, 164, 165,* 243, *270*
Heitner S, 156, *165*
Heizoq RW, 6, *24*
Helenius A, 262, *289*
Hemmi S, 120, *138*
Henderson DR, 158, *166*
Henderson GA, 158, *166*
Henderson GS, 207, *218*
Henderson RA, 324, *353,* 422, *441*
Henegariu O, 320, *350*
Hengartner H, 247, 248, *275*
Hengstermann A, 151, *164,* 243, *270*
Henig NR, 376, *382*
Hennebel V, 429, *448*
Henry CJ, 60, *83*
Henry LJ, 129, *142*
Henry S, 459, *469*
Henson PM, 174, *186*
Herbst RS, 258, *286*
Herena J, 320, *351*
Hermiston T, 147, 150, *162, 164*
Hermonat PL, 52, 62, 67, *79, 85, 88*
Hernandez YJ, 66, *87,* 333, *359,* 413, *417*
Hernandez-Alcoceba R, 157, *165*
Hernan LJ, 432, *449*
Herrick SE, 104, *115*
Herrmann R, 242, *270,* 306, *317*
Herscovici J, 331, *358*
Herscowitz HB, 149, *163*
Hertz MI, 460, *469, 470*
Herve P, 437, *453,* 464, *472*
Herzog RW, 14, *26,* 110, *117*
Hewick RM, 195, *210*
Hewlett B, 177, 179, *188, 189,* 222, *229*
Hewlett BR, 436, *451*
Hicklin DJ, 258, *286*
Hicks G, 320, *350*
Hidaka C, 120, *138*
Hieshima K, 255, *283*
Hieter P, 36, *45*
Higenbottam T, 459, *469*
Higgins CF, 320, 321, *351,* 387, *394*
High KA, 6, *24,* 51, *78,* 110, *117*
Hilaris BS, 293, *312*

Hildinger M, 6, *24,* 66, 68, *87, 89*
Hill AV, 207, *217*
Hilleman MR, 32, *44*
Hillery E, 439, *454*
Hilliard J, 439, *454*
Hillinger S, 466, *473*
Himbeck R, 306, *317*
Hinton DR, 136, *144*
Hirai Y, 65, *86*
Hiraki A, 247, 253, *274, 281*
Hirano N, 157, *165*
Hirao M, 249, *277*
Hirata RK, 375, *381*
Hiratsuka M, 461, 463, 464, *470, 471, 472*
Hirohashi S, 240, *268*
Hirose S, 135, *144*
Hirrata T, 346, *364*
Hirsch-Lerner D, 99, *113*
Hirschl RB, 432, *449*
Hirsch R, 433, *450*
Hirsh AJ, 322, *352*
Hirth P, 403, *406*
Hitt MM, 177, 184, *188, 191,* 250, *279*
Hjerrild K, 249, *278*
Ho LP, 320, 321, *351*
Ho SB, 176, *187*
Hodge SE, 126, *141*
Hodgeman BA, 9, *25*
Hodson ME, 103, 104, 106, 111, *116,* 320, 321, *350, 351*
Hoekstra D, 100, *113*
Hoenes C, 320, 321, *351*
Hoffman EP, 51, 69, *78, 89*
Hoffman JW, 3, *24*
Hoffmann RM, 458, *468*
Hofland H, 331, *358*
Hofland HE, 102, *115*
Hofman C, 136, *144*
Hofman CR, 107, *117,* 400, *405*
Hogan SP, 177, *188*
Hoganson D, 240, 244, 245, 261, *269, 271, 289*
Hoganson DK, 120, 122, 124, *138, 140,* 294, *313,* 435, *451*
Hoganson S, 240, *269*

Hoggan MD, 53, 54, 65, *79*, *87*, 365, *377*, 411, *416*
Hogness DS, 19, *27*
Hohneker KW, 13, *26*, 38, *46*, 320, *350*, *351*, 373, *380*, 387, *395*, 427, *446*
Hoidal JR, 458, *468*
Holash J, 255, *283*
Holden EP, 432, *449*
Holgate ST, 181, *190*
Holland TC, 7, *25*
Hollenbaugh D, 346, *364*
Holm M, 384, *393*
Holmberg E, 429, *447*
Holmes KV, 343, *363*
Holmgren L, 255, 256, 257, *283*, *285*
Holscher C, 65, *86*
Holt PG, 251, *280*
Homer RJ, 172, 183, *185*, *190*, 220, *229*
Hong JS, 103, 104, 106, 111, *116*, 120, 122, *137*, 326, *355*, 425, 426, *440*, *445*
Hong KU, 320, *350*
Hong SS, 132, *143*
Hong TM, 257, *285*
Hong WK, 15, *26*, 151, *165*
Hoogeland S, 127, *142*
Hoogerbrugge P, 262, *289*
Hopkins C, 458, *468*
Hoque M, 60, *82*
Horbburgh B, 157, *165*
Horer M, 65, *86*
Horgan MJ, 458, *468*
Horita K, 244, *271*
Horn MV, 458, *467*
Horn S, 151, *164*
Horowitz AD, 420, 432, *441*
Horswood RL, 325, *354*
Horton MA, 176, *187*
Horvath J, 147, *162*
Horwitz MA, 207, *217*
Horwitz MS, 32, *44*, 120, 122, *137*, 326, *355*
Hosenpud JD, 457, *467*
Hosford D, 196, *211*

Hoshino H, 197, *213*
Hosoda Y, 135, *144*
Hotfidler M, 258, *286*
Houghton AN, 247, *275*
Houssin D, 296, *313*
Hovis JF, 32, *45*
Howard A, 207, *217*
Howard B, 174, 179, *185*, 201, *215*
Howard M, 100, 103, 105, *114*, 196, *212*
Howe JA, 150, 151, *164*
Howe TS, 425, *444*
Howorth SG, 126, 135, *141*
Hromas R, 255, *282*
Hruban RH, 235, *266*, 460, *469*
Hsieh CL, 158, *166*
Hsieh JT, 121, *138*
Hsu DH, 197, *212*
Hu J, 102, 104, *115*, 135, *144*, 435, *450*
Hu PC, 13, *26*, 320, *350*, 428, *446*
Huang AYC, 253, *281*
Huang J, 238, *267*, 366, *377*
Huang L, 93, 99, 100, 101, 102, 103, 104, 107, 108, 109, 110, *112*, *113*, *114*, *115*, *117*, 136, *144*, 320, 321, 322, 331, *351*, *352*, *358*, 384, *393*, 399, *405*, 422, 425, 426, 429, 439, *440*, *445*, *447*, 454, 461, *471*
Huang M, 247, 249, 250, *275*, *278*, *279*
Huang SK, 10, *25*, 174, *185*
Huang W, 197, *213*, 333, *360*
Huang XH, 466, *473*
Huard J, 7, *25*, 36, 37, *45*, 428, *447*
Hubbard RD, 207, *217*
Huber BE, 294, *312*
Hudak S, 255, *283*
Hue C, 12, *26*
Hue H, 367, *378*
Huebner RJ, 32, *44*, 146, *161*
Huehns TY, 127, *141*
Huffman JA, 176, *187*
Huffman Reed JA, 176, *187*
Huffnagle GB, 175, 182, *186*, *190*
Hughes BJ, 429, *447*
Hughes J, 301, *315*

Hughes JV, 66, *87*
Hughes WT, 198, *214*
Hughey R, 324, *353*, 422, *441*
Hugle-Dorr B, 54, *80*
Hui L, 120, *137*
Hulbert WC, 336, *360*
Huleihel M, 249, *276*
Hull WM, 39, 43, *47*, 176, *187*
Hunninghake GW, 178, *188*
Hunt BH, 249, *277*
Hunter DN, 459, *468*
Hunter L, 6, *24*
Hunter WD, 148, 149, *163*
Hurley CM, 320, *350*
Hurst HC, 134, *143*, 158, *167*
Husain AN, 460, *469*
Husband AJ, 175, *186*
Huser A, 136, *144*
Hussell T, 207, *218*
Husser RC, 420, 426, 431, 437, *441*,
    453
Hutchins B, 37, *46*
Hutchins GM, 184, *191*
Hutchinson G, 304, *316*
Huygen K, 207, *217*
Hwang HC, 245, *272*, 296, 297, *314*
Hwang S, 320, *350*
Hwang TH, 338, *361*, 367, *379*
Hwang Y, 198, *214*
Hyde SC, 320, 321, *351*, 387, 389, *394*,
    395

I

Iacomini J, 461, *470*
Ichioka M, 244, *271*
Idell S, 223, *229*
Igboaka G, 459, *469*
Iggo R, 158, *167*
Ihle J, 249, *278*
Iida A, 346, *364*
Ikawa S, 243, *270*
Ikeda E, 135, *144*
Ikegami M, 224, *230*, 420, 426, 431,
    441

Ikegaya K, 180, *189*
Ilson DH, 246, *273*
Im DS, 55, 62, *80*, *84*
Imai E, 180, *189*
Imai T, 255, *283*
Imai Y, 247, *274*
Imaizumi K, 244, *271*
Imaizumi T, 247, *274*
Imler JL, 43, *49*, 263, *290*, 326, *355*,
    429, 435, *448*, *451*
Imperiale MJ, 34, 35, *45*, 311, *318*
Imrie M, 320, 321, *351*
Imro MA, 247, *275*
Imundo L, 371, *380*
Inase N, 244, *271*
Ingram L, 308, *318*
Ingram LA, 107, 109, *117*
Inman MD, 177, *187*
Innes BA, 70, *90*
Innes JA, 320, 321, *351*
Inoue K, 260, *287*
Inoue N, 375, *381*
Irish P, 178, *188*
Ironside J, 151, *165*
Irvine KR, 198, *214*
Isaka Y, 180, *189*
Ischiropoulos H, 126, *141*
Ishai-Michaeli R, 256, *284*
Ishihara H, 251, *280*
Ishii I, 296, *313*
Ishizu K, 60, *82*
Isner JM, 16, 17, *27*
Isom OW, 333, *359*
Israel BF, 125, *140*
Itano H, 175, *186*, 437, *452*, 463, *472*
Itaya T, 247, 249, *275*, *277*
Itoh K, 247, *274*
Ittensohn M, 148, *163*
Iuliano S, 68, *89*, 366, *377*
Iuzzolino P, 303, *316*
Ivics Z, 110, *118*
Iwakawa S, 437, *453*
Iwaki Y, 61, 64, *84*
Iwamoto I, 180, *189*, 225, *230*
Iwamoto O, 247, *274*

Iyengar T, 245, *272*, 300, *315*
Iyer A, 157, *165*
Izsvak Z, 110, *118*

J

Jablons DM, 309, 310, *318*
Jacks T, 237, *267*
Jackson CK, 61, *83*
Jackson JC, 74, *92*, 426, 429, 432, *444*, 449
Jacob CO, 196, *211*
Jacobs F, 198, *214*
Jacobson M, 304, *316*
Jacoby D, 67, *88*
Jacquet C, 197, *212*
Jadeja L, 201, *215*
Jaenisch R, 238, *267*
Jaffe A, 13, *26*, 103, 104, 106, 111, *116*, 320, 321, *351*, 427, 439, *446*, 455
Jaffe E, 249, *276*
Jaffe HA, 38, *47*, 410, *415*, 426, *444*
Jaffee EM, 15, *26*, 253, *281*
Jager D, 247, *274*
Jager E, 247, 254, *274*, *282*
Jagneaux V, 320, *350*, 430, *448*
Jain RK, 256, 258, 261, *284*, *286*, *288*
Jaio S, 9, *25*
James KK, 223, *229*
Jamieson SW, 466, *473*
Janeway CA, 427, *445*
Jani A, 8, *25*, 36, 37, *45*, 428, *447*
Janssens SP, 402, *405*
Jantscheff P, 306, *317*
Jay FT, 59, *82*
Jefferson DM, 319, *349*
Jeffery PK, 103, 104, 106, 111, *116*, 178, *189*, 320, 321, 345, *350*, *351*, *364*
Jehan A, 305, *317*
Jenkins RG, 104, *115*
Jenks S, 251, *280*
Jensen G, 240, *268*
Jensen K, 207, *218*
Jensen-Pergakes K, 136, *144*

Jeppsson A, 463, 464, *472*
Jerome J, 429, *447*
Jerome V, 127, *142*
Jet J, 233, 234, 249, *265*
Jiang C, 93, 100, 103, 105, *112*, *115*, 205, *216*, 333, 334, *359*, *360*, 425, *443*
Jiang Q, 93, 99, *112*
Jiang Y, 245, *273*
Jiao S, 461, *471*
Jia SF, 175, *186*
Jia XC, 326, *354*
Jia Z, 158, *166*
Jicha DL, 249, *278*
Jie T, 346, *364*
Jimenez B, 258, *286*
Jobe AH, 224, *230*, 420, 426, 431, *441*
Joh K, 195, *210*
Johnson CL, 107, 109, *117*
Johnson DE, 150, 151, *164*
Johnson F, 6, 14, *24*, *26*
Johnson GR, 15, *26*
Johnson JG, 319, *349*
Johnson KJ, 432, *449*
Johnson LG, 13, *26*, 120, 123, *137*, *139*, 150, *164*, 239, *268*, 320, 322, 323, 327, 331, 333, 336, 338, 341, *351*, *352*, *353*, *355*, *358*, *360*, *362*, 366, 373, *377*, *380*, 391, 392, *395*, *396*, 423, 424, 426, 427, *442*, *444*, *446*
Johnson PR, 65, 67, 68, *86*, *88*
Johnson RP, 333, *358*, 425, *443*
Johnston J, 135, *144*
Johnston JC, 330, *357*
Johnston KM, 67, *88*
Johnston SA, 128, *142*
Jolicoeur FC, 197, *213*
Jolly DJ, 3, *24*, 123, *139*, 323, 330, 336, 341, 343, *353*, *357*, *360*, *363*, 420, 423, *441*
Jolly DL, 423, *442*
Jones D, 245, *273*
Jones KD, 258, *286*, 320, *351*, 373, *380*
Jones KR, 13, *26*, 320, *350*, 373, *380*
Jones L, 207, *218*

Jones LA, 65, 73, *87*, 333, 334, *359*, 370, *379*
Jones M, 401, *405*
Jones OW, 3, *24*
Jooss K, 40, *48*, 64, 66, *86*, *88*, 346, *364*, 425, *444*
Jordan JL, 181, *190*
Jordana M, 173, 174, 175, 177, *185*, *186*, *187*, *188*, 197, *212*, 433, 436, *450*, *451*, *452*
Jorgensen C, 197, *212*
Joseph B, 241, *269*
Joshi B, 366, *377*, 429, *447*
Joshi MS, 183, *190*, 202, *215*
Jovanovic DV, 197, *213*
Judd DV, 70, *90*, 308, *318*, 345, *364*, 385, *394*, 422, 425, 426, 427, *440*, *445*
Judy K, 249, *272*
Juers D, 196, *211*
Juillard V, 39, 43, *47*, *48*, 461, *470*
Jurim O, 197, *212*

K

Kadan MJ, 40, *48*
Kaetzel CS, 332, 335, *358*
Kafri T, 341, *363*
Kagawa S, 244, *271*
Kageshita T, 249, *277*
Kahlos K, 303, *315*
Kahn A, 461, *471*
Kahn ML, 251, *280*
Kaiser LR, 108, 111, *117*, 150, 156, *163*, *165*, 246, *273*, 293, 294, 296, 297, 300, 302, 303, 307, 308, *312*, *313*, *314*, *315*, *316*, *317*, *318*, 327, *355*
Kaji EH, 461, *470*
Kalachikov S, 126, *141*
Kalayoglue M, 458, *468*
Kaleko M, 40, *48*
Kaliberova L, 134, *143*
Kalla M, 55, *80*
Kallmeyer G, 320, 321, *351*
Kaludo N, 338, *362*

Kamath AT, 207, *217*
Kamb A, 235, *266*
Kameya T, 240, *268*
Kameyama T, 247, *274*
Kamholz SL, 458, *467*
Kamidono S, 158, *166*
Kan Y, 262, *289*
Kan YW, 119, 128, *137*, 337, *361*, 367, *378*
Kanaan SA, 463, 465, *472*, *473*
Kanaly S, 197, *213*
Kanda T, 337, *361*
Kaneda Y, 180, *189*, 222, 225, 226, *229*, *230*, 392, *395*
Kaner RJ, 120, *138*, 438, 439, *454*
Kaneshige T, 253, *281*
Kang AH, 178, *188*
Kang E, 243, *270*, 300, *315*
Kang W, 250, *279*
Kang WK, 251, *280*
Kao AW, 57, *82*
Kao C, 158, *166*, 238, *267*
Kapanci Y, 178, *188*, *189*
Kapikian AZ, 65, *87*, 207, *218*, 365, *377*, 411, *416*
Kaplan J, 308, *318*, 425, *443*
Kaplan JD, 459, *468*
Kaplan JM, 322, 326, 333, 346, *352*, *354*, *358*, *359*, *360*, *364*, 421, 422, 424, 426, 429, *441*, *445*, *448*
Kaplan L, 105, *115*
Kapler J, 249, *278*
Kaplitt MG, 68, 69, *89*, *90*
Kaplon RJ, 458, *468*
Karabin GD, 256, *284*
Karbach J, 247, 254, *274*, *282*
Karpati G, 428, *447*
Kasahara N, 119, 128, *137*, 148, *163*, 262, *289*, 337, *361*
Kasahara Y, 403, *406*
Kashentseva E, 120, 128, 129, 131, *137*, *142*, 337, *361*
Kashiwara M, 254, *282*
Kashiwazaki H, 158, *167*
Kasid A, 249, *276*
Kaslow R, 203, *215*

Kasono K, 120, *138*
Kaspar-Konig W, 458, *468*
Kass-Eisler A, 39, 43, *48*, 346, *364*
Katkin JP, 420, 426, 430, 431, 437,
 441, *448*, *453*
Kato A, 345, 346, *364*
Kato J, 256, *284*
Katsel PL, 94, *112*
Katz A, 249, *276*
Kaufman SA, 429, *447*
Kawabata K, 101, *114*
Kawabe T, 244, *271*, 296, *313*
Kawakami Y, 253, *281*
Kay MA, 6, 14, *24*, *26*, 36, *45*, *46*, 51,
 52, 61, 63, 64, 66, 69, 74, 75, *78*, *84*,
 85, *89*, 110, *118*, 147, *162*, 262, *289*,
 326, 346, *355*, *364*, 375, *381*, 409,
 415
Kaye SB, 151, *165*
Kazui T, 459, *469*
Keagy BA, 458, *468*
Keane MP, 256, 261, *284*, *288*
Kearney M, 16, *27*
Kearns WG, 61, 63, 64, 65, 66, *84*, *85*,
 87, 333, *359*, 368, *379*
Keck BM, 457, *467*
Keefer R, 321, *352*
Keenan RJ, 459, *468*
Keighern MA, 70, *90*
Keith RL, 235, *266*
Keller JR, 337, *361*
Kellermann SA, 255, *283*
Kelley C, 207, *217*
Kelley T, 338, *361*
Kelly BP, 207, *217*
Kelly D, 103, 104, 106, 111, *116*
Kelly FJ, 120, 123, *138*
Kelly J, 179, *189*
Kelly K, 460, *470*
Kelly MM, 336, *360*
Kelsen DP, 246, *273*
Kelso A, 15, *26*
Kemp BL, 15, *26*, 424, *442*
Kennedy MT, 99, *113*
Kennedy TP, 458, *468*

Kennel SJ, 429, *447*
Kennell S, 429, *447*
Kennell W, 205, *216*
Kenney SC, 125, *140*
Keogh CV, 197, *213*
Kerem B, 38, *46*, 366, *377*
Kerem BS, 386, *394*
Keriakian CB, 172, *184*
Kerkol T, 428, *446*
Kern A, 55, 60, 67, 68, *80*, *82*, *88*, 412,
 416
Kern DH, 151, *164*
Kern JA, 235, *266*
Kern S, 241, *269*
Kerr KM, 235, *266*
Keshavjee S, 57, 74, *81*, 330, 339, *357*,
 362, 376, *381*, 424, *443*, 463, 466,
 472, *473*
Keshavjee SH, 461, *471*
Kessler DA, 22, *27*
Kessler T, 259, *287*
Kesten S, 460, 466, *470*, *473*
Ketner G, 36, 37, *45*
Keyes LD, 320, 333, *350*, *358*, 425, *443*
Khalil N, 178, *189*
Khan TZ, 322, *352*
Khanna A, 198, *214*
Kharasch VS, 431, *449*
Khuntirat B, 57, 62, 72, *81*, *85*
Khuri FR, 151, *164*
Kibbelaar R, 235, *266*
Kicuchi T, 158, *166*
Kida H, 222, *229*
Kiefer M, 308, *318*
Kiertscher SM, 253, *281*
Kikuchi T, 202, *215*
Kim CH, 255, *282*
Kim F, 376, *381*
Kim HW, 207, *218*
Kim IH, 42, *49*
Kim JH, 156, *165*, 245, *272*
Kim KC, 324, *353*
Kim KS, 69, *90*
Kim M, 132, *143*, 243, *270*
Kim RW, 244, *271*

Kim SH, 238, 245, 260, *267, 272, 287*
Kim SJ, 69, *90*
Kimar CC, 259, *287*
Kindler V, 193, *208*
King G, 235, *266*, 399, *404*
King GA, 411, *416*, 439, *454, 455*
King I, 148, *163*
King JA, 55, 60, *80*
King TE, 178, *188*, 220, *229*
King VV, 370, *379, 380*
King-Biggs MB, 459, *469*
Kingston HD, 389, *395*
Kinnon C, 104, *115*
Kinnula K, 303, *315*
Kinnula VL, 303, *315*
Kinrade E, 100, *114*
Kinsella AR, 296, *313*
Kinzler K, 241, *269*
Kirchner KK, 322, *352*
Kirik D, 68, *89*
Kirillova I, 326, *355*
Kirioka T, 296, *313*
Kirk CJ, 254, *282*
Kirlappos H, 11, *25*, 391, *395*
Kirn D, 146, 150, 151, *161, 164, 165,*
    243, *270*
Kirn DH, 146, *162*, 243, *270*
Kirthivas A, 120, 122, *137*
Kiselyov K, 367, *379*
Kishimoto T, 225, 226, *230*
Kita Y, 459, *469*
Kitamura M, 326, *354*
Kitamura Y, 337, *361*
Kitson C, 70, *90*, 111, *118*, 345, *364,*
    385, *394*, 422, 425, 426, 427, *440,*
    445, 461, *470*
Kitten O, 337, *361*
Kiura K, 253, *281*
Kiyono H, 333, *358*
Klatzmann D, 296, *313*
Klebanoff SJ, 196, *211*
Kleckner AL, 69, *89*
Klein E, 245, *273*
Klein H, 12, *26*
Klein JS, 376, *382*

Klein TW, 196, *212*
Kleine LJ, 333, *358*
Kleinerman ES, 175, *186*
Kleinman HK, 257, *285*
Kleinschmidt J, 136, *144*
Kleinschmidt JA, 54, 55, 59, 60, 65, 67,
    68, *80, 82, 86, 88*, 338, *362*, 412, *416*
Klemsz M, 255, *282*
Klibanov A, 429, *447*
Kline JN, 323, *353*, 420, 423, *441*
Klinger KW, 319, *349*
Klink DT, 345, *364*
Klinman D, 427, *445*
Klump W, 369, 373, *379*
Kmiec EB, 414, *418*
Knechtle S, 8, *25*
Knechtle SJ, 458, 461, *468, 471*
Knight A, 124, *140*
Knowles JA, 126, *141*
Knowles MR, 13, *26*, 38, *46*, 320, *350,*
    351, 373, *380*, 386, 387, *394*
Knox L, 301, *315*
Knuth A, 254, *282*
Kobayashi A, 195, *210*
Kobayashi M, 195, *210*, 250, *279*
Kobinger GP, 4, *24*, 344, *363*
Kobzik L, 174, *185*, 235, *266*
Koch AE, 259, *287*
Koch PE, 120, 122, *138*
Kochanek S, 263, *290*, 326, 333, *355,*
    359, 411, *415*
Kochi A, 206, *216*
Kockanek S, 411, *416*
Koeberl DD, 110, *118*
Koehler DR, 102, 104, *115*
Koehler G, 175, *186*
Koeplin DS, 296, *313*
Koh DR, 240, *269*
Kohl NE, 243, *270*
Koivunen E, 129, *142*
Kojima H, 36, *45*
Koki AT, 253, *281*
Kokorina N, 52, *79*
Kokoris MS, 303, *315*
Kolansky DM, 13, *26*

Kolb M, 179, 180, *189*, 222, 226, *229*, 230
Kollef MH, 434, *450*
Kollen WJ, 322, 344, *352*, *363*, 392, 395
Koller BH, 240, *269*
Kolls JK, 182, 183, *190*, *191*, 194, 196, 201, 204, 206, *209*, *212*, *215*, *217*, 294, 304, 305, *312*, *316*, *317*, 433, 437, *449*, *453*
Koltover I, 94, 99, *112*, *113*
Komada F, 437, *453*
Komaki R, 15, *26*
Komatsu K, 459, *469*
Kong HL, 425, *444*
Konishi H, 459, *469*
Kontermann E, 127, *142*
Koo J, 324, *353*
Koomagi R, 257, 259, *285*, *286*
Koopmans SC, 411, *416*
Kopf M, 175, *186*
Kopolovitc Y, 134, *143*
Koretzky G, 427, *445*
Korfhagen TR, 172, *184*
Korn WM, 151, *164*
Kornberg A, 2, *23*
Kornbluth RS, 198, *214*
Korokhov N, 132, *143*
Korst RJ, 439, *454*
Kos FJ, 249, *278*
Kosai KI, 304, *316*
Koshikawa T, 241, *269*
Kotenko SV, 436, *452*
Kothakota S, 255, *282*
Kotin RM, 6, *24*, 55, 56, 60, 61, 62, 65, 80, *81*, *83*, *84*, *85*, *86*, 339, *362*, 376, *381*, 438, *454*
Kouyama K, 320, *351*, 371, *380*, 412, *417*
Kovesdi I, 120, 122, 125, 127, 129, 132, *137*, *138*, *140*, *141*, *142*, 158, *166*, 269, *291*, 325, 333, 337, 346, *354*, *359*, *361*, *364*
Koyama H, 64, *86*
Kozarsky KF, 5, 13, *24*, *26*, 39, *47*, 296, *314*, 325, *354*, 425, *443*

Kozelsky TW, 121, *138*
Kozin SV, 258, *286*
Koziol J, 305, *317*
Kozlosky CJ, 197, *213*
Kozower BD, 463, 465, *472*, *473*
Kraeger S, 433, 437, *450*
Krahenbuhl JL, 196, *212*
Krantz QT, 320, *350*
Krasnykh V, 120, 128, 129, 130, 131, 132, *137*, *138*, *142*, *143*, 150, *164*, 337, *361*
Krasnykh VN, 119, 128, *137*
Kratzke RA, 309, *318*
Krause DS, 320, *350*
Kreda S, 338, *362*
Kreda SM, 126, *140*, 338, *362*
Kren BT, 414, *418*
Krieg AM, 106, *115*, 427, *445*
Krithivas A, 326, *355*
Kropf DA, 120, *138*
Krougliak V, 5, *24*
Kubba S, 425, *444*
Kube DM, 57, 62, *81*, 371, *380*
Kucharczuk JC, 296, 297, *313*, *314*
Kufe DW, 158, *166*, 254, *282*
Kugler A, 246, *273*
Kuhn C, 172, *185*, 220, *229*
Kukowska-Latallo JF, 427, *445*
Kuliszewski MA, 398, *404*
Kulkarni AB, 207, *218*
Kuma H, 346, *364*
Kuman M, 183, *190*
Kumano K, 180, *189*, 225, *230*
Kumar R, 259, *286*, 384, *393*
Kumar V, 193, *209*
Kuniyasu H, 260, *288*
Kunkel HG, 198, *214*
Kunkel SL, 175, 178, 184, *186*, *188*, *191*, 195, 196, 197, *211*, *213*, 256, 259, 260, 261, *284*, *287*, *288*, 436, *452*
Kunzelmann K, 367, *379*
Kuo SH, 258, *286*
Kupiec-Weglinski JW, 459, *469*
Kuppuswamy M, 150, *164*
Kurachi K, 39, 43, *47*

Kurahashi K, 197, *213*, 436, *452*
Kurcharczuk JC, 150, *163*
Kurie JM, 234, 249, *266*
Kurihara T, 158, *166*
Kurioshi T, 241, *269*
Kurochkina LP, 127, *142*, 337, *361*
Kuroiwa A, 193, *209*
Kurt-Jones EA, 120, 122, *137*, 326, *355*
Kuzu I, 235, *266*
Kwiatkowski PA, 458, *468*
Kwon-Chung KJ, 195, *211*
Kwon HJ, 58, *82*
Kyasapura BL, 202, *215*, 436, *452*
Kylander JE, 330, *357*
Kyosito SR, 56, 60, *81*
Kyotani S, 403, *406*
Kyriazis AP, 240, *268*
Kyritsis AP, 150, *164*

L

La Face D, 437, *452*
La Monica N, 61, 65, 67, *84*
La R, 197, *213*
Laan M, 197, *213*
Labat-Moleur F, 384, *393*
Lachapelle A, 127, 135, *141*, *144*
Lachapelle AL, 68, *89*, 338, *362*, 425, *444*
Lachmann S, 148, *163*
Lackie PM, 181, *190*
Ladetto JV, 438, *454*
Ladner M, 424, *442*
Lagarde C, 64, 75, *85*, 375, *381*
Lahm H, 136, *144*
Lai WC, 193, *209*
Laichalk LL, 196, *211*
Laipis PJ, 64, *86*, 413, *417*
Lake R, 294, *312*
Lake RA, 306, *317*
Lam S, 234, 249, *266*
Lamartina S, 61, 65, 67, *83*, *84*, *86*
Lamb D, 235, *266*
Lambright ES, 108, 111, *117*, 150, 156, *163*, *165*, 243, *270*, 302, 307, *315*, *317*

Lampe MF, 205, *216*
Lamy D, 320, *350*
Lancaster HE, 438, *454*
Lancaster JR, 183, *190*, 202, *215*
Lancon A, 304, *316*
Landis SH, 233, 249, *265*
Landrum MJ, 413, *417*
Lane DJ, 320, 321, *351*
Lane HC, 203, *215*
Lane KB, 126, 135, *141*
Lane MB, 93, 100, 103, *112*, 334, *360*
Lane MD, 103, 106, *116*
Langer S, 36, 37, *45*
Langhorne J, 193, *209*
Langle-Rouault R, 391, *395*
Langston C, 39, 43, *47*, 333, *359*, 411, *415*, *416*, 420, 425, 426, 430, 431, *441*, *443*, *444*, *448*
Lankford EB, 69, *89*
Lantuejoul S, 243, *271*
Lanuti M, 108, 111, *117*, 156, *165*, 300, 301, 302, 307, *315*, *317*
Lapuz C, 103, *113*
Larocca D, 136, *144*
Larsimont D, 148, *163*
Larson KA, 176, *187*
Larson PJ, 6, *24*
Lasic DD, 10, *25*, 99, *113*, 429, *447*
Lasson PJ, 14, *26*
Latoche J, 324, *353*, 422, *441*
Latoche JD, 347, *364*, 426, *444*
Lattime EC, 146, *162*
Lauffenburger DA, 429, *447*
Laughlin CA, 6, *24*, 59, *82*
Launspach J, 123, *139*, 320, 321, 336, *351*, *360*, 421, 425, 427, 431, *441*, *446*
Laurent GJ, 104, *115*, 178, *189*
Laurent JC, 305, *317*
Laurino L, 303, *316*
Lausier J, 384, *393*
Lawlor PA, 69, *90*
Lawrence DD, 15, *26*, 242, *269*, 424, *442*
Layani MP, 320, *350*
Lazarowski ER, 126, *140*, 338, *362*

Lazenby AJ, 15, *26*, 249, *276*
Le Boulaire C, 264, *290*
LeClair C, 5, *24*
Le Deist FL, 12, *26*
Le Gal FA, 264, *290*
Le Gall C, 107, *117*
Le Gros G, 249, *278*
Leach CL, 74, *91*, 432, *449*
Leahy KM, 253, *281*
Leapman SB, 256, *284*
Leclerc T, 103, *115*
Lecocq JP, 410, *415*
Leder P, 249, 260, *276*, *287*
Lederberg J, 1, 2, *23*
Ledley FD, 331, *358*
Lee CS, 238, *267*
Lee CT, 252, *280*
Lee CY, 427, *445*
Lee DC, 100, *113*, 197, *213*
Lee DS, 247, 248, *275*
Lee ER, 93, 95, 96, 100, 103, 105, *112*,
    113, *115*, 333, 334, *359*, *360*, 384,
    393
Lee FS, 41, *48*
Lee GM, 125, 127, 129, *140*, *141*, *142*,
    337, *361*
Lee HC, 69, *90*
Lee JG, 120, 122, *137*
Lee JH, 123, *139*, 425, 430, 431, *444*,
    448, *449*, 459, *468*
Lee JJ, 15, *26*, 176, *187*
Lee JS, 234, 249, *266*
Lee KC, 148, *163*
Lee KH, 459, *468*
Lee MG, 367, *379*
Lee NA, 176, *187*
Lee PJ, 437, *453*
Lee PS, 150, *164*, 250, *279*, 341, 342,
    363, 424, *442*
Lee PW, 146, 147, 150, *161*, *162*,
    163
Lee R, 429, *447*, 461, 463, 464, *471*,
    472
Lee TC, 461, *471*
Lee WM, 251, *280*
Lee YL, 102, *115*

Lee YS, 346, *364*
Lefebvre M, 304, *316*
Lefer AM, 458, *468*
Lefer DJ, 458, *468*
Leff T, 61, *83*
Legendre JY, 331, *358*
Legler DF, 255, *283*
Legrand V, 122, 132, *138*
LeGuern C, 461, *470*
Lehmann JR, 333, *360*
Lehmann M, 422, *441*
Lehn JM, 103, *115*
Lehn P, 103, *115*
Lehr J, 431, *449*
Lehrman S, 263, *290*
Leibovich SJ, 256, *284*
Lei D, 183, *190*, *191*, 194, 198, 201,
    202, 204, *209*, *213*, *215*, 245, *272*,
    304, *316*, 422, *441*
Lei XF, 174, 177, *185*, *187*, *188*
Leiden JM, 39, 43, *47*, 440, *455*, 461,
    470
Leiferman KM, 15, *26*
Leigh MW, 13, *26*, 320, 330, 333, *350*,
    351, *357*, *360*, 373, *380*
Leikauf GD, 176, *187*
Leike K, 136, *144*
Leinonen M, 205, *216*
Leinwand LA, 39, 43, *48*, 346, *364*
Leissner P, 122, 132, *138*
Leitman S, 194, *209*
Leiva LE, 198, *214*
Lejarreta M, 411, *416*
Leland F, 409, *415*
Lelkes PI, 257, *285*
Lemarchand P, 401, *405*, 437, *453*, 464,
    472
Lemione NR, 147, *162*
Lemkine GF, 94, *112*
Lemoine NR, 134, *143*, 158, *167*
Leng EC, 100, *113*
Leonard P, 101, 102, *114*, 429, *447*
Leone P, 68, 69, *89*, *90*
Leong C, 294, *312*
Leong CC, 305, 307, *317*
Leong KW, 392, *395*

Leopold PL, 120, 135, *138*, *144*, 323, *353*, 420, 425, 430, 439, *441*, *448*, *454*
Lepore JJ, 440, *455*
Lespagnard L, 148, *163*
Lethe B, 246, 247, *274*
Letterio JJ, 179, *189*
Leung BP, 193, *209*
Levame M, 175, *186*, 438, *454*
Levanon K, 134, *143*
Leventis R, 384, *393*
Lever AM, 424, *442*
Levin VA, 150, *164*
Levine AJ, 238, *268*
Levine AM, 433, *450*
Levine AS, 311, *318*
Levine SM, 460, *469*
Levitsky HI, 15, *26*, 253, *281*
Levitt HJ, 158, *166*
Levkovitz H, 134, *143*
Levrero M, 38, *46*
Levrey H, 320, *350*
Levy LB, 245, *272*
Levy S, 177, *188*
Lewensohn R, 241, *269*
Lewis C, 457, *467*
Lewiston NJ, 370, *379*
Li C, 424, *443*
Li Chen XH, 304, *316*
Li CL, 15, *26*, 193, *209*
Li D, 103, 104, 106, 111, *116*, 320, 321, *351*
Li E, 122, 132, *138*
Li H, 131, *142*, 259, *287*, 302, *315*
Li HO, 346, *364*
Li J, 52, 55, 57, 67, 68, 69, 74, 75, *78*, *81*, *89*, 244, *271*
Li M, 367, *379*
Li Q, 39, *47*, 57, *82*, 252, 262, *280*, *289*, 333, *359*, 409, *415*
Li S, 101, 102, 104, 107, 108, 109, 110, *114*, *115*, *117*, 136, *144*, 158, *166*, 399, *405*, 426, *445*, 461, *471*
Li XK, 459, *469*
Li Y, 120, 121, 122, 129, *137*, *138*, *142*, 337, *361*

Li Z, 107, 108, *117*, 148, *163*, 207, *217*, 400, *405*, 426, *445*
Liang H, 177, *188*
Liang X, 11, *25*, 101, *114*
Liao F, 259, *287*
Liao Q, 458, *468*
Libby DM, 194, *210*
Libermann TA, 41, *48*, 263, *290*
Lieber A, 326, *355*
Liggitt D, 123, *139*
Liggitt HD, 74, *92*, 102, 103, 108, 110, *115*, *116*, *117*, 194, 195, *210*, 263, *290*, 399, *404*, *405*, 425, 426, 427, 429, 430, 433, *444*, *446*, *449*, *450*
Lim HY, 158, *166*
Lima O, 461, *470*
Lima VM, 207, *217*
Limper AH, 178, *189*, 224, *230*
Lin AJ, 94, *112*
Lin CM, 259, *287*
Lin J, 158, *166*, 326, *355*, 425, *444*
Lin SL, 148, *163*
Lin Y, 238, 253, *267*, *281*
Linden A, 197, *213*
Linden RM, 54, 56, 59, 60, 61, 65, *79*, *81*, *83*, *84*, *87*, 411, *416*
Lindenmeyer F, 259, *287*
Lindholm L, 132, *143*
Ling YH, 111, *118*
Linnainmaa K, 303, *315*
Linnoila R, 238, *268*
Linsely P, 346, *364*
Linzonova A, 129, *142*
Lipari P, 245, *272*
Lipner EM, 151, *164*
Lipps BV, 54, *79*
Lis D, 102, 104, *115*
Lisby DA, 74, *91*, 433, *449*
Littlewood JM, 320, 321, *351*
Litzinger DC, 429, *447*
Litzky LA, 150, *163*, 245, *272*, 294, 296, 297, 300, 301, *312*, *314*, *315*, 326, *354*
Liu C, 333, *358*
Liu D, 102, 103, 109, 110, *115*, *117*, 262, *289*

Liu F, 102, 103, 104, 107, 108, *115, 117,* 400, *405,* 426, *445*
Liu H, 260, *287*
Liu J, 435, *451*
Liu JJ, 102, *115*
Liu L, 9, *25*
Liu M, 461, 463, 466, *471, 472, 473*
Liu N, 258, *286*
Liu R, 245, *273*
Liu SL, 414, *418*
Liu T, 409, *415*
Liu TJ, 409, *415*
Liu W, 258, *286*
Liu XL, 67, 68, *88*
Liu YJ, 67, *88,* 255, *283,* 424, *443*
Lizonova A, 120, 122, 127, *137, 141,* 337, *361*
Llamas-Saiz AL, 54, *80*
Lleonart M, 156, *165*
Lo SK, 439, *455*
Lochmuller H, 36, 37, *45,* 428, *447*
Lockey RF, 183, *190*
Locksley RM, 205, *216*
Lodish HF, 225, *230*
Lodish S, 439, *454*
Loeb LA, 303, *315*
Loeffert EJ, 110, *117,* 426, *445*
Loetscher M, 255, *283*
Loetscher P, 255, *283*
Logan JJ, 100, 103, 105, *114*
Logan M, 101, 102, *114*
Logg A, 148, *163*
Logg CR, 148, *163*
Loh S, 252, *281,* 305, *317*
Lohmann-Metthes ML, 195, *210*
Loiler S, 66, *87,* 333, *359,* 413, *417*
Loisel S, 107, 109, *117,* 399, *404*
Lok S, 366, *377*
London WT, 207, *218*
Long SD, 105, *115,* 426, *445*
Longenecker G, 38, *47*
Longo DL, 203, *215*
Lonnemann G, 436, *452*
Look DC, 333, *358,* 425, *440*
Lorence RM, 148, *162*
Loskutoff DJ, 223, *229*

Losordo DW, 17, *27*
Lotvall J, 177, *187,* 197, *213*
Lotze MT, 194, *209,* 249, 253, *277, 278, 282*
Louis B, 42, *49*
Loulmet DF, 458, *467*
Louzier V, 403, *406,* 438, *454*
Love RB, 458, *468*
Low KB, 148, *163*
Lowe S, 158, *166*
Lowenthal A, 2, *23*
Lowrie DB, 207, *217,* 307, *317*
Lowry OH, 461, *470*
Lowry SF, 194, 197, *209, 213*
Lozonschi L, 251, *280*
Lu S, 60, *83*
Lu W, 249, *277*
Lu X, 207, *218*
Lu Z, 135, *144,* 255, *283,* 435, *451*
Ludewig B, 247, 248, *275*
Ludkovski O, 100, *113*
Ludwig SL, 32, *45*
Luedke C, 194, *209*
Luedke GH, 244, *271*
Lui MA, 207, *217*
Luistro L, 250, *279*
Lukacs KV, 206, *217,* 307, 308, *317, 318*
Lukacs NW, 175, 177, 184, *186, 188, 191,* 195, *211,* 436, *452*
Lukason M, 123, *139*
Lukason MJ, 103, 106, *115, 116,* 320, 336, *350, 360,* 421, 425, 429, 430, 433, *441, 448, 450*
Lunardi-Iskandar Y, 399, *404*
Lundholm-Beauchamp U, 325, *354*
Luo J, 238, 253, *267, 281*
Luo X, 148, *163*
Luo Y, 255, *283*
Lupien PJ, 13, *26*
Lupton S, 249, *278*
Lurquin C, 246, 247, *274*
Lusby E, 55, *81*
Luster AD, 251, 259, 260, *280, 287, 288*
Lutz KL, 335, *360*

Luykx-de Bakker SA, 124, *140*
Lympany PA, 178, *189*
Lynch C, 367, 369, 373, *378*, *379*
Lynch CM, 424, *443*
Lynch JP, 256, *284*, 460, *469*
Lyrene RK, 103, 104, 106, 111, *116*

M

Maat C, 197, *213*
Mabbs R, 149, *163*
Macdonald I, 68, *89*
Macdonald M, 207, *217*
MacDonald RC, 99, *113*
MacDougall RH, 151, *165*
Macduff BM, 198, *214*
Machado RD, 126, 135, *141*
Machemer T, 151, *164*
Macher AM, 203, *215*
MacIntyre N, 434, *450*
Mack CA, 333, *359*
Mackall CL, 249, *278*
Macke M, 343, *363*
Mackman N, 223, *229*
MacLean A, 149, *163*
MacLean AR, 150, *163*
MacVinish LJ, 320, 321, *351*
Madrenas J, 459, *469*
Madrid L, 245, *273*
Magdaleno S, 239, *268*
Magee DM, 205, *216*
Magliocco AM, 302, *315*
Magnuson M, 399, *404*
Magnusson MK, 132, *143*
Magosin S, 54, 65, *79*, 333, *360*
Magovern CJ, 333, *359*
Maguire AM, 65, 73, *87*
Mah C, 57, 58, 62, 72, *81*, *82*, *85*, 328, *356*, 375, *381*
Mahan LC, 101, 102, *114*
Mahato RI, 101, 102, *114*, 429, *447*
Mahfouz I, 131, *143*
Mahvi DM, 251, *280*
Maino V, 254, *282*
Maisonpierre PC, 255, *283*
Maisto L, 308, *318*

Mak TW, 240, *269*
Makeh I, 38, *47*
Makela PH, 205, *216*
Malanga CJ, 175, *186*
Malcus C, 320, *350*, 430, *448*
Malerba M, 158, *167*
Malik AB, 458, *468*
Malipiero U, 466, *473*
Malkinson AM, 236, 237, *267*
Malkowski M, 259, *287*
Mall M, 367, *379*
Malone RW, 8, *25*
Manchester JK, 461, *470*
Mandel M, 54, 63, *79*
Mandel RJ, 68, *89*, 329, 330, 341, *357*
Mandelboim O, 247, *274*
Mandeli J, 259, *286*
Mane M, 52, *79*
Maneval D, 151, *164*
Manley S, 320, *351*, 371, *380*
Manly S, 412, *417*
Manning JK, 240, *268*
Manning L, 306, *317*
Manning LS, 305, *317*
Manno CS, 6, 14, *24*, *26*, 69, *89*
Manor O, 16, *27*
Man SF, 336, *360*
Mantell LL, 437, *453*
Manthorpe M, 94, 101, *112*, *114*
Mantovani A, 249, *276*
Mao JT, 247, *275*
Mao L, 234, 235, 249, *266*
Mao MW, 245, *273*
Mao Q, 131, *143*
Maordomo JI, 253, *282*
Maragoudakis ME, 257, *285*
Marchant A, 196, 197, *212*, *213*
Marchetti A, 235, *266*
Marchevsky A, 460, *469*
Marchisio C, 244, *271*
Marchisio PC, 244, *271*
Marconi P, 7, *25*
Margetts PJ, 179, 180, *189*, 222, 226, *229*, *230*
Margitich D, 148, *163*
Marguilies S, 99, *113*

Marino CR, 320, *350*
Markakis D, 327, *356*, 366, *378*
Markert JM, 149, *163*
Marks RM, 256, *284*
Marley J, 294, *312*
Marley JV, 305, *317*
Maron DJ, 249, *277*
Marrack P, 249, *278*
Marriott C, 111, *118*, 322, *352*
Marrogi A, 304, *316*
Marrogi AJ, 294, 305, *312*, *317*
Marr RA, 177, 179, *188*, *189*, 222, *229*, 436, *451*
Marsh J, 6, *24*
Marsh JA, 366, *377*
Marshall BC, 178, *188*
Marshall DJ, 440, *455*
Marshall FF, 15, *26*
Marshall J, 93, 94, 95, 96, 98, 100, 101, 103, 105, 106, 110, *112*, *113*, *114*, *115*, 148, *162*, 304, 308, *316*, *318*, 320, 321, 333, 334, 346, *351*, *359*, *360*, *364*, 384, *393*, 426, 427, *445*
Martel-Pelletier J, 197, *213*
Martich GD, 459, *468*
Martin FD, 15, *26*
Martin FJ, 10, *25*
Martin L, 246, *273*
Martin TR, 195, *210*
Martinet O, 259, *286*
Martinez C, 156, *165*
Martinez J, 322, *352*
Martini N, 293, *312*
Martuza RL, 146, 148, 149, 157, *161*, *163*, *165*, 249, *277*
Maruyama K, 429, *447*
Marvin SA, 319, *349*, 366, *377*
Masaki I, 345, *364*
Masferrer JL, 253, *281*
Mason CM, 196, *212*
Mason E, 412, *416*, 437, *453*
Mason SJ, 338, *361*
Masroor S, 458, *468*
Massacrier C, 198, *214*
Masse C, 438, *453*

Mastrangeli A, 13, *26*, 146, *162*, 249, *276*, 320, 333, *350*, *359*, 401, *405*
Mastruzzo C, 177, *188*
Masur H, 203, *215*
Matalon S, 100, 103, 105, *114*, 425, *440*
Mathias P, 122, *139*, 262, *289*, 326, *355*
Matson S, 427, *445*
Matsubara S, 134, *143*, 158, *166*
Matsui H, 70, *91*, 120, *137*, 240, 245, 249, *269*, *276*, 322, 327, *352*, *355*, 391, *395*, 425, 427, *443*, *446*
Matsumoto A, 60, *82*, 101, *114*
Matsumoto K, 249, *277*
Matsumoto N, 225, 226, *230*
Matsumoto O, 101, *114*
Matsumura A, 461, *470*
Matsumura R, 180, *189*, 225, *230*
Matsumura T, 257, *285*
Matsuoka H, 222, 226, *229*, *230*
Matsuse H, 183, *190*
Matsushita T, 52, 68, *78*
Mattern J, 257, 259, *285*, *286*
Matthaei KI, 175, 177, *186*, *187*, *188*
Matthay MA, 437, 438, *453*, *454*
Matthews T, 294, *313*
Mattila K, 205, *216*
Mattson K, 303, *315*
Matzinger P, 106, *117*
Mavier IM, 175, *186*
Mayo M, 245, *273*
Mayo MS, 120, 123, *137*
Mayordomo JI, 247, 253, *274*, *282*
Mayor HD, 53, 54, 63, *79*
Maysky M, 17, *27*
Mazmanian M, 464, *472*
Mazzolini G, 251, *280*
McAnulty RJ, 104, *115*, 178, *189*
McArthur JG, 66, *87*
McBride W, 245, 249, 253, *272*, *276*, *281*
McBride WH, 247, 249, *275*, *278*
McCabe C, 60, *83*
McCann JD, 319, *349*
McCarthy AM, 7, *25*, 437, *452*
McCarthy KE, 305, *317*

McCarthy TJ, 175, *186*, 465, *473*

McCarty D, 68, 70, 72, 74, *88*, *91*, 120, *137*, 327, 333, *355*, *360*, 425, *443*

McCarty DM, 55, 60, 61, *80*, *83*

McCarty JM, 172, *184*

McClarrion M, 102, 110, *115*, 429, *448*

McCleland ML, 110, *117*

McClelland A, 6, 14, *24*, *26*, 40, *48*

McCormack PM, 293, *312*

McCormick F, 147, 151, *162*, *164*, 243, 270, 309, *318*

McCown TJ, 367, *378*

McCoy KS, 38, *46*, 429, *448*

McCoy RD, 175, *186*, 224, *230*, 263, *290*

McCray PB, 52, 57, 70, 71, 73, *78*, 123, *139*, 323, 324, 330, 336, 341, 342, 343, 344, *353*, *357*, *360*, *363*, 375, *381*, 420, 423, 424, 425, 426, *441*, *442*, *443*, *444*, *445*

McCullough B, 338, *362*

McDevitt HO, 196, *211*

McDonald DM, 101, 102, 107, *114*

McDonald GA, 129, *142*

McDonald JA, 178, *189*, 224, *230*

McDonald R, 369, *379*

McDonald RJ, 103, *116*, 429, *448*

McDonald TD, 126, 127, *141*

McDonald WF, 62, *84*

McDonnell TJ, 15, *26*, 150, *164*, 310, *318*

McDougall JC, 460, *469*

McElkvaney N, 263, *290*, 320, *350*, *351*

McElkvaney NG, 13, *26*, 38, *46*, 387, *394*

McEvoy LM, 255, *283*

McFadden G, 199, *214*

McGarry MP, 176, *187*

McGhee JR, 103, 104, 106, 111, *116*, 333, *358*

McGill G, 241, *269*

McGillicuddy DC, 196, *211*

McGrath JP, 68, *88*

McGrath SA, 327, *356*, 365, 368, *377*, 413, *417*

McGregor CG, 463, 464, *472*

McGuire SE, 121, *138*

McIlwrath A, 245, *273*

McKenzie FN, 458, *468*

McKie E, 149, *163*

McKinley DR, 39, *47*

McKinney TG, 250, *279*

McLachlan G, 100, 102, 103, 105, *114*, 320, 321, *351*, 387, *394*

McLaughlin SK, 67, *88*

McLean JW, 101, 102, 107, *114*, 429, *447*

McMahan L, 7, *25*

McNeilly D, 98, 110, *113*, 427, *445*

McShane H, 207, *217*

McVeigh U, 70, *90*, 368, *379*

McVey DL, 346, *364*

Meaney C, 101, 102, *114*, 429, *447*

Mechtler K, 11, *25*

Medock MD, 149, *163*

Medrano FJ, 65, *87*

Meegalla RL, 71, *91*

Meehan KR, 149, *163*

Meeker DP, 103, 104, 106, 111, *116*, 320, 321, *351*, 387, *394*, 427, 429, *446*, *448*

Meerzaman D, 324, *353*

Mehrad B, 183, *190*, 200, *215*, 436, *451*

Mehrotra PT, 249, *278*

Mehta JG, 336, *360*

Mehtali M, 39, 43, *48*, 122, 132, *138*, 306, *317*

Meko J, 250, *279*

Melani C, 249, *276*

Melcher A, 304, *316*

Melcher AA, 304, *316*

Melchert P, 70, *91*, 330, *357*, 423, *442*

Mello C, 440, *455*

Melnick JL, 54, 63, 65, *79*

Melton SM, 432, *449*

Memento M, 158, *166*

Menard O, 305, *317*

Mendell J, 69, *89*

Mendez M, 426, 430, 432, *444*

Meneses P, 56, 60, *81*

Meng QH, 104, *115*

Menkis AH, 458, *468*

Menninger JC, 61, *84*
Menon M, 156, *165*
Mercer K, 239, *268*
Mercola KE, 2, *23*
Merkow LP, 60, *83*
Meropol NJ, 148, *162*
Merryweather J, 194, *209*
Mesnil M, 296, 304, *313*, *316*
Mesri M, 244, *271*
Messina M, 398, *404*
Messner AH, 64, 76, *86*, 92, 320, 339, *351*, *362*, 370, 371, *380*, 412, *416*, *417*
Mesyanzhinov VV, 127, *142*, 337, *361*
Meuse L, 110, *118*
Mew DJ, 311, *318*
Mewshaw JP, 331, 341, *358*, 424, *442*
Meyers BF, 459, *469*
Meyers C, 52, *79*
Meylan PR, 198, *214*
Meyn RE, 245, *272*
Meyrick BO, 399, *404*, 411, *416*, 439, *455*
Mezzacasa A, 120, *138*
Mi Lee G, 122, 132, *138*
Miao CH, 64, *86*, 375, *381*
Michael JG, 240, *268*
Michael SI, 123, *139*, 269, *291*, 337, *361*
Michel-Calemard L, 320, *350*, 430, *448*
Michaelis U, 320, 321, *351*
Michiel D, 337, *361*
Michler RE, 458, *468*
Michou AI, 39, 43, *48*
Middleton PG, 320, 321, *350*, *351*, 387, *394*, 395
Midoux P, 344, *363*, 428, *446*
Midthun PE, 460, *469*
Mignot P, 305, *317*
Migueres J, 305, *317*
Mihaud B, 103, *113*
Mikhak B, 252, *281*
Mikheeva G, 120, 129, 131, 132, *137*, *142*, *143*, 337, *361*
Mikos AG, 94, *112*
Milan S, 177, *187*

Milano E, 120, *138*
Miletich DJ, 126, 127, *141*
Miller AD, 3, 12, *24*, *26*, 38, *46*, 61, 65, 69, 70, 72, 74, *83*, 87, *90*, *91*, 110, *118*, 197, *213*, 224, *230*, 328, 329, 330, 333, 334, *356*, *357*, *359*, 368, 369, 376, *379*, *381*, *382*, 423, 429, *442*, *448*
Miller AR, 249, *278*
Miller CR, 120, 123, 124, 129, 131, 132, *137*, *138*, *139*, *142*, *143*, 337, *361*
Miller DG, 330, *357*
Miller DW, 127, *142*, 429, *447*
Miller LF, 32, *44*
Miller N, 262, *290*
Miller PW, 233, 238, 245, 249, *265*, *267*
Miller VM, 463, 464, *472*
Miller YE, 235, *266*
Milliken CE, 17, *27*
Milsark IW, 194, *209*
Mineta T, 148, *163*
Minna JD, 150, *163*, 258, *286*
Minson AC, 198, *214*
Minter RM, 437, *452*
Miozzo M, 234, 249, *266*
Mireles V, 239, *268*
Mishra L, 59, *82*
Misko IS, 15, *26*
Mitani K, 263, *290*, 326, *355*
Mitchell RH, 207, *218*
Mitlianga P, 150, *164*
Mitsudomi T, 235, *266*
Mittereder N, 333, *359*
Miyake H, 249, *277*
Miyake S, 244, *271*
Miyatake S, 157, *165*
Miyazaki Y, 178, *189*
Miyazono K, 180, *189*, 225, *230*
Mizuguchi H, 36, *45*, *46*
Mizuguchi Y, 193, *209*
Mizukami H, 57, *82*
Mizuno M, 249, *277*
Modesti A, 244, *271*
Mofford KA, 320, 321, *351*, 387, *394*

Mohanakumar T, 175, *186*, 437, *452*, 460, 463, 464, 465, *469*, *470*, *471*, *472*, *473*
Mohapatra SS, 183, *190*
Mohr L, 127, *141*
Molema G, 100, *113*
Molina PL, 376, *382*
Molinier-Frenkel V, 264, *290*
Mollenkopf FP, 458, *467*
Molnar-Kimber KL, 150, *163*, 245, 261, *272*, *289*, 297, 298, 300, 301, 303, *314*, *315*, *316*
Molto L, 251, *280*
Momand J, 238, *268*
Monahan PE, 461, *471*
Mona M, 151, *164*
Monciotti A, 61, 65, 67, *84*
Monck M, 100, *113*
Monesano R, 256, *284*
Moninger T, 54, *80*, 332, *358*, 427, *446*
Moninger TO, 96, *113*, 123, *139*, 338, *362*, 430, 431, *449*
Monnet I, 305, *317*
Monsigny M, 344, *363*, 428, *446*
Montefusco C, 458, *467*
Montgomery A, 257, *285*
Montgomery DL, 207, *217*
Montgomery GL, 320, *350*
Montier T, 103, *115*
Monzo M, 244, *271*
Moolten FL, 296, *313*, *314*
Moore A, 435, *451*
Moore GW, 184, *191*
Moore KJ, 126, *141*
Moore KL, 366, *377*
Moore KW, 196, *212*
Moore MA, 202, *215*, 432, *449*
Moore TA, 183, *190*, 196, *211*
Mora BN, 175, *186*, 461, 463, 464, 465, *470*, *471*, *472*, *473*
Moralee S, 320, 321, *351*
Morales MM, 367, *378*
Moran ML, 76, *92*, 320, 339, *351*, *362*, 370, 371, *379*, *380*, 412, *416*, *417*
Moran P, 337, *361*

Mordenti J, 101, 102, *114*
Morel Y, 320, *350*
Morell NW, 126, 135, *141*
Morey S, 294, 306, *312*, *317*
Morgan CJ, 459, *468*
Morgan M, 413, *417*
Morgan RA, 12, *26*
Mori M, 222, 226, *229*, *230*
Morling FJ, 123, *139*, 337, 338, *361*
Moro E, 384, *393*
Morral N, 39, 40, 42, 43, *47*, *48*, *49*, 333, *359*, 411, *415*, *416*, 425, *443*, *444*
Morris JC, 156, *165*, 245, *272*, 302, *315*
Morris JE, 103, 104, 106, 111, *116*, 320, 321, *351*
Morris KG, 126, *141*
Morris R, 466, *473*
Morris S, 207, *217*, 261, *288*
Morris SL, 207, *217*
Morse HC, 207, *218*
Morse JH, 126, *141*
Morse KM, 343, *363*
Morse MA, 238, *267*
Morsy MA, 263, *290*, 326, *355*, 425, *444*
Moscicki RA, 320, *351*
Moser B, 259, *287*
Moser KM, 223, *229*
Moses MA, 258, *286*
Moskalenko M, 54, 65, 66, *80*
Mosmann TR, 196, *212*
Moss B, 147, *162*
Moss DJ, 15, *26*
Moss RB, 320, 339, *351*, *362*, 370, 371, 373, *379*, *380*, *381*, 412, *416*, *417*
Mosselmans R, 257, *285*
Motulsky AG, 145, *161*
Motzel S, 263, *290*, 326, *355*, 425, *444*
Mountz JD, 421, *441*
Mroz PJ, 296, *313*
Muallem D, 367, *379*
Muallem S, 367, *379*
Mueller GM, 341, *363*, 423, *442*
Muhle C, 124, *140*

Mukherjee S, 252, *281*, 306, *317*
Mukherjee SA, 294, *312*
Mukhopadhyay T, 15, *26*, 241, 243, 269, *270*, 424, *442*
Mularo F, 439, *454*
Mulbacher A, 249, *278*
Mulberg AE, 322, *352*, 392, *395*
Mule JJ, 249, 254, *276*, *278*, *282*
Mullen CA, 12, *26*, 244, *271*
Mullen JB, 461, *471*
Muller DW, 13, *26*, 250, *279*
Muller R, 127, *142*
Mulligan R, 3, *24*, 176, *187*, 329, 330, 341, *357*
Mulligan RC, 15, *26*, 341, *363*, 461, *470*
Munk ME, 182, *190*
Munkonge F, 387, *395*
Munoz A, 203, *215*
Munshi NC, 60, *83*
Munson K, 367, 369, 373, *378*, *379*
Munson KL, 424, *443*
Munz PL, 36, 37, *45*
Muraishi A, 392, *395*
Murali R, 33, *45*
Muramatsu T, 134, *143*
Murata M, 247, *275*
Murdin AD, 206, *216*
Murphy BR, 207, *218*
Murphy JW, 205, *216*
Murphy PM, 199, *214*
Murray DR, 147, *162*, 194, *210*
Murray HW, 103, 106, *115*, *116*, 194, *209*
Murray T, 233, 234, 249, *265*
Muruve DA, 41, *48*, 263, *290*
Musatov SA, 64, 75, *85*
Musk AW, 294, 305, 306, *312*, *317*
Muslow HA, 302, *315*
Mutlu G, 426, 430, 432, *444*
Muul L, 12, *26*
Muul LM, 194, *209*
Muzcyzka N, 6, *24*, 54, 55, 59, 60, 62, 67, 77, *79*, *80*, *83*, *84*, *88*, *92*, 365, 366, *377*, 412, 413, *416*, *417*

Muzykantov VR, 126, *141*
Myers MW, 59, 60, *82*

N

Nabel EG, 249, *277*, 401, *405*
Nabel GJ, 16, 18, *27*, 249, *277*, 401, *405*
Nabioullin R, 251, *280*
Nafziger D, 156, *165*
Nagahiro I, 461, 464, *471*, *472*
Nagai H, 249, *277*
Nagai Y, 345, 346, *364*
Nagao Y, 247, *274*
Nagaraju K, 51, *78*
Nagaya N, 403, *406*
Nagira M, 255, *283*
Nagy D, 102, *115*, 329, 330, 341, *357*
Nahm MH, 198, *214*
Nair SK, 253, *282*
Nairn R, 35, *45*
Nakai H, 52, 61, 63, 64, 74, 75, *78*, *84*, *85*, 375, *381*
Nakakes A, 307, *317*
Nakanishi-Matsui M, 251, *280*
Nakanishi Y, 122, *139*, 258, *286*
Nakao A, 180, *189*, 225, *230*
Nakao M, 247, *274*
Nakayama D, 341, *363*, 423, *442*
Nakazaki Y, 250, 252, *280*, *281*
Nakazato H, 249, *276*
Naldini L, 3, 7, *24*, *25*, 51, 66, *78*, 147, *162*, 262, *289*, 329, 330, 331, 341, *357*, *358*
Namen AW, 249, *278*
Nanney L, 260, *288*
Nanni P, 244, 249, *271*, *275*
Narita M, 461, *470*
Narumi K, 158, *166*
Narvaiza I, 251, *280*
Nash AA, 193, *209*
Nastala CL, 250, *279*
Nathan CF, 193, 194, *208*, *209*
Nathans D, 19, *27*
Natsume A, 249, *277*

Nau MM, 235, *266*
Naujoks K, 320, 321, *351*
Naume B, 250, *279*
Naundorf S, 384, *393*
Naviaux RK, 305, *317*
Negrini M, 235, *266*
Neigh GS, 177, *188*
Nelson AL, 324, *353*
Nelson D, 252, *281*
Nelson JA, 296, *313*
Nelson S, 183, *190*, *191*, 194, 196, 197, 202, 206, *209*, *212*, *213*, *215*, *217*, 422, *441*
Nelson WG, 15, *26*, 158, *166*
Nemerow GR, 122, *138*, *139*, 262, *289*, 326, *355*
Nemunaitis J, 151, *164*, 242, 243, *269*, *270*
Nepomuceno IB, 76, *92*, 339, *362*, 370, *379*, 412, *417*
Neri M, 308, *318*
Nesbitt JC, 15, *26*
Nestle F, 253, *281*
Nettesheim P, 324, *353*
Nettlebeck DM, 127, *142*, 429, *447*
Neugebauer SE, 150, *164*
Neugeboren BA, 341, *363*
Neumann K, 240, *268*
Neutzel S, 320, *350*
Neuzil KM, 207, *218*
Nevins JR, 150, *164*
Newcomb TG, 303, *315*
Newman PJ, 257, *285*
Newman W, 146, *161*
Newstead MW, 196, 202, *211*, *215*, 436, *452*
Ng L, 151, *164*
Nguyen CM, 100, *113*
Nguyen D, 15, *26*, 242, *269*, 424, *442*
Nguyen DM, 247, *274*
Nguyen H, 103, *113*
Nguyen HT, 102, 110, *115*
Nguyen N, 158, *166*
Ni H, 331, 341, *358*, 424, *442*
Ni TH, 62, *84*

Nichols MR, 93, 100, 101, 103, *112*, *114*, 334, *360*
Nicklee T, 258, *286*
Nicklin SA, 128, 134, *142*, *143*, *144*
Nickoloff BJ, 252, 254, 256, *280*, *282*, *284*
Nicoletti G, 244, *271*
Nicoll J, 149, *163*
Nicolo G, 308, *318*
Niedbala W, 193, *209*
Nielsen L, 245, *272*
Nieminen MS, 205, *216*
Nienhuis AW, 65, *86*, 341, *363*
Nieroda CA, 16, *27*
Nietupski JB, 93, 95, 96, 99, 100, 101, 103, 107, 109, *112*, *113*, *114*, *117*, 334, *360*, 461, *471*
Nijitsu Y, 158, *166*
Nijman HW, 242, *269*
Nikaido Y, 193, *209*
Nilius B, 367, *379*
Nishida Y, 256, *285*
Nishiguchi K, 437, *453*
Nishino K, 222, *229*
Nishioka T, 101, *114*
Nishioka Y, 249, *277*
Nishio M, 241, *269*
Nishizaki M, 242, 245, *269*, *272*
Niven RW, 433, *449*
Noah TL, 13, *26*, 320, 322, *350*, *351*, 352, 373, *380*
Noble NA, 178, 180, *188*, *189*
Nochumson S, 105, *115*
Nocken F, 337, *361*
Noelle RJ, 333, *360*, 422, *441*
Noguchi M, 157, *165*
Noguchi PD, 22, *27*
Noma T, 249, *276*
Nong Z, 402, *405*
Noone PG, 320, *351*, 373, *380*, 387, *395*, 427, *446*
Norbash AM, 320, 339, *351*, *362*, 370, 371, *379*, *380*, 412, *417*
Norberg JE, 235, *266*
Nordstrom JL, 105, *115*, 426, *445*

Norman J, 101, 102, 104, *114*, *115*
Norman KL, 146, *161*
Normolle DP, 252, *280*
Norrby E, 32, *45*
Norris J, 158, *166*
Norton J, 250, *279*
Nosakowski J, 343, *363*
Noteboom JL, 297, *314*
Novelli M, 239, *268*
Novick RJ, 457, 458, 459, *467*, *468*
Nowak-Gottl U, 258, *286*
Nu PC, 373, *380*
Nukiwa T, 158, *166*
Nunes FA, 5, *24*, 39, 41, *47*, *48*, 326, *354*
Nusbaum P, 12, *26*
Nussbaum E, 305, *317*
Nye JA, 151, *164*

O

Oakley RE, 308, *318*
Obo H, 461, *470*
O'Brien JM, 14, *26*, 464, *472*
O'Brien T, 463, *472*
Obrocka M, 320, *350*
O'Brodovich H, 101, 102, 103, *114*, 461, *471*
O'Carroll SJ, 151, *164*, 243, *270*
Ochoa L, 458, *467*
Ochsenbein AF, 247, 248, *275*
O'Connell BC, 438, *454*
O'Connor E, 68, *89*
O'Connor RN, 178, *189*
O'Connor W, 259, *287*
Odaka M, 249, *277*, 303, 308, *316*, *318*
Odom G, 183, *190*
O'Donovan DJ, 437, *453*
Oesch F, 254, *282*
Offringa R, 242, *269*
O'Garra A, 196, 207, *212*, *218*
Ogata K, 260, *288*
Ogata M, 255, *282*
Ogston P, 77, *92*
Oh J, 158, *166*
Ohara M, 197, *213*, 436, *452*

Ohba M, 459, *469*
Ohira T, 247, *275*
Ohishi N, 36, *45*
Ohkawara Y, 173, 175, 176, 177, *185*, *186*, *187*, *188*, 197, *212*, 436, *452*
Ohori NP, 460, *469*
Ohri E, 243, *270*
Ohta Y, 257, *285*
Oka H, 327, *356*, 365, 368, *377*, 413, *417*
Oka K, 42, *49*
Okegawa T, 121, *138*
Okuda A, 101, *114*
Okumura K, 437, *453*
Okunaka T, 249, *277*
Old L, 246, *273*
Oldfield EH, 296, *313*
Oldham ER, 255, *283*
Olek K, 101, 102, 103, *114*
Olie RA, 244, *271*
Oliff A, 243, *270*
Olman MA, 223, *229*
Olsen JC, 13, *26*, 120, 122, *138*, 240, 244, 261, *269*, *271*, 289, 294, *313*, 319, 320, 330, 331, 338, 341, 343, 346, *349*, *350*, *357*, *358*, *362*, *363*, 366, 373, *377*, *380*, 392, *396*, 423, 424, *442*
Olson N, 54, *80*
Olthoff KM, 197, *212*
O'Malley BW, 109, *117*
Omori F, 64, *86*
O'Neal W, 39, 42, 43, *47*, *49*, 425, *443*
O'Neal WK, 40, *48*, 333, *359*
O'Neill MA, 425, *444*
Ono T, 249, *277*
Ooserom R, 306, *317*
Openshaw PJ, 207, *218*
Opolon P, 425, *444*
Orci L, 256, *284*
Ordway DJ, 207, *217*
O'Reilly EM, 246, *273*
O'Reilly MS, 255, 256, 257, 258, *283*, *285*, *286*
Oreve S, 55, *81*

O'Riordan CR, 68, *89*, 126, 127, 128, 135, *140, 141, 144*, 338, *361, 362*, 425, *444*
Orkin SH, 145, *161*
Ornelles DA, 156, *165*
Orosz CG, 459, *469*
O'Rourke MG, 15, *26*
Orte C, 126, 135, *141*
Ortega MA, 258, *286*
Ory D, 3, *24*, 329, 330, 341, *357*
Ory DS, 341, *363*
Osakada M, 157, *165*
Osaki T, 222, *229*, 244, *271*
Osburn WO, 98, 110, *113*, 461, *471*
Oshikawa K, 251, *280*
Oskam R, 306, *317*
Ostapchuk P, 40, *48*
Ostrand-Rosenberg S, 278, 249
O'Sullivan C, 333, *359*
Otake K, 333, *358*, 425, *440*
Otsuki T, 135, *144*
Ottenhoff TH, 207, *217*
Otterbein LE, 437, *453*
Otulana B, 459, *469*
Oudrhiri N, 103, *115*
Ouyang L, 341, *363*
Overholser JP, 258, *286*
Overturf K, 134, *143*
Overwijk WW, 247, 248, *275*
Owens AH, 15, *26*
Owens RA, 56, 60, 61, 64, 65, *81, 84, 86*, 327, *356*, 366, *378*, 424, *443*
Owusu I, 193, *209*
Oyer PE, 466, *473*
Oz HS, 198, *214*
Ozaki I, 414, *418*
Ozols R, 243, *270*

P

Paakko PK, 366, *377*, 410, *415*
Pacilio C, 460, *470*
Packman CH, 296, *313*
Paczan PR, 432, *449*
Padmabandu G, 103, *115*
Padmanabhan R, 326, *355*

Pahud DR, 197, *212*, 436, *452*
Paielli DL, 156, *165*
Paillard F, 338, *361*
Paillard JC, 305, *317*
Pakes SP, 193, *209*
Pal PG, 207, *217*
Palasis M, 440, *455*
Palmer GA, 146, *162*
Palmer K, 174, 175, 177, *185, 187*
Palombo F, 61, 65, 67, *84*
Palumbo P, 55, *80*
Panelouris EM, 240, *268*
Pang MC, 413, *417*
Panis Y, 296, *313*
Papagianis D, 205, *216*
Papahadjopoulos D, 10, *25*
Papaioannou SP, 257, *285*
Papanastassious V, 149, *163*
Papo MC, 432, *449*
Paradis IL, 459, 460, *469, 470*
Paradis TJ, 260, *288*
Paradiso AM, 338, *361*
Parashar B, 414, *418*
Pardo A, 178, *188*, 220, *229*
Pardo M, 60, *83*
Pardo OE, 308, *318*
Pardoll DM, 15, *26*, 246, 247, 253, *274, 275, 281*
Parham GP, 62, *85*
Park C, 250, 251, *279, 280*
Park HS, 239, *268*
Park MS, 158, *166*
Parker RE, 400, *405*, 439, *455*
Parker SE, 102, 104, *115*
Parkes V, 135, *144*, 338, *362*, 425, *444*
Parkins DA, 111, *118*
Parks RJ, 42, *49*, 61, 65, 67, *84*, 326, 333, *354, 355, 359*, 411, *415, 416*, 425, *444*
Parks WP, 54, 65, *79*
Parmiani G, 249, *276*
Parr M, 135, *144*
Parry CM, 198, *214*
Parry G, 15, *26*
Parsons D, 322, *352*

Parsons DW, 123, *139*, 323, *353*, 426, *444*
Parsons PG, 15, *26*
Partovian C, 175, *186*, 403, *406*
Pascual DW, 333, *358*
Pasqualini R, 128, 129, *142*
Pass HI, 311, *318*
Pastan I, 11, *25*, 303, *316*, 326, *355*
Pastore JN, 427, *445*
Pastore L, 42, *49*
Pastorino U, 234, 249, *266*
Pataer A, 310, *318*
Patapoff T, 101, 102, *114*
Patrone L, 247, *275*
Pattengale P, 249, *276*
Patterson GA, 175, *186*, 458, 459, 460, 461, 463, 465, *467*, *468*, *469*, *470*, *471*, *472*, *473*
Patton JH, 432, *449*
Paubert-Braquet M, 196, *211*
Pauciulo MW, 126, *141*
Paul S, 319, *349*
Paulauskis JD, 174, *185*
Paulin C, 320, *350*
Paulin D, 247, 248, *275*
Paull DE, 458, *468*
Pauls K, 126, *141*
Pavirani A, 39, 43, *47*, *48*, 122, 132, *138*, 320, 326, *350*, *355*, 410, *415*, 425, *444*, 461, *470*
Pavlakis GN, 99, *113*, 429, *447*
Pawelek J, 148, *163*
Peabody J, 156, *165*
Pearlman R, 101, 102, 107, 110, *114*, *115*, 320, *351*, 429, *447*
Pearson AS, 120, 122, *138*
Pechacek TF, 234, 249, *265*
Pechan PA, 67, *88*
Peck K, 257, *285*
Peckinpaugh RO, 54, 65, *79*
Pecora AL, 148, *162*
Peeira GMB, 249, *278*
Peeples ME, 148, *162*, 343, *363*
Pegg J, 156, *165*
Pei XH, 122, *139*

Pellegrini C, 463, 464, *472*
Pellegrini S, 235, *266*
Peng B, 101, 102, *114*
Peng S, 100, 103, 105, *114*
Pennington L, 458, *468*
Pennington SE, 326, 333, 346, *354*, *358*, *364*, 425, *443*
Pentenazzo A, 384, *393*
Pentice HG, 68, *89*
Penttila T, 205, *216*
Pepper MS, 256, *284*
Perales JC, 10, *25*, 332, *358*, 439, *454*
Pereboev A, 131, *143*
Pereboeva L, 131, *143*
Pereira DJ, 55, *80*
Peretti SW, 322, *352*
Perez A, 371, *380*
Perez-Cruet MJ, 296, *314*
Perez-Diez A, 251, *280*
Perez-Soler R, 111, *118*
Perlman S, 343, *363*
Pernis B, 325, *354*
Peronne C, 197, *212*
Perraud F, 320, *350*, 428, 429, *446*, *447*
Perricaudet M, 38, *46*, *47*, 131, *143*, 325, *354*, 410, *415*, 425, *443*
Perricone MA, 103, 104, 106, 111, *116*, 320, 321, 322, *351*, *352*, 387, 389, *395*, 426, 427, *445*, *446*
Perrin S, 200, *215*
Perrotte P, 260, *287*
Perry ST, 150, *164*
Perry-Lalley D, 247, *275*
Pertl U, 251, *280*
Perussia B, 250, *279*
Pesce AJ, 240, *268*
Peschon JJ, 197, *213*
Pessin JE, 57, *82*
Pestka S, 436, *452*
Peter I, 120, *138*
Peters GE, 120, *137*, *138*
Peters J, 320, *350*
Peters SG, 460, *469*
Petersen DM, 320, *350*
Petersen G, 54, *80*

Peterson D, 254, *282*, 461, *471*
Peterson EM, 195, *210*
Peterson PA, 326, 333, *354, 358*
Petrak K, 103, *115*
Petrak KL, 105, *115*
Petrella JM, 70, *91*, 120, 125, *137*, 324, *353*, 425, *440*
Pettaway C, 249, *277*
Pettenazzo A, 345, *364*
Petty R, 149, *163*
Petzelbauer P, 257, *285*
Peuchmaur M, 103, *115*
Pezzella F, 235, *266*
Pfaffenenbach D, 256, *284*
Phair J, 203, *215*
Phan SH, 178, *188*
Phelan DL, 460, *469*
Phelps SF, 76, *92*
Philip M, 102, *115*
Philip R, 102, *115*, 436, *452*
Philipson L, 120, 122, *137*
Phillips HS, 147, *162*
Phillips J, 103, 104, 106, 111, *116*, 320, 321, *351*, 427, *446*
Phillips JA, 126, *141*
Phillips MI, 64, *86*
Phillips P, 306, *317*
Phipps ML, 326, *354*
Phupakdi W, 156, *165*
Pian M, 427, *446*
Piantadosi S, 15, *26*, 293, *312*
Picarella DE, 172, 176, *184, 187*
Picat-Joossen D, 305, *317*
Piccione D, 240, *269*
Piche A, 125, *140*
Picher M, 322, *352*
Picker L, 254, *282*
Pickles R, 120, *137*, 240, *269*, 333, 343, *360, 363*
Pickles RJ, 70, *91*, 120, 122, 125, 126, *137, 138, 140*, 320, 324, 326, 338, *352, 353, 355, 362*, 373, *380*, 425, *440, 443*
Pidwell DJ, 459, *469*
Pieczek A, 16, *27*

Piedimonte G, 333, *360*
Piedrafita D, 193, *209*
Pier GB, 367, *378*
Pier MV, 376, *382*
Pierce BK, 300, *315*
Pierce GF, 124, 125, *140*, 435, *451*
Pierce WE, 32, *44*, 54, 65, *79*
Pieroni L, 61, 65, 67, *84*
Pierre A, 461, *471*
Pierre L, 458, *468*
Pierrot D, 326, *355*, 435, *451*
Pierson RN, 458, *468*
Pietenpol J, 241, *269*
Piguet PF, 178, *188, 189*, 193, *208*
Pihalja M, 157, *165*
Piillai R, 103, *115*
Pike J, 148, *163*
Pike SE, 258, *286*
Pike-Cavalcoli M, 7, *25*
Pilewski J, 297, *314*
Pilewski JM, 324, 327, 341, 347, *353, 355, 363, 364*, 423, 426, *442, 444*
Pinedo HM, 124, 127, 132, *140, 142, 143*
Piquet PF, 196, *211*
Piraino ST, 55, 67, *81*
Pisters KM, 15, *26*
Pitard B, 331, *358*
Pitcher C, 254, *282*
Pitossi F, 179, *189*, 222, *229*
Pitt BR, 104, 107, 109, 110, *115, 117*, 136, *144*, 341, 347, *363, 364*, 423, *442*
Pizer L, 62, *85*
Pizzorno G, 158, *166*
Platt JL, 458, *468*
Platzer E, 194, *209*
Plavsic N, 366, *377*
Plent MM, 3, *24*
Plewe M, 101, *114*
Plitman JD, 411, *416*, 439, *454*
Plotz P, 51, *78*
Pluda JM, 255, 256, *283*
Plumb J, 135, *144*, 435, *451*
Podrazik RM, 398, *404*

Podsakoff G, 61, 64, *84*
Poellinger KA, 332, *358*, 427, *446*
Pohl MS, 458, 459, *467*, *469*
Poirier A, 66, 70, *87*, *91*, 323, 333, *353*, *359*, 412, 413, *416*, *417*, 421, 424, *441*
Poitevin F, 320, *350*, 430, *448*
Pokorny W, 409, *415*
Pokreisz P, 402, *405*
Polak JM, 126, 135, *141*
Polakowski I, 256, *284*
Polverini PJ, 259, 260, 261, *287*, *288*
Pomerantz R, 414, *418*
Pompetti F, 311, *318*
Ponder KP, 409, *415*
Pong RC, 121, *138*
Ponnazhagan S, 57, 61, 62, 65, *81*, *84*
Pope HA, 319, *349*, 366, *377*, 386, 387, *394*
Pope IM, 296, *313*
Popescu NC, 64, *86*
Poplonski L, 247, *275*
Porgador A, 249, *276*
Porteous DJ, 100, 102, 103, 105, *114*, 320, 321, *351*, 366, *378*
Porter CD, 308, *318*
Porteus DJ, 387, *394*
Post M, 101, 102, 103, 104, *114*, *115*, 427, *445*
Poston GJ, 296, *313*
Potter M, 412, *416*
Potter TA, 108, *117*, 263, *290*
Poulard K, 336, *360*, 375, *381*
Povlsen CO, 239, 240, *268*
Powell S, 66, *87*
Pozharshi EV, 99, *113*
Prasad B, 172, *184*
Prasad G, 176, *187*
Prasad KM, 55, 60, *80*
Prawling J, 247, *275*
Prayssac P, 437, *453*
Prendergrast TJ, 194, *209*
Prevec L, 37, *46*, 147, *162*
Price JE, 260, *288*
Prince A, 371, *380*
Prince GA, 325, 326, *354*

Printz MA, 124, *140*
Prockop DJ, 320, *350*
Procopio A, 310, 311, *318*
Propert KJ, 54, 65, *79*, 156, *165*, 333, *360*
Prussin C, 198, *214*
Przybylska M, 106, 109, 110, *115*, *117*, 426, 427, *445*
Puchelle E, 326, *355*
Puddicombe SM, 181, *190*
Puente XS, 122, *138*
Puga AP, 70, *91*, 120, 123, *137*, *139*, 320, 327, *350*, *355*
Puliti M, 194, *210*
Punt CJ, 306, *317*
Purkerson JM, 198, *214*
Putnam JB, 15, *26*
Puurula V, 205, *216*
Pyles G, 207, *218*

Q

Qi H, 102, 103, *115*
Qian Q, 260, *288*
Qian R, 5, *24*, 54, 65, *79*, 333, *360*, 429, *447*
Qian Y, 54, 65, *79*, 333, *360*
Qiang D, 157, *165*
Qin L, 175, *186*, 197, *212*, 262, *289*, 421, 425, 436, *440*, *441*, *452*, 464, 465, *472*, *473*
Qing K, 57, 58, 62, 72, *81*, *82*, *85*, 328, 337, *356*, *360*, 375, *381*
Qiu J, 57, *82*
Qu G, 67, 68, *88*, *89*, 366, *377*
Qu X, 56, *81*
Quan ZM, 201, *215*
Quiao HJ, 303, *315*
Quinn PM, 250, *279*
Quinn TJ, 389, *395*
Quinones J, 411, *415*, 425, *444*
Quintana A, 427, *445*
Quintanilla M, 156, *165*
Quinton PM, 367, *378*
Quiquerez AL, 306, *317*

Quirk JG, 62, *85*
Quiroz D, 330, *357*

R

Raabe O, 369, *379*
Raabe OG, 102, 110, *115*, 429, *448*
Raben D, 120, 123, *137*
Rabinovich P, 101, 102, *114*
Rabinowitz JE, 54, *80*, 328, *356*, 424, *443*
Rabkin SD, 148, 149, 157, *163*, *165*, 249, *277*
Rabreau M, 51, *78*
Raczka E, 427, *445*
Rader DJ, 13, *26*
Radler JO, 99, *113*
Raffer PW, 95, 96, *113*
Raffestin B, 175, *186*, 403, *406*, 438, *454*
Raghow R, 178, *188*
Raghuram V, 322, *352*
Ragni MV, 6, 14, *24*, *26*, 69, *89*
Rahemtulla A, 240, *269*
Rahman A, 422, *442*
Raivio KO, 303, *315*
Raj K, 77, *92*
Rakhmanova VA, 99, *113*
Rakmilevich AL, 251, *280*
Ralston R, 151, *164*
Ram Z, 296, *313*
Ramachandra M, 151, *164*, 422, *442*
Ramagopal M, 376, *382*
Ramakrishna N, 158, *166*
Ramakrishnan R, 7, *25*
Ramalingam R, 120, *138*
Ramesh R, 262, *289*, 294, 304, *312*, *316*
Rampling R, 149, *163*
Ramsay AJ, 177, *188*, 436, *452*
Ramsey BW, 320, *351*, 373, *381*, 429, *448*
Ramsey WJ, 12, *26*, 156, *165*, 175, *186*, 302, *315*
Ramshaw I, 294, *312*

Ranapathi M, 245, *273*
Rancourt C, 125, 129, *140*, *142*
Randazzo B, 150, *163*
Randell SH, 70, *91*, 120, *137*, 320, 322, 324, 327, *350*, *352*, *353*, *355*, 391, *395*, 425, 427, *443*, *446*
Randlev B, 151, *165*
Rankin JA, 172, 176, *184*, *187*
Ranshaw IA, 175, *186*, 306, *317*
Rao NV, 458, *468*
Rao SP, 198, *214*
Raper SE, 5, 13, *24*, *26*, 39, 41, *47*, *48*, 297, *314*
Rasmussen UB, 428, *446*
Ratcliff R, 320, 321, *351*
Ratcliff RA, 425, *443*
Ratner AJ, 371, *380*
Ratnoff OD, 10, *25*
Rauch CT, 197, *213*
Rautonen N, 205, *216*
Ravetch JV, 260, *288*
Raviglione MC, 206, *216*
Ray JM, 69, *89*, 257, *285*
Ray M, 239, *268*
Ray P, 172, *185*, 220, *229*
Rayman P, 251, *280*
Read ML, 100, *113*
Recchia A, 61, 65, 67, *84*
Recio A, 300, 301, *315*
Rectenwald JE, 437, *452*
Reddy P, 197, *213*
Reddy RC, 202, *215*, 436, *452*
Reddy S, 240, *269*
Redman BD, 252, *280*
Reed JA, 433, *450*
Reed JC, 244, *271*
Reed ND, 240, *268*
Rees DD, 322, *352*, 421, 424, *441*
Rehg JE, 198, *214*
Reichard KW, 148, *162*
Reichenspurner H, 466, *473*
Relvink PW, 127, *141*
Remick D, 436, *452*
Remington JS, 194, *209*
Remold HG, 194, *209*

Remy JS, 392, *395*
Ren DR, 247, *275*
Ren J, 56, *81*
Rendahl KG, 424, *442*
Rengaraju M, 250, *279*
Repetto G, 9, *25*
Rerko RM, 195, *210*
Restifo NP, 253, *281*
Reynolds HY, 193, *208*
Reynolds PN, 120, 123, 124, 126, 130,
    131, 134, *137, 138, 139, 140, 143,
    144,* 150, *164,* 402, *405,* 429, *447*
Reynolds SD, 320, *350*
Reynolds T, 7, *25,* 58, 76, *82, 92,* 320,
    351, 369, 370, 373, *379, 380, 381,*
    412, *416, 417*
Reynolds TC, 333, 334, *359,* 368, 370,
    379, 424, *442*
Reznikoff CA, 238, *267*
Rhoades ER, 195, *211*
Rhys CM, 366, *377*
Ribas A, 253, *281*
Rice K, 42, *49*
Rice WR, 176, *187*
Richards CA, 294, *312*
Richards CD, 174, 175, *185, 186,* 436,
    452
Richards SM, 320, *351*
Richardson G, 458, *467*
Richardson WD, 6, *24*
Rich DP, 319, 325, *349, 354,* 387, *394*
Rich SS, 304, *316*
Riches DW, 322, *352*
Richter CA, 131, *142*
Ridge K, 426, *444*
Riedemann N, 367, *379*
Ried M, 54, *80,* 136, *144*
Ries SJ, 151, *164*
Riese RJ, 183, *190*
Rijswijik A, 124, *140*
Rimoldi R, 308, *318*
Rinaldo C, 203, *215*
Rinaudo D, 61, 65, *84, 86*
Ring CJ, 134, *143*
Ringhoffer M, 254, *282*
Ringold GM, 9, *25*

Riordan JR, 366, *377,* 386, *394*
Risau W, 256, *283, 284*
Ritchie T, 64, 75, *85,* 375, *381*
Ritter JH, 175, *186,* 437, *452,* 460, 465,
    469, 472
Ritter JK, 464, 465, *472*
Ritter JM, 465, *473*
Rittner K, 67, 68, *88,* 412, *416*
Ritz SA, 177, *188*
Rivadeneira ED, 64, *86*
Rivera VM, 109, *117*
Rizk NP, 150, *163*
Rizvi N, 148, *162*
Rizzo MA, 399, *405*
Rizzo P, 311, *318*
Rizzuto G, 60, 61, *83*
Robaye B, 257, *285*
Robbins PD, 249, 250, *277, 279,* 341,
    363, 423, *442*
Roberts AB, 179, *189*
Roberts AD, 195, 207, *211, 217*
Roberts B, 304, *316*
Roberts DD, 99, *113,* 429, *447*
Roberts HR, 424, *442*
Roberts JR, 297, *314*
Robin R, 19, *27*
Robinson BW, 294, 305, 306, *312, 317*
Robinson BWS, 305, 307, *317*
Robinson CB, 38, *46,* 429, 438, *448,*
    453
Robson ND, 197, *212,* 436, *452*
Rocco JW, 150, *164*
Roche AC, 102, 110, *115,* 344, *363*
Roche E, 103, *113*
Roche L, 102, 110, *115*
Rochlitz C, 306, *317*
Roder C, 246, *273*
Rodillon L, 320, *350*
Rodman DM, 401, *405,* 429, 436, *447,*
    451
Rodolfo M, 249, *276*
Rodriguez FH, 197, 206, *213, 217*
Rodriguez R, 158, *166*
Roelvink P, 269, *291*
Roelvink PW, 120, 122, 129, 132, *137,*
    138, 142, 337, *361*

Roessler BJ, 39, 43, *47*, 175, *186*, 263, *290*
Roger S, 2, *23*
Rogers BE, 123, 124, 125, 126, 128, *139*, *140*, *142*, 269, *291*, 337, *361*, 429, 435, *447*, *451*
Rogulski KR, 156, *165*
Rogy MA, 436, *452*
Rohan MC, 255, *282*
Roizman B, 148, *163*
Rojanasakul Y, 175, *186*
Rolland A, 101, 102, *114*
Rolland G, 103, *115*
Rom WN, 156, *165*, 182, *190*, 245, *273*
Romanczuk H, 126, 128, *140*
Romano G, 460, *470*
Romel L, 151, *164*
Romer M, 428, *446*
Rommelaere J, 148, *163*
Rommens JM, 38, *46*, 319, *349*, 366, *377*, 386, *394*
Rook AH, 203, *215*
Rosato K, 458, *467*
Roscilli G, 61, 65, *84*, *86*
Rose JA, 59, *82*
Rosell R, 244, *271*
Rosen I, 32, *45*
Rosenbaum MJ, 54, 65, *79*
Rosenberg M, 103, 104, 106, 111, *116*
Rosenberg SA, 12, *26*, 194, *209*, 246, 247, 249, *274*, *275*, *278*
Rosenblad C, 68, *89*
Rosenfeld MA, 13, *26*, 38, *46*, 249, 257, 263, *276*, *285*, *290*, 319, 320, *349*, *350*, 387, *394*, 410, *415*, 425, 437, *443*, *453*
Rosenfeld ME, 123, *139*, 269, *291*, 337, *361*
Rosenfeld MR, 148, *163*
Rosengart T, 333, *359*
Rosenstein B, 7, *25*, 412, *416*
Rosenthal ER, 319, *349*, 425, *443*
Rosenthal KL, 175, *186*
Rosman GJ, 329, *357*
Ross G, 245, *273*

Rosseels V, 207, *217*
Rosser LE, 195, *210*
Rossman MG, 54, *80*
Rosso R, 308, *318*
Rosychuk MK, 336, *360*
Roth DA, 14, *26*
Roth JA, 15, *26*, 120, 122, *138*, 195, *210*, 241, 242, 243, *269*, *270*, 310, *318*, 424, *442*
Roth MD, 253, *281*
Rothenberg S, 409, *415*
Rothermel CD, 194, *210*
Rothery S, 422, 425, 427, *440*
Rothman BS, 376, *382*
Rothmann T, 151, *164*, 243, *270*
Rottenberg ME, 205, *216*
Rousculp MD, 435, *450*
Rousset F, 197, *212*
Rowe WP, 32, *44*, 53, 54, 65, *79*, *87*, 146, *161*, 365, *377*, 411, *416*
Roy S, 40, *48*
Royston I, 305, *317*
Rozmahel R, 366, *377*
Ruan S, 201, *215*
Rubenstein RC, 70, *90*
Rubenstein RD, 74, *91*
Rubenstein SD, 432, *449*
Rubin BY, 194, *209*, *210*
Rubinchik S, 158, *166*
Rubins JB, 309, *318*
Rubsam LZ, 296, *313*
Rudge JS, 255, *283*
Rudginsky S, 108, 111, *117*, 307, 308, *317*, *318*
Rudginsky SA, 95, 96, *113*
Rudnicki MA, 326, *354*
Rudolph C, 384, *393*
Rudolph M, 136, *144*
Ruffing M, 59, 60, *82*
Ruiz FE, 103, 104, 106, 111, *116*, 387, 389, *395*, 426, *445*
Ruoslahti E, 128, 129, *142*
Ruscetti FW, 337, *361*
Rusch V, 293, *312*
Rusch VW, 293, *312*
Russell DG, 206, *216*

Russell DW, 61, 64, 65, 70, 72, *84*, *87*,
  91, 328, 333, 334, 338, *356*, *359*,
  362, 365, 368, 375, 376, *377*, *379*,
  381
Russell SJ, 123, *139*, 147, *162*, 337,
  338, *361*
Russell WC, 35, *45*, 146, *161*
Rutledge EA, 61, 64, 65, *84*, *87*, 338,
  362, 365, 376, *377*, *381*
Rux JJ, 33, *45*
Ryan A, 101, 102, *114*
Ryan M, 195, *210*, 250, *279*
Rygaard J, 239, 240, *268*
Rymaszewski M, 427, *445*
Rytel M, 32, *44*
Ryuke Y, 249, *277*

S

Saahet A, 203, *215*
Saavedra A, 296, *313*
Sabo P, 303, *315*
Sachar J, 109, *117*
Sacks CR, 322, 333, *352*, *359*, 421,
  424, *441*
Saeki T, 262, *289*
Saeki Y, 157, *165*
Safinya CR, 94, 99, *112*, *113*
Saida T, 249, *277*
Saigon Y, 158, *166*
Saijadi N, 37, *46*
Saikku P, 205, *216*
Saito H, 101, *114*, 296, *313*
Saito I, 225, 226, *230*, 436, *451*
Saito Y, 180, *189*
Sakatani M, 225, 226, *230*
Sakharov I, 126, *141*
Sakimura L, 249, *278*
Sakuma J, 225, 226, *230*, 436, *451*
Sakuma-Mochizuki J, 226, *230*
Sakuragawa N, 64, *86*
Sakurai F, 101, *114*
Salas SD, 205, *215*
Saldias F, 426, *444*
Salditt T, 99, *113*
Salgia R, 234, *265*

Salhany KE, 251, *280*
Sallenave JM, 173, *185*, 438, *454*
Salser W, 2, *23*
Saltz LB, 246, *273*
Salusto F, 255, *283*
Salvati F, 308, *318*
Salvetti A, 55, *81*
Salzmann JL, 296, *313*
Sampson-Johannes A, 150, 151, *164*,
  243, *270*
Samuel CE, 94, *112*
Samulski RJ, 6, *24*, 52, 54, 55, 57, 58,
  60, 62, 63, 67, 68, 72, 74, *78*, *79*, *80*,
  81, *82*, *83*, *85*, 88, 89, *91*, 136, *144*,
  328, 338, *356*, *362*, 367, 375, *378*,
  381, 412, *416*, 424, *443*, 461, *471*
Samulski T, 328, *356*
Samways JM, 320, 321, *351*
San H, 401, *405*, 429, *447*
Sanchez-Prieto R, 156, *165*
Sanda MG, 311, *318*
Sanders DA, 343, *363*
Sanders LC, 257, *285*
Sanford MA, 304, *316*
Sang N, 71, *91*
Sankar U, 326, *354*
Sanlioglu S, 58, 62, 63, *82*, *85*, 424,
  443
Santana A, 178, *188*
Santin AD, 62, *85*
Santoli D, 250, *279*
Santoro L, 39, 43, *48*
Santosuosso M, 176, *187*
Sany J, 197, *212*
Sappino AP, 178, *188*, 193, *208*
Sarkadi B, 319, *349*, 366, *377*, 392,
  396, 423, *442*
Sarraf C, 127, *141*
Sarvas M, 205, *216*
Sasaki Y, 157, *165*
Sato N, 256, *284*
Sato TA, 198, *214*
Satoh W, 65, *86*
Saudan P, 62, *85*
Sauter BV, 259, *286*
Sauter SL, 330, 343, *357*, *363*

Sauthoff H, 156, *165*
Savil J, 174, *186*
Sawa T, 103, *113*, 197, *213*, 436, *452*
Saxena B, 178, *188*
Scallan C, 6, 14, *24*, *26*, 110, *117*
Scallan M, 103, 104, 106, 111, *116*,
  320, 321, *351*
Scanlin TF, 322, 345, *352*, *364*
Scaravilli F, 124, *140*
Scaria A, 333, *360*, 422, *441*
Scarpa M, 100, 111, *114*, *118*, 345, *364*
Schaack J, 36, 37, *45*
Schaerli P, 255, *283*
Schaffer PA, 7, *25*
Schall TJ, 174, *185*
Schatten WE, 146, *161*
Schatz C, 306, *317*, 425, *444*
Schea R, 15, *26*
Scheffner M, 151, *164*, 243, *270*
Scheid P, 345, *364*, 439, *454*
Schembri FM, 322, *352*
Schenkel FA, 458, *467*
Scheonberger S, 254, *282*
Scheper RJ, 124, *140*
Scherman D, 331, *358*
Scherrer P, 100, *113*
Scheule RK, 93, 95, 96, 100, 103, 105,
  106, 107, 108, 109, 111, *112*, *113*,
  115, *116*, *117*, 123, *139*, 175, *186*,
  307, 308, *318*, 333, 334, 336, *359*,
  360, 421, 425, 426, 430, *441*, *445*,
  448, 461, 464, 465, *470*, *471*, *472*,
  473
Schichijo S, 247, *274*
Schiedner G, 411, *415*, *416*, 425, *444*
Schiemann WP, 225, *230*
Schilham M, 240, *269*
Schiller J, 425, *444*
Schilz R, 39, 43, *48*
Schlehofer JR, 51, *78*
Schlesinger Y, 122, 132, *138*
Schlom J, 16, *27*
Schlossberg H, 70, *90*
Schluger NW, 182, *190*
Schmid RA, 461, 466, *470*, *473*
Schmidt CW, 15, *26*

Schmidt M, 65, *86*, 180, *189*
Schmidt MC, 367, *378*
Schneider H, 124, *140*
Schneiderman RD, 341, *363*
Schnell MA, 5, *24*, 41, *48*, 66, *87*, 263,
  290
Schnurr DP, 32, 40, *45*
Schoenhaut DS, 195, *210*
Schoumacher RA, 103, 104, 106, 111,
  116
Schowalter DB, 64, *86*, 346, *364*
Schreier H, 337, *361*
Schrieber RD, 195, *210*
Schroeder JA, 175, *186*, 436, *452*
Schroth MK, 120, 126, *137*, 324, *353*
Schrump DS, 247, *274*, 311, *318*
Schughart K, 428, 429, *446*, *447*
Schultz H, 429, *448*
Schultz L, 177, *187*
Schulze-Osthoff K, 256, *284*
Schurr J, 197, *213*, 422, *442*
Schuster DP, 434, *450*, 459, *468*
Schuur ER, 158, *166*
Schwartz AG, 234, *265*
Schwartz AL, 461, *470*
Schwartz DA, 235, *266*, 389, *395*
Schwartz M, 181, *190*
Schwartz PE, 158, *166*
Schwartzbach C, 320, *351*, 373, *380*
Schwarzenberger P, 183, *190*, 197, *213*,
  245, *272*, 294, 304, *312*, *316*, 337,
  361
Schwarzenberger PO, 201, *215*, 305,
  317
Schwarz MA, 341, *363*, 423, *442*
Schwiebert EM, 338, *361*, 367, *379*
Scollard D, 196, *212*
Scolnick EM, 3, *23*
Sconocchia G, 125, *140*, 337, *361*
Scott B, 294, 306, 307, *312*, *317*
Scott J, 459, *469*
Scott JP, 460, *469*
Scott MO, 69, *89*
Scudeletti M, 247, *275*
Scully TA, 64, 75, *85*
Sears AE, 148, *163*

Seaver S, 37, *46*
Seddon T, 320, 321, *351*
Seegmiller JE, 3, *24*
Seemuller E, 72, *91*
Segal DM, 125, 127, *140*, *141*, 337,
   338, *361*, *362*
Segal S, 249, *276*
Sehgal A, 70, *90*
Seiler M, 70, 74, *90*, 339, *362*, 376,
   381
Selden RF, 14, *26*
Sellak H, 464, 465, *472*
Seller TA, 234, 249, *265*
Selman M, 178, *188*, 220, *229*
Selz F, 12, *26*
Semenkovich J, 458, *467*
Sene C, 320, *350*, 429, *448*
Seng M, 158, *166*
Sesholtz D, 68, *89*, 366, *377*
Seth P, 11, *25*, 262, *289*
Sethi T, 234, 249, *265*
Setoguchi Y, 410, *415*
Severs NJ, 422, 425, 427, *440*
Seymour A, 241, *269*
Seymour LW, 100, *113*
Sferra TJ, 429, *448*
Sgadari C, 260, *287*
Shaffer TH, 74, *91*, 432, 433, *449*, *450*
Shah AS, 458, *468*
Shah N, 76, *92*, 339, *362*, 370, *379*
Shahbazian M, 320, *350*
Shahzeidi S, 178, *189*
Shaish A, 134, *143*
Shaked A, 197, *212*, 436, *452*
Shalinksy DR, 259, *287*
Shanafelt AB, 259, 260, *287*
Shao J, 123, *139*, 330, 336, 343, *357*,
   360, *363*, 421, 425, 431, *441*
Shapiro GI, 235, *266*
Shapiro L, 436, *452*
Shapiro MJ, 251, *280*
Shapiro N, 156, *165*
Shapiro PS, 324, *353*
Shapiro SD, 183, *190*
Sharkis SJ, 320, *350*

Sharma P, 63, 64, *85*
Sharma SK, 183, *190*, 233, 234, 238,
   239, 245, 247, 249, 250, 253, *265*,
   266, *267*, *268*, *275*, *278*, *281*
Shaszeidi S, 178, *189*
Shattuck-Eidens D, 235, *266*
Shaw DR, 131, *142*
Shawler D, 305, *317*
Shean MK, 183, *190*, 201, 204, *215*,
   422, 433, *442*, *449*
Shearer G, 12, *26*
Shears LL, 129, *142*, 337, *361*
Shedlock DJ, 200, *215*
Sheehan JK, 324, *353*
Sheehy MJ, 18, *27*
Shell R, 429, *448*
Shellito JE, 183, *190*, 194, 195, 201,
   210, *215*, 422, *441*, *442*
Shen S, 110, *118*
Shen T, 224, *230*
Shenk TE, 32, 33, 34, *45*, 54, 62, 63,
   67, *79*, *85*, *88*, 120, 122, *137*, 328,
   356
Shepard BA, 427, *445*
Shepherd D, 403, *406*
Shepherd F, 258, *286*
Sher A, 195, *210*
Sherman DH, 300, *315*
Sherry B, 196, *211*
Sherwin RS, 69, *90*
Shevach EM, 249, *278*
Shewach DS, 296, *313*
Shi F, 61, *84*, 251, *280*
Shi Q, 158, *167*
Shi X, 175, *186*
Shi YX, 150, *164*
Shimada T, 65, *86*
Shimizu K, 254, *282*
Shimokata K, 296, *313*
Shimonishi M, 403, *406*
Shimosata Y, 240, *268*
Shimotono K, 3, *23*
Shin DM, 15, *26*
Shin HC, 69, *90*
Shine HD, 296, *314*

Shing Y, 257, *285*
Shinkin MB, 237, *267*
Shinoda JY, 422, *442*
Shinohara H, 258, *286*
Shirakura Y, 436, *452*
Shirley PS, 40, *48*
Shopland DR, 234, 249, *265*
Shorthouse R, 466, *473*
Showell HJ, 256, *284*
Shridhar V, 311, *318*
Shuler M, 242, *270*
Shvedoff RA, 207, *218*
Siahaan TJ, 335, *360*
Sibille Y, 193, *208*
Sibley RK, 460, *469*
Siders W, 308, *318*
Siders WM, 108, 111, *117*
Sidransky D, 150, *164*, 235, *266*
Siegal G, 100, 103, 105, *114*, 243, *270*
Siegal GP, 123, 125, *139*, *140*, 435, *451*
Siegel CS, 93, 95, 96, 100, 103, *112*,
    113, *115*, 334, *360*
Siegel JP, 22, *27*, 249, *278*
Siegfried W, 38, *46*, 410, *415*
Siegling A, 422, *441*
Sieling PA, 249, *278*
Sieve MC, 195, *211*
Sikora C, 433, *450*
Silletti S, 259, *287*
Silski C, 428, *446*
Silverstein RL, 258, *286*
Silvius JR, 384, *393*
Simari R, 401, *405*, 429, *447*
Simas JP, 198, *214*
Simecka JW, 333, *358*
Sime PJ, 173, 176, 179, 180, 181, 182,
    185, *187*, *189*, *190*, 222, 225, 226,
    229, *230*, 436, *451*, 466, *473*
Similo S, 459, *469*
Simoes-Wust AP, 244, *271*
Simon RH, 175, *186*, 220, 224, 228,
    229, *230*, 429, *448*
Simons JW, 15, *26*, 158, *166*, 252, *281*
Simons K, 331, *357*
Simpson AJ, 438, *454*

Simpson K, 175, *186*
Sindel L, 103, 104, 106, 111, *116*
Singh R, 120, *138*, 202, *215*, 438, 439,
    454
Siniscalco M, 60, *83*
Siniscalco R, 6, *24*
Sinkovics JG, 147, *162*
Sinn PL, 341, 343, *363*
Sirninger J, 367, *378*
Sisson TH, 183, *190*, 200, *215*, 224,
    230, 436, *451*
Sivack JG, 7, *25*
Sjoberg T, 458, *468*
Sjostrand M, 197, *213*
Skarin AT, 234, *265*
Skarsgard E, 6, *24*
Skerrett SJ, 195, *210*
Skipper J, 246, 247, *274*
Skoogh BE, 197, *213*
Skulimowski A, 54, *79*
Slack JL, 197, *213*
Slack NL, 94, *112*
Slager SL, 126, *141*
Slaton J, 260, *287*
Slebos R, 235, *266*
Slepushkin V, 330, 341, *357*, *363*, 426,
    445
Slepushkin VA, 330, *357*, 423, *442*
Slingerland R, 306, *317*
Sloan DL, 68, *89*, 366, *377*
Slovis B, 425, *444*
Slutsky AS, 197, *212*, 433, *450*, 458,
    461, 463, 466, *468*, *471*, *472*, *473*
Smale ST, 367, *378*
Smiley J, 35, *45*
Smirnow VN, 126, *141*
Smith AE, 38, *46*, 93, 100, 101, 103,
    104, 105, 106, 111, *112*, *114*, *115*,
    116, 135, *144*, 319, 320, 321, 325,
    326, 333, 334, 338, 346, *349*, *350*,
    351, *354*, *358*, *359*, 360, *362*, *364*,
    422, 425, *441*, *444*
Smith CV, 437, *453*
Smith DE, 458, *468*
Smith DH, 65, *87*

Smith DR, 260, *288*, 294, 306, *312*, *317*
Smith GL, 198, *214*
Smith KA, 322, *352*, 421, 424, *441*
Smith MA, 460, *469*
Smith MJ, 435, *450*
Smith MP, 333, *359*
Smith R, 146, *161*
Smith RH, 55, *80*
Smith SN, 103, 104, 106, 111, *116*, 320, 321, *351*, 366, *378*
Smith VP, 198, *214*
Smithies O, 240, *269*
Smyth R, 459, *469*
Smyth SE, 320, *351*
Smythe JA, 54, *79*
Smythe WR, 245, *272*, 296, 297, 310, *314*, *318*
Snider D, 177, *188*
Snider DP, 177, *188*
Snyder D, 253, *282*
Snyder RO, 62, 64, 75, *84*, *85*, *86*, 375, *381*
So S, 320, *350*
Sobol RE, 305, *317*
Sodoyer R, 206, *216*
Sogn JA, 247, *275*
Sollinger HW, 458, *468*
Solodin I, 399, *404*
Solow R, 74, *92*, 319, 327, *349*, *356*, 365, 366, 367, 368, *377*, *378*, 413, *417*, 424, *443*
Somia N, 51, 66, *78*
Sondel PM, 251, *280*
Sone S, 251, *280*
Song A, 106, *117*, 426, *445*
Song S, 64, *86*, 413, *417*
Song WR, 135, *144*, 262, *289*, 333, *359*, 425, *444*
Song YK, 102, 104, *115*
Sonnenberg MG, 207, *217*
Sookdeo CC, 326, 333, *354*, *359*
Soong S, 320, *350*
Sorensen RU, 198, *214*
Sorg C, 256, *284*

Sorgi FL, 100, *114*, 320, 321, 322, *351*, 352, 384, *393*, 422, 425, *440*
Sorscher EJ, 103, 104, 106, 111, *116*, 333, *358*, 425, *440*
Sosnowski BA, 123, 124, 125, *139*, *140*, 435, *451*
Sotnikov AV, 207, *218*
Soubrier F, 331, *358*
Southam CM, 146, 147, *161*, *162*
Southern KW, 320, 321, *351*, 387, 389, *394*, *395*
Souza DW, 36, *45*
Sozzani S, 255, *283*
Sozzi G, 234, 235, 249, *266*
Sparer TE, 326, *354*
Spear PG, 3, *23*
Speich R, 460, *470*
Spence SE, 337, *361*
Spencer F, 36, 37, *45*
Spender LC, 207, *218*
Spink CH, 99, *113*
Sporeno E, 61, *83*
Spragg RG, 439, *454*
Spratt K, 102, *115*
Spray DC, 296, *313*
Spriggs MK, 198, *214*
Springer K, 122, *138*
Sridhar CN, 384, *393*
Srinivasan R, 57, 62, *81*, 247, *275*
Srivastava A, 57, *81*, 82, 328, 337, *356*, *360*, 375, *381*
Srivastava R, 424, *442*
Staber PD, 341, 342, 343, *363*, 426, *445*
Stahel RA, 244, *271*
Stahlman M, 238, *268*
Stamler J, 434, *450*
Stammberfer U, 466, *473*
Stampfli MR, 173, 177, *185*, *187*, *188*
Standaert TA, 65, 70, *87*, 320, 333, 334, *351*, *359*, 368, 369, *379*, 429, *448*
Standiford TJ, 182, 183, 184, *190*, *191*, 197, 200, 202, *213*, *215*, 436, *451*, *452*
Standjord TP, 433, *450*
Stang HD, 2, *23*

Stanley ER, 194, *209*
Stark H, 100, *113*
Starnbach MN, 205, *216*
Starnes VA, 458, *467*
Starr S, 250, *279*
Stastny VA, 258, *286*
Stavropoulos E, 206, 207, *217*
Stedman H, 69, *89*
Stedman M, 106, *115*, 427, *445*
Steel RM, 111, *118*, 308, *318*, 345, *364*
Steen S, 458, 459, *468*
Steer BM, 102, 104, *115*, 135, *144*, 435, *451*
Steer CJ, 414, *418*
Steffan AM, 384, *393*
Steinberg H, 195, *210*
Steinberg SM, 235, *266*, 311, *318*
Stein EA, 13, *26*
Steinhorn DM, 432, *449*
Steinman RM, 253, *281*
Steinmuller C, 195, *210*
Stenmark KR, 126, *141*
Stepan T, 367, *378*
Stephan D, 401, *405*, 429, *447*
Stephens LC, 15, *26*
Sterman D, 148, *162*, 245, *272*, 293, 297, *312*, *314*
Sterman DH, 150, *163*, 246, 249, 261, *273*, 277, *289*, 294, 301, 308, *312*, *315*, *318*
Stern M, 103, 104, 106, 111, *116*, 320, 321, 322, *351*, *352*, 387, 389, *395*, 422, 425, 427, 438, *440*, *446*, *453*
Sternberg B, 384, *393*
Stetler-Stevenson WG, 257, 258, *285*, *286*
Steutermann D, 193, *209*
Stevens DA, 204, *215*
Stevenson BJ, 100, 102, 103, 105, *114*, 320, 321, *350*, *351*
Stevenson MM, 195, *210*
Stevenson SC, 147, *162*
Stewart AK, 259, *287*
Stewart AS, 439, *455*
Stewart CA, 198, *214*

Stewart CE, 207, *218*
Stewart D, 158, *166*
Stewart DJ, 398, *404*
Stewart S, 459, 460, *469*, *470*
Stewart TA, 206, *216*, 217
Stewart WE, 196, *212*
St George JA, 103, 105, 106, *115*, *116*, 123, *139*, 320, 322, 326, 333, 336, 346, *350*, *352*, *354*, *358*, *359*, *360*, *364*, 421, 424, 425, 426, 433, *441*, *443*, *445*, *450*
Stickle RI, 245, *273*
Stier LE, 319, *350*, 410, *415*
Stillman IE, 41, *48*
Stocker CJ, 127, *141*
Stockholm D, 336, *360*, 375, *381*
Stocking KL, 197, *213*
Stoeckel F, 42, *49*
Stolina M, 238, 239, 245, 250, 253, *267*, *268*, *278*, *281*
Stolz D, 183, *190*, 201, 202, *215*
Stolz DB, 101, 102, *114*, 399, *405*
Stolze E, 120, *138*
Stoner GD, 237, *267*
Stoppacciaro A, 249, *276*
Storkus WJ, 247, 250, 253, *274*, *279*, *282*
Storm TA, 52, 63, 74, 75, *78*, *85*, 375, *381*
Stoter G, 306, *317*
Stotter H, 249, *278*
Strandjord TP, 74, *92*, 424, 426, 429, 433, *443*, *444*, *449*
Stratford-Perricaudet LD, 38, 39, *46*, *47*, 70, *91*, 319, 325, *350*, *354*, 410, *415*, 425, *443*
Strayer DS, 414, *418*
Strey HH, 99, *113*, 429, *447*
Stribling R, 427, 430, *446*
Stricker H, 156, *165*
Strict CA, 260, *288*
Strieter RM, 174, 175, 184, *185*, *186*, *191*, 195, 196, 197, *211*, *213*, 255, 256, 257, 259, 260, *283*, *284*, *285*, *287*, 436, *452*

Stripp B, 172, *184*
Stripp BR, 176, *187*, 320, *350*
Strizzi L, 310, *318*
Strockbine L, 198, *214*
Stromblad S, 257, *285*
Strom SRB, 255, *283*
Strong JE, 147, *162*
Strong T, 302, *315*
Strong TV, 120, 131, *138*, *142*
Strous GJ, 72, *91*
Stuhler G, 246, *273*
Stupack DG, 122, *138*
Stutts MJ, 319, *349*, 423, *442*
Su J, 249, *277*
Su LT, 69, *89*
Su Q, 39, 43, *47*, *48*, 326, *355*, 425, *444*
Subauste CS, 198, *214*
Suda T, 461, 463, 465, *470*, *472*, *473*
Sudre P, 206, *216*
Sugenoya Y, 157, *165*
Sugita M, 322, *352*
Suit HD, 258, *286*
Sukhatme VP, 129, *142*
Sukhu L, 94, 101, *112*, *114*
Sullivan D, 422, *442*
Sullivan R, 256, *284*
Sullivan SM, 102, *115*
Sumimoto H, 250, *280*
Sumimoto R, 461, *471*
Summerford C, 52, 57, 62, 68, *78*, *81*, *82*, 328, *356*, 375, *381*, 412, *416*
Summer WR, 183, *190*, *191*, 194, 196, 197, 198, *209*, *212*, *213*, 294, 304, *312*, *316*
Sun L, 52, 74, 75, *78*
Sunamura M, 151, *164*, 251, *280*
Sundaresan P, 149, *163*
Sundaresan S, 458, 460, 461, *467*, *469*, *470*
Sundaresan V, 235, *266*
Sunderkotter C, 256, *284*
Sundt TM, 459, *469*
Sung RS, 262, *289*, 421, *441*
Sunnarborg SW, 197, *213*
Surman DR, 247, *275*

Surosky RT, 55, *80*
Sutherland R, 245, *272*
Suzuki F, 256, *285*
Suzuki K, 130, 131, *143*, 150, *164*, 249, *276*, 459, *469*
Suzuki S, 459, *469*
Suzuki Y, 195, *210*
Svanholm C, 205, *216*
Swanson GM, 234, *265*
Swanstrom R, 319, *349*, 366, *377*, 423, *442*
Swantz RJ, 172, *184*
Swartz DR, 376, *382*
Sweeney HL, 439, *455*
Sweeny TD, 431, *449*
Sweet M, 193, *209*
Swisher SG, 242, *269*, 310, *318*
Symes CW, 69, *90*
Symes JF, 17, *27*
Symons JA, 198, *214*
Sypek J, 195, *210*
Szabo P, 60, 61, *83*
Sznajder JI, 437, 438, *453*
Sznol M, 148, *163*
Szoka FC, 102, 103, 104, *115*, 331, *358*, 385, *394*

T

Tabata M, 245, *273*
Tabata R, 245, *273*
Tabibi S, 371, *380*
Tabin CJ, 3, *24*
Tachibana I, 222, *229*, 244, *271*
Tada H, 249, *277*
Taga T, 101, *114*
Tagawa T, 463, 465, *472*
Tagliaferri F, 101, 102, *114*, 429, *447*
Tahara H, 249, 250, *277*, *279*
Tai C, 148, *163*
Tai SJ, 6, 14, *24*, *26*
Tainsky M, 243, *270*
Takahashi K, 157, *165*
Takahashi M, 158, *166*, 247, *275*
Takahashi T, 249, *277*
Takaki T, 247, *274*

Takakura Y, 101, *114*
Takakuwa T, 436, *452*
Takayama K, 122, *139*, 258, *286*
Takeda K, 177, *187*
Takeuchi E, 251, *280*
Takeuchi Y, 123, *139*, 262, *290*, 337, 338, *361*
Takigawa M, 256, *285*
Takita H, 240, *269*
Tam MF, 195, *210*
Tam P, 100, *113*
Tamatani M, 436, *452*
Tamayose K, 65, *86*
Tamura A, 459, *469*
Tamura T, 437, *453*
Tan Y, 104, 107, 108, 109, *115*, *117*, 136, *144*, 400, *405*, 426, *445*
Tanabe S, 255, *283*
Tanaka M, 244, 257, *271*, *285*
Taner CB, 463, *472*
Tang K, 333, *359*
Tang W, 172, *185*, 220, *229*
Tang YW, 207, *218*
Tanghe A, 207, *217*
Tani K, 250, 252, *280*, *281*
Tanida T, 242, *269*
Tanigawara Y, 437, *453*
Tanio Y, 244, *271*
Tannahill CL, 437, *452*
Tanner F, 401, *405*, 429, *447*
Tannock IF, 151, *164*, 256, *284*
Tanswell AK, 101, 102, 103, *114*, 458, 461, *468*, *471*
Tao N, 135, *144*
Tarallo A, 172, *184*
Taraseviciene-Stewart L, 403, *406*
Tarran R, 322, *352*
Tartour E, 306, *317*
Tascon RE, 206, 207, *217*
Tateda K, 196, 202, *211*, *215*, 436, *452*
Tatsuta M, 157, *165*
Tattersall P, 54, *80*, 146, *162*
Tatum EL, 2, *23*
Taub DD, 260, *287*
Tawa NE, 14, *26*
Taylor G, 7, *25*, 32, *44*, 412, *416*

Taylor MD, 439, *455*
Tazawa R, 158, *166*
Tazelaar HD, 460, 463, 464, *469*, *472*
Tazelaar J, 5, *24*, 41, *48*, 66, *87*, 263, *290*
Tchou-Wong K, 245, *273*
Teague TK, 249, *278*
Teasdale R, 427, *445*
Teftt JD, 181, *189*, *190*
Temann UA, 172, 176, *184*, *187*
Temin HM, 3, *23*, 262, *289*
Templeton NS, 99, *113*, 262, *289*, 429, *447*
Ten DG, 206, *216*
Tepper R, 249, *276*
Tepper RS, 320, *350*
Teramoto S, 72, 74, *91*, 333, *360*
Terheggen HG, 2, *23*
Terwilliger EF, 64, *86*
Tew DN, 458, *468*
Tewari RP, 195, *211*
Tezak Z, 51, *78*
Thacker JD, 249, *276*
Thakur A, 249, *278*
Theise ND, 320, *350*
Themis M, 124, *140*
Theodore J, 466, *473*
Theodossiou C, 294, 304, *312*, *316*
Thiagalingam S, 241, *269*
Thielemans K, 198, *214*
Thierry AR, 101, 102, *114*, 399, *404*
Thomas D, 198, *214*
Thomas E, 198, *214*
Thomas EK, 198, *214*
Thomas LB, 146, *161*
Thomas P, 341, *363*
Thomas PJ, 367, *379*
Thome U, 438, *453*
Thompson AR, 375, *381*
Thompson JJ, 196, *212*
Thompson S, 369, 373, *379*
Thomson A, 320, 321, *351*
Thomson JR, 126, *141*
Thorne PS, 389, *395*, 425, *444*
Thorpe PE, 258, *286*
Thouvenot D, 320, *350*, 430, *448*

Thurner B, 246, *273*
Thurston G, 101, 102, 103, 107, *114, 115*
Tiberghien P, 294, *312*
Tiffany HL, 199, *214*
Till GO, 432, *449*
Tiller R, 320, *350*
Tillman BW, 124, 125, *140*
Timmons T, 242, *269*
Tiruppathi C, 439, *455*
Titus JA, 125, *140*, 337, *361*
Tjandrawan T, 253, *282*
Tobias J, 247, *275*
Tobiasch E, 51, *78*
Tockman M, 235, *266*
Toda M, 249, *277*
Todisco T, 194, *210*
Todo T, 149, *163*
Todryk S, 304, *316*
Toes R, 254, *282*
Tohyama M, 436, *452*
Tolan MJ, 458, *467*
Tollefson AE, 150, *164*
Tolley E, 458, *468*
Tolstoshev P, 12, *26*
Toman C, 409, *415*
Tomko RP, 120, 122, *137*
Tonelli MR, 376, *382*
Tong A, 243, *270*
Toniatti C, 61, 65, *83, 84, 86*
Top FH, 32, *45*
Topf N, 439, *454*
Torchilin VP, 429, *447*
Torikai K, 54, 63, *79*
Torrent C, 42, *49*
Torry DJ, 174, *185*
Tosi M, 323, *353*, 425, *440*
Toth K, 150, *164*
Tough TW, 249, *278*
Touraine-Moulin F, 320, *350*
Tousignant JD, 103, 106, *115, 116, 117*, 426, 430, *445, 448*
Townsend A, 247, *274*
Toyoizumi T, 150, *163*
Tracey KJ, 194, *209*
Trakht IN, 126, *141*

Traktman P, 425, *444*
Transwell AK, 102, 104, *115*
Trapnell BC, 38, *46*, 224, *230*, 319, 333, *349, 358, 359*, 366, *377*, 420, 425, 426, 431, 439, *440, 441, 443, 454*
Trask TW, 296, *314*
Travis E, 433, 437, *450*
Trazelaar HD, 460, *469*
Treat J, 245, *272*, 294, 297, 300, *312, 314, 315*
Treco DA, 14, *26*
Tremblay GM, 176, *187*, 436, *451*
Trempe JP, 52, 55, 56, 60, 68, *78, 80, 81*
Trenthem LL, 432, *449*
Trentin JJ, 32, *44*
Trepel M, 128, *142*
Triantafillou AN, 459, *469*
Triebold KJ, 195, 206, *210, 217*
Trinchieri G, 39, *47*, 196, *211*, 250, 251, *279, 280*, 333, *360*
Tripathy SK, 39, 43, *47*
Tripp RA, 207, *218*
Trono D, 3, *24*, 262, *289*, 328, 329, 330, 341, *356, 357*, 463, *471*
Trulock EP, 458, 459, 460, *467, 468, 469, 470*
Truong-Le, 392, *395*
Tsai MS, 258, *286*
Tsai SY, 109, *117*
Tsai V, 422, 437, *442, 452*
Tsai WC, 196, *211*
Tsai YJ, 94, 100, 101, *112, 113, 114*
Tsan GL, 427, 432, *446*
Tsan MF, 427, 432, *445, 446*
Tsang KY, 16, *27*
Tsao YP, 69, *89*
Tseng WC, 101, 102, *114*, 399, *405*
Tseng YY, 56, *81*
Tsui LC, 101, 102, 103, *114*, 319, *349*, 366, *377*, 435, *450*
Tsui LV, 440, *455*
Tsujii M, 253, *281*
Tsujimura K, 249, *277*
Tsukuda K, 303, *316*

Tsung K, 250, *279*
Tsunoda H, 64, *86*
Tsuruta N, 260, *288*
Tubb J, 39, 43, *47*
Tucker AL, 430, *448*
Tufaro F, 157, *165*
Tugenderiech S, 36, 37, *45*
Turka LA, 346, *364*
Turley H, 235, *266*
Turnbull AE, 54, *79*
Turnell AS, 151, *164*
Turnier J, 148, *163*
Tursz T, 264, *290*, 425, *444*
Tuveson DA, 237, *267*
Tuyunder M, 148, *163*
Tyler RC, 400, *405*, 429, *448*
Tymen G, 103, *115*
Tzehoval E, 249, *276*
Tzeng E, 129, *142*, 337, *361*, 425, *440*

U

Ueda T, 224, *230*, 420, 426, 431, *441*
Ueda Y, 346, *364*
Uematsu K, 310, *318*
Uenaka A, 247, *274*
Ueno H, 122, *139*, 258, *286*
Ulrich JT, 240, *268*
Ulrich K, 438, *453*
Umemoto EY, 101, 102, 107, *114*
Umetsu DT, 177, *188*
Unfer RC, 400, *405*, 429, *448*
Unkeless JC, 260, *288*
Unruh H, 178, *189*
Upton C, 304, *316*
Urabe M, 55, 65, 66, *80, 88*
Usual K, 158, *166*
Usuda J, 249, *277*
Uy G, 465, *473*
Uyechi LS, 102, 103, *115*
Uyemura K, 249, *278*

V

Vadas MA, 196, *211*
Vahanian NN, 156, *165*

Vaidai E, 247, *274*
Vaillancourt MT, 150, *164*
Vale PR, 17, *27*
Valerio D, 100, *114*, 297, *314*
Valiante NM, 250, *279*
Valsesia-Wittmann S, 262, *289*
Valyi-Nagy T, 196, *211*
van Bekkum DW, 297, *314*
Vanbervliet B, 198, *214*, 255, *283*
van Beusechem VV, 119, 127, 128, 132, *137, 142, 143*
VanBuskirk AM, 459, *469*
van B V, 199, *214*
Vandenabeele P, 196, *212*
van der Bruggen P, 246, *274*
Vanderplasschen A, 198, *214*
van der Poel HG, 158, *166*
van der Poll T, 197, *213*
Vandershceuren R, 305, *317*
van der Velde I, 37, *46*
van der Voort E, 254, *282*
Vanderwaak TJ, 129, *142*
van Es HH, 132, *143*, 330, 341, *357, 363*
van Es HHG, 423, *442*
Van Ginkel FW, 103, 104, 106, 111, *116*, 333, *358*
Van GY, 429, *447*
Van Hazel G, 306, *317*
van Heeckeren A, 323, *353*, 425, *440*
Vanhook MK, 336, *360*
Vanin EF, 65, *86*, 341, *363*
Van Itallie CM, 335, *360*
Vankeerberghen A, 367, *379*
Van Kessel A, 466, *473*
Van Kooten C, 198, *214*
Vannier E, 436, *452*
Van Pacherbeke C, 148, *163*
Van Pel A, 246, *273*
Van Pelt N, 402, *405*
van Praag H, 341, *363*
van Raaij M, 122, 132, *138*
van Rijswijk AL, 132, *143*
Van Roey M, 54, 65, 66, *80, 87*
Van Roijen N, 135, *144*, 323, *353*, 420, 425, *441*

van Rooijen N, 262, *289*
Vanrroijen N, 135, *144*
van Someren GD, 297, *314*
van't Hof W, 120, 126, *137*, 324, *353*
VanZandwijk N, 305, *317*
Varda-Blooom N, 134, *143*
Varga CM, 429, *447*
Varki NM, 251, *280*
Varlet F, 305, *317*
Varnavski AN, 5, *24*
Vasey P, 245, *273*
Vassalli JD, 194, *209*
Vassalli P, 178, *188*, *189*, 193, 194, 196, *208*, *209*, 211
Vassaui JD, 256, *284*
Vassaux G, 134, *143*, 158, *167*
Vazquez C, 183, *190*, 204, *215*
Vazquez F, 258, *286*
Vecchiarelli A, 194, *210*
Veith FJ, 458, *467*
Vella A, 249, *278*
Venet A, 39, 43, *47*
Venetos G, 126, *141*
Venetsanakos E, 307, *317*
Verma IM, 3, *24*, 51, 66, *78*, 262, *289*, 329, 330, 333, 341, *357*, *359*, *363*
Veronese ML, 235, *266*
Verwaerde C, 197, *212*
Vesin C, 178, *189*
Vezzio N, 197, *212*
Viale G, 303, *316*
Viallat JR, 305, *317*
Viallet J, 258, *286*
Vianale G, 310, *318*
Vicari A, 255, *283*
Vick RN, 120, *137*, 320, *352*, 373, *380*
Vieira P, 196, *212*
Viellard-Baron A, 403, *406*
Vierboom MP, 242, *269*
Vigne E, 42, *49*, 131, *143*
Vigneron JP, 103, *115*
Vijayasarathy C, 439, *455*
Vikis HG, 243, *270*
Vile RG, 147, *162*, 296, 304, *313*, *316*
Villefroy P, 39, 43, *47*
Vincent AJ, 297, *314*

Vincent KA, 55, 67, 68, *81*, *89*
Vincent-Lacaze N, 64, 75, *85*, 375, *381*
Virella-Lowell I, 70, *91*, 323, *353*, 412, 413, *416*, *417*, 421, 424, 437, *441*, *453*
Viroonchatapan E, 104, *115*, 136, *144*, 400, *405*
Visfeldt J, 240, *268*
Vliegenthart JF, 322, *352*
Vlodavsky I, 256, *284*
Vogelstein B, 241, 249, *269*, *277*
Vogler C, 77, *92*
Vogt P, 303, *316*
Volk HD, 422, *441*
Volm M, 257, 259, *285*, *286*
Volpert OV, 258, *286*
von Bonsdorff CH, 331, *357*
Von Hoff D, 243, *270*
Voulgaropoulou F, 65, *86*
Vreim CE, 459, *468*
Vukusic B, 247, *275*
Vuola JM, 205, *216*

W

Wada Y, 158, *166*
Waddell BE, 320, *351*
Wadhwa MS, 101, 102, *114*, 429, *447*
Wadsworth SC, 55, 67, 68, *81*, *89*, 93, *112*, 126, 128, 135, *140*, *144*, 326, 333, 338, 346, *354*, *358*, *359*, *360*, *362*, *364*, 422, 425, *441*, *443*, *444*
Wagener JS, 322, *352*
Wagner E, 11, *25*, 122, *139*, 391, *395*, 428, *446*
Wagner JA, 76, *92*, 320, *351*, 370, 372, *379*, *380*, 412, *417*
Wagner RD, 195, *210*
Waheed I, 247, *274*, 311, *318*
Wainwright BJ, 111, *118*, 366, *378*
Waitze A, 207, *218*
Wala I, 429, *447*
Walbridge B, 296, *313*
Walden P, 246, *273*
Walden S, 7, *25*, 412, *416*
Waldrep JC, 428, *446*, *447*

Waldrop S, 254, *282*
Waldschmidt TJ, 427, *445*
Walker GR, 457, *467*
Walker LC, 100, 103, 105, *114*
Walker SL, 65, *86*
Wall NR, 244, *271*
Wallace WA, 320, 321, *351*
Wallbridge S, 296, *313*
Wallwork J, 458, 459, *468*, *469*
Walsh CE, 424, *443*
Walsh GL, 15, *26*
Walsh K, 16, *27*
Walsh SM, 333, 334, *359*, 370, *379*
Waltenberger J, 258, *286*
Walter DM, 177, *188*
Walter RJ, 148, *162*
Walter S, 249, *276*
Walters RW, 54, 57, 69, 70, 71, 73, 74,
  80, *81*, *90*, *91*, 120, 123, 126, 131,
  137, *139*, 262, *289*, 324, 338, 339,
  347, *353*, *362*, *364*, 376, *381*, 420,
  424, 425, 430, 431, *440*, *443*, *449*
Waltz D, 373, *381*
Walz J, 72, *91*
Wandeler AI, 147, *162*
Wands JR, 127, *141*
Wang B, 69, *89*
Wang C, 245, *273*
Wang CY, 198, *214*, 245, *273*
Wang D, 76, *92*, 333, *358*, 367, *378*
Wang F, 54, *80*, 249, *276*
Wang G, 70, *91*, 123, *139*, 239, *268*,
  323, 330, 336, 341, 342, 343, *353*,
  357, *360*, *363*, 385, *394*, 420, 421,
  423, 425, 426, 431, *441*, *442*, *445*
Wang J, 177, 182, 183, *187*, *188*, *190*,
  206, *216*, 249, 250, *278*, *279*, 322,
  333, *352*, *359*, 413, *417*, 461, *471*
Wang KX, 93, 98, 99, 100, 103, 105,
  106, 110, *112*, *113*, *115*, 333, 334,
  359, *360*, 427, *445*
Wang L, 6, *24*, 66, *87*, 110, *117*, 426,
  445
Wang M, 120, 125, 129, 131, *137*, *140*,
  142, 337, *361*
Wang MH, 126, *141*

Wang P, 172, *185*, 220, *229*
Wang Q, 42, *49*, 326, *354*
Wang S, 367, *379*, 438, *454*
Wang XS, 57, 62, *81*
Wang Y, 109, *117*, 243, 255, *270*, *282*,
  304, *316*
Wan NC, 93, 100, 103, *112*, 334, *360*
Wan Y, 174, 179, *185*, 201, *215*
Wantroba Z, 438, *453*
Warburton D, 181, 182, *189*, *190*
Ward DC, 61, *84*
Ward P, 65, *87*, 150, *164*
Ward PA, 178, *188*
Ward TG, 32, 41, *44*
Ware LB, 437, 438, *453*
Warmington K, 175, *186*
Warrier RR, 250, *279*
Warth R, 367, *379*
Wasfi DS, 302, *315*
Watchko JF, 69, *89*
Watkins SC, 7, *25*, 101, 102, 110, *114*,
  117, 324, *353*, 422, 426, *441*, *445*
Watkins SJ, 127, 128, *142*, 337, *361*,
  429, *447*
Watral V, 102, 110, *115*
Watson JD, 19, *27*
Weatherly MR, 103, 104, 106, 111, *116*
Weaver TE, 439, *454*
Webb AK, 320, 321, *351*
Webb S, 366, *378*
Webb WR, 457, *467*
Weber CE, 15, *26*
Weber PS, 220, 228, *229*, *230*
Weber-Pendleton S, 429, *448*
Webster P, 262, *289*
Weder W, 460, 466, *470*, *473*
Weger S, 55, 60, *80*, *82*
Wei CM, 3, *23*
Wei D, 136, *144*
Wei L, 367, *379*
Wei XQ, 193, *209*, 322, *352*, 392, *395*
Weibel ER, 174, *185*
Weinacker A, 294, 304, *312*, *316*
Weinberg RA, 3, *24*
Weindler FW, 59, *82*
Weiner DB, 200, *215*

Weiner DJ, 4, *24*, 71, *91*, 344, *363*

Weiser TS, 247, *274*

Weiss DJ, 69, 74, *90, 92*, 224, *230*, 376, *382*, 424, 425, 426, 429, 430, 433, *443, 444, 448, 449, 450*

Weiss RA, 123, *139*, 262, *290*, 337, 338, *361*

Weissman S, 19, *27*

Weitzman MD, 56, 60, 62, 65, *81, 85*, 87, 128, *142*

Wells JM, 296, *313*

Wells WJ, 458, *467*

Welsh MJ, 38, *46*, 69, 70, 71, 73, *90, 91*, 93, 101, *112, 114*, 120, 122, 123, 126, 131, *137, 139, 140*, 262, *289*, 319, 320, 321, 324, 325, 327, 332, 338, 339, 347, *349, 351, 353, 354, 355, 358, 361, 362, 364*, 376, *381*, 386, *394*, 424, 425, 427, 430, 431, *443, 445, 446, 448, 449*, 465, *473*

Welty SE, 420, 426, 431, *441*

Wen SF, 422, *442*

Wen XY, 259, *287*

Wen Y, 102, 104, *115*, 135, *144*, 435, *451*

Werner JH, 32, *44*

Wert SE, 39, 43, *47*, 172, 176, *184, 187*, 330, 333, *357, 359*, 423, 439, *442, 454*

Wessendarp M, 198, *214*

West DC, 257, *285*

West JD, 70, *90*, 436, *451*

Westphal H, 6, *24*

Westra WH, 235, *266*

Wetzel R, 7, *25*, 412, *416*

Whartenby KA, 242, *269*, 296, *313*

Wheeler CJ, 94, 101, 102, 104, *112, 114, 115*

Whelan J, 262, *290*

Whitaker NJ, 151, *164*, 243, *270*

White DE, 247, *275*

White DJ, 458, *468*

White GC, 424, *442*

White JE, 427, 432, *445, 446*

White SJ, 128, 134, *142, 144*

Whitehead SS, 207, *218*

Whitehill TA, 398, *404*

Whiteway A, 68, *89*

Whitley M, 136, *144*

Whitmore M, 110, *117*, 400, *405*, 426, *445*

Whitsett J, 172, *184*, 238, 244, *268, 272*, 333, *359*

Whitsett JA, 172, 176, 178, *184, 187, 189*, 224, *230*, 330, *357*, 420, 423, 426, 431, 432, 439, *441, 442, 454*

Whitt MA, 341, *363*

Wicha MS, 157, *165*

Wickham TJ, 119, 120, 122, 125, 127, 129, 132, *136, 137, 138, 139, 140, 141, 142*, 147, *162*, 262, 269, *289, 291*, 325, 326, 333, 337, *354, 355, 359, 361*, 429, *447*, 461, 462, *471*

Widdicombe JH, 93, 99, *112*, 367, *378*

Wiebe ME, 194, *209*

Wiederschain D, 258, *286*

Wiegand GW, 437, *453*

Wiegand SJ, 255, *283*

Wiener-Kronish JP, 103, *113*, 197, *213*, 436, *452*

Wiewrodt R, 156, *165*, 249, *277*, 308, *318*, 425, *444*

Wigzell H, 205, *216*

Wikenheiser K, 238, 244, *268, 272*

Wilcher R, 57, 58, *82*

Wilcox BR, 458, *468*

Wildner O, 147, 156, *162, 165*, 245, 272, 302, *315*

Wiletts M, 262, *289*

Wiley JA, 198, *214*

Wiley R, 177, *187*

Wiley RE, 177, *188*

Wilkowski JM, 183, *190*, 200, *215*, 436, *451*

Willemot JM, 429, *448*

William Davis C, 324, *353*

Williams A, 150, 151, *164*, 243, *270*

Williams JP, 296, *314*

Williams P, 8, 9, *25*

Williams PM, 430, *448*

Williamson R, 100, *114*

Willimann K, 255, *283*

Willingham M, 11, *25*
Willingham MC, 326, *355*
Willis RC, 3, *24*
Willson AP, 108, *117*
Wilmott RW, 333, *359*
Wils P, 331, *358*
Wilson AP, 263, *290*
Wilson CB, 205, *216*, 346, *364*, 369, *379*, 429, *448*
Wilson GL, 385, *394*
Wilson HMP, 303, *315*
Wilson JM, 4, 5, 6, 13, *24*, *26*, 37, 39, 40, 41, 42, 43, *46*, *47*, *48*, *49*, 54, 59, 62, 65, 66, 68, 69, 70, 71, *79*, *82*, *85*, *87*, *88*, *89*, *91*, 109, *117*, 120, 135, *137*, *144*, 220, 228, *229*, *230*, 262, 263, *289*, *290*, 294, 296, 297, 300, 308, *312*, *314*, *315*, *318*, 319, 320, 325, 326, 327, 333, 338, 341, 342, 344, 346, 347, *349*, *350*, *352*, *354*, *355*, *359*, *360*, *362*, *363*, *364*, 366, 373, *377*, *380*, 392, *396*, 423, 424, 425, *442*, *444*
Wilson LA, 196, *212*, 369, 373, *379*
Wilson SJ, 181, *190*
Wimmer E, 148, *163*
Wine JJ, 320, 339, *351*, *362*, 370, 371, *379*, *380*, 412, *416*, *417*
Wing L, 103, 104, 106, 111, *116*
Wingo PA, 233, 234, 249, *265*
Winocour E, 56, 60, 62, *81*, *83*, *85*
Wiseman DM, 256, *284*
Wistuba A, 60, *82*
Wistuba II, 150, *163*, 234, 249, *266*
Witschi H, 237, 238, *267*
Wivel NA, 67, *88*
Wlesh MJ, 120, 126, *137*, 420, 425, *440*, *444*
Wobus C, 54, *80*, 136, *144*
Wobus CE, 54, *80*
Woffendin C, 18, *27*
Wolchok JD, 247, *275*
Wold WS, 150, *164*, 325, *354*
Wolf S, 195, *210*
Wolf SF, 195, *210*
Wolfert MA, 100, *113*

Wolff G, 127, 135, *141*, *144*, 262, *289*, 323, *353*, 420, 425, *441*, *443*
Wolff JA, 1, 8, 9, *23*, *25*, 461, *471*
Wolff JE, 258, *286*
Wolff K, 257, *285*
Wolfson MR, 74, *91*, 197, *213*, 432, 433, *449*, *450*
Wolgamot GM, 328, *356*
Wolitzky AG, 250, *279*
Wollenberg GK, 436, *452*
Wolpe S, 194, *209*
Wolpe SD, 196, *211*
Wonderling RS, 61, 64, 65, *84*, *86*
Wong CP, 177, *188*
Wong KK, 61, 64, *84*
Wong NC, 263, *290*
Wood KJ, 461, *471*
Woodcock J, 22, *27*
Woodworth LA, 346, *364*
Woo SC, 304, *316*
Woo SL, 121, *138*, 259, *286*, 409, *415*
Woo SLC, 296, *314*
Worgall S, 120, 127, 135, *138*, *141*, *144*, 202, *215*, 262, *289*, 323, *353*, 420, 425, 439, *441*, *443*, *454*
Worth LL, 175, *186*
Wright NA, 239, *268*
Wright SD, 458, *468*
Wu A, 149, *163*
Wu CH, 11, *25*
Wu CY, 198, *214*
Wu GY, 11, *25*
Wu-Hsieh B, 195, *210*
Wu IH, 106, *117*, 426, *445*
Wu KK, 94, *112*
Wu L, 197, *212*, 436, *452*
Wu P, 54, 64, *80*, *86*
Wu SP, 101, 102, 110, *114*, *117*, 400, *405*, 426, *445*
Wu SQ, 238, 252, *267*, *280*
Wu XY, 437, *453*
Wu Y, 411, *416*
Wwinacker A, 245, *272*
Wyllie AH, 235, *266*
Wynn SG, 326, *354*
Wysocka M, 251, *280*

Wysokenski DM, 98, 110, *113*, 427, *445*

X

Xia D, 129, *142*
Xia H, 131, *143*, 330, *357*
Xiao W, 54, 57, 66, 67, 71, *80*, *81*, 87, 88, *91*, 338, *362*
Xiao X, 52, 55, 57, 60, 61, 64, 67, 68, 69, 72, 74, 75, *78*, *81*, *83*, *84*, 88, 89, *91*
Xie J, 194, *209*
Xin KQ, 66, *88*
Xing Z, 173, 174, 175, 177, 179, 180, 181, 183, *185*, *186*, *187*, *188*, *189*, *190*, 197, *212*, 222, 225, 226, *229*, *230*, 433, 436, 438, *450*, *451*, *452*, *454*, 466, *473*
Xiong M, 120, 122, *138*
Xu B, 428, *446*, *447*
Xu H, 458, *468*
Xu K, 15, *26*
Xu L, 18, *27*
Xu N, 439, *455*
Xu R, 69, *90*, 120, 122, *137*
Xu X, 437, *453*
Xu Y, 224, *230*, 385, *394*
Xue Y, 260, *287*

Y

Yabe Y, 32, *44*
Yacoub M, 459, *468*
Yacoub MH, 126, 135, *141*
Yagi K, 36, *45*
Yajima T, 337, *361*
Yamada I, 401, *405*
Yamamoto M, 134, *143*, 333, *358*
Yamamoto S, 225, 226, *230*
Yamamoto T, 243, *270*
Yamamura H, 157, *165*
Yamasaki H, 296, *313*
Yamashita F, 101, *114*
Yamashita K, 256, *285*
Yan Z, 52, 57, 58, 59, 63, 64, 66, 69, 70, 71, 73, 74, 75, 76, *78*, *85*, 88, *92*, 324, 328, 339, *353*, *356*, *362*, *363*, 375, *381*, 424, *443*
Yanagawa H, 251, *280*
Yancopoulos GD, 255, *283*
Yang AD, 150, *163*
Yang C, 309, 310, *318*
Yang CC, 61, 64, *84*
Yang JC, 52, 57, 58, 59, 63, 64, 66, 69, 70, 71, 73, 74, 75, 76, *78*, 82, *85*, 88, 247, *275*, 328, *356*, 375, *381*
Yang JP, 100, *113*
Yang JS, 341, 342, *363*, 424, *442*
Yang L, 376, *381*
Yang NS, 18, *27*, 251, *280*
Yang P, 234, *265*, 421, *441*
Yang PC, 261, *288*
Yang Y, 5, *24*, 39, 40, 42, 43, *47*, *48*, *49*, 65, 66, 70, *86*, 88, *91*, 220, 228, *229*, *230*, 262, *289*, 300, *315*, 320, 325, 326, 333, 341, *350*, *354*, *359*, *360*, *363*, 425, 429, *443*, *444*, *448*
Yang ZY, 18, *27*, 249, *277*, 401, *405*, 429, *447*
Yankaskas JR, 70, *90*, 93, 99, *112*, 120, *137*, 319, 320, 322, 325, 330, *349*, *350*, *352*, *354*, *357*, 373, *380*, 423, *442*
Yano M, 461, 463, 464, 465, *470*, *471*, *472*, *473*
Yano S, 258, *286*
Yano T, 247, *275*
Yant SR, 110, *118*
Yao J, 70, *90*, 333, *359*
Yao L, 258, *286*
Yao SN, 39, 43, *47*
Yarosh OK, 147, *162*
Yatsunami J, 122, *139*, 260, *288*
Yawman AM, 207, *217*
Yazaki T, 148, *163*
Ye C, 64, *86*
Ye H, 120, *137*, 320, 326, *352*, *355*, 373, *380*
Ye L, 435, *450*
Ye P, 183, *190*, 197, 198, 201, *213*, *215*, 294, 304, *312*, *316*

Ye X, 41, *48*, 109, *117*, 326, *354*
Yee D, 121, *138*
Yee JK, 330, *357*
Yeh C, 309, 310, *318*
Yeh P, 131, *143*
Yei S, 40, *48*, 333, *359*, 439, *454*
Yen N, 15, *26*
Yesner R, 237, *267*
Yeung S, 157, *165*
Yew NS, 93, 98, 100, 103, 105, 106, 109, 110, *112*, *113*, *115*, *117*, 175, *186*, 333, 334, *359*, *360*, 426, 427, 437, *445*, *452*, 464, 465, *472*, *473*
Yewdell JW, 247, *274*
Yi AK, 427, *445*
Yi SM, 57, 74, *81*, 120, 126, 128, *137*, *140*, 324, 338, 339, *353*, *361*, *362*, 376, *381*, 424, *443*
Yie T, 245, *273*
Yim J, 250, *279*
Yin Z, 259, *287*
Ying W, 435, *451*
Ying WB, 123, 124, *139*, *140*
Yip A, 344, *363*
Yoden T, 157, *165*
Yokoyama C, 403, *406*
Yokoyama M, 436, *452*
Yoneda J, 259, 260, *286*, *288*
Yonemitsu Y, 345, *364*, 392, *395*, 426, *445*
Yoneyama K, 319, *349*, 410, *415*, 425, *443*
Yong L, 399, *404*
Yoo JH, 437, *453*
Yoon H, 250, *279*
Yoon HL, 251, *280*
Yoon JW, 69, *90*
Yoon M, 65, *87*
Yoon SK, 127, *141*
Yoon SS, 259, *287*
Yoshida J, 249, *277*
Yoshida M, 222, 225, 226, *229*, *230*, 436, *451*
Yoshida S, 193, *209*
Yoshiike K, 337, *361*

Yoshimura K, 38, *46*, 319, *349*, 366, *377*, 410, *415*, 425, *443*
Yoshino I, 247, *275*
Yoshizawa Y, 244, *271*
You L, 309, 310, *318*
Young CS, 36, 37, *45*
Young D, 69, *90*
Young IG, 177, *188*
Young KR, 103, 104, 106, 111, *116*
Young SM, 60, 61, *83*
Young VK, 458, *468*
Yousem SA, 459, 460, 466, *469*, *470*, *473*
Yu CJ, 258, 261, *286*, *288*
Yu DC, 158, *166*
Yu QC, 4, 5, *24*, 344, *363*, 366, *377*
Yu R, 310, *318*
Yu Y, 260, *288*
Yuan A, 258, 261, *286*, *288*
Yue H, 367, *379*
Yue Y, 52, 57, 58, 59, 63, 64, 66, 69, 70, 71, 73, 74, 75, 76, *78*, *82*, *85*, *88*, *90*, *92*, 324, 328, 339, *353*, *356*, *363*, 375, *381*, 424, *443*
Yung WK, 150, *164*
Yurt RW, 196, *211*
Yvon E, 12, *26*

Z

Zabner J, 38, *46*, 70, 74, *90*, *91*, 93, 101, *112*, *114*, 120, 123, 126, 128, 131, *137*, *139*, *140*, 262, *289*, 320, 321, 323, 324, 327, 330, 332, 333, 336, 338, 339, 341, *350*, *351*, *353*, *355*, *357*, *358*, *359*, *360*, *361*, *362*, *363*, 376, *381*, 387, *394*, 420, 421, 423, 425, 426, 427, 429, 430, 431, *440*, *441*, *443*, *444*, *445*, *446*, *448*, *449*
Zacchello F, 345, *364*
Zager J, 157, *165*
Zahm JM, 326, *355*, 435, *451*
Zaidi TS, 367, *378*
Zangemeister-Wittke U, 244, *271*
Zanta MA, 100, *114*

Zar HJ, 371, *380*
Zaremba S, 16, *27*
Zatloukal K, 11, *25*
Zayek N, 440, *455*
Zebrowski BK, 258, *286*
Zeevi A, 459, *469*
Zeh HJ, 247, 250, *275, 279*
Zeiher BG, 70, *90*, 327, 332, *355, 358*,
    425, 427, *443, 446*
Zeitlin PL, 63, 70, 74, *85, 90*, 319, 327,
    349, 356, 365, 366, 367, 368, 373,
    377, 378, 379, 380, 413, *417*, 424,
    443
Zelphati O, 11, *25*, 100, *113*
Zeng X, 196, *211*
Zenke M, 391, *395*
Zentgraf H, 59, 60, 65, *82, 86*
Zepeda M, 220, 228, *229, 230*, 429, *448*
Zern MA, 414, *418*
Zganiacz A, 176, 183, *187, 190*
Zhai Y, 459, *469*
Zhang G, 8, *25*
Zhang H, 158, *166*
Zhang HB, 296, *313*
Zhang HG, 421, *441*
Zhang L, 76, *92*, 244, *272*, 343, *363*,
    367, *378*
Zhang M, 197, *213*
Zhang MQ, 55, *81*
Zhang P, 201, *215*
Zhang W, 175, *186*, 437, *452*, 461, 463,
    471, 472
Zhang WJ, 259, *286*
Zhang WW, 55, *80*
Zhang Y, 5, *24*, 41, *48*, 52, 64, 66, 69,
    74, 75, *78, 85, 88, 90*, 93, 99, *112*,
    135, *144*, 193, *209*, 243, 255, 263,
    270, 282, 290, 308, *318*, 339, 347,
    362, 364, 429, *447*
Zhang YB, 122, *138*
Zhang Z, 198, *213*
Zhao H, 106, *117*, 426, *445*
Zhao J, 181, *189, 190*, 326, *355*, 425,
    444
Zhau HE, 158, *166*
Zheng LM, 148, *163*

Zheng T, 172, 183, *185, 190*
Zheng X, 224, *230*
Zhivotovsky B, 241, *269*
Zhoa J, 182, *190*
Zhong G, 195, *210*
Zhou H, 39, 40, 42, 43, *47, 48, 49*, 333,
    359, 411, *415*, 425, *443, 444*
Zhou JX, 121, *138*, 309, *318*
Zhou MY, 439, *455*
Zhou P, 195, *211*
Zhou S, 57, *82*, 328, *356*, 375, *381*,
    424, *442*
Zhou T, 421, *441*
Zhou W, 64, 70, 75, *85, 90*
Zhou X, 60, *83*, 331, *358*
Zhou Z, 13, *26*, 38, *46*, 175, *186*, 320,
    350, 351, 373, *380*, 387, *395*, 427,
    446
Zhu G, 129, *142*
Zhu HL, 439, *455*
Zhu J, 345, *364*
Zhu L, 239, 253, *268, 281*
Zhu MZ, 16, *27*
Zhu N, 102, *115*, 399, *404*
Zhu NL, 136, *144*
Zhu XD, 6, *24*, 60, 61, 64, *83, 84*
Zhu YF, 346, *364*
Zhu Z, 183, *190*
Ziaday A, 345, *364*
Ziady AG, 321, 338, *352, 361*, 439,
    454
Zidon T, 64, 75, *85*, 375, *381*
Ziegler A, 244, *271*
Ziegler RJ, 93, 98, 100, 103, 109, 110,
    112, 113, 117, 334, *360*, 427, *445*
Ziegler SF, 249, *278*
Zielenski J, 366, *377*
Zier K, 249, *276*
Zieske A, 197, *213*
Zimonjic DB, 64, *86*
Zinder ND, 19, *27*
Zinkernagel RM, 247, 248, *275*
Zinn KR, 126, *140*, 402, *405*, 429, *447*
Zitvogel L, 250, 253, *279, 282*
Zlotnik A, 196, *212*, 255, *282, 283*
Zoller M, 249, *276*

Zolotukhin I, 62, *84*, 366, *377*
Zolotukhin S, 67, *88*, 366, *377*, 412, *416*
Zong G, 111, *118*
Zoon KC, 22, *27*
Zorina T, 247, *274*
Zou H, 259, *287*
Zou Y, 111, *118*
Zsengeller ZK, 39, 43, *47*, 176, *187*, 330, *357*, 423, 433, *442*, *450*
Zuckerman JB, 38, *46*, 425, 429, *444*, *448*
Zufferey R, 329, 330, 341, *357*

Zuhl F, 72, *91*
Zuidam NJ, 99, *113*
Zullo TG, 459, *469*
zur Hausen H, 54, 65, *79*, 151, *164*, 243, *270*, 365, *377*
Zusman B, 413, *417*
Zuzarte M, 127, *142*
Zuzart M, 429, *447*
Zwacka R, 433, 437, *450*
Zwacka RM, 437, *453*
Zwart R, 341, *363*
Zweibel JA, 147, *162*
Zwiebel J, 146, *161*

SUBJECT INDEX

A

AAV
  AAV-hAAT, 413–414
  administration, 374
  aerosolized vector, 369
  antibody response to, 370
  assembly of, 59
  barriers to infection, 71–73, 328
  biodistribution studies of, 413–414
  Cap proteins, 55, 327
  cellular and molecular biology of,
    57–65
  CFTR vector development, 366–
    367
  circular intermediates, 64
  clinical studies, 76, 370–374
  delivery to the lung, 367–370
  gene transfer, 323
  immunology of, 65, 66
  infectious entry pathways, 57–59

[AAV]
  integration, 55
    sequence (AAVS1), 60
  inverted terminal repeats (ITRs), 55–
    57, 366
  life cycle, 6
  lysogenic life cycle, 60
  lytic life cycle, 59–60
  mediated transduction
    barriers, 71–73, 328
  molecular structure of, 55–57
  neutralizing antibodies to, 65, 369, 373
  nuclear entry of, 58
  packaging limitations of, 74
  packaging systems, 67
  physical properties of, 52–54
  production of, 67–68
  receptors, 57
  Rep (replication) proteins, 55, 61
  retargeting of, 136

545

[AAV]
  rodent models, 69–76
  safety of, 77
  serotypes, 54, 73
  serum neutralizing antibodies (*see*
    Neutralizing antibodies)
  toxicology studies, 413–414
  transduction in the lung with, 69–76
  trans-splicing, 75
  vector dissemination, 368
  vectors, 13, 72, 136, 324, 327–328,
    334, 338–340, 402, 424
AAV-2, 339, 365, 375
AAV-5, 339, 376
AAV-6, 339, 376
Acute inflammation, 105
Acute lung injury (ALI), 434
Acute respiratory distress syndrome
    (ARDS), 174, 434
Adaptive immune responses, 108
Ad CEA460, 160
Ad delta24 mutant, 150
Adeno-associated virus (*see* AAV)
Adenosine deaminase deficiency
    (ADA), 2, 12
Adenoviral vectors, 4–5, 228, 242, 263
  Ad.AAT, 410
  conjugate-based retargeting ap-
    proaches, 123–128
  EIA-deleted mutants, 150
  first-generation vectors (*see also*
    Helper-dependent Ad vectors),
    325, 333
  fully deleted vectors (*see also* Helper-
    dependent Ad vectors), 42
  genetic capsid modifications, 128–132
  genetic fiber modification, 129
  gutless (*see also* Helper-dependent
    vector), 263, 326, 402
  helper-dependent vectors, 326, 333
  high-capacity, 326
  humoral immune responses, 333
  immunogenic responses, 333
  production, 31–37
  replication-competent adenovirus, 36,
    37, 300, 309
  retargeting, 337

[Adenoviral vectors]
  second-generation E2a-defective vec-
    tors, 325, 333
  third-generation Ad vectors, 326
Adenovirus(es), 31–44, 147, 221, 296,
    324, 401
  conserved region 2 (CR2), 150
  E1A gene, 33, 35
  E1B gene, 33, 35, 151
  E2 gene, 34
  E3 gene, 34
  E4 gene, 34
  fiber, 33, 120, 122, 129, 337
  hexon protein, 127
  immune response to, 4–5
  infections with, 32, 120–123
  life cycle of, 409
  pathway of infection, 120–123
  penton-base proteins, 120
  serotypes of, 12, 32, 338
  structure of, 33–34
  subgroups, 32
  toxicity of, 5
  transcription, 33
AdHSV*tk* (*see also* Herpes simplex thy-
    midine kinase), 297
AdIFN, 206
Ad knob domain (*see* Adenovirus, fiber)
Adoptive immunotherapy, 15
β₂-Adrenergic receptor, 438
Aerosolized cationic lipid:pDNA com-
    plexes, 103
Aerosolized vector, 430
AIDS, 17–18
Airway cells, 322
Airway epithelial cells, 38, 427
Airway gene delivery barriers, 420–422
Airway gene transfer, vectors for, 321
Airway surface liquid, 323
Allergic airway response, 176
Allograft rejection, 459
Allograft survival, 436
Alveolar atypical hyperplasia (AAH),
    235
Alveolar macrophage(s) (*see also* Macro-
    phages), 102, 135, 193, 194,
    323, 420, 423, 425

Alveolar proteinosis, 176, 433
Amphotropic receptor, 330
Angiogenesis, 242, 255, 256
    inhibitors, 258
Angiogenic squamous dysplasia, 235
Angiopoietin, 257
Angiostatin, 258
Angiotensin-converting enzyme (ACE),
    126, 402
Anionic liposomes, 9
Anti-adenoviral antibodies, 421
Anti-adenoviral neutralizing antibodies,
    198
Antibiotic resistance gene, 98
Anti-CD40, 123
Anti-EpCAM, 123
Anti-epidermal growth factor receptor
    (EGF-R), 123
Antigen-loss variants, 254
Antigen-presenting cells (APCs) (see
    also Dendritic cells), 40, 109
Antioxidants, 437, 439
Antisense inhibition, 244, 311
Anti-TAG-72, 123
α_1-Antitrypsin (α_1AT), 76, 38, 323, 438
α_1 Anti-trypsin therapy
    adenoviral vectors for, 409–410
    recombinant adeno-associated vectors
        for, 411–414
    retrovirus vectors for, 408–409
Apical cell membrane, 327, 391
Apoptosis, 156, 174, 241, 309, 334, 400
Aquaporin water channels, 438
Arg-Gly-Asp (RGD), 122
Arginemia, 2
Arteriosclerosis, 17
    obliterans, 16
Asialoglycoprotein receptor, 11
Asilomar conference, 19
Atrial natriuretic peptide, 438
Autonomous parvovirus, 148

B

B lymphocytes, 39
Bacteria, 148
Bacterial plasmids, 36

Bak (see also Apoptosis), 310
Ballistic gene transfer, 411
Basolateral cell surface membrane recep-
    tors, 426
Bcl-2 (see also Apoptosis), 244, 310
Biosafety, 51
Biotechnology Science Board (BSB), 21
Bispecific adapter molecules, 123
Bispecific antibody(-ies), 127, 337, 402
Bleomycin, 227, 433
Bleomycin-induced pulmonary fibrosis,
    219
Bronchial secretions, 421
Bronchiolitis obliterans, 457, 460, 466
Bronchoalveolar lavage (BAL), 322
Bronchopulmonary dysplasia (BPD),
    182
Bystander effect, 15, 242, 244, 296

C

Calcium phosphate, 430–431
    coprecipitation, 347
Calretinin, 303
Canavan's disease, 68
CAR (see Coxsackie-adenoviral re-
    ceptor)
Carcinogens, 234
Cardiovascular disease, 16–17
CAR-EGF fusion molecule, 128
Catalase, 437, 439
β-Catenin, 159
Cathepsin G, 407
Catheter-directed instillation, 429–430
Cationic lipid(s), 344, 384, 411
    colipids, 96
    formation of, 99–100
    headgroup domain, 95
    in vivo potency of, 100
    lipid:cationic lipid ratio, 96–97
    structure of, 94–96
Cationic lipid:pDNA complexes, 9,
    123, 263, 331, 426, 427–428
    aerosolized, 103
    biodistribution of, 101–102
    first-generation cationic lipid:DNA
        complexes, 99

[Cationic lipid:pDNA complexes]
  inflammatory response to, 334–335
  luminal administration of, 102
  persistence of expression, 109–111
  targeted complexes, 104
  tissue-specific expression, 104–105
  toxicities of, 105–108
Cationic polymers, 400
CC10 promoter, 172
CC-10Tag transgenic mice, 239
CD4 T-lymphocytes (T-cells), 39, 43,
  247
CD8$^+$ T-lymphocytes, 204, 308
CD40 ligand, 198, 202, 208
CD69, 399
Cell cycle, 241
Cell-based gene delivery, 398–399
Cell-mediated immune responses, 298,
  346
293 Cells, 35
Cellular *transformation*, 241
Center for Biologicals Evaluation and
  Research (CBER), 22
Cesium chloride (CsCl), 67
CFTR (*see* Cystic fibrosis transmem-
  brane conductance regulator
  gene)
Charge-charge interaction, 99
Chemoattractants, 254
Chemokines, 259
Chemotherapy, 151, 219
Chlamydia pneumoniae, 205
Chloroquine, 10, 345
Cholesterol, 96, 331, 399
Chromatographic purification methods, 68
Chronic granulomatous disease, 12
Chronic rejection, 457
CMV immediate early gene enhancer re-
  gion, 110
CMV immediate early gene promoter,
  109
c-myc, 235
CN706, 158
Coccidioides immitis, 204
Collagen, 222–224
Collagen vascular diseases, 219
Concatemers, 375

Coronavirus, 343
Coxsackie-adenoviral receptor (CAR),
  33, 121, 122, 324, 326, 424–425
CpG bacterial sequences, 107, 307, 335,
  308, 389, 402, 411, 427
Cross presentation, 254
CsCl density gradient ultracentifugation,
  37, 67
CV787, 158
CXC chemokines, 259
CXCR2, 260
Cystic fibrosis, 13, 38, 76
  liposome/plasmid complexes, 387
  surrogate endpoints, 376
Cystic fibrosis transmembrane conduc-
  tance regulator gene (CFTR), 38,
  319, 366–368
Cytokeratin, 104
Cytokine(s), 15, 107, 193, 222, 248,
  305
Cytokine-induced neutrophil chemo-
  attractant (KC), 174
Cytokine-inducible cyclooxygenase
  (COX-2), 253
Cytomegalovirus promoter (*see also*
  CMV), 8
Cytosine deaminase (CDA), 156, 244,
  294
Cytosine-guanosine deoxynucleotides
  (CpG), 106
Cytotoxic (CD8) T lymphocytes, 39, 66,
  304, 333
Cytotoxic lymphocytes, 304

                              D

DEAE-dextran, 347
Decorin, 180, 226
Dendritic cells (DCs), 125, 202, 250,
  253
  transfected, 253
Detergent, 431
Dexamethasone, 108, 400, 426
Dioleylphosphatidyl-ethanolamine
  (DOPE) (*see also* Cationic lip-
  ids), 96, 331
Diphytanoyl PE, 96

dl922/947, 150
DMRIE (*see also* Cationic lipids), 384
DNA immunization, 205
DNA-ligand-polymer complexes, 331
DNA polymerase gamma, 62
DNA-protein complexes, 10–11
DNA vaccination, 205
DNA vaccines, 199, 207
DNAse, 422
DOTAP (*see also* Cationic lipids), 94, 95, 384
DOTMA (*see also* Cationic lipids), 384

Endotoxin, 436
env (*see also* Retrovirus), 328
Envelope glycoprotein (G) of VSV, 331
Envelope glycoproteins, 330
Epidermal growth factor receptor, 338
Epithelial neutrophil-activating protein-78 (ENA-78), 260
ErbB2-neu, 235, 243
Escherichia coli, 182
Estrogen receptors (ERs), 159
Exosurf, 431–432
Extracellular matrix, 225, 257

E

E1A (*see also* Adenovirus), 33, 35
    gene product, 157
E1B 19kD gene (*see also* Adenovirus), 156
E1B 55kD gene (*see also* Adenovirus), 156
E1B (*see also* Adenovirus), 33, 35
E2 (*see also* Adenovirus), 34
E2F, 150, 159, 303
E3 (*see also* Adenovirus), 32
E3-adenoviral death protein (ADP) (*see also* Adenovirus), 156
E4 34kD protein (*see also* Adenovirus), 156
E4 proteins (*see also* Adenovirus), 34, 156
Ebola virus, 344
Edema clearance, 438
EGTA, 123, 336, 421, 431
Electroporation, 14
Embryonic epithelium, 181
ENA-78, 261
Endocytosis, 326, 331
Endosome, 122
    escape, from, 385
    lysis of, 122
    processing, 337
    shunting, 9
Endostatin, 259
Endothelial cell specific promoter, 402
Endothelial cells, 102, 256
Endothelium, 429

F

Familial hypercholesterolemia, 13
Fas ligand, 466
FDA, 20, 21–23
Federal Coordinating Council for Science Engineering and Technology (FCCSET), 21–22
Feline immunodeficiency virus (FIV), 328
α-Fetoprotein, 158
FHIT locus, 235
Fibrin, 223
Fibritin, 132
Fibroblast(s), 223, 224, 225
Fibroblast growth factor(s) (FGF), 123, 229, 328, 435
Fibroblast growth factor receptor 1 (FGFR1), 57, 125
Fibrosis, 178
Filoviridae, 344
Folate, 123
Fowlpox virus, 16
Fungus, 204
Fusogenic peptides, 345

G

G207, 149
gag, 328
Ganciclovir (GCV), 15, 294, 297
Gene transfer, 261
    limitations of, 227
Gene-modified tumor cells, 252
Genetic immunotherapy, 245–255

Genome conversion, 62
GL-67 (*see also* Cation lipid), 94, 384
Glutathione reductase, 437
Glycocalyx, 125, 323, 324
  proteins, 425
Goblet cell hyperplasia, 176
Graft dysfunction, 459
Gram-negative bacterial infection, 436
Granulocyte-macrophage colony-stimulating factor (GM-CSF), 15, 175, 177–179, 249, 251, 436
Growth factors, 241
Growth-related genes (GRO-α, -β, and $-\gamma$), 260
Gutless Ad vectors (*see also* Adenovirus), 263, 326, 402

H

Heat shock protein, 307
Heat shock protein 60 (pHSP-60), 205
Heat shock protein 65, 307
Heat shock protein 70/nitric oxide synthase, 464
Helper (CD4$^+$) T-lymphocyte, 333
Helper virus contamination, 68
Helper-dependent Ad vectors (*see also* Adenoviral vectors), 326, 410–411, 425
Heme oxygenase, 437
Hemophilia A, 12
Hemophilia B, 13, 69
Heparan sulfate proteoglycan (HSPG), 57, 327
Hepatic dysfunction, 301
HER-2/neu, 243
Herpes simplex thymidine kinase (HSV*tk*), 15, 33, 294–303
Herpes simplex virus (HSV), 7, 149–150, 157, 243
  ICP4, 157
  ICP6 (ribonuclease reductase), 149
  ICP34.5 protein, 149
Hexon protein (*see also* Adenovirus), 33, 131
  HI loop, 129, 131

High-capacity Ad vectors (*see also* Adenoviral vectors), 326
HIV infection, 203
Homologous gene conversion, 375
Homologous recombination, 36
Human airway epithelial (HAE) cell cultures, 324
Human bronchial xenograft system, 70
Humoral immune response, 262, 346
Hydroxyproline, 222, 223, 225
Hyper-IgM syndrome, 198
Hypersensitivity pneumonitis, 219

I

ICAM-2, 134
ICP34.5 protein (*see also* Herpes virus), 149
ICP4 (*see also* Herpes virus), 157
Idiopathic pulmonary fibrosis (IPF) (*see also* Fibrosis), 178, 219, 221
Interleukin(s), 249
Interleukin-1 (IL-1), 178
  receptor antagonist (IL-IRA), 175
Interleukin-1β (IL-1β), 174, 179, 222, 322
Interleukin-2 (IL-2), 194, 248, 304, 305, 306
Interleukin-4 (IL-4), 175, 176
Interleukin-5 (IL-5), 176, 436
Interleukin-6 (IL-6), 41, 105, 174, 175, 176, 322, 436
Interleukin-7 (IL-7), 249
Interleukin-8 (IL-8), 198, 260, 322, 372
Interleukin-10 (IL-10), 175, 177, 196–197, 222, 436, 464, 465, 466
Interleukin-11 (IL-11), 176
Interleukin-12 (IL-12), 150, 175, 177, 184, 194, 195, 200, 249, 251, 306, 347, 436
Interleukin-17 (IL-17), 197, 201
Interleukin-18 (IL-18), 177
Immune responses (*see also* Cellular immune responses)
  cell-mediated, 346
  humoral, 346
Immune suppression, 248

Immunosuppressive agents, 263
Inflammatory response, 228
Influenzavirus, 343
INK4a/ARF, 309
Innate immune response, 183, 420
Insulator sequences, 134, 158
αVβ5 Integrin (*see also* Integrins), 57
$α_v$-Integrins (*see also* Integrins), 338
$α_vβ_{3/5}$ Integrins (*see also* Integrins), 326,
    424–425
$α_vβ_5$ Integrins (*see also* Integrins), 328
Integrins (*see also* αvβ$_5$, αv-Integrins,
    αvβ$_{3–5}$ Integrins), 57, 131, 122,
    326, 328, 338, 424–425, 435
Interferon(s), 249
Interferon-β (IFN-β), 249, 251, 305
Interferon-γ (IFN-γ), 105, 182, 194–
    195, 203, 205, 208, 305, 347,
    399, 400, 420
  IFN-γ gene, 201
  IFN-γ knockout mice, 206
Interferon-γ–inducible protein (IP-10),
    174, 251, 255, 260–261
Intratracheal delivery, 224
Intravenous (IV) administration, 428
Intron, 98
Inverted terminal repeats (ITRs) (*see
    also* AAV), 59, 412
Ischemia reperfusion injury, 464

J

Jaagsiekte sheep retrovirus (JSRV), 343
Jet nebulization, 103

K

Keratinocyte growth factor (KGF), 330,
    336, 342, 423
Klebsiella pneumoniae, 196, 200
K-ras oncogene, 235, 243
Kupffer cells, 5, 102, 127, 135, 429

L

Lactosylated poly-L-lysine, 332, 344
Large T antigen, 311

Leber's congenital amaurosis, 68
Legionella pneumonia, 196
Lentivirus(es), 3, 328, 329
  Lentiviral vectors, 262, 341, 342
Lesch-Nyhan syndrome, 3
Leukocyte adherence deficiency, 12
Leupeptin, 10
Lewis lung cancer cells (*see also* Lung
    cancer), 238
Lewis lung carcinoma cells (3LL), 238,
    247
Line 1 alveolar carcinoma (LIC2), 238
Lipid/DNA complexes, 307, 384 (*see
    also* Cationic lipids)
Lipid-protamine-DNA complexes (*see
    also* Cationic lipids), 399
Lipoplex(es), 311, 399
Liposomes (*see also* Cationic lipids), 9,
    10, 411
Liquid ventilation, 432
Lung cancer
  human, 236–240
  murine models, 236–240
  pathogenesis, 234–236
Lung endothelial cells, 400
Lung fibrosis (*see also* Idiopathic pulmo-
    nary fibrosis), 436
Lung transplantation
  acute rejection, 459–460
  adenovirus, 461
  airway transfection, 463
  chronic rejection, 460
  clinical overview of, 457–458
  delivery routes, 463
  ex vivo gene transfer, 463
  indications for, 458
  ischemia reperfusion injury, 458–
    459
  liposomes, 462
  naked plasmid, 462
  other vectors, 462
  survival, 457
Lymphocytes, 305
Lymphokine-activated killer (LAK)
    cells, 249, 305
Lysine, 322

Lysogenic integration, 64
Lysosomal degradation, 326

M

M3 protein, 198
Macrophage-activation genes, 206
Macrophage inflammatory protein-2
    (MIP-2), 174, 179, 196, 200
Macrophages (see also Alveolar macro-
    phages), 105, 323
Major histocompatibility complex class
    proteins (MHC), 183
    MHC class I, 346
    MHC class I pathway, 247
    MHC class II-dependent epitopes,
        247
    MHC class II expression, 250
    MHC expression, 253
    MHC genes, 249
Malignant mesothelioma, 245, 293–
    312
Malignant pleural effusions, 258
Manganese superoxide dismutase
    (MnSOD), 303
Marburg virus, 344
Matrix (see also Extracellular matrix),
    225
Matrix metalloproteinases, 256
Maxillary sinus, 370
MDM2, 309
Mesothelin, 303
Mesotheliomas (see also Malignant
    mesothelioma), 294–312
Metalloproteinases MMP-2, 260
Minigenes, 76
MIP-1α, 198
Molecular conjugates, 332
Moloney murine leukemia virus
    (MMLV), 408
Monocrotaline, 403
Monocyte chemoattractant protein-1
    (MCP-1), 198, 222, 249
Monogenic deficiency diseases, 12–
    14
Monokine induced by IFN-γ (MIG),
    174, 254, 260, 261

Mouse fibroblasts, 409
Mucin glycoproteins, 324, 420, 422
    hypersecretion, 176
    MUC1, 324
    MUC-1, 421
    MUC4, 324
    MUC5ac, 324
Mucolytic agents, 70, 391
Mucous layer, 391
Murine leukemia virus (MLV), 328
Mycobacterium tuberculosis, 182, 196,
    206
Myofibroblasts, 179

N

n-acetylysteine, 322, 434
Na+, K+-ATPase, 437
Nacystelyn, 322
Naked DNA, 107, 344, 399, 427
Nanospheres, 392
Nasal deposition, 429
Nasal epithelium, 387
Nasal gene transfer, 373
Natural killer (NK) cells, 194, 204, 305
Neuraminidase, 421
Neurogenic inflammation, 334
Neutral carrier lipid (see also Lipids),
    399
Neutralizing antibodies (see also Adeno-
    viral vectors), 40, 66
Neutrophil(s), 322, 458
Neutrophil elastase (NE), 322, 407
    inhibitor, 438
Neutrophil inhibitory factor, 439
Newcastle disease virus (NDV), 147,
    148
Nitric oxide, 421, 426
    NOS2, 403
    NOS3 gene, 402
    synthase (NOS3), 398
Nonviral gene delivery (see also Cat-
    ionic lipids), 399–401
Nonviral vectors, 8–11
Nuclear entry, 332, 385
Nuclear factor kappa B (NF-κB), 245,
    439

Nuclear-localizing signal (NLS), 385
Nuclease sensitivity, 100
Nude mice, 240

O

Office of Therapeutics Research and Review (OTRR), 22
ONYX-015/Cl-042 replicating adenovirus, 151, 242, 309
Ovarian cancer, 120
Oxidant gas injury, 341

P

p14^{ARF}, 151, 309
p16^{INK4a}, 235, 309
P2Y$_2$ receptor, 126, 338
p5 promoter, 367
p53, 15, 151, 235, 241–242, 309, 310
PA1-STK cells, 304
Paracellular permeability, 335–336
Paramyxoviruses, 345
Penton (*see also* Adenovirus), 33
Perflubron, 432
Perfluorochemical (PFC) liquid(s), 74, 123, 376, 426, 432, 438
Persistence of transgene expression, 108
Phage panning, 128
Plaque, 35
Plaque-forming assay, 37
Plasmid DNA, 8, 97–98, 308, 331
Plasmin, 223
Plasminogen activator inhibitor-1 (PAI-1), 223, 224
Plasminogen activator system, 229
Platelet-derived growth factor (PDGF), 226, 257
Platelet-derived growth factor beta receptor, 227
Platelet endothelial cell adhesion molecule (PECAM-1), 104, 136, 257, 400
Platelet factor-4 (PF4), 260
Pneumocystis carinii, 183, 196, 203–204
pol (*see also* Retrovirus), 328

Polidocanol, 336
Polio, 148
Polyadenylation signal, 98
Polyamidoamine dendrimers, 384
Polybrene, 347
Polycations, 347
Polyethylene glycol (PEG), 103, 135, 263, 338, 347, 425
Polyethyleneimine (PEI), 384, 392, 428
polymers, 345
Poly-L-lysine, 10, 332, 347
Polylysine-plasmid DNA, 11
Polyplexes, 344, 428
Positron emission tomography, 301
Prodrug, 15, 294
Promoters, 133, 435
Prostaglandin E2 (PGE2), 253
Prostaglandin G/H synthase, 400, 403, 439
Prostate-specific antigen (PSA), 157
Protamine sulfate, 347
Proteasome, 72, 375
Proteasome inhibitors, 72, 337
Protein kinase R (PKR), 147
Proteinase-3, 407
Proteinase activity, 256
Pseudomonas aeruginosa, 182, 201–202, 323, 372, 389, 426
Pseudotypes, 330, 338, 343
Public oversight, 18–21
Pulmonary artery catheter, 401
Pulmonary circulation, 401
Pulmonary edema, 437
Pulmonary endothelium, 126
Pulmonary graft endothelium, 458
Pulmonary hypertension, 402–404
Purine nucleoside phosphorylase deficiency, 12

R

Rabies virus, 147
Radiation therapy, 219, 245
Radiation-induced acute pneumonitis, 437
Ralginase, 322
RANTES, 174, 199
Ras-signaling pathway, 147, 235

rb (retinoblastoma), 150, 241, 309
  rb mutations, 235
  rb phosphorylation, 244
Real-time PCR analysis, 374
Receptor for AAV-2 (*see also* AAV),
      327–328
Recombinant DNA Advisory Committee
      (RAC), 2, 19–21
Reimplantation response, 459
Reolysin, 147
Reovirus, 147
Rep gene (*see also* AAV), 65, 327
Rep proteins (*see also* AAV), 55
Replication-competent adenovirus (*see
      also* Adenovirus), 36, 37, 300,
      309
Replication-competent virus(es), 36,
      145–161, 242
Respiratory syncytial virus (RSV), 207,
      343, 346
Reticuloendothelial cells, 262
Reticuloendothelial system, 135
Retrovirus, 148, 323, 423–424
  retargeting, 135, 136
  transduction, 324
  vectors, 3, 135, 262, 296, 328–331,
      340–344
RGD domain, 104, 131
Rhesus macaque, 368
Ribonucleotide reductase (RR, ICP6)
      (*see also* Herpes virus), 149

S

Salmonella typhimurium (VNP200009),
      148
Sarcoidosis, 219
Secondary lymphoid chemokine (SLC),
      254
Sendai virus (SeV), 345
Serotype switching, 346
Serpin enzyme complex receptor (SEC-
      R), 338
Serum transaminases, 107
Severe combined immunodeficiency
      mice (SCID mice), 240
Sialic acid, 339

Silencer, 158
Simian virus 40 (SV40), 310
  simian virus-40 large T-Ag (SV40-
      TAg), 238
Single chain antibody (scFv), 127
  scFv-fusion proteins, 337
Single-strand D sequence binding pro-
      tein (ssD-BP), 62
Site-specific integration, 60
Smads, 225
  smad2, 225
  smad3, 225
  smad7, 180, 225
Solvoplexes, 428
Spermine, 95
Sputum, 322
  viscosity, 322
Stabilized plasmid-lipid particles, 100
"Stealth" liposomes, 10
Stem cell, 320
Stem cell factor receptor, 338
Strand elongation, 59
Stromal inflammatory cells, 253
Submucosal glands, 320, 390
Suicide gene therapy, 244, 252, 294–303
Suicide gene variations, 303–305
Sulfur dioxide (SO$_2$), 336, 341
Superoxide dismutase (SOD), 437
Surfactant, 439
Surfactant-B protein promoter, 160
Surfactant-C protein (SPC) promoter,
      172
Survanta, 431–432
Survivin, 244, 303
SV40 (*see also* Simian virus 40), 311
  SV40-derived vectors, 414
Synthase gene, 400

T

T lymphocytes, 194, 459
Targeted synthetic vectors, 104
T-cell alpha chemoattractant (I-TAC),
      260
T-cell costimulatory pathways, 347
T-cell receptors, 338
Tetanus toxin fragment, 123

TH1 cytokine response, 400
β-Thalassemia, 2
Therapeutic vaccination, 246
Thrombospondin-1, 258
Thymidine-cytosine deaminase (tk-CD), 156
Thymidine kinase (tk) (*see also* Herpes simplex thymidine kinase), 149, 156, 244
Tight junctions, 71, 420
Tissue inhibitor of metalloproteinase-1 (TIMP-1), 403
Tissue remodeling, 180
Tissue-specific promoters, 172
TNF-α converting enzyme (TACE), 197–198
Tobacco smoke, 238
Tolerance, 254
Toxicity, 399
Toxicity studies, 297
Transcription factor Tcf4, 159
Transcriptional regulation, 133, 156–157
Transduction in the lung, 69–76
Transductional targeting, 7
Transepithelial potential difference (TEPD), 371, 387
Transforming growth factor-β (TGF-β), 175, 178–179, 180, 181, 222, 224, 226, 249, 253, 257, 436, 465
Transgenic animal lines, 220
Transgenic mice, 224
Transient immunosuppression, 346
Translation initiation factor, eIF2α, 147
Trans-splicing, 339
Tumor antigens, 246, 247, 248, 254
Tumor cell vaccines, 246
Tumor necrosis factor (TNF)-related apoptosis ligand (TRAIL), 244
Tumor necrosis factor-α (TNF-α), 105, 174, 178, 179, 183, 194, 196, 200, 202, 222, 249, 322, 400, 421, 436
Tumor rejection, 247
Tumor-induced immunosuppression, 246

U

Ubiquitin, 72
Ubiquitination, 57, 337
Ubiquitin B promoter, 110
Unmethylated CpG dinucleotide sequences (*see also* CpG bacterial sequences), 335
Urokinase plasminogen activator (uPA), 223
Urokinase plasminogen activator receptor (uPA-R), 338

V

Vaccine(s), 147, 311
Vaccinia virus (VV), 16, 147, 306
Vascular endothelial growth factor (VEGF), 16, 17, 175, 256, 257, 403, 438
Vascular endothelial growth factor (VEGF-R) receptors, 258
  VEGFR-1 (flt-1), 134, 258
  VEGF receptor 2 (VEGF-R2 or Flk-1), 256
Vascular endothelium, 439
Vascular smooth muscle cells, 398
Vasculogenesis, 256
Vector instillation, 429
Vectors, airway gene transfer, 321
Vero cells, 306
Viral vectors, 401
Virosomes, 392
Von Willebrand factor, 134
VSV-G-pseudotyped MLV, 341

W

Wild-type vesicular stomatitis virus (VSV), 330

X

Xenogenetic models, 236
Xenotransplantation, 239, 458
X-linked SCID, 12

Z

Zeta potential, 100